Essentials of Food Science and Nutrition

Essentials of Food Science and Nutrition

Editor: Lisa Jordan

Callisto Reference
www.callistoreference.com

Callisto Reference,
118-35 Queens Blvd., Suite 400,
Forest Hills, NY 11375, USA

Visit us on the World Wide Web at:
www.callistoreference.com

ISBN: 978-1-63239-842-0 (Hardback)

Printed in China.

Cataloging-in-publication Data

Essentials of food science and nutrition / edited by Lisa Jordan.
p. cm.
Includes bibliographical references and index.
ISBN 978-1-63239-842-0
1. Food--Research. 2. Nutrition. 3. Food animals. I. Jordan, Lisa.
TX357 .E87 2017
641.3--dc23

Table of Contents

Preface

Food science refers to the study of quality, processing, chemical traits and physical traits and deterioration of food. It unifies the elements of biochemistry, microbiology and chemical engineering for a better understanding for the traits of food. In this book using case studies and examples, constant effort has been made to make the understanding of the difficult concept of food science and nutrition as easy and informative as possible, for the readers. This book provides thorough information about food science and nutrition. It gives insights into the role of nutrition in food and how it is essential for the human body. The aim of this text is to present researches that have transformed this discipline and aided its advancement. It will help the readers in keeping pace with the rapid changes in this field.

Various studies have approached the subject by analyzing it with a single perspective, but the present book provides diverse methodologies and techniques to address this field. This book contains theories and applications needed for understanding the subject from different perspectives. The aim is to keep the readers informed about the progress in the field; therefore, the contributions were carefully examined to compile novel researches by specialists from across the globe.

Indeed, the job of the editor is the most crucial and challenging in compiling all chapters into a single book. In the end, I would extend my sincere thanks to the chapter authors for their profound work. I am also thankful for the support provided by my family and colleagues during the compilation of this book.

Editor

1

Underperformance of African Protected Area Networks and the Case for New Conservation Models: Insights from Zambia

Peter A. Lindsey[1,2]*, Vincent R. Nyirenda[3], Jonathan I. Barnes[4], Matthew S. Becker[5,6], Rachel McRobb[7], Craig J. Tambling[8], W. Andrew Taylor[9], Frederick G. Watson[6,10], Michael t'Sas-Rolfes[11]

1 Panthera, New York, New York, United States of America, **2** Mammal Research Institute, Department of Zoology and Entomology, University of Pretoria, Pretoria, Gauteng, South Africa, **3** Zambia Wildlife Authority, Chilanga, Lusaka, Zambia, **4** Design & Development Services, Windhoek, Namibia, **5** Department of Ecology, Montana State University, Bozeman, Montana, United States of America, **6** Zambian Carnivore Programme, Mfuwe, Zambia, **7** South Luangwa Conservation Society, Mfuwe, Zambia, **8** Centre for African Conservation Ecology, Department of Zoology, Nelson Mandela Metropolitan University, Port Elizabeth, South Africa, **9** Centre for Veterinary Wildlife Studies, Faculty of Veterinary Science, University of Pretoria, Pretoria, South Africa, **10** Division of Science and Environmental Policy, California State University Monterey Bay, Seaside, California, United States of America, **11** Cape Town, South Africa

Abstract

Many African protected areas (PAs) are not functioning effectively. We reviewed the performance of Zambia's PA network and provide insights into how their effectiveness might be improved. Zambia's PAs are under-performing in ecological, economic and social terms. Reasons include: a) rapidly expanding human populations, poverty and open-access systems in Game Management Areas (GMAs) resulting in widespread bushmeat poaching and habitat encroachment; b) underfunding of the Zambia Wildlife Authority (ZAWA) resulting in inadequate law enforcement; c) reliance of ZAWA on extracting revenues from GMAs to cover operational costs which has prevented proper devolution of user-rights over wildlife to communities; d) on-going marginalization of communities from legal benefits from wildlife; e) under-development of the photo-tourism industry with the effect that earnings are limited to a fraction of the PA network; f) unfavourable terms and corruption which discourage good practice and adequate investment by hunting operators in GMAs; g) blurred responsibilities regarding anti-poaching in GMAs resulting in under-investment by all stakeholders. The combined effect of these challenges has been a major reduction in wildlife densities in most PAs and the loss of habitat in GMAs. Wildlife fares better in areas with investment from the private and/or NGO sector and where human settlement is absent. There is a need for: elevated government funding for ZAWA; greater international donor investment in protected area management; a shift in the role of ZAWA such that they focus primarily on national parks while facilitating the development of wildlife-based land uses by other stakeholders elsewhere; and new models for the functioning of GMAs based on joint-ventures between communities and the private and/or NGO sector. Such joint-ventures should provide defined communities with ownership of land, user-rights over wildlife and aim to attract long-term private/donor investment. These recommendations are relevant for many of the under-funded PAs occurring in other African countries.

Editor: Danilo Russo, Università degli Studi di Napoli Federico II, Italy

Funding: The funding for this research was provided by the Wildlife Producers Association of Zambia. CJT was funded with a Claude Leon Fellowship. The funders had no role in study design, data collection and analysis, decision to publish, or preparation of the manuscript.

Competing Interests: JB is employed by Design and Development Services. PL was employed as a consultant during the research which provided the data used to compile this paper. There are no patents, products in development or marketed products to declare. This does not alter the authors' adherence to all the PLOS ONE policies on sharing data and materials.

* E-mail: plindsey@panthera.org

Introduction

Many African countries have designated generous proportions of their land surface as protected areas. Such protected areas vary greatly in their makeup, from strictly protected areas with no human settlement to areas that have resident communities where multiple uses of wildlife are permitted. African governments find it difficult to fund protected area networks adequately and are facing severe threats from poaching and human encroachment [1,2]. These problems are pronounced where human settlement is permitted or tolerated inside protected areas, as occurs in parts of Ethiopia, Mozambique, Tanzania and Zambia, for example [3,4].

Zambia has a vast wildlife estate encompassing 20 national parks (~64,000 km^2), 3 wildlife and bird sanctuaries (33.5 km^2), 36 GMAs (167,000 km^2) and several other protected area categories, comprising ~40% of the nation's land area [5] (Figure 1). Human settlement is not permitted in national parks, and land use is limited primarily to photo-tourism. National parks have generally not suffered from human encroachment, but are subject to widespread poaching, regular uncontrolled burning (which sometimes emanates from areas outside of the park boundaries) and in some cases, informal mining [6]. With the exception of Lusaka and Mosi-oa-tunya national parks, no protected areas in Zambia are fenced and most are simply demarcated with cut-lines or rivers, and in some cases, beacons.

GMAs were established as buffer-zones for national parks and have been used primarily for trophy hunting in recent years [7]. Unlike in the national parks, settlement is permitted in GMAs and there are large and expanding human populations in many of them, which is accompanied by widespread habitat loss. Habitat destruction is exacerbated by shifting agriculture, charcoal production and in some cases, mining [7,8,9]. In both national parks and GMAs, wildlife is under severe pressure from poaching, both for bushmeat and for trophies such as ivory [10].

In the 1980s, there was recognition of a need for greater community participation in wildlife-based land uses in GMAs [8]. In the early 1980s, subsidiary legislation was introduced to partially decentralize authority over wildlife to communities [8]. The Zambia Wildlife Act of 1998 provided for establishment of ZAWA as a parastatal responsible for managing protected areas [9]. The Wildlife Act identified Community Resource Boards as the institutions for communities to co-manage and benefit from

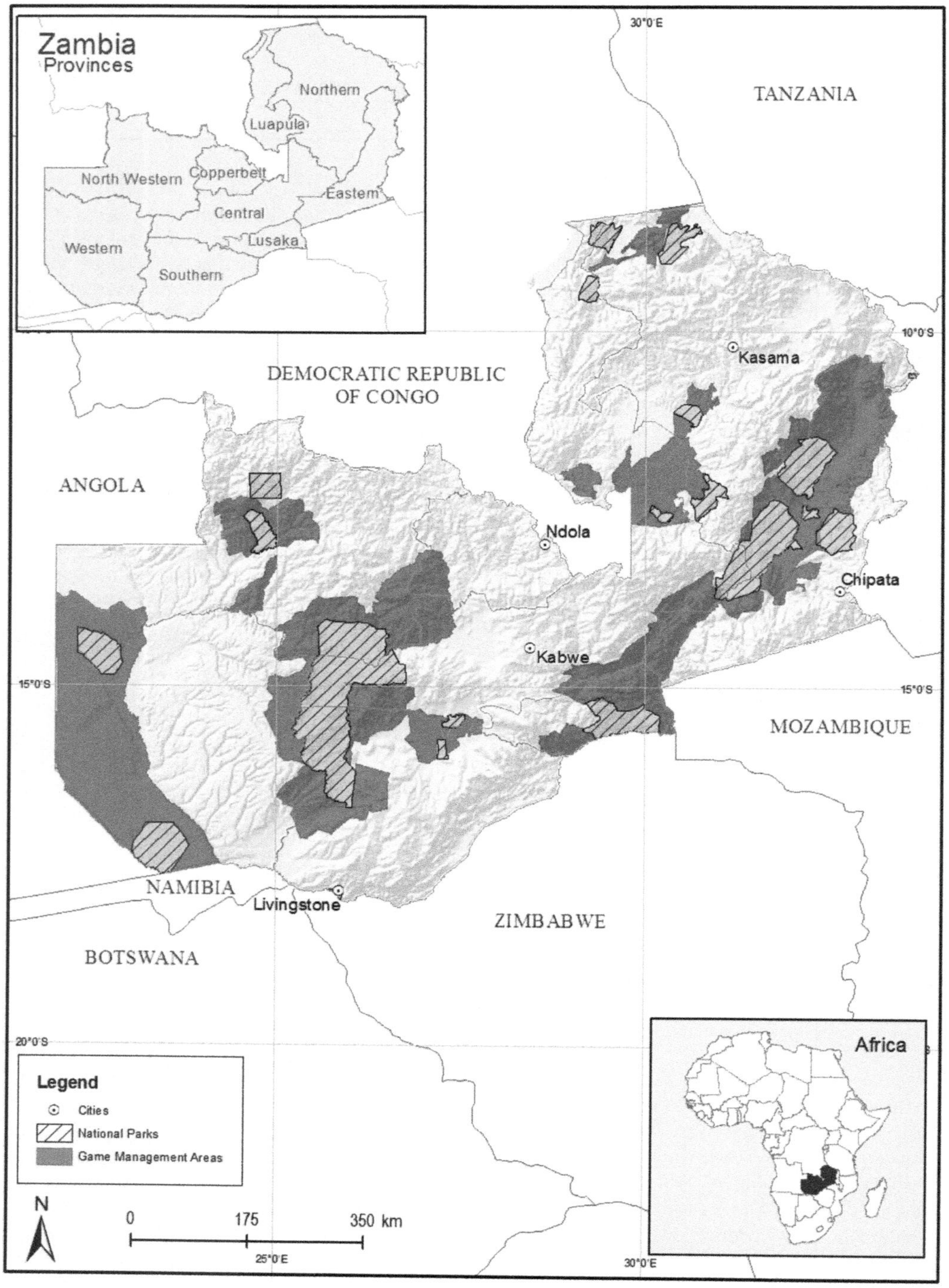

Figure 1. The Zambian protected area network.

wildlife in GMAs [9] though no mechanisms were created to enable communities to benefit from wildlife in national parks.

Wildlife-based land uses in the PA network have potential to improve livelihoods significantly for communities. People in GMAs are poorer and less educated than the national average, and GMAs have low agricultural potential and offer few alternative livelihood opportunities [11]. Trophy hunting in the GMAs has potential to generate significant incomes for communities if wildlife populations are allowed to recover and systems are put in place to ensure equitable benefit sharing and best-practices [12]. Similarly, national parks have potential to benefit rural communities through tourism-related employment and business opportunities. The PA network as a whole has enormous potential to contribute to rural and national economic growth by providing the basis for development of a major tourism industry [13]. However, wildlife populations are waning in many GMAs and national parks, and incomes from both trophy hunting and photo-tourism are limited to fractions of the GMAs and national parks [7]. In addition, mechanisms to enable communities to benefit legally from the PA area network are limited. Consequently the PA network is under-performing in ecological, economic and social terms.

There have been several attempts by the Zambian government to address the underperformance of the protected area network. For example, in 2006, the Zambian Government embarked upon a reclassification programme for protected areas [5] and in early 2013, a moratorium was imposed on hunting in GMAs. In addition, two protected areas have been added to the estate in recent years: the ~50 km^2 Lusaka National Park and the 5,104 km^2 Mukungule GMA. However, key challenges with regards to the functioning and effectiveness of Zambia's PA network remain.

In this paper we provide evidence of the under-performance of the Zambian protected area network, give reasons for that performance and suggest interventions needed to make the system more effective in ecological, economic and social terms. These recommendations have relevance for the PA networks of many other African countries.

Results and Discussion

Ecological Indicators of Protected Area Performance

Human encroachment of protected areas in Zambia is worse than in most other African countries [14], and ~2,500–3,000 km^2 of land are deforested annually [15]. Human population growth rates in GMAs (2.49±0.18%) are higher than elsewhere (2.31±0.24%, T-test 0.577, d.f. = 70, p = 0.566) [16]. Almost 40% of the total area of GMAs is now comprised of human-modified habitat (c.f. 71.2% outside of the protected area network) [6]. By contrast, habitat loss in national parks is limited (2.1%) (Table 1). The rate of habitat loss in GMAs (0.69% conversion per year) is faster than in national parks (0.05%) or outside protected areas (0.51%) (Table 1, Figure 2, [6]). Extrapolating from [6]'s sample area (Table 1, Figure 2), ~82 hectares of habitat are lost per daylight hour in GMAs on a national level. Human encroachment in GMAs is advancing from main roads towards national parks at a rate of up to 2 km per year ([6]). In some protected areas, and most notably Lukusuzi National Park [17], mining activity is evident and has potential to affect wildlife populations adversely through habitat degradation and bushmeat poaching [18]. In addition to habitat loss, human encroachment undermines the buffer zone role of GMAs for national parks, jeopardizes ecological connectivity among PAs and the concept of transfrontier conservation areas ([6]).

Table 1. Estimates of the extent and rate of habitat conversion in GMAs (from natural to human-modified habitat), national parks and land outside the protected area network in Zambia (taken from data extracted from [6]).

		~1970		~1985		~2010		~1970–~1985		~1980–~2010	
Land type	Total in study area (km^2)	Area human (km^2)	% human	Area human (km^2)	% human	Area human (km^2)	% human	Increase per year (km^2)	% increase per year	Increase per year (km^2)	% increase per year
Whole study area	159805	58926	36.9%	60935	38.1%	80157	50.2%	134	0.08%	769	0.48%
NPs	27098	252	0.9%	257	1.0%	571	2.1%	0	0.00%	13	0.05%
GMAs	47430	9468	20.0%	10616	22.4%	18744	39.5%	77	0.16%	325	0.69%
Non-NP, Non-GMA	85277	49206	57.7%	50061	58.7%	60841	71.3%	57	0.07%	431	0.51%
Luangwa Valley GMAs	26502	6815	25.7%	6190	23.4%	8878	33.5%	−42	−0.16%	108	0.41%
Southern Kafue GMAs	20928	2652	12.7%	4427	21.2%	9866	47.1%	118	0.57%	218	1.04%

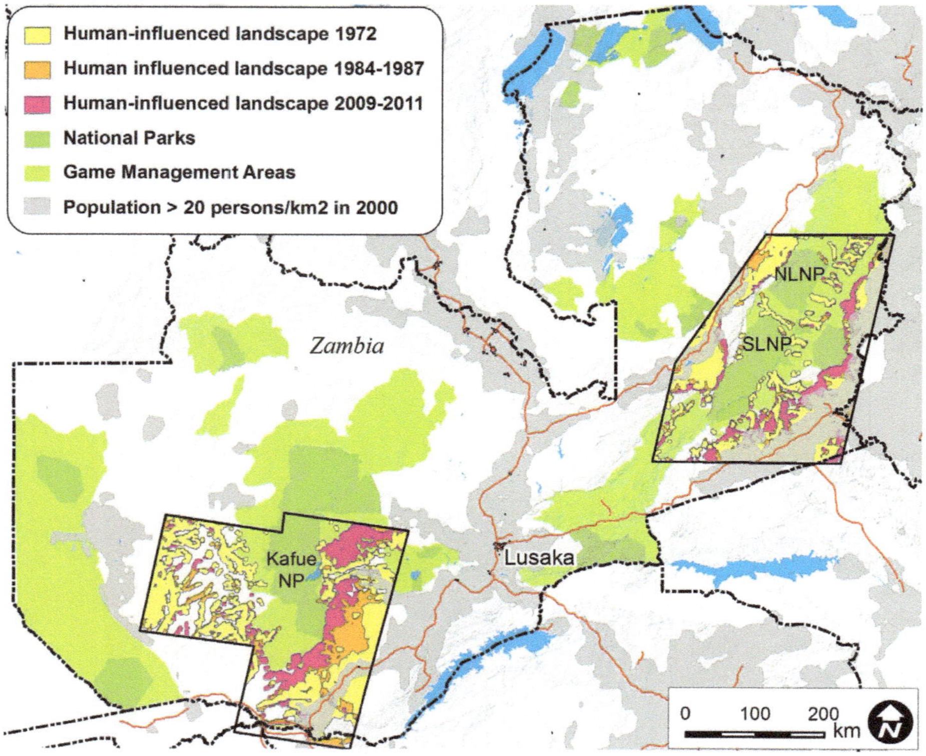

Figure 2. The extent of human encroachment of natural habitat in two focal areas in Zambia extracted from [6].

Data from aerial censuses indicate that wildlife populations in Zambian protected areas are relatively low (Table 2): ~169,000 wild ungulates occur in the ~61,000 km^2 of Zambian national parks for which data are available (excluding species of the size of a bushbuck or smaller and hippos) and ~143,000 in the ~160,000 km^2 of GMAs for which data were available. By contrast, ~63,000 ungulates occur on <6,000 km^2 of game ranches in Zambia [19]. Country-level population data for wildlife in other countries are scarce, but to provide a coarse comparisons, 1.8–2.8 million wild ungulates occur on 287,000 km^2 of Namibian wildlife ranches ~841,000 ungulates occurred on 27,000 km^2 of Zimbabwean game ranches prior to the land seizures [20] and ~215,000 ungulates occur in the ~20,000 km^2 Kruger National Park in South Africa [21,22].

The biomass of large wild ungulates is lower in GMAs (mean 212±59 kg/km^2) and national parks (791±240 kg/km^2) than in extensive game ranches (2,424±305 kg/km^2) (which are devoid of human settlement and rely primarily on trophy hunting for income) (Figure S1a) [19]. The diversity of wild ungulates is also lower in GMAs (4.7±0.58 species) and national parks (7.2±0.9 species) than on extensive unfenced game ranches 11.1±0.86 species) (Figure S1b) [19]. The higher biomass and diversity on private ranches is likely to be primarily due to the availability of greater resources for anti-poaching than in state protected areas. These findings reinforce the suggestion that trophy hunting need not have a negative impact on wildlife populations given appropriate land tenure arrangements [23].

Combining data from GMAs, national parks and extensive game ranches, wildlife ungulate biomass was negatively related to the presence of human settlement (in areas with settlement mean biomass was 268±70.8 kg/km^2 c.f. 1,755±281 kg/km^2), as was wild ungulate diversity (5.20±0.61 species c.f. 9.68±0.7) (F Ratio 26.2, d.f. = 2, p<0.001). Wild ungulate biomass was positively related to investment by the private sector/NGOs (in areas with such support, mean biomass was 1,592±222 kg/km^2 c.f. 233±113 kg/km^2 in areas without such investment, as was wild ungulate diversity (9.1±0.71 species c.f. 5.0±0.65) (F Ratio = 37.0, d.f. = 2, p<0.01) (Figures S2a, S2b).

Observed biomasses of large mammals in Zambian protected areas were lower than potential maximum carrying capacities by 93.7% in GMAs and 74.1% in national parks (Figures 3a, 3b). Wildlife densities are suppressed in some of Zambia's 'flagship' national parks and GMAs. For example, biomasses in Kafue, South Luangwa and Lower Zambezi national parks are 29%, 16% and 23% of potential carrying capacity, whereas that in Lupande GMA (which has in the recent past been categorised as a 'super-prime' concession), stands at 11% of carrying capacity. Depressed prey populations means that predator populations are almost certainly also occurring well below historic densities.

Population trend data are generally not available for Zambian protected areas. An exception is the Luangwa ecosystem, where the biomass of wildlife declined significantly in all five GMAs and four national parks during 2011–2012, and 80% of species showed declining trends during 2009–2012 [24]. By contrast, in Liuwa Plains (co-managed by African Parks/ZAWA since 2003), wildlife populations have recovered and large mammal biomass (excluding hippos and species of bushbuck size and smaller) increased from 966 kg/km^2 in 2003 to 1,921 kg/km^2 in 2013 [25].

Declining wildlife populations in GMAs have been reflected in changes to the way ZAWA classifies GMAs. In 2008, 24 GMAs were classified as depleted or secondary whereas in 1997, only 16 were categorized as such [7].

Table 2. Estimated wildlife populations in National Parks (data available for 61,462 km^2 of the ~64,000 km^2), Game Management Areas (GMAs, data available for 159,654 km^2 of the ~167,000 km^2) and game ranches (5,829 km^2) in Zambia (excluding species of bushbuck size and smaller, and hippopotamuses for which count data were not available) (data taken from [19]).

Species	National parks	GMAs	Game ranches	Total
Lechwe	9,737	75,808	1,513	87,058
Impala	27,820	13,507	27,998	69,325
Wildebeest	47,815	4,069	630	52,514
Buffalo	21,301	15,938	2,107	39,346
Puku	16,838	7,529	4,904	29,271
Elephant	10,830	8,094	1,710	20,634
Sable	8,172	4,895	3,682	16,749
Zebra, plains	8,375	1,050	2,060	11,485
Waterbuck	5,254	2,333	2,987	10,574
Kudu	1,908	1,976	6,287	10,171
Hartebeest	4,429	3,952	2,051	10,432
Roan	2,384	1,632	1,647	5,663
Reedbuck	1,137	852	2,735	4,724
Eland	1,069	237	1,558	2,864
Tsessebe	990	88	410	1,488
Giraffe	579	178	321	1,078
Sitatunga	40	369	328	737
Nyala	0	0	95	95
	168,678	142,507	63,023	374,208

Economic Indicators of Park Performance

Zambia attracts fewer tourists than other African countries known for wildlife: South Africa (~9.2 million), Botswana (~2.3 million), Zimbabwe (~2.2 million), Kenya (~1.8 million), Mozambique (~1.6 million), Tanzania (~1.25 Million), Namibia (~1.1 million), Zambia (~0.9 million) (www.wttc.org, accessed July 2013). In 2005 (when the latest data on tourist visitation to parks were available), just 59,350 tourists visited Zambia's national parks and 95% of those visited just five parks (Kafue, South Luangwa, Mosi-oa-Tunya, Lower Zambezi and Lochinvar): the remaining 15 parks comprising ~32,000 km^2 attracted just 1,384 tourists [26,27]. Most national parks thus fail to attract enough tourists to support viable photo-tourism [27]. Earnings from national parks and GMAs in Zambia are low. Photo-tourism generated USD9.1 million for ZAWA in 2011 (USD142/km^2) and UDD9.4 million in 2012 (USD146/km^2) (ZAWA unpublished data). The majority of those earnings (96.9%, USD154/km^2) were from four parks (South Luangwa – 44.4%, Mosi-o-tunya – 23.7%, Kafue – 14.7% and Lower Zambezi – 14.1%), which comprise 36,681 km^2 (57.3%) of the national parks network (ZAWA unpublished data). The remainder of the parks generated just USD182,229 (USD6.7/km^2) due to the relative (or actual) absence of tourism operators. Photo-tourism operations exist in only 10 of 36 GMAs [7] and in a marginal capacity given they currently are unable to bid for concessions in GMAs. Photo-tourism operations in GMAs are generally limited to lodges on national park boundaries with little investment or activity in the GMAs.

From trophy hunting income, ZAWA only earned concession fees from ~51% of the GMA estate in 2012 (ZAWA unpublished data). ZAWA earned a total of USD4.34 million from trophy hunting and resident hunting respectively in 2012 (equating to USD26/km^2) (ZAWA unpublished data). We estimate that an additional USD16.1 million was earned by operators from trophy hunting in GMAs, yielding total earnings of USD97/km^2 (averaged across all GMAs including those not hunted, Table 3). Earnings per km^2 from trophy hunting (when excluding hunting areas that do not generate any income to allow for comparison with other countries) (US$291±116/km^2) are lower than most other SADC countries: Zimbabwe – USD1,028/km^2; Tanzania – USD424/km^2; Namibia – USD378/km^2; Mozambique – USD130/km^2, [28] (F-Ratio 11.0, *d.f.* = 1, p = 0.001). Within Zambia, gross earnings per km^2 from trophy hunting in GMAs (USD97/km^2) are markedly lower than on extensive game ranches (USD878±226) (F Ratio 15.9, d.f. = 1, p<0.001) [19]. Contributing to the low earnings from hunting in Zambia in 2012 was the fact that 19 leases for hunting concessions ended prior to the end of the hunting season, and resident hunting was halted by the Zambian government (ZAWA unpublished data).

Social Indicators

The primary benefit to communities from national parks is employment and the development of wildlife-based economies around tourism hubs such as the growth point of Mfuwe, adjacent to South Luangwa National Park. Tourism generates an estimated 19,000 jobs in Zambia [27], though the proportion derived specifically from parks is not clear. In Mfuwe, ~900 jobs are created and such workers receive mean salaries of US$450/month, ~3x the minimum wage (A. Coley, pers. comm.). Tourism-related employment is significant because it can result in improved attitudes towards wildlife conservation [29]. However, most parks generate virtually no employment for communities due to the lack or small-scale of tourism operations.

In GMAs, benefits accruing to communities from trophy hunting include income generation for Community Resource

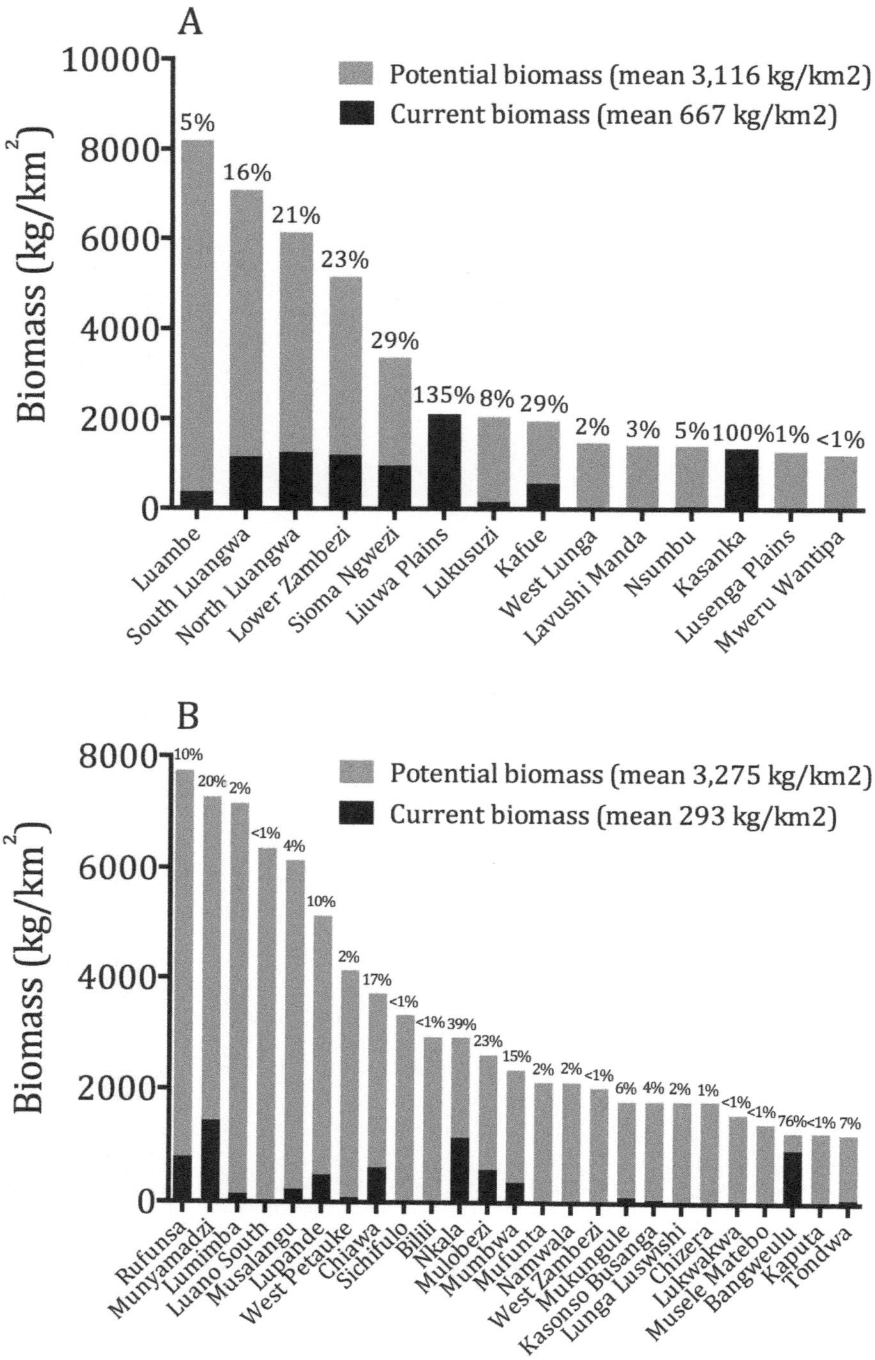

Figure 3. Observed large mammal biomass versus potential carrying capacity in Zambian (a) national parks and (b) GMAs.

Boards, employment and in some cases, various forms of development assistance from hunting operators. In some GMAs, such as those in the Luangwa Valley and Bangweulu system, livelihood improvements associated with income from trophy hunting are significant [30]: families in the most wildlife-rich GMAs are ~17% better off than those outside of the GMAs, and have a 7.8% higher chance of obtaining employment [8]. However, no earnings whatsoever are generated in half of the GMAs, and average earnings accruing to communities across all GMAs are low (USD11.9/km^2) (ZAWA unpublished data, Table 3). Concurrently, communities incur significant costs as a result of living with wildlife and ~50 people are killed annually by wild animals [31]. Overall, communities living in GMAs are 30% poorer than the national rural average [32].

Reasons for the Under-performance of Protected Areas

1. Community-related issues. There are no legal mechanisms to enable communities to benefit financially from photo-tourism in PAs. Furthermore, photo-tourism is under-developed and is practiced in a small fraction of the PA estate where the

Table 3. Gross earnings in USD from trophy hunting and non-resident hunting in Game Management Areas in 2012 (excluding land under 99 year lease within or near to GMAs) (NB that operators' net earnings are markedly lower than the gross income, due to the costs associated with paying concession and animal license fees to ZAWA, the costs of running and marketing safaris, and the costs of managing the concessions).

	Total	Operators*	ZAWA*	Community Resource Boards*	Chiefs*
Trophy hunting					
Concession fees	N/A	N/A	580,572	108,857	36,286
Animal license fees	N/A	N/A	1,697,878	1,528,090	169,788
Operators license fees	N/A	N/A	80,500	0	0
PH license fees	N/A	N/A	65,621	0	0
Daily rates	N/A	11,655,430	N/A	N/A	N/A
Trophy fees	N/A	4,506,987	N/A	N/A	N/A
Sub total	16,162,417	16,162,417	2,424,571	1,636,947	206,074
Resident hunting					
Total earnings	88,932	N/A	44,489	40,040	4,449
Non resident hunting earnings/km^2	0.6	N/A	0.3	0.3	0.0
Total earnings	16,251,349	16,162,417	2,469,060	1,676,988	210,522
Total earnings/km^2	97	N/A	14.8	10.0	1.3

*NB Operators were assumed to generate the total gross income from trophy hunting, from which the ZAWA and community income is derived. This income excludes that generated from extensive game ranches, which are on 99 year lease.

resource and existing conditions are suitable. For example, photo-tourism operations exist in only 10 of the 36 GMAs [7] and the existing legal framework does not require photo-tourism operators to pay Community Resource Boards [9]. Consequently, communities are only able to derive legal benefits from wildlife via trophy hunting in GMAs and through employment in national parks and GMAs.

The Wildlife Act fails to recognize communities as the rightful owners of the land or wildlife in GMAs (in contradiction to the Lands Act of 1995, [33]). There are no mechanisms for specific communities to obtain exclusive rights over land in GMAs or over the wildlife resources therein. Consequently, mechanisms to prevent in-migration of external communities into GMAs are weak. Immigration is likely fuelled by the availability of bushmeat, firewood and other natural resources, and in some cases, due to potential employment opportunities from tourism in adjacent national parks. Clearing of lands for settlement and shifting agriculture and tree-cutting for charcoal production all contribute to habitat loss in GMAs [9,15]. Uncontrolled immigration means that land use planning is difficult to enforce [6] and creates an open-access system whereby it pays communities to occupy land or kill wildlife before someone else does.

ZAWA collects revenues from trophy hunting and remits 20% of the concession fees to communities and 50% of animal license fees for wildlife shot as trophies in GMA [8]. ZAWA thus retains most of the income from hunting in GMAs even though the land is under customary tenure and belongs to the community. Wildlife-based land uses are effectively heavily taxed, whereas livestock production, small-scale agriculture and others are not (Table 3). Furthermore, income from wildlife is often paid late and as hand-outs that do not create a clear link between conservation and earnings [9,30]. Earnings for communities from trophy hunting are lower than estimated earnings from illegal bushmeat hunting and create weak incentives for conservation [34].

Communities living in GMAs are also marginalized from the decision-making relating to wildlife management. The concession agreements that are signed between ZAWA, hunting operators and Community Resource Boards on the leasing of GMAs favour ZAWA. ZAWA retain most of the income, delegate numerous responsibilities to other stakeholders, allocate minimal rights, are able to dismiss Community Resource Boards or to cancel the leases of hunting operators, and are not obliged to make their financial records available [11]. There is widespread resentment towards ZAWA, hunting and tourism operators (anon survey respondent, pers. comm.).

The make-up and functioning of Community Resource Boards is also problematic. More affluent community members benefit disproportionately from trophy hunting [30]. There is a lack of appropriately educated or skilled community members to form Community Resource Boards, which limits their ability to negotiate effectively with ZAWA or operators [9]. Skills shortages are exacerbated by the fact that the Community Resource Boards are re-formed each 2–3 years [35]. Furthermore, local chiefs can dismiss board members and 'village scouts' (community members employed by the community resource boards for anti-poaching) at their discretion, making Community Resource Boards unstable. There are frequent financial irregularities associated with CRB income from wildlife and funding allocated to resource protection is inadequate [9]. The 850 village scouts employed throughout Zambia are poorly and irregularly paid, insufficiently trained or equipped and are too few in number to effectively patrol the vast GMA estate [11].

2. ZAWA-related issues. When ZAWA was formed in 2000, a key objective was to increase efficiency and financial self-sufficiency [35]. ZAWA was meant to retain government support, but in practise funding was reduced to just 15% of operational budget. Including the ~USD4.6 million generated from trophy hunting, ZAWA's resources equate to USD20–60/km^2/year, which compares poorly with the USD358–USD455/km^2 required to manage protected areas effectively [36] ZAWA has a field staff complement of 1,179 to protect 231,000 km^2, which equates to 1/196 km^2 and compares poorly with the southern African regional average of 1/40 km^2 [1]. As little as 8% of the ZAWA budget is spent on GMAs even though they generate >50% of ZAWA earnings and comprise >70% of land under their jurisdiction [7]. Furthermore, ZAWA is encumbered by large numbers of sick and poorly trained staff, and an increasing proportion of ZAWA funds have been accruing to head office (anonymous survey respondent pers. comm.). Consequently, field capacity is low when the threat to wildlife from the bushmeat trade and is unprecedented and that from ivory poachers resurgent [2,37]. Funding shortages mean that ZAWA's mandate of protecting the vast wildlife estate is impossible to achieve.

To rectify this situation, ZAWA have allocated partial responsibility for resource protection to Community Resource Boards and hunting operators with the effect that roles are blurred and none of the stakeholders contribute sufficiently. This is despite the fact that responsibility for anti-poaching falls on ZAWA according to the Wildlife Act [11]. Technical support to Community Resource Boards from ZAWA is inadequate and communication between Community Resource Boards and ZAWA is limited [9].

Forced to generate their own funding, ZAWA rely on safari hunting in GMAs for ~45–67% of their revenue [11,35]. This reliance means that ZAWA are sometimes forced to make decisions to achieve financial survival at the expense of the wildlife they are mandated to conserve. For example, in 2003, ZAWA increased quotas and reduced the size of hunting blocks [7]. In addition, ZAWA have imposed high 'fixed-quotas' (of 60–100%) whereby operators are forced to pay for animal license fees before commencement of hunting [7,11]. Such quotas create a perverse incentive, forcing operators to harvest wildlife regardless of sustainability. Due to lack of funds, there is a lack of monitoring of wildlife populations or of trophies. Trophy quotas are established arbitrarily, quota utilization is low (averaging 40%) and prior to the ban trophy quality was falling, implying that quotas were not sustainable [7]. Quotas of lions have been particularly excessive [38,39].

The requirement for ZAWA to generate their funds means that it is not in their best interests to devolve user-rights over wildlife to communities in GMAs or to private landowners on extensive wildlife ranches (who are forced to pay license fees for animals hunted to ZAWA), as that would reduce income in the short-term and create perceived competition [19]. A similar conflict arose when the Zimbabwe Parks and Wildlife Management Authority became a parastatal responsible for generating their own revenue [40]. In Zimbabwe, that shift resulted in a gradual shift towards centralized authority over wildlife and gradual reversal of the devolution that made the wildlife ranching industry in that country such a success [40].

Wildlife in GMAs is affected by several other forms of legal harvest including resident hunting conducted by Zambian citizens and residents. Resident hunting licenses cost ~1/3 the meat value of the animals hunted, and consequently resident hunters often shoot wildlife specifically to obtain meat to sell, and in many cases, quotas are exceeded (Table 4). Such abuses are made possible by inadequate supervision of resident hunts and corruption. Prior to the hunting ban, a varying amount of wildlife was also killed under 'special licenses' allocated on a discretionary basis by the Minister of Tourism and Arts [35]. Special licenses and non-resident hunting licenses strip the value of wildlife and create minimal incentives for conservation by communities. The multiple forms of legal off-take compound the effects of habitat loss, predation and poaching and confer heavy depletion of wildlife in most GMAs (Figure 3b).

3. Operator-related issues. In national parks, tourism operators are not required to conduct anti-poaching and input is generally limited to sporadic provision of support for NGOs involved in resource protection [41]). In GMAs, the concession allocation system created disincentives for investment and good practice by hunting operators. Leases are granted for 10 years (or 15 for depleted blocks), which is not sufficient to encourage adequate investment in the area or to a sense of ownership of the areas [42]. Where wildlife populations are depressed, 15 years does not allow for sufficient time for operators to recoup the investments needed to allow wildlife populations to recover [43].

The hunting concession agreements (which outline commitments to anti-poaching and community outreach) are not effectively enforced [9]. Furthermore, operators typically vacate the hunting blocks during the rainy season, leaving their areas vulnerable to poachers. Some of the hunting blocks in GMAs are extremely large, and several operators complained that their size renders effective enforcement impossible. Some operators appear to invest a significant amount in anti-poaching and others virtually nothing. However, there is no system to link past performance of hunting operators to the prospects of them obtaining an extension of a lease or a new area. Consequently, responsible operators are not adequately rewarded, and unscrupulous operators not adequately punished, reducing incentives for good practice and allowing abuses (including alleged over-shooting of quotas by some operators) to continue [44]. In general, declining wildlife populations have resulted in falling incomes [7] and thus declining resources available protect the resource.

In early 2013, ZAWA imposed a moratorium on hunting in GMAs in response to alleged corruption in the tender process and due to concern over wildlife population trends. Consequently, hunting operators have vacated the GMAs, resulting in loss of their contribution to anti-poaching and creating a vacuum in which illegal activities are more likely to proceed unhindered. Evidence from Kafue National Park suggests that the simple presence of operators has a significant deterrent effect for poachers [41]. Furthermore, there have been extended periods in 2013 when village scouts went without pay, and many likely relied on poaching for income (Anon survey respondent, pers. comm.). While government has subsequently stepped in to pay the salaries of village scouts, it is not clear as to how such payments will be sustained in the absence of hunting income. There have been few proposals from the photo-tourism industry to take over GMAs in the wake of the hunting ban. The hunting moratorium is thus likely to fuel wildlife declines by reducing: anti-poaching effort and presence in GMAs; working capital for ZAWA; and incentives for conservation by communities.

4. Other factors. There are multiple authorities in GMAs with jurisdiction over the management of different resources [35]. In addition, conflicting legislation precludes effective land use planning. For example, the wildlife act states that ZAWA is responsible for wildlife resources in the area, and by implication habitat, whereas the Local Government Act says that local councils are responsible for planning and development [35]. Consequently development-related decisions are sometimes made in GMAs with little consideration of their impacts on wildlife or the potential for wildlife-based land uses. Furthermore, chiefs are able to allocate land to private investors in the middle of GMAs without consulting Community Resource Boards [9].

Changes Needed to Improve the Functioning of the Protected Area Network

In this section we outline a number of key steps that we consider to be necessary to improve the functioning of the Zambian PA

Table 4. The price of citizen licenses for hunting in GMAs, the meat value of those species and the value of the meat relative to the price of citizen licenses.

	Citizens	Meat value*	Meat value relative to license fee
Buffalo	493	1398	3
Bushbuck	40	142	4
Bush pig	16	146	9
Duiker	32	40	1
Eland	592	1425	2
Hartebeest	158	355	2
Impala	40	150	4
Kudu	493	551	1
Oribi	59	33	1
Puku	69	159	2
Reedbuck	79	159	2
Warthog	79	185	2
Waterbuck	158	615	4
Wildebeest	158	593	4
Zebra	296	757	3
Average ± S.E.			3±0.75

*Assuming male animals are hunted, a meat price of USD4.3/kg (the price paid by Lusaka butchers for dressed meat) and assuming the mean mass of dressed carcasses presented by [72].

network, many of which are likely to apply to PAs in various other parts of Africa.

1. Empowering communities to benefit more from the PA network. There is a need to develop systems to enable communities to benefit more from PAs so as to enhance their social and economic value. Potential models to for such community engagement are discussed in the next section.

2. Re-defining the role of ZAWA. The role of ZAWA should be re-defined so that the organisation focuses primarily on national parks, and elsewhere plays more of a hands-off coordinating role to facilitate the development of wildlife-based land uses by community, private, and NGO partners. There is need for recognition from government that unless earnings are vastly higher than they have been in the past, the GMAs cannot be used to fund other parts of the PA network or to support ZAWA headquarters. If ZAWA continue to extract revenues from GMAs, then a commensurate reinvestment in law enforcement and wildlife management in those areas is required.

3. Greatly increasing funding from government for ZAWA. Drastically increasing government funding for ZAWA. Such funding should be seen as an investment in the development of the tourism industry rather than as a cost (as discussed further below). Even at current rates of funding for ZAWA, there is evidence of impressive returns on investment: in 2005, the government of Zambia received USD8 million from wildlife-related tourism from an investment of just USD1 million [32]. The tourism industry in Zambia comprises just 5% of GDP compared to a global mean of 14%, and creates just 3.6% of national employment compared to a regional mean of 7.2% [13,45,46]. In addition, there has been relatively minimal capital investment in the tourism industry in Zambia (1.7% of GDP c.f. a regional average of 6.9%) [13]. There is thus major scope for growth in the Zambian tourism industry, particularly given projections of rapid increases in visitor arrivals to the SADC region [13]. To achieve that growth, however, there is a need for much greater investment in protecting the wildlife product.

4. Harnessing international willingness to pay for conservation. There is a need for greater international support for PA management in Zambia. The Zambian PA network constitutes ~40% of the country's land area, compared to a global average of 12% [47]. A developing country such as Zambia cannot reasonably be expected to pay for all of the costs of the maintenance of that global asset in addition to bearing the associated opportunity costs. Furthermore, tourism and trophy hunting (in the case of GMAs) may never generate enough income to cover the costs needed for effective protected area management. There are numerous potential avenues for harnessing international willingness to pay for wildlife conservation, including *inter alia*:

a) Encouraging co-management agreements for PA management. In national parks, ZAWA could pursue the development of co-management agreements with NGOs and the private sector to share the burden of PA management and attract additional technical capacity. Encouragingly, there has been an increasing trend towards development of such agreements in Zambia in recent years [5,48]. There are official co-management agreements in place for five national parks and two GMAs (ZAWA unpublished data). In addition, there is significant NGO involvement in resource protection in several other national parks (e.g. Kafue, South Luangwa, Lower Zambezi, Sioma Ngwezi, and Nyika) and 11 other GMAs. If ZAWA could focus primarily on coordinating and regulating the management of PAs by partner organisations, the effectiveness and cost-effectiveness of parks could be greatly enhanced. NGOs and the private sector could be encouraged to take over the management of entire PAs or of concessions within PAs. Such a set up also would provide NGOs that are opposed to trophy hunting with the opportunity to reduce the prevalence of the practice by making payments in lieu of hunting revenues in the GMAs.

b) Attracting funding for the development of a national CBNRM programme. In addition to funding ZAWA and the PA network, there is a need for funding to allow for a national community-based natural resource management (CBNRM) programme to facilitate the capture of a greater proportion of benefits from the PA network by communities. Such funding could build on the progress made by the Administrative Management Design for Game Management Areas (ADMADE) during the 1990s. The successes of the Namibian community conservancy programme and the Zimbabwean CAMPFIRE programme have been dependent on long-term and substantial injections of technical capacity and funding (USD173 million and USD35 million respectively) ([49], C. Weaver pers. comm.). Likewise, the community conservancies in the northern Kenyan rangelands are supported by a coordinating NGO with funding of ~USD1.2 million annually [50]. A similarly well funded, supported and coordinated national CBNRM programme is needed in Zambia.

c) Encouraging allocation of a greater portion of overseas development aid towards PAs. There is a strong case for donors to direct a portion of international development aid towards PA management, capitalizing ZAWA and/or co-management agreements between ZAWA and NGOs, and/or developing a national CBNRM programme. Recent estimates suggest that for every 1% increase in tourism-related investment in the SADC region, a 0.3% increase in GDP per capita accrues [13]. An allocation of just 2–3% of the ~USD1 billion of overseas development aid that Zambia receives annually [51] would cover the costs of managing the national parks effectively and of protecting the main tourism asset [32]. However, there is a need for checks and balances to ensure efficient use of donor funds by ZAWA.

A potentially cost-effective way of using donor funds to achieve both conservation and development objectives (ideally in the context of a coordinated national CBNRM programme) is through schemes that channel payments to communities living in or near PAs for the provision of ecosystem services. For example, communities could be paid an annual fee for desisting from converting habitat or for protecting wildlife from poaching. In the Maasai steppe in Tanzania for example, such an approach has achieved notable conservation gains for a cost of just USD48/km^2 [52], which compares favourably with the costs of traditional PA management. A key potential value of PES approaches is that they can help correct 'market failures' whereby wildlife that is valuable to the nation as a whole is not valuable to the people living with it, who thus over-exploit the resource or invest little in protecting it [50]. PES approaches could be combined with efforts to provide communities with stable markets and fair prices for livestock and crops, as is being conducted in the Kenyan community conservancies, and as part of the community markets for conservation approach in parts of Zambia [50,53]. However, the latter approaches are only likely to be successful if combined with efforts to actively protect wildlife populations via anti-poaching.

d) Other options. Capturing the willingness of international philanthropists to pay for conservation represents another potential means of funding PAs [54]. Several precedents for such investment exist, such as that provided in Gorongosa National Park in Mozambique and the Grumeti Game Reserve in Tanzania. Additionally, attracting carbon-related investment via projects such as REDD+ could potentially generate funds for the protection of woodlands and associated biodiversity, notwithstanding the constraints currently associated with that programme [55]. Further, government could potentially generate additional revenue by taxing stakeholders who benefit substantively from ecological services provided by PAs, such as commercial farmers and power-generating or mining companies.

5. Attracting significant private investment. To develop tourism and hunting businesses in national parks and GMAs, and to protect and manage wildlife in GMAs (assuming that ZAWA focuses their efforts on national parks) would require substantial private and/or donor investment. Rehabilitating a single depleted GMA is predicted to cost millions of dollars and such investments would likely take many years to recoup [43]. Attracting such investment is most likely under the following circumstances: an enabling policy environment; simple safe and standardized processes for investing; long leases (of at least 40 years for depleted areas [43]); attractive terms (e.g. as would be conferred if ZAWA desisted from taxing wildlife-based land uses in GMAs); minimal red-tape or interference from ZAWA, a functioning national programme for the development of community wildlife conservancies (see below) and knowledge that communities are supportive of wildlife investments on their land. In GMAs, investors and community partners should be able to choose any forms of wildlife-based land uses and the combinations that will yield the best returns for their particular spatial setting. Consequently, hunting bans or bans on the hunting of high-value species are to be avoided so long as hunting can be managed in a manner that ensures sustainability [12]. Finally, resident hunting should not be allowed to undermine private investments in GMAs and should only be permitted if desired by the community and investor partners and if priced appropriately.

6. Addressing key conservation threats decisively. For the PA networks to function better, there is a need to decisively address key threats such as human encroachment, bushmeat and other forms of poaching. Human encroachment could be addressed through linking the allocation of leases to communities with agreed land use plans (see below). Alternatively, portions of GMAs close to national parks could be re-gazetted as 'buffer-zones' where human settlement is not permitted (though the leases for such areas could still be leased to communities to enable them to benefit from legal wildlife-based land uses, see below). In such instances and at the edge of community conservancies (see below), fencing external boundaries (if supported by communities) may play a significant role in reducing edge-effects, reducing human-wildlife conflict, demarcating boundaries and helping to prevent further encroachment [58,59]. Where human settlement has reached right up to the boundaries of national parks, the fencing of such sections may be justified if appropriate materials are used and if adequate funding for maintenance exists.

Addressing poaching requires elevated opportunities for communities to benefit legally from wildlife, stiffer legal frameworks relating to poaching (with penalties that reflect the value of wildlife and the threat posed by poachers to the life of PA staff) and improved anti-poaching are required [2]. To achieve professional, well-funded anti-poaching requires either a much greater investment from ZAWA, and/or significant investments from the private and/or NGO sector.

7. Prioritising conservation efforts. Zambia's PA network is vast and funding limited. Furthermore, some of the GMAs are probably damaged beyond repair due to heavy human settlement and habitat modification. Given these factors plus the high human population growth rates, conserving the entire PA network in the long term is unlikely. There is a case for a scientific priority setting exercise to identify the PAs that should be the priority for investment of available funding.

Potential Models for Achieving Elevated Community Participation in the PA Network

The degree of involvement of communities in national parks versus GMAs should arguably differ as people reside the latter but generally not the former. For national parks, one option would be to allocate ownership of PAs, shareholdings of PAs, or tourism concessions within parks to neighbouring communities for them to lease out to tourism operators. Precedents for such arrangements have been established in South Africa, for example, through the creation of contractual parks [56]. Such changes would require clear definition on who comprises 'the community' as at present, membership is poorly defined, compromising effective plan implementations and revenue sharing.

In the GMAs, we recommend changes that empower communities and enable them to participate in and benefit from wildlife-based land uses through the formation of Community Wildlife Conservancies (CWCs). Precedents for such conservancies have been developed in both Namibia and the northern rangelands of Kenya, both of which have achieved significant conservation and livelihood gains [50,57]. While there are many potential variants of such models that could applied to the GMAs, there are a few general principles that we believe should be adhered to: a) communities should be allocated the maximum permissible degree of ownership over land and wildlife; b) that ownership should be structured such that it is exclusive for specific communities to avoid perpetuation of the tragedy of the commons; c) communities should accrue benefits from wildlife directly, and not via remittances from ZAWA; d) communities must actively participate in wildlife management decisions and not be passive recipients of hand-outs; e) community structures that are used to administer finances relating to wildlife must be democratic, transparent and regularly audited to ensure equitable distribution of benefits and avoid elite capture; and f) there must be mechanisms to ensure funding for high-quality anti-poaching security given the level of threat in GMAs. Two examples of potential models for the establishment and functioning of CWCs in GMAs are as follows:

1. Complete devolution model. Here CWCs in the GMAs would be established as community conservancies based on joint ventures between communities and the private sector. ZAWA would not extract income from the CWC and would play a purely regulatory, facilitating and over-seeing role. ZAWA currently earn nothing from half of the GMAs as it is and so in such areas this kind of arrangement would not cause loss of revenue for ZAWA. The community would create a democratic, accountable and transparent body or trust to administer the area as a conservancy. A long lease would then be allocated by government to that community conservancy trust, the validity of which should be contingent on a land use plan that ensures that a particular area is set aside for wildlife only. Communities would then sub-lease the land to or engage in business partnerships with private or NGO investors, ideally for long periods to attract significant investment. That leasing process could follow either a public auction or an open tender process. The communities and successful bidding investors would then form a second body or trust with the mandate of managing wildlife in the GMA, ensuring professional anti-poaching and effective communication and cooperation between the community and investors. Alternatively, the investors could gain representation on the community conservancy trust after signing a partnership agreement, and then that body would coordinate wildlife management. Investors would then pay: a) an annual land rental to communities (which means they would derive some income without waiting years for wildlife populations to recover); b) an annual resource use fee (e.g. bed night levies or licence fees for animals hunted) (which means that communities would receive income proportional to their conservation 'performance'); and, c) an annual levy to capitalize the body with the responsibility for managing wildlife. Investors could generate income either by acting as their own hunting or tourism operators, by auctioning hunting packages to the highest bidding operator, or sub-leasing tourism concessions.

2. Partial devolution model. In this model, GMAs would be administered as community conservancies based on tripartite public-private-community-partnerships involving communities, ZAWA and private investors. As in the previous model, the communities would form a body that obtains a lease for the land, and would sub-lease the land to investors (or engage in a long term business partnership). A largely independent not-for-profit body would be established with representation from ZAWA, investors/ participating NGOs and communities with the mandate of managing the wildlife in the area. The fees that have traditionally been paid to ZAWA by operators would be paid into that not-for-profit body to ensure that they are reinvested in the area.

Re-designating GMAs as CWCs would confer multiple benefits: CWCs would secure land rights for communities and protect against the loss of land and natural resources that would arise from the current open access system; CWCs could provide an effective buffer role for national parks; communities would generate significant and sustainable incomes, meat supplies and employment; if wildlife populations were successfully rehabilitated, CWCs could generate economic outputs at least 20x greater than currently being earned in GMAs [43]; CWCs would attract external investment by a wide-spectrum of donors; CWCs would create scope for communities to sell carbon and biodiversity credits by securing land rights [15]; and ZAWA would be relieved of the burden and costs of protecting wildlife in GMAs.

Legislative Changes Needed to Allow CWCs to Happen

Ownership of wildlife in Zambia is vested in the President on behalf of the country [19]. On private land, user-rights over wildlife can be conferred to landowners via certificates of ownership, but there is no such provision for communities. Similarly, there is scope for investors, but not communities, to alienate land [9]. New legislation is required to enable communities to obtain 99-year leases for their land in GMAs following formation of a CWC, and to enable them to obtain full-user rights over wildlife.

At present, fencing is a pre-requisite for obtaining ownership over wildlife on wildlife ranches in Zambia [19]. In some contexts, as discussed, fencing can confer clear benefits [58,59]. However, fencing can also reduce ecological connectivity and provide massive supplies of snare-material if inappropriate wires are used [58,60]. Fencing should not be a pre-requisite for communities to obtain user-rights over wildlife and should not be permitted between adjacent CWCs or between CWCs and national parks. If needed, fencing should also be composed of kinked wire mesh to prevent snare construction, and should be accompanied by an environmental impact assessment and a clear long-term maintenance plan and budget.

Conclusions

Wildlife populations are faring poorly in many African protected areas [61] and many of the challenges and solutions highlighted in this paper occur in other African countries. The under-funding of protected area networks is a widespread problem and parks agencies are often required to generate their own income, which creates the kinds of conflicts of interest outlined in this paper. There is a need for vastly elevated funding for PA management from both African and international governments and institutions. There is the need for improved mechanisms to enable communities to participate in and benefit more from wildlife in many African countries. In addition, creating frameworks for safe and secure private and NGO investment in PA management is an intervention with widespread applicability. Strong measures to address unplanned human encroachment in PA networks are also needed in many areas, as are efforts to tackle high levels of ivory and bushmeat poaching. The net result of these interventions is likely to be significant improvements in the effectiveness of parks networks, substantial job creation and economic gains due to growth in tourism industries. In the absence of such changes, wildlife populations in protected areas in Zambia and many other countries are likely to continue to wane due to on-going poaching and human encroachment.

Methods

Insights into the Performance of Protected Areas

We provided insights into the performance of PAs using: a) a literature review; b) data obtained from ZAWA and other sources; c) and, semi-structured interviews with key stakeholders, including the highest-ranking ZAWA officials (n = 7); representatives from relevant NGOs (n = 14); wildlife industry experts/photo-tourism operators (n = 11); and trophy hunting operators (n = 13). The literature review was conducted using key words such as 'Zambia', 'GMAs', 'wildlife policy', 'CBNRM', 'ADMADE', 'trophy hunting', 'wildlife ranching', 'co-management', 'bushmeat', 'and encroachment', etc. We included both published papers and unpublished consultancy reports. We searched for references using Google and Google Scholar. Selection of survey respondents was conducted by contacting and meeting as many individuals from each group that we could during our fieldwork period (September–November, 2012). Refusal rate was zero.

1. Ecological performance of protected areas. We assessed ecological performance of protected areas by looking at the degree of human encroachment and the size and diversity of wildlife populations. Data on human encroachment were obtained from [6]. The 2010 Zambian census was used to obtain district-level estimates of human population growth rates [16].

Data on wildlife abundance in protected areas were derived from aerial census reports [17,24,25,62–67]. The most recent reports were used, though some abundance estimates were made using census reports as old as 2003, and for some PAs no census data were available at all. Census data were available for 39 Zambian PAs (14 National Parks comprising 61,812 km^2 and 25 GMAs comprising 152,122 km^2) (or ~93% of the national park and GMA estate). Estimates of mammalian biomass were made by removing species of bushbuck *Tragelaphus scriptus* size or smaller, hippopotamuses *Hippopotamus amphibius* and predators as most reports did not provide estimates for those species. The typical mass of an individual in a population for each species following [68] was multiplied by population sizes to estimate biomass.

We used rainfall, soil nutrient status and large herbivore biomass for 28 wildlife areas in eastern and southern Africa [69] to create five regression curves for predicting herbivore biomass for: 1) medium soil nutrient areas for moist-adapted species; 2) medium soil nutrient areas for arid-adapted species; 3) low soil nutrient areas for moist-adapted species; 4) low soil nutrient areas for arid-adapted species with annual rainfall <700 mm; 5) low soil nutrient areas for arid-adapted species with annual rainfall > 700 mm. In each case, herbivore biomass was plotted against rainfall using the software programme GraphPad Prism. These five regression curves were then used to predict *potential* herbivore standing crop biomasses (kg/km^2) for protected areas in which annual rainfall and soil nutrient data were available. Estimates for annual rainfall were determined from literature and internet sources, while soil nutrient status was determined using a combination of two sources: 1) soil maps [70] and 2) vegetation types identified from the literature and vegetation maps [71].

In protected areas where there was more than one soil or vegetation type, we estimated the proportion of each type within the area, and used these to calculate an average soil nutrient status. In many cases, the soil nutrient status estimated from soil and vegetation types corresponded well, but in cases when they differed, the lower estimate was selected for the sake of conservatism.

2. Economic performance of protected areas. Data on earnings from photo-tourism in national parks, and from trophy and resident hunting in GMAs were obtained from ZAWA to assess economic performance of protected areas. Earnings of safari operators in GMAs were estimated using trophy off-takes for 2012 obtained from ZAWA, following [28] and using the mean 2013 pricing for Zambian trophy hunts (from a survey of $n = 10$ websites). Current per km^2 earnings from trophy hunting in Zambia were compared with regional estimates derived from [28]. Further insights into the performance of the hunting and tourism industries were obtained from the literature.

3. Social performance. Insights into the social performance of protected areas were obtained from the literature and through surveys. Comprehensive community surveys in GMAs have been completed by other authors recently (e.g. [8,9,30] and their findings provided insights into community-related issues.

Ethics Statement

The University of Pretoria Ethics Committee approved this research, and approved the procedure for obtaining consent for the surveys conducted during the research. We were issued with written consent for this study from the Wildlife Producers' Association of Zambia. In addition Zambia Wildlife Authority provided verbal approval and participated in the research. From respondents we obtained verbal consent prior to conducting the surveys. Written consent from individual respondents was not considered practical or necessary and the requirement for written consent was waived by the University of Pretoria. We documented any cases where respondents did not wish to participate in order to calculate refusal rates.

Supporting Information

Figure S1 The (a) biomass and (b) diversity of wild ungulates (excluding species of bushbuck size and smaller and hippos, for which data were unavailable for state protected areas) in GMAs, national parks and extensive (unfenced) private game ranches [19].
(TIFF)

Figure S2 The (a) biomass and (b) diversity of wild ungulates (excluding species of bushbuck size and smaller and hippos, for which data were unavailable for state protected areas) in protected areas and extensive game ranches with and without NGO or private investment in law enforcement.
(TIFF)

Acknowledgments

Thanks to ZAWA for permission to conduct the study, for participating in surveys and for provision of information, thanks to the Wildlife Producers Association of Zambia, Don Stacey and to the ranchers and other respondents.

Author Contributions

Conceived and designed the experiments: PL WAT VN JB MT CT. Performed the experiments: PL WAT VN JB MT CT. Analyzed the data: PL WAT VN JB MT MB RM FW CT. Contributed reagents/materials/analysis tools: PL WAT VN JB MT MB RM FW CT. Wrote the paper: PL WAT VN JB MT MB RM FW CT.

References

1. Cumming D (2004) Performance of parks in a century of change. In: Child B, editor. Parks in Transition: Biodiversity, Rural Development, and the Bottom Line. UK: Earthscan.
2. Lindsey PA, Balme G, Becker M, Begg C, Bento C, et al. (2013) The bushmeat trade in African savannas: Impacts, drivers, and possible solutions. Biol Conserv 160: 80–96.
3. Caro TM, Pelkey N, Borner M, Campbell K, Woodworth B, et al. (1998) Consequences of different forms of conservation for large mammals in Tanzania: Preliminary analyses. Afr J Ecol 36: 303–320.
4. Nelson F, Lindsey P, Balme G (2013) Trophy hunting and lion conservation: a question of governance? Oryx 47: 501–509.
5. Government of Zambia (2010) Reclassification and effective management of the national protected areas system. Lusaka, Zambia: Ministry of Tourism, Environment and Natural Resources.
6. Watson FGR, Becker MS, Nyirenda MA (In press) Human encroachment into protected area networks in Zambia: Implications for large carnivore conservation. Environmental Change.
7. Simasiku P, Simwanza H, Tembo G, Bandyopadhyay S, Pavy J (2008) The impact of wildlife management policies on communities and conservation in game management areas in Zambia. Zambia: Natural Resources Consultative Forum.
8. Fernandez A, Richardson RB, Tschirley DL, Tembo G (2010) Wildlife conservation in Zambia: Impacts on rural household welfare. Michigan State University: Food Security Collaborative Working Papers.
9. Chemonics International Inc (2011) Situational and livelihoods analysis study in nine Game Management Areas, surrounding the Kafue National Park, Zambia. Washington DC, USA: Millenium Challenge Corporation.
10. Becker M, McRobb R, Watson F, Droge E, Kanyembo B, et al. (2013) Evaluating wire-snare poaching trends and the impacts of by-catch on elephants and large carnivores. Biol Conserv 158: 26–36.
11. Manning I (2011) Wildlife conservation in Zambia and the Landsafe customary commons. Natural Resources Journal 52: 195–214.
12. Lindsey P, Balme G, Funston P, Henschel P, Madzikanda H, et al. (2013) The trophy hunting of African lions: Scale, current management practices and factors undermining sustainability. Plos One 8(9): e73808.
13. Makochekanwa A (2013) An analysis of tourism contribution to economic growth in SADC countries. Botswana Journal of Economics 11(5): 42–56.
14. Pfeifer M, Burgess ND, Swetnam RD, Platts PJ, Willcock S, et al. (2012) Protected areas: Mixed success in conserving east Africa's evergreen forests. Plos One 7: e39337.
15. Vinya R, Syampungani S, Kasumu EC, Monde C, Kasubika R (2011) Preliminary study on the drivers of deforestation and potential for REDD+ in Zambia. Lusaka, Zambia: FAO/Zambian Ministry of Lands and Natural Resources.
16. Zambia Central Statistical Office (2011) 2010 census of population and housing: Preliminary population figures. Lusaka, Zambia: Government of Zambia.
17. Simukonda C (2011) Wet season survey of the African elephant and other large herbivores in selected areas of the Luangwa Valley. Chilanga, Zambia: Zambia Wildlife Authority.
18. Poulsen JR, Clark CJ, Mavah G, Elkan PW (2009) Bushmeat supply and consumption in a tropical logging concession in northern Congo. Conserv Biol 23: 1597–1608.
19. Lindsey P, Barnes J, Nyirenda V, Pumfrett B, Taylor A, et al. (2013) The Zambian wildlife ranching industry: Scale, associated benefits, and limitations affecting its development. Plos One 8(12): e81761.
20. Bond I (2009) CBNRM as a mechanism for addressing global environmental challenges. In: Roe D, Nelson F, Sandbrook C, editors. Community management of natural resources in Africa: impacts, experiences and future directions. London, UK.: International Institute for Environment and Development. 95–104.
21. Owen-Smith N, Ogutu J (2003) Interactions between biotic components. In: Du Toit J, Rogers K, Biggs H, editors. The Kruger experience: ecology and management of savanna heterogeneity. Washington DC: Island Press. 310–331.
22. Whyte I, van Aarde R, Pimm S (2003) Kruger's elephant population: Its size and consequences for ecosystem heterogeneity. In: Du Toit J, Rogers K, Biggs H, editors. The Kruger experience: ecology and management of savanna heterogeneity. Washington DC: Island Press. 332–348.
23. Lindsey PA, Roulet PA, Romañach SS (2007) Economic and conservation significance of the trophy hunting industry in sub-Saharan Africa. Biol Conserv 134: 455–469.
24. Frederick H (2013) Aerial survey report: Luangwa valley, 2012. Chilanga, Zambia: Zambia Wildlife Authority.
25. ZAWA (2013) Liuwa Plain National Park aerial wildlife survey results 2013. Lusaka, Zambia: ZAWA.
26. ZAWA (2013) Kafue National Park general management plan. Chilanga, Zambia: Zambia Wildlife Authority.
27. Hamilton K, Tembo G, Sinyenga G, Bandyopadhyay S, Pope A, et al. (2007) The real economic impact of nature tourism in Zambia. Lusaka, Zambia: Natural Resources Consultative Forum.
28. Lindsey P, Balme G, Booth V, Midlane N (2012) The significance of African lions for the financial viability of trophy hunting and the maintenance of wild land. Plos One : e29332.
29. Snyman SL (2012) The role of tourism employment in poverty reduction and community perceptions of conservation and tourism in southern Africa. Journal of Sustainable Tourism 20: 395–416.
30. Bandyopadhyay S, Tembo G (2010) Household consumption and natural resource management around national parks in Zambia. Journal of Natural Resources Policy Research 2: 39–55.
31. Chomba C, Senzota R, Chabwela H, Mwitwa J, Nyirenda V (2012) Patterns of human–wildlife conflicts in Zambia, causes, consequences and management responses. Journal of Ecology and the Natural Environment 4: 303–313.
32. World Bank (2007) Economic and poverty impact of nature-based tourism. Lusaka, Zambia: World Bank.
33. Manning I (2011) Wildlife conservation in Zambia and the landsafe customary commons. Pretoria: University of Pretoria, PhD thesis.
34. Lindsey P, Taylor A, Nyirenda V, Barnes J (2014) Through severe impacts on wildlife populations and net negative economic and food security impacts, bushmeat poaching is a market failure. Harare, Zimbabwe: FAO/Panthera/IUCN SULi/ZSL report.
35. Sichilongo M, Mulozi P, Mbewe B, Machala C, Pavy J (2013) Zambian wildlife sector policy: Impact analysis and recommendations for the future policy. Lusaka, Zambia: Africa Technical Environment and Natural Resources Unit, World Bank.
36. Cumming DH (2008) Large scale conservation planning and priorities for the Kavango-Zambezi Transfrontier Conservation Area. Unpublished report commissioned by Conservation International.
37. Douglas-Hamilton I (2009) The current elephant poaching trend. Pachyderm 45: 154–157.
38. Yamazaki K (1996) Social variation of lions in a male-depopulated area in Zambia. The Journal of Wildlife Management 60: 490–497.
39. Becker M, Watson F, Droge E, Leigh K, Carlson R, et al. (2012) Estimating past and future male loss in three Zambian lion populations. Journal of Wildlife Management DOI:10.1002/jwmg.446.
40. Wels H (2003) Private wildlife conservation in Zimbabwe: Joint ventures and reciprocity. Leiden, Netherlands: Brill.
41. Lindsey P, Midlane N, Sayer E, van der Westhuizen H (2013) Kafue National Park resource protection strategy review. New York: Panthera/Frankfurt Zoological Society.
42. Lindsey P, Balme G, Funston P, Henschel P, Hunter L, et al. (2013) The trophy hunting of African lions: Scale, current management practices and factors undermining sustainability. Plos One 8(9): e73808.
43. Lindsey P, Nyirenda V, Barnes J, Becker M, Taylor A, et al. (2013) The reasons why Zambian Game management areas are not functioning as ecologically or economically productive buffer zones and what needs to change for them to fulfill that role. Lusaka, Zambia: Wildlife Producers Association of Zambia.
44. Leader-Williams N, Baldus RD, Smith RJ (2009) The influence of corruption on the conduct of recreational hunting. In: Dickson B, Hutton J, Adams W, editors. Recreational Hunting, Conservation and Rural Livelihoods. Oxford, UK: Wiley-Blackwell. 296–316.
45. WTTC (2013) Economic impact of travel and tourism: Mid-year update, October 2013. London, UK: World Travel and Tourism Council.
46. WTTC (2012) Travel and tourism, economic impact 2012 Zambia. London, UK: World Travel and Tourism Council.
47. Secretariat of the Convention on Biological Diversity (2008) Protected areas in today's world: Their values and benefits for the welfare of the planet. Montreal, Canada: CBD.
48. Nyirenda VR, Nkhata BA (2013) Collaborative governance and benefit sharing in Liuwa Plain National Park, western Zambia.
49. Taylor RD (2009) Community based natural resource management in Zimbabwe: The experience of CAMPFIRE. Biodiversity and Conservation 18(10): 2563–2583.
50. Pye-Smith C (2013) The story of the northern rangelands trust. Isiolo, Kenya: Northern Rangelands Trust.
51. OECD (2013) Development aid at a glance. Paris, France: Organisation for Economic Co-operation and Development.
52. Ingram J, Wilkie D., Clements T, McNab R, Nelson F, et al. (In press) Evidence of payments for ecosystem services as a mechanism for supporting biodiversity conservation and rural livelihoods. Ecosystem Services.
53. Lewis D, Bell SD, Fay J, Bothi KL, Gatere L, et al. (2011) Community markets for conservation (COMACO) links biodiversity conservation with sustainable improvements in livelihoods and food production. Proceedings of the National Academy of Sciences 108: 13957–13962.

54. Spierenburg M, Wels H (2010) Conservative philanthropists, royalty and business elites in nature conservation in southern Africa. Antipode 42: 647–670.
55. Phelps J, Webb EL, Koh LP (2011) Risky business: An uncertain future for biodiversity conservation finance through REDD+. Conservation Letters 4: 88–94.
56. Reid H (2001) Contractual national parks and the Makuleke community. Hum Ecol 29: 135–155.
57. Jones B, Weaver C (2008) CBNRM in Namibia: Growth, trends, lessons and constraints. In: Suich H, Child B, Spenceley A, editors. Evolution and innovation in wildlife conservation in southern Africa. London, UK: Earthscan. 223–242.
58. Lindsey PA, Masterson CL, Beck AL, Romañach S (2012) Ecological, social and financial issues related to fencing as a conservation tool in Africa. In: Somers MJ, Hayward M, editors. Fencing for Conservation.: Springer New York. 215–234.
59. Packer C, Canney S, Loveridge A, Garnett S, Zander K, et al. (2013) Effective conservation of large carnivores. Ecological Letters 16: 635–641.
60. Lindsey PA, Romañach SS, Tambling CJ, Chartier K, Groom R (2011) Ecological and financial impacts of illegal bushmeat trade in Zimbabwe. Oryx 45: 96–111.
61. Craigie ID, Baillie JEM, Balmford A, Carbone C, Collen B, et al. (2010) Large mammal population declines in Africa's protected areas. Biol Conserv 143: 2221–2228.
62. Simwanza H (2004) Aerial survey of large herbivores in West Lunga National Park, Chizera, Musele Matebo, Lukwakwa and Chibkwika Ntambo Game Management Areas. Chilanga, Lusaka: Zambia Wildlife Authority.
63. Simwanza H (2004) Aerial survey to establish the status of large herbivores in the Upper Luano hunting block. Chilanga, Lusaka: Zambia Wildlife Authority.
64. Simwanza H (2005) Aerial survey of large herbivores in the Zambezi heartland, Zambia: October 2005. Kariba, Zimbabwe: African Wildlife Foundation.
65. Simukonda C (2008) A country-wide survey of large mammals in Zambia. Chilanga, Zambia: Zambia Wildlife Authority.
66. Frederick H (2011) Aerial survey of Kafue ecosystem 2008. Lusaka, Zambia: Zambia Wildlife Authority.
67. Viljoen P (2013) Liuwa plain national park and adjacent Game Management Area, Zambia: Aerial wildlife survey April 2013. Johannesburg: African parks network report.
68. Coe M, Cumming D, Phillipson J (1976) Biomass and production of large African herbivores in relation to rainfall and primary production. Oecologia 22(4): 341–354.
69. East R (1984) Rainfall, soil nutrients status and biomass of large African mammals. African Journal of Ecology 22: 245–270.
70. Jones A, Breuning-Madsen H, Brossard M, Dampha A, Deckers J, et al. (2013) Soil atlas of Africa. Luxembourg: European Commission.
71. Wild H, Fernandes A (1967). Vegetation map of the Flora Zambesiaca area. Salisbury, Rhodesia: Collins.
72. du P Bothma J, du Toit JG (2010) Game ranch management. Pretoria, South Africa: Van Schaik.

2

Mapping Large-Area Landscape Suitability for Honey Bees to Assess the Influence of Land-Use Change on Sustainability of National Pollination Services

Alisa L. Gallant[1]*, Ned H. Euliss Jr.[2], Zac Browning[3]

1 United States Geological Survey, Earth Resources Observation and Science Center, Sioux Falls, South Dakota, United States of America, **2** United States Geological Survey, Northern Prairie Wildlife Research Center, Jamestown, North Dakota, United States of America, **3** Browning's Honey Company, Inc., Jamestown, North Dakota, United States of America

Abstract

Pollination is a critical ecosystem service affected by various drivers of land-use change, such as policies and programs aimed at land resources, market values for crop commodities, local land-management decisions, and shifts in climate. The United States is the world's most active market for pollination services by honey bees, and the Northern Great Plains provide the majority of bee colonies used to meet the Nation's annual pollination needs. Legislation requiring increased production of biofuel crops, increasing commodity prices for crops of little nutritional value for bees in the Northern Great Plains, and reductions in government programs aimed at promoting land conservation are converging to alter the regional landscape in ways that challenge beekeepers to provide adequate numbers of hives for national pollination services. We developed a spatially explicit model that identifies sites with the potential to support large apiaries based on local-scale land-cover requirements for honey bees. We produced maps of potential apiary locations for North Dakota, a leading producer of honey, based on land-cover maps representing (1) an annual time series compiled from existing operational products and (2) a realistic scenario of land change. We found that existing land-cover products lack sufficient local accuracy to monitor actual changes in landscape suitability for honey bees, but our model proved informative for evaluating effects on suitability under scenarios of land change. The scenario we implemented was aligned with current drivers of land-use change in the Northern Great Plains and highlighted the importance of conservation lands in landscapes intensively and extensively managed for crops.

Editor: Dennis vanEngelsdorp, University of Maryland, United States of America

Funding: The United States Geological Survey; the United States Department of Agriculture, Farm Service Agency; and the United States Department of Agriculture, Natural Resources Conservation Service, Conservation Effects Assessment Project—Wetlands jointly supported this project. Other than policy review by the United States Geological Survey and a general editorial review the authors solicited from a colleague at the United States Department of Agriculture's Farm Service Agency, the funders had no role in study design, data collection and analysis, decision to publish, or preparation of the manuscript.

Competing Interests: Zac Browning is a co-owner and operator of Browning's Honey Company, Inc. There are no patents, products in development or marketed products to declare. This does not alter the authors' adherence to all the PLOS ONE policies on sharing data and materials.

* E-mail: gallant@usgs.gov

Introduction

Maintaining human prosperity and quality-of-life standards requires landscapes that sustainably deliver ecosystem services valued by society. Decisions that improve the sustainability of landscapes call for information on the simultaneous responses of multiple ecosystem services to changes in land use and climate as a more comprehensive approach to safeguard against unintended, and potentially negative, outcomes of land management or policy actions [1]. Changes in land use and climate clearly alter how ecosystems function within any given landscape [2], affecting all ecosystem services, from supporting to cultural, provisioning, and regulating services [3]. Socioeconomic factors cause dynamic, often unforeseen, fluctuations and shifts in land use, so adaptive modeling systems that are quantitatively linked to monitoring activities provide both the feedback on landscape responses needed to inform decision makers and the basis for continued model improvement [2].

Socioeconomic factors are exerting considerable influence on decisions affecting land use in the Northern Great Plains of North America, a region of major agricultural production [4] and the most important area for production of continental waterfowl populations [5], [6]. The area's significance for conservation in the United States has influenced various federal, state, and nongovernmental entities to protect lands in the region from agricultural development. The U.S. Department of Agriculture administers various programs that target delivery of ecosystem services, through traditional agricultural crop programs to voluntary conservation programs. The Conservation Reserve Program (CRP) [7] is the largest of the latter and has received considerable recognition from an array of conservation interests [8], [9], [10]. The program enables landowners to enroll or re-enroll eligible farmland for 10- or 15-year contracts during specified sign-up periods or on a continuous basis for priority conservation practices, such as to support pollinators and wetlands.

Euro-American settlement of the Northern Great Plains brought conversion of vast tracts of grassland to cropland, and while grasslands continue to be converted to cropland, periods in recent decades have seen some reversal of that land-change dynamic [11], [12], [13], [14], [15]. Satellite imagery revealed a notable return of cropland to grassland in years following inception of the CRP [11], as landowners realized increased land values resulting from enrollment in the program [16]. Land conversion since the mid-2000s has favored cropland over grassland, likely influenced by the convergence of technological advances in agriculture, a push for renewable energy from biofuels, and rising commodity prices [17], [18], as well as crop insurance and disaster relief programs [12].

As incentives have risen for landowners to maximize crop acreages, Congress has reduced total allowable acreage enrollments for the CRP. The highest cap allocated for the program was 39.2 M acres (15.9 M ha; note, we report here the measurement units used in the legislation and federal reports) during 2002–2007 [19]. From 2008–2013 the cap was lowered about 20% to 32 M acres (12.9 M ha) [20]. Actual acres enrolled in CRP nationally have dropped more than 27% since the peak of the program in 2007. Reductions in enrollment in the Northern Great Plains exceeded national rates. North Dakota's peak enrollment was 338.9 K acres (137.1 K ha) in 2007, dropping 53% by 2013. The latest Farm Bill [21] specifies further, annual decrements of total allowable acres, from 27.5 M acres (11.1 M ha) in 2014 to 24 M acres (9.7 M ha) by 2017.

Concurrent interests in achieving national energy independence [22], new technology (e.g., genetically modified crops) [23], and strong economic incentives for production of agricultural crops in recent years have resulted in many private landowners converting expiring CRP acreage back into agricultural production, especially for biofuel and feedstock crops. The impact of a land-use shift of this magnitude on the ecosystem services delivered from the Northern Great Plains has been the subject of recent investigations on carbon sequestration [8], [9], wildlife habitat provisioning [10], [24], sediment reduction [9], and others. Several studies underway in the Northern Great Plains are evaluating the importance of the region for meeting the needs of national pollination services, an industry now valued at $29B (USD) annually, with about $19B attributable to honey bees [25]. No quantitative evaluations have been conducted, however, to assess how future land-use shifts may affect national pollination services.

There have been increasing concerns about declines in pollinators over past decades [26], [27], but it was the major loss of honey bees to Colony Collapse Disorder in 2007 that brought pollination services into national focus and caught the attention of the U.S. Congress and the public [28], [29]. Approximately 70% of the world's flowering plants rely on pollinators [30]. In the United States, the agricultural industry depends heavily on the pollination services of honey bees, a commercially managed insect [31], and the Nation is the world's most active market for their pollination services [32]. Numbers of managed honey bee colonies in the United States have declined by 60% since the 1940s [29], [33], while the proportion of crops in the agricultural industry that rely on their pollination services has increased [33]. In recent years rates of overwintering losses in colonies have been around 30% in the United States [34], much higher than the 18% loss rate beekeepers anticipate on average [35], and there is a concomitant perception of waning bee health [36]. Annual reports dating back to the mid-1980s also show a downward trend in national honey production [37], [38], [39], [40], [41], [42], [43], [44], [45].

A principal contributor to declines in honey bees (as well as native bees) is the loss of floral sources of pollen and nectar in the landscape [30], [46], [47]. Worldwide, conversion of land cover has been extensive, typically to support agriculture [48]. These shifts, along with trends in using synthetic fertilizers rather than rotations of nitrogen-fixing cover types (e.g., clover, alfalfa) that are beneficial to bees, challenge bees to find sufficient floral sources [30]. Understanding how land-use change affects honey bees and other pollinators is one element needed to inform decisions affecting development of sustainable management paradigms for delivering ecosystem services to society.

The Northern Great Plains carries great importance for U.S. honey production and pollination services. Commercial beekeepers from states as far away as coastal areas transport honey bees to the prairies each summer to produce honey, a crop valued at more than $256.5M nationally in 2011, with about 50% of the contribution coming from the Northern Great Plains [49]. The region typically produces most of the Nation's honey [37], [38], [39], [40], [41], [42], [43], [44], [45], but the importance of the area extends far beyond the honey crop. In 2011, over one million colonies of bees were maintained in the region during the summer, representing nearly 40% of the total number of colonies in the United States. Essentially, all of these bees are transported throughout the Nation at other times of the year to pollinate a large variety of crops, often making multiple stops in different geographic locations. Although there have been no quantitative assessments, honey bees that spend the summer in the Northern Great Plains are thought to provide 60–85% of the pollination needs for the entire Nation (Dr. Jeff Pettis, U.S. Department of Agriculture-Agricultural Research Service, personal communication). The summer locations beekeepers use for honey production in the Northern Great Plains have tremendous influence on the nutritional status and health of honey bees because foods, especially pollen, collected and stored in hives during the summer are the primary sources for nutrition during winter and other times when natural foods are unavailable. Land-cover types with abundant supplies of polyfloral and nutritious pollen are known to positively influence honey bee health through improved immune system function [50].

Although CRP lands in the Northern Great Plains have abundant polyfloral sources of pollen for pollinators, there is little information available to quantify the magnitude of that ecosystem service across large geographic extents or its contribution to national pollination services. Government policies and programs that target land resources exert influence on land-management decisions at the local level. Decisions are made parcel by parcel, but tend to accumulate to regional patterns of change [51] and can have substantial influence on ecosystem services over broad scales. Agencies that manage land resources or administer policies and programs focused on land resources seek consistent ways to evaluate outcomes of land management for ecosystem services. Ideally, these evaluations also could be conducted in a proactive context to inform decisions about policies, programs, and management actions. Within the context of developing sustainable management paradigms for landscapes, ecosystem services that are provided in one geographic location but are dependent upon conditions from other locations require special attention because they are subject to different interests and support groups [52]. Provisioning national pollination services for agricultural crops is a good example because most beekeepers are migratory and transport honey bees from pastoral locations used for honey production to distant locations for pollinating a variety of agricultural crops [53].

We describe here a prototype model we developed to quantify the influence of land use on honey bees in the Northern Great Plains to inform decisions affecting conservation programs that target delivery of national pollination services. Our objectives were to (1) develop an approach to map regional-scale habitat suitability for honey bees based on their nutritional needs from the local landscape, (2) evaluate the efficacy of available land-cover data for monitoring effects of interannual land-cover change on landscape suitability for honey bees, and (3) demonstrate how our approach can be used to assess outcomes for honey bees from drivers of land-cover and land-use change. These objectives are the foundation for a module on honey bees in a larger, integrated assessment tool developed to evaluate effects of policies, programs, climate, and other drivers of land change simultaneously across multiple ecosystem services [54].

Materials and Methods

We prototyped our approach for North Dakota, the Northern Great Plains state with the highest production of honey among all 50 states in most years [37], [38], [39], [40], [41], [42], [43], [44], [45]. We identified local landscape criteria for honey bees and designed a spatially explicit model to locate places in the North Dakota landscape that could meet these land-cover requirements. We used available land-cover data to map interannual changes in landscape suitability, then applied our model to these maps as well as to maps we developed to fit a scenario based on recent drivers of land-use change.

Landscape criteria for honey bees

We specified landscape criteria based on industry standards professional beekeepers use to place hives in the Northern Great Plains. These criteria consider the potential of sites to produce honey crops and to provide the nutrition needed to ensure the health of honey bees. We developed landscape criteria to support apiaries of 100 hives (Table 1, "original criteria"). This is approximately twice the number of hives a commercial beekeeper would maintain in an average apiary setting for this part of the country; however, competition for locations to place hives in the summer is high, and it is common to find multiple apiaries of 40–48 or more hives placed within overlapping forage ranges by multiple beekeepers. In many cases the cumulative stocking rate for a local landscape may exceed 100 hives.

Modeling approach

Apiaries in the Northern Great Plains typically are maintained in grassland settings within proximity of roads so hives can be transported. Therefore, we first identified grassland settings sufficient in size to place commercial numbers of hives. We merged information from two sources to develop a map of grassland cover. We used proprietary data on lands with graminoid/herbaceous land treatments enrolled in the CRP [7]. These data were delineated by the Farm Service Agency with orthoimagery of high spatial resolution (typically one to several meters), and boundaries were very accurate for our type of application. For non-CRP lands we relied on grassland cover mapped from satellite data by the North Dakota Gap Analysis Program (NDGAP) [55]. The NDGAP data had lower spatial resolution (30 m) and only a fair level of mapping accuracy for grasslands (somewhat better than 50%), but provided wall-to-wall data on land cover with sub-classes that allowed us to exclude saline and sand prairie grasslands, which we deemed unlikely to provide good floral conditions for honey bees. We merged NDGAP and CRP grasslands into a single map, then fragmented the resulting grassland areas by intersecting them with the road network for North Dakota [56] to measure accessibility for transporting hives.

North Dakota requires beekeepers to register locations of their apiaries by the "quarter section" designation from the United States public land survey system [57]. We used the areal extent of a quarter section, approximately 65 ha (160 ac in the U.S. land system), as a minimum size threshold for eliminating grassland polygons that were less likely to support 100 bee colonies. We also eliminated grassland polygons that were too far from road access via information from a national gridded layer representing Euclidean distance to the nearest road [58], [59]. The road network across North Dakota largely is laid out as a grid of north-south and east-west routes, with road spacings of a mile (1620 m; although, many farms also have field access roads every half-mile or quarter-mile). We rationalized that grassland areas more than a mile from the nearest public road would be infeasible for a beekeeper to place hives; thus, we removed grassland areas having centroids (approximate centers) farther than 1620 m (1 mi) from a road. Only 0.6% of the area of the state was farther than a mile from the nearest public road, and most of this area was associated with badlands, river breaks, and large expanses of water (e.g., reservoirs). In total this criterion removed of 0.2% of the grassland centroids from further consideration as potential apiary sites. Remaining grassland polygons were at least 65 ha in size and had edges within reasonable proximity to road access. We considered the locations of centroids of these remaining polygons as potential apiary sites, though in reality an apiary could be sited anywhere within a grass polygon.

We needed to quantify acreages of desired land-cover types (per Table 1, "original criteria") within forage distance from potential apiary sites. Forage distance for honey bees varies based on floral availability, landscape structure, and ambient conditions, such as from wind (e.g., [60], [61], [62]), but beekeepers typically look for sites providing good cover types within a distance of about 3.2 km from the hive [63], defining a forage area of 3255 ha around an apiary. We developed a separate map layer for each land-cover class of interest, determining that we needed to use a common spatial resolution of 10 m across all layers to retain certain important features (see section on "Compiling annual maps of land cover").

Conceptually, we wanted to move a circular forage window across North Dakota to summarize land-cover classes at each potential apiary location. This is a challenge for geospatial analytical software at the 10-m spatial resolution we used because each land-cover layer is well over 47,000 rows by 77,100 columns, and a circular forage window would encompass about 325,500 cells and require geometric calculations to determine which cells fell within the forage radius around an apiary centroid. We overcame these challenges with a modified moving-window approach (Figure 1). First, we applied a 10×10 rectangular moving window over each 10-m binary map to calculate the proportion per hectare of the respective land-cover type, then saved the results at a 100-m (one ha) cell size, yielding output layers having 0.01 times the number of cells of the original, binary layers. For example, if the original maps showed that a 10-cell×10-cell area contained 30 cells of grassland, 35 cells of non-suitable cover (such as corn and roads), 20 cells of alfalfa, and 15 cells of sunflowers, the resulting ha-sized cell would carry the information of 30% grassland, 20% alfalfa, 15% sunflowers, and 35% other (although the information for each cover type would be stored as a separate map layer, as shown in Figure 1). Second, we applied a 57×57 rectangular moving window (dimensions needed to survey acreage comparable to the forage area around an apiary) across each 100-m raster layer to calculate the amount of each cover type within forage distance from the center of the window, advancing the window one cell (100 m) at a time. We avoided the compute-intensive, circular moving window with a square window of the closest possible areal match to the size of the desired forage

Table 1. Landscape criteria used to identify potential locations for apiaries that would ensure sources of pollen and nectar throughout the growing season in the Northern Great Plains.

Typical timing of flowering for major beneficial cover types in the Northern Great Plains
Deciduous trees/shrubs[a]: Second half of May
Canola: First 3 weeks in June
CRP[b] grassland and comparable mixed grass/forb: 3rd week of June through end of growing season (sometime in September)
Oilseed sunflowers: 3rd week of July through end of August
Second-crop[c] alfalfa: Mid-July through end of growing season (sometime in September)
Original criteria:
≥65 ha (160 ac[d]) deciduous trees/shrubs
≥130 ha (320 ac) CRP[b] grassland or comparable mixed grass/forb cover
≥65 ha (160 ac) alfalfa
≥65 ha (160 ac) oilseed sunflowers
≥65 ha (160 ac) canola
presence of surface water[e]
Relaxed criteria:
≥130 ha (320 ac) CRP[b] grassland or comparable mixed grass/forb cover
≥130 ha (320 ac) any combination of alfalfa, oilseed sunflowers, and canola

[a]Occurrence of deciduous trees and shrubs in the Northern Great Plains generally is limited to windbreaks, fence lines, riparian corridors, and landscaping around houses.
[b]Land enrolled in the Conservation Reserve Program. Of particular interest for honey bees are grasslands rich in leguminous species because they offer long-flowering land cover with good sources of pollen and nectar.
[c]The first cutting of alfalfa for hay typically is done prior to blooming, but flowers are present following re-growth between subsequent cuttings.
[d]Acres (ac) are the unit of measure for the property system in the United States and are provided here because they relate to multiples of standard crop field sizes.
[e]Bees collect water for evaporative cooling in the hive, so our criteria recognize this landscape requirement in addition to sources of pollen and nectar.

area. Given the imprecision of land-cover data and forage behavior by bees (influenced by wind, air temperature, and floral density, in addition to land cover type), having a round, rather than square, window was not worth the extra processing burden for a statewide application. Third, we summarized acreages across land-cover types within forage distances around all 100-m cells that had been identified as potential apiary locations to determine which sites met the areal thresholds for required land-cover types (per Table 1).

Compiling annual maps of land cover

We compiled annual land-cover maps from multiple sources, as no single source provided all information needed to assess landscape suitability for bees. We encountered expected differences in data vintages, resolutions, and origins (see Table S1 for information sources), as well as product quality. We used the Cropland Data Layer produced annually by the National Agricultural Statistics Service (NASS) [64] for information on alfalfa (*Medicago sativa*), canola (a group of cultivars developed from *Brassica napus* and *B. campestris*), and sunflowers (*Helianthus annuus*), the three crop types needed for our analysis. All three types have been distinguished annually in map products in North Dakota since 2002, prior to which alfalfa was aggregated with grassland hay crops not nutritious for bees. We used information on woody cover types from the same two sources we used for grassland cover, the CRP and NDGAP products. The dataset for CRP-enrolled lands contained information on the years for which the conservation treatments were under contract, which enabled us to update our land-cover maps annually for both woody and grassland parcels. The NDGAP data we used for the remainder of the landscape was a single, static map derived from a collection of Landsat imagery spanning 1992–1998. We amended the NDGAP information with the relatively high-resolution wetland cover delineated by the National Wetlands Inventory (NWI) [65], as bees need sources of water and wetlands typically are poorly represented in land-cover products generated from the mid-resolution satellite data used by NDGAP [66]. The NWI map was derived from high resolution orthoimagery, but similar to the NDGAP product, represented a static depiction of wetlands derived from a collection of different orthophoto dates mosaicked across North Dakota.

The annual maps we assembled spanned 2002, the earliest year for which we could distinguish all three crop types of interest, through 2006, the latest year for which we had annual data on CRP-enrolled lands (although, we later received updated data on CRP enrollments that enabled the example application we describe in the next section). We filled the remainder of the landscape each year with data from the static NDGAP and NWI product sources. We processed all geospatial data in an equal-area map projection (following parameters used by the U.S. Geological Survey for the conterminous United States, see [67]) to maintain appropriate areal properties. All land-cover information was converted to raster layers of 10-m cell size, the spatial resolution needed to retain features from the finest-grained sources, the CRP and NWI data. We developed binary maps ("1" for presence and "0" for absence) for each land-cover type of interest, including alfalfa, canola, oilseed sunflowers, grasslands (CRP grasslands and NDGAP [non-saline and non-sandy] grasslands), wetlands, and woodlands (CRP and NDGAP woodlands).

Assessing outcomes from a scenario of land change

We used a scenario that captured contemporary drivers of change in the Northern Great Plains to evaluate if our model could reflect influences from programs and policies on landscape

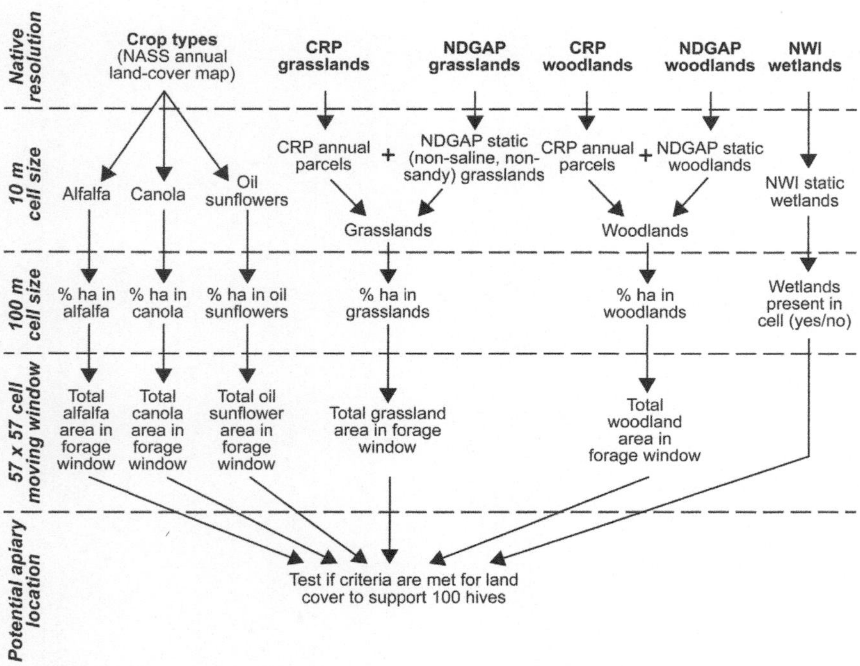

Figure 1. Geospatial processing schematic for compiling annual land-cover maps. We extracted land-cover components needed to meet criteria shown in Table 1 and saved them as separate gridded layers at 10-m cell resolution to retain needed spatial detail. We then summarized the proportion of area per hectare for each land-cover type (except wetlands, for which we recorded only presence/absence) and saved results as separate gridded layers at 100-m cell resolution to reduce the dimensions of the data layers. We used a moving filter of 57×57 cells to tally land-cover elements over an area comparable with the forage zone for honey bees, and queried the tallies for grassland locations we previously had identified as potential sites for placing apiaries. Figure abbreviations: NASS – National Agricultural Statistics Service, CRP – Conservation Reserve Program, NDGAP – North Dakota GAP Analysis Program, NWI – National Wetlands Inventory.

suitability for honey bees. Owners of agricultural lands in North Dakota have been avid participants in the CRP. Nationwide, approximately 28 million acres (11.3 M ha) under CRP contract were set to expire between 2007 and 2010 [68]. During that same time frame, production pressures for corn-based ethanol and soybean biodiesel, the two major crops used to produce biofuels in the United States [69], [70], were on the rise [71], [72] from requirements for substantial increases in national use of renewable fuels [22]. In addition, commodity prices for corn and soybeans have been trending upwards since the mid-2000s [73]. We therefore compiled land-cover maps for 2002 and 2010 to capture conditions before and after the convergence of these pivotal influences of land-use change.

Initial results from the analysis of landscape suitability (discussed in the "Results" section) motivated us to modify some of the source information for this scenario application. We used CRP land-cover information, as before, but changed the second source of data on grasslands and woody cover from NDGAP to the 2001 National Land Cover Database (NLCD) [74]. The NLCD offered notably better mapping accuracy [75] than the NDGAP product [55] (Table S2), though did not provide information distinguishing sandy and saline grassland subtypes. For cropland information we extracted pixels from NASS maps for 2002 and 2010 across all crop types to obtain general extent of cropland for each of the years, and used specific information for canola and sunflowers to distinguish those two cover types. The accuracy for alfalfa on the NASS cropland maps was not very high; total acreages represented for alfalfa departed considerably from statistics reported from ground-based surveys conducted by NASS. Mapped alfalfa was 16x the acreage reported from ground-based surveys for 2002 and 5x the acreage reported for 2010 [76]. In addition, the distribution of alfalfa pixels tended to have a "shotgun" appearance, with many isolated pixels scattered across the landscape, rather than occurring in contiguous patches as would be expected for agricultural fields.

We developed our own maps of potential alfalfa distribution with remotely sensed data from the Landsat Enhanced Thematic Mapper sensor obtained through the Web Enabled Landsat Data (WELD) online distribution site [77], [78]. WELD data are terrain corrected and spectrally calibrated to top-of-atmosphere reflectance. We used the data layer for the Normalized Difference Vegetation Index, a data transformation that highlights photosynthetic activity in plants [79]. We targeted the WELD composite for October because it is a month in which alfalfa remains green in the Northern Great Plains after other cover types (with the exception of some grasses) have senesced for the season. For 2010 we used the WELD composite for November to fill any data gaps in the October composite. The year 2002 was exceptionally cloudy for North Dakota overpasses, so we substituted data from 2003, with the rationale that alfalfa is managed on a four- to eight–year rotation cycle in the Northern Great Plains [80], therefore minimizing potential differences in the distribution of alfalfa between 2002 and 2003. We filled data gaps in the WELD October composite for 2003 with information from the WELD Autumn composite for that year, as the November composite was contaminated with widespread clouds and snow. To generate distributions of alfalfa we simply selected thresholds of green biomass response that resulted in relatively comparable total acreages reported from the 2002 and 2010 NASS ground-based surveys. We had no means to determine the accuracy of our results, but were satisfied we had usable examples for the scenario application, given total acreage tallies and the fact our maps had

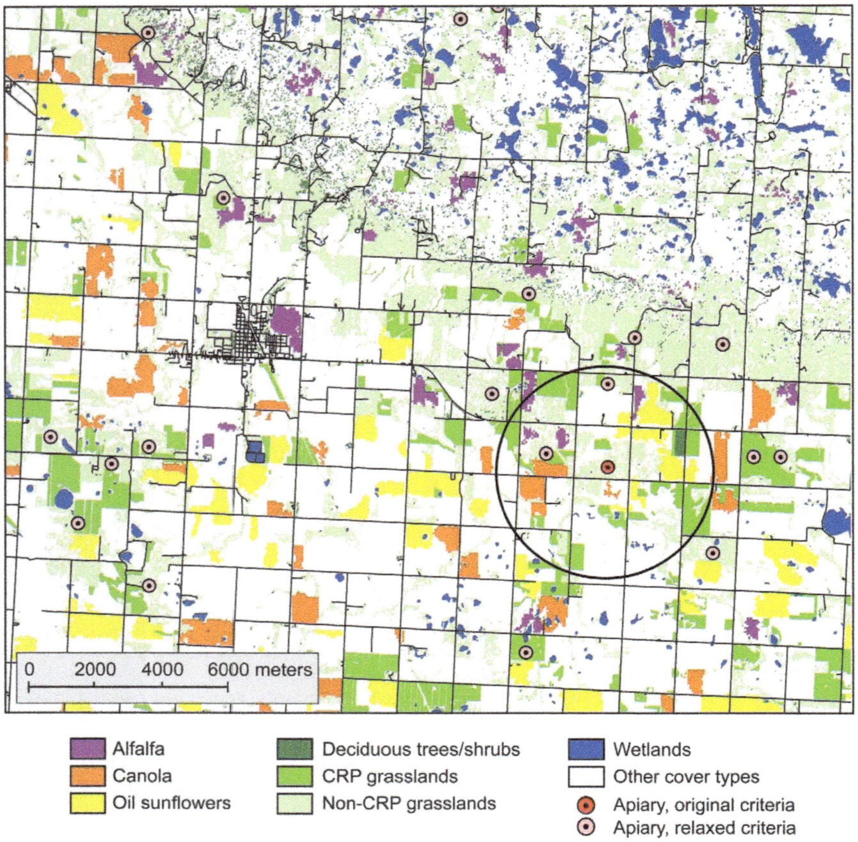

Figure 2. Predicted apiary locations resulting from original versus relaxed criteria for 2006. The original criteria resulted in only one apiary site identified (circle shows forage zone for this apiary), but relaxed criteria resulted in many more potential sites. Beekeepers often install apiaries in close proximity to one another in good landscapes such that forage zones are overlapping, as would be the case in this figure.

much more contiguous patches of alfalfa than did the NASS cropland maps. Still, our alfalfa maps also captured grassy areas that remained green late in the year, such as along drainage courses, in other depressional areas, and in urban settings. We make no claim as to how well our land-cover compilations represented actual North Dakota land-cover patterns for 2002 and 2010 (other than the CRP data would have been fairly accurate), but our maps did provide total acreages of key land-cover types in amounts approximating those reported by NASS.

Results

Output from the modeling approach

A relatively sparse number of locations met our initial land-cover criteria. We found the requirements likely were challenged by limitations in the source information we used for the annual land-cover maps. Less than half the woodlands in the landscape actually had been mapped correctly as woodlands in the NDGAP product [55], which made it hard to meet the acreage criterion for early season flowering shrubs and trees. Meeting certain crop requirements also was difficult. For example, in 2006, only 20% of the alfalfa was mapped accurately in the cropland data layer [81], meaning that 80% of the alfalfa in the actual landscape was not classified as alfalfa in the crop map. We relaxed the land-cover criteria to overcome these limitations in the source data (see Table 1, "Relaxed criteria"), then re-ran the landscape model. The model was able to find many additional locations that could meet the relaxed criteria (Figure 2), though these locations might not support apiaries as large as the 100 colonies our original criteria were defined to support.

North Dakota requires that all apiaries be registered with the state by quarter-section legal units, so we obtained (from the North Dakota Department of Agriculture, Beekeepers Association) and mapped annual registered locations of apiaries for visual comparison with potential apiary locations produced by our model (Figure 3). We did not perform a quantitative comparison between modeled and registered sites because registered apiary sites can contain any number of beehives (based on the discretion of the beekeeper), and our model was parameterized to identify landscapes that could support large apiaries. Also, once a beekeeper registers an apiary location, they tend to re-register that same location over time, regardless if they stock it with bees, as most beekeepers do not own the property on which their hives are located and are motivated to maintain ongoing agreements with landowners. To validate this assumption we constructed a time series of registered apiary locations for North Dakota from 1981 (90 registered sites) to 2010 (10,054 registered sites). We found that the total number of sites increased every year (e.g., Figure 3B-C shows registered sites in 2002 and 2010, respectively), and rarely did any site drop from the registry. We selected 2002 to compare the distribution of locations identified with our model and registered locations for apiaries (Figure 3) because that year had the highest rates of mapping accuracy in the cropland maps for the three crop types of interest. An informal visual comparison

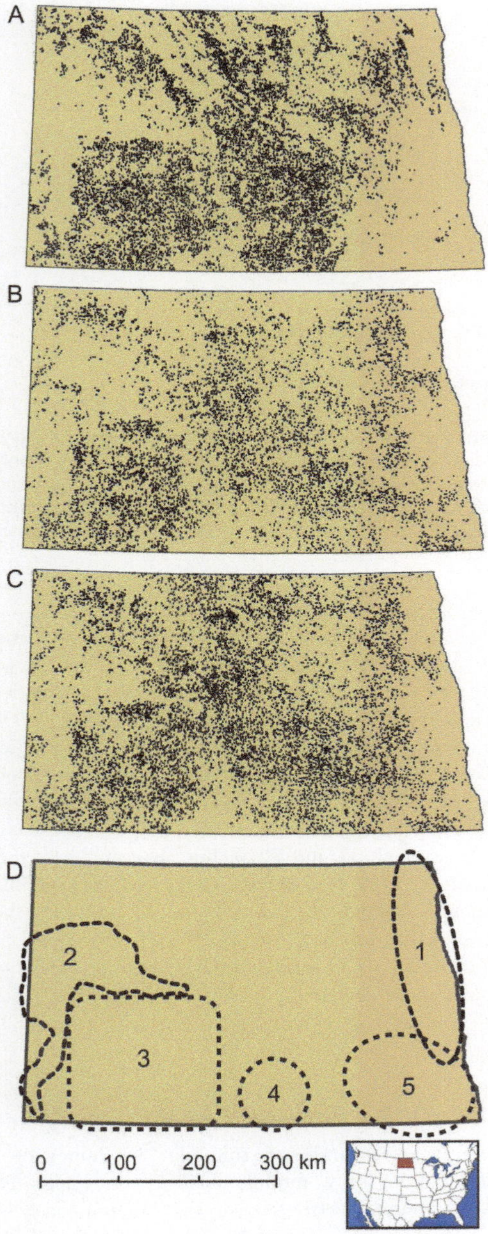

Figure 3. Predicted versus registered apiary locations (note: 1 dot = 1 apiary location). The cropland data we used had the highest mapping accuracies for the three crops of interest in 2002 (metadata on accuracy for all years is available through [82]). The distribution of sites we predicted to support large apiaries in 2002 (A) shares general similarities with apiaries registered for 2002 (B). Distribution of registered sites has grown more dense over time, as shown by a map of sites registered for 2010 (C). Hand-delineated areas of particular agreement (1, 2, and 3) and disagreement (4 and 5) of point distribution patterns between predicted and registered apiaries in 2002 (D), as described in the Discussion.

revealed general similarities in statewide patterns of predicted locations and locations registered by beekeepers, but a notable difference is our model did not identify many locations for large apiaries in the southeastern part of North Dakota, though many apiary sites have been registered there (Figure 3D, area 5).

Annual maps of land cover

Our annual series predicting potential apiary locations revealed a legacy of patterns from the mosaic of Landsat imagery used by NASS to develop the crop-type maps, particularly for years 2002–2004 (Figure 4). Despite such issues associated with satellite image boundaries, many suitable locations were identified throughout the central swath of the state in all years. In contrast, we found few locations in the eastern, southeastern, and central-west parts of the state for any year (Figure 3D, areas 1, 2, and 5). Interestingly, our model consistently predicted a dense distribution of potential locations in south-central North Dakota that is not echoed by the record of registered apiaries (Figure 3D, area 4).

Assessing outcomes from a scenario of land change

An important motivation to evaluate effects of land change on honey bees is to provide information on how resource manage-

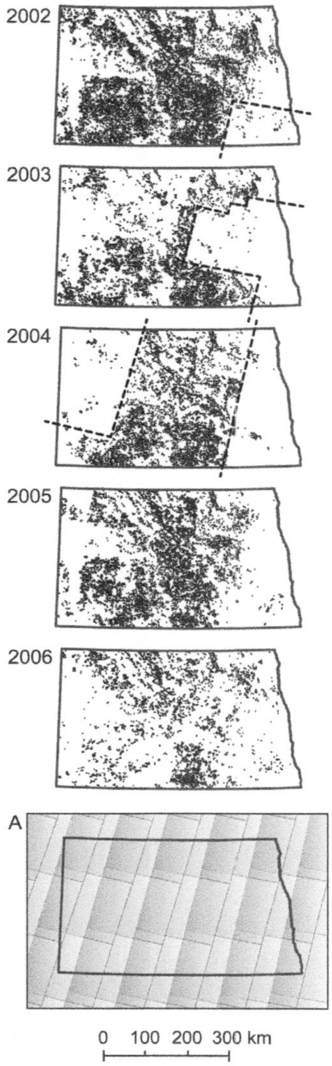

Figure 4. Effects of mosaicking satellite images for mapping crop types on subsequent application of resulting crop maps (note: 1 dot = 1 apiary location). Annual predicted apiary sites for 2002–2006 and Landsat scene boundaries (map A) from (side-lapping) north-south orbital paths. The influence of satellite scene boundaries on the crop-type maps derived from the set of Landsat overpasses needed to provide statewide coverage of cloud-free data are most apparent in our apiary predictions for 2002–2004 (note dashed lines). The various dates of imagery pieced together to provide statewide coverage of data often represent differences in phenological timing or other environmental conditions, making it difficult for image analysts or algorithms to detect comparable cover types across scenes [66]. This example highlights limitations of current large-area land-cover products for applications such as ours that rely on local-scale landscape components.

ments programs and policies can influence pollination services. We highlighted predicted locations that depended on CRP-enrolled lands to meet criteria for siting apiaries (Figure 5). Landowners throughout North Dakota participate in the CRP, but the benefits for honey bees may best be realized in the eastern/southeastern part of the state, where our model found few locations outside of CRP-enrolled lands to meet the criteria for siting large apiaries.

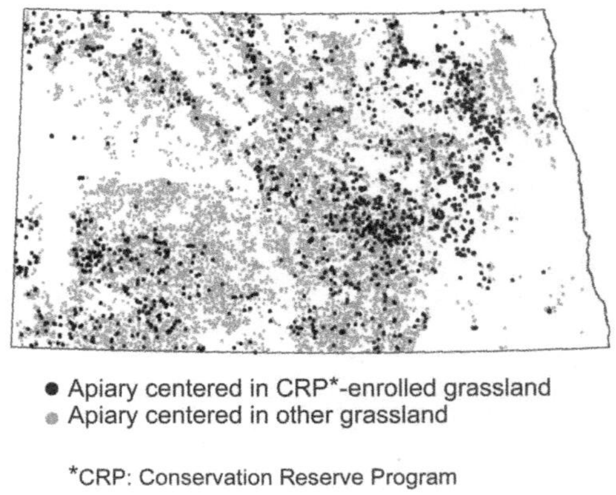

Figure 5. Influence of the Conservation Reserve Program (CRP). In this map we distinguish potential apiary sites that met criteria only because CRP-enrolled grasslands provided a suitable place for locating hives. This example shows how our model could be used to distinguish contributions to apiary-friendly landscapes from different sources of land management.

Our results for the scenario application representing pre- and post-incentive years to expand production of biofuel crops revealed a reduction in landscape suitability for large apiaries between 2002 and 2010 (Figure 6). The model identified 10% fewer locations for large apiaries in 2010 than in 2002 across all potential grassland centroids, but the decrease in centroids located in CRP parcels was 60%. The number of CRP-enrolled polygons available as potential apiary centroids in North Dakota declined by about 15% between 2002 and 2010, but geographically this decrease represented 24% less surface area enrolled in the program in North Dakota. Coupled with changes in the surrounding land cover, much of the CRP land remaining in 2010 was unable to meet the local landscape criteria for large apiaries. This was most evident in eastern North Dakota, but substantial reduction in CRP-related sites was evident throughout most of the state.

Discussion

Our approach to assess landscape suitability for honey bees provides the foundation for a module in a larger, integrated framework to assess multiple ecosystem services simultaneously to inform decisions on land management and policy, as well as evaluate outcomes from government conservation investments [54]. Competing drivers of change in the agricultural industry can have substantial influence on the Nation's ability to sustain the annual demand for pollination services by honey bees. For example, conservation programs supported by the Food, Conservation, and Energy Act of 2008 [20], which generally amended the conservation programs from earlier farm legislation (e.g., the CRP was in the Food Security Act of 1985 [83], have encouraged increased acreage of floral sources beneficial for bees. Conversely, the Energy Independence Security Act of 2007 [22] laid requirements for considerable increases in the volume of biofuels produced over the next decade, which currently encourages expansion of acreage in corn and soybeans, crops that provide little nutritional value for bees in the Northern Great Plains. The model we developed enables assessing outcomes from such competing influences on landscape suitability for honey bees.

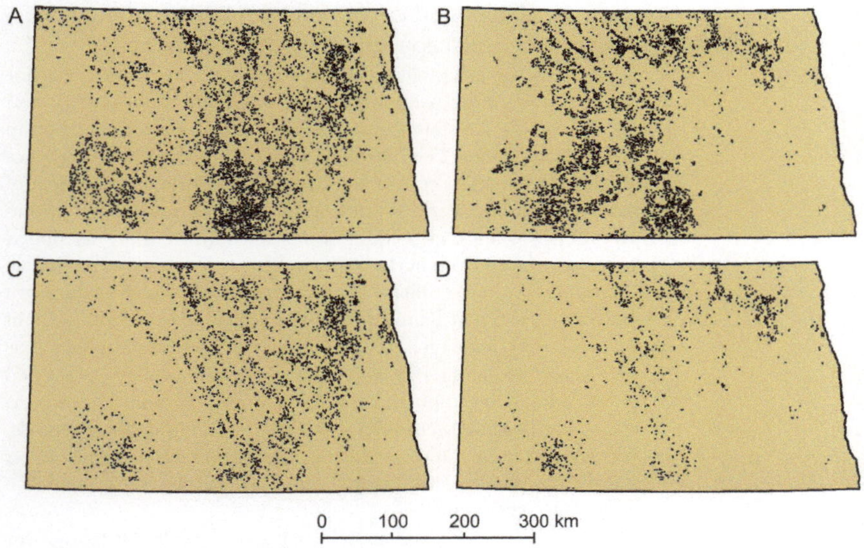

Figure 6. Results from a scenario of land-use change (note: 1 dot = 1 apiary location). A scenario influenced by high commodity prices and incentives to expand production of biofuel crops resulted in a loss of local landscapes suitable for apiaries. The distribution of all grassland centroids meeting criteria to support large apiaries in 2002 (A), prior to land-change incentives, is more extensive than in 2010 (B), subsequent to incentives. The same is true for the distribution of CRP centroids that met the apiary criteria in 2002 (C) versus 2010 (D).

Output from the modeling approach

Informal visual comparison of the distribution of locations predicted by our model for 2002 with registered locations of apiaries for that year exhibited some general similarities (Figure 3). Both maps depict ample landscape opportunities for apiaries throughout the central swath of the state. Both maps agree the arid, erosional landscapes of the badlands and river breaks in western North Dakota and the crop types of the wall-to-wall cropland in the Lake Agassiz Plain in eastern North Dakota hold lower value for honey bees (Figure 3D, areas 1 and 2, respectively), and the maps show a strong pattern of agreement for the distribution of good apiary locations in the Missouri Plateau (Figure 3D, area 3). The maps differ most in the southeastern part of the state (Figure 3D, area 5), where our model found few locations for supporting large apiaries, yet many apiary sites are registered. It is likely these apiaries support far fewer colonies than in more floristically diverse landscapes elsewhere in the state, though this has not always been the case. According to beekeepers who have operated in southeastern North Dakota for many decades, it was rare to see corn or soybean crops in this area a decade ago, but now there is extensive cropland planted in corn, soybeans, and wheat, which are not very nutritious for bees (although, soybean varieties grown elsewhere in the United States can be beneficial for honey bees at times). In previous decades, southeastern North Dakota had many more acres of CRP, alfalfa, sunflowers, and canola (Doug Ruby, Ruby's Apiaries, personal communication). Data from the Farm Service Agency show that land enrollment in the Conservation Reserve Program for southeastern counties of North Dakota totaled 103,856 ha in 1990, rose to 163,472 ha by 2000, then dropped to 135,553 ha by 2010, and continues to drop (120,874 ha by 2013) [84]. Maps produced by the U.S. Department of Agriculture for the agricultural census series show the distribution of alfalfa has been decreasing in southeastern North Dakota since at least 1978 (though we note there is no indication canola or oilseed sunflowers were grown in much quantity in this part of the state during the past few decades [85], [86], [87], [88], [89]. Migratory beekeepers have little flexibility for shifting their operations to new regions of North Dakota to accommodate changes in land cover and instead adjust the sizes and numbers of colonies per apiary to compensate for diminished acres of forage. Given the current cropland types grown wall-to-wall in southeastern North Dakota, the benefits of land enrolled in conservation programs there can be especially important for supporting honey bees, an outcome highlighted by our model results (Figure 6). Beekeepers in that area have experienced sharp declines in honey yields as a result of these changing cropping trends, and have been required either to reduce per-site hive allotments or to abandon sites (Doug Ruby, Ruby's Apiaries, personal communication). In contrast, our model found more locations for supporting apiaries than were reflected by the distribution of registered sites in the southern part of the Prairie Coteau Slope region (see Figure 3D, area 4). The distribution of registered apiaries is not very dense in this area, but our model found plenty of locations suitable for apiaries across all years (Figure 4) because the area had many CRP-enrolled parcels, abundant acreage in oilseed sunflowers, and moderate acreages in alfalfa and mixed grass prairie.

Results from our analyses helped us identify several ways to refine our model. First, the approach we developed to identify potential apiary locations was successful in implementing local landscape requirements across a statewide extent, but the all-or-nothing recipe for 100 hives is limiting. A shift from a model based completely on expert opinion to one developed statistically from data on number of hives and honey production relative to landscape setting would enable predicting suitability across a range of apiary sizes, as well as contribute information towards understanding how land-cover changes in the Northern Great Plains could affect the supply of honey bee colonies for national pollination needs. Second, we also should incorporate seasonal influences from weather into our model because of effects on plant flowering and nectar flow. Even if land-cover types were held constant across years, different weather conditions would provide substantially more or substantially less pollen and nectar because of variations in moisture and growing degree days. Third, we used

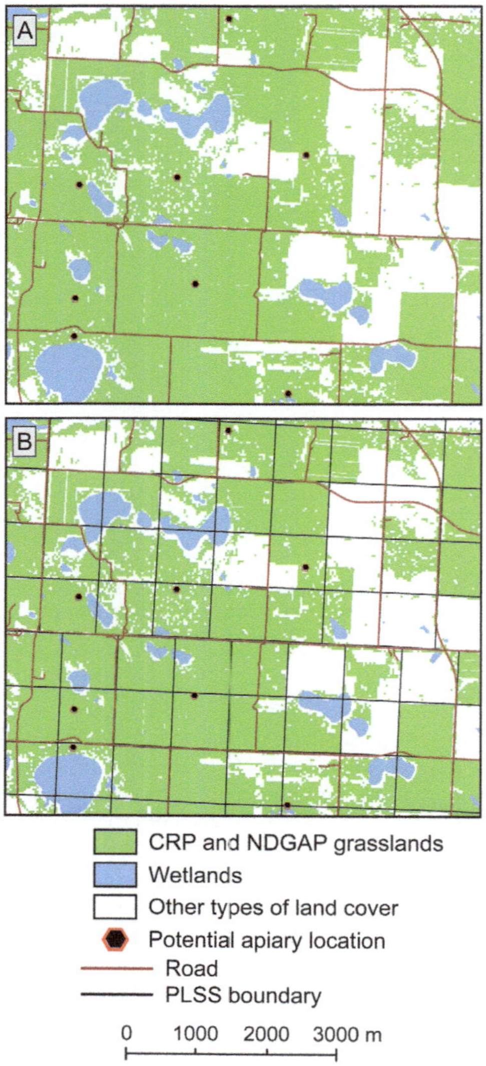

Figure 7. Approach we used versus future algorithm modification for identifying potential grassland sites for placing apiaries. We identified centroids (grassland locations for potential apiary sites) based on criteria for minimum extent of grassland acreage and proximity to roads (A). Density of potential site locations would increase if, instead of using grassland centroids, we applied the spatial framework of the U.S. Public Land Survey System used for registering apiary locations (B). We could maintain our same criteria for grassland extent and road access, but could have multiple apiaries within a large grassland patch, a situation that often occurs in the actual landscape. Figure abbreviations: CRP – Conservation Reserve Program, NDGAP – North Dakota GAP Analysis Program, PLSS – Public Land Survey System.

centroid locations within grassland patches that met criteria for areal extent and proximity to roads to identify potential apiary sites. For future model refinement we could retain the areal and proximity requirements for grasslands, but instead use centroids from the legal mapping units (quarter sections) that beekeepers register. This would densify the number of point locations around which we could analyze land-cover components (Figure 7) and would better mimic the concentration of overlapping forage areas we have observed *in situ* with commercial apiaries.

Using available land-cover data to monitor annual changes in landscape suitability for honey bees

The data we assembled to compile a land cover time series for North Dakota were a mix of annual and static information, and the vintages of the static sources were not always well matched to the annual sources. The Northern Great Plains have had low rates of annual land-cover conversion (typically a fraction of a percent of the total area per year) [11] during the years of our analysis and in preceding decades, providing some reassurance our assembled landscapes were relatively representative of this rather stable region of the United States. The principal land-change dynamic in the Northern Great Plains during this period was the influence of the CRP [11], for which we did have temporally dynamic data, as well as annual changes in crop types, for which we had the annual NASS data. One implicit assumption in our approach, however, was that grasslands were suitably rich in season-long floral sources. We know of no data on the floral components of land cover (except for isolated, local cases) and currently have no means to refine this assumption.

For initial trials of our model we used the NDGAP land-cover product because it offered an array of grassland and woodland subclasses that allowed us to discard those we expected to be poor for bees. The downside to using this product was relatively low rates of mapping accuracy for grassland and woodland classes. For that reason we used non-cropland land-cover information from the NLCD for our subsequent example application because NLCD had a better rate of accuracy for mapping woodland and grassland cover (Table S2) [75], [90], [91]. In addition, the NLCD provided land-cover products for 1992, 2001, and 2006 [74], which we could more easily crosswalk (than the single NDGAP product) to the vintages of our other land-cover information, and the NLCD continues to provide new national maps of land cover.

Until recently, annual mapping of land cover for the United States has been untenable at mid-resolution spatial scales. Improvements in technology and free access to Landsat data [92] have advanced this capability, as evidenced by national-scale annual products from NASS [64]. The methods employed to classify land-cover types across extensive geographic areas, however, produce maps better suited for applications that summarize outcomes at regional scales, rather than applications like ours that rely on local-scale accuracy. The results we generated based on annual land-cover maps compiled from NASS, NLCD, and NDGAP data inherited patterns of inaccuracies from those maps (e.g., Figure 4) that underscore limitations in the current state of operational development of large-area land-cover products. These maps fall short of the accuracy and precision needed for local-scale applications such as ours, an observation that has been noted elsewhere (e.g., [93]). Our algorithm relies on tallying land-cover components within a 3.2-km radius around each potential apiary site throughout the state. Local errors in individual pixels therefore can have strong influence on our results. We conclude that current operationally produced land-cover maps do not provide sufficient local accuracy for monitoring landscape suitability for honey bees. This finding underscores the need for those conducting similar habitat assessments to exercise caution in reporting shifts in landscape suitability and to evaluate if they signal mapping inaccuracies, rather than true landscape change.

There are legitimate reasons for the errors in operational-scale land-cover products. Spatiotemporal ambiguities in the spectral characteristics of land cover make it difficult to optimize a classification system for all cover types at once for all places in the landscape [66], [94], as demonstrated by image pattern effects on our annual results (Figure 4). For this reason, NASS focuses on

Table 2. Comparison of acreage planted in 2002 and 2010 in North Dakota for corn and soybeans, the major crop types used to produce biofuels in the United States, versus other cover types that provide important sources of pollen and nectar for bees.

Commodity	Hectares planted in 2002 (reported acres[c])	Hectares planted in 2010 (reported acres[c])	Change in hectares (change in acres[c])
Alfalfa[a]	44,515 (110,000)	32,375 (80,000)	−12,140 (−30,000)
Canola[a]	526,095 (1,300,000)	518,000 (1,280,000)	−8095 (−20,000)
Sunflowers[a]	554,420 (1,370,000)	358,150 (885,000)	−196,270 (−485,000)
CRP-enrolled lands[b]	1,346,345 (3,326,883)	1,100,510 (2,719,413)	−245,835 (−607,470)
Corn[a]	497,765 (1,230,000)	829,610 (2,050,000)	331,845 (820,000)
Soybeans[a]	1,080,515 (2,670,000)	1,659,220 (4,100,000)	578,705 (1,430,000)

[a]Data are from probability-based surveys of farmers conducted by the U.S. Department of Agriculture [76].
[b]Data are total acres enrolled, provided online by the U.S. Department of Agriculture [97].
[c]Acres are the unit of measure for the property system in the United States and are reported in the literature we accessed for U.S. agricultural statistics.

optimizing their annual land-cover algorithms for a handful of important crops, though their maps do distinguish numerous other crop types. NASS assesses mapping accuracy for all crop types, but not for other classes of land cover. Hence, although the availability of annually updated, wall-to-wall maps of land cover is attractive for a growing population of users, the NASS maps are best employed for applications centered on the land-cover classes NASS maps with high accuracy. The metadata for the NASS cropland data layers we used (via [95]) showed the accuracy for mapping alfalfa in 2002, for example, ranged from 19% to 95% for different parts of North Dakota, and for 2004, ranged from 40% to 97%. The accuracy for mapping canola across North Dakota ranged from 88% to 97% in 2002 and from 86% to 99% in 2004. Likewise, the accuracy for mapping sunflowers varied from 80% to 99% in 2002 and 63% to 99% in 2004. The best rates of mapping accuracy at the statewide level across all years were achieved in 2002 (77% accuracy for alfalfa, 93% for canola, and 90% for sunflowers). However, even in this year when 77% percent of the land area planted in alfalfa was correctly mapped as alfalfa, the commission rate for that cover type was 55%, meaning that over half the time a pixel was called "alfalfa" it was not really alfalfa on the ground. This type of error likely contributed to the great density of locations we identified as suitable for large apiaries in 2002 compared with other years (Figure 4). We found far fewer locations that met our landscape criteria in 2006, which likely was more an artifact of a change in mapping methods used by NASS than a change in crop distribution. The NASS product for 2006 is much cleaner in appearance than in previous years, but does not provide improved mapping accuracy (alfalfa in 2006 had 80% omission error and 39% commission error; see [82]). One way NASS might improve mapping accuracy for alfalfa is to extend the range of seasonal dates of Landsat imagery they use. Alfalfa, along with some grasses, in the Northern Great Plains is one of the earliest cover types to become green in the spring, and remains green into the fall after other cover types have senesced.

Using the model to assess outcomes for honey bees from a scenario of land-cover change

Although we found that the land-cover products currently available lack sufficient local accuracy to enable monitoring of actual landscape suitability for honey bees, our model does achieve the goal to provide a way to evaluate how different policies, programs, and market incentives could influence land cover and alter landscape suitability for honey bee colonies. Land-cover maps can be developed to meet various scenario criteria (e.g., [96]), and our model then could be applied to assess how distribution patterns of apiary locations would be affected.

The scenario we employed showed marked differences in landscape suitability prior and subsequent to agricultural and energy drivers currently influencing change in the Northern Great Plains (Figure 6). The landscapes we assembled met reported abundances of crop types important for bees in amounts comparable to those reported by NASS from ground-based sources. Ground-based statistics for 2002 and 2010 indicated decreases in acreages for alfalfa, canola, sunflowers, and CRP-enrolled land, and corresponding increases in acreages of corn and soybeans, the two major crop types associated with biofuels (Table 2) [98]. Further corroboration for shifts in land cover that affected landscape suitability is offered by the U.S. Department of Agriculture's findings that native grasslands were converted to croplands in the Northern Great Plains at a rate of about 1% (311,610 ha) per year from 1997–2007 [12], and that acreage in principal crops for North Dakota increased 117,765 ha between 2002 and 2010 [71], [99]. Also, as of 2010, North Dakota was among the top ten U.S. states for production of ethanol and biodiesel, and the amount of corn used for production of biofuels has increased sharply since 2002 [100].

Conclusions (and Future Directions)

We developed a modified moving-window approach to tally land-cover components within local-scale proximity to potential apiaries for statewide or larger regional assessments of landscape suitability for honey bees. Our work responds to a need to estimate effects from various scenarios of land change that can result from major drivers such as market values, shifts in climate, or how national programs and policies for land resources are implemented. Because the approach is sensitive to local-scale information, results based on existing land cover time series generated from remotely sensed data may reveal more about limitations in land-cover products than about actual land-cover change. Our model therefore currently is more valuable for assessing outcomes from different scenarios of land-use change than for monitoring actual changes in landscape suitability. New approaches for monitoring land-cover change with remotely sensed data are emerging (e.g., [101], [102]) that eventually will enable our model to be used as a monitoring tool in addition to a scenario-assessment tool.

Our model was parameterized based on expert opinion for a set of land-cover criteria sufficient in floral sources to support apiaries of approximately 100 hives. These criteria highlighted the best landscapes for bees in North Dakota, but is not very representative of the range of numbers of hives commercial beekeepers typically place in apiaries. Having demonstrated a method that successfully implements local-scale criteria across a large geographic extent, our future efforts will focus on developing a more sophisticated model to provide predictions covering a more realistic spectrum of apiary sizes and environmental conditions. This would be a move towards estimating the number of colonies that could be contributed from the Northern Great Plains to meet national pollination demands under different land-change scenarios.

Our motivation to develop an approach to assess landscape suitability for honey bees is to support a larger, integrated effort to evaluate multiple ecosystem services in concert. This capability is needed to provide information for land resource agencies and policy makers on potential outcomes for ecosystem services from drivers of change. Our initial efforts already have highlighted the importance of conservation lands for honey bees in landscapes extensively cropped in cover types having little pollen or nectar value for bees. Incorporating our model into the larger, integrated framework of ecosystem service models [54] will provide a more balanced assessment to support decisions related to policy, programs, and other drivers of land-use and land-cover change.

Supporting Information

Table S1 Information on source data.
(DOCX)

Table S2 Accuracy of grassland and woody land cover in maps from the National Land Cover Database and the North Dakota GAP Analysis Program.
(DOCX)

Acknowledgments

We benefitted from reviews by S. Hyberg, J. Walker, D. vanEngelsdorp (PLOS ONE academic editor), and two anonymous reviewers on earlier versions of this paper.

Author Contributions

Conceived and designed the experiments: NHE ALG ZB. Performed the experiments: ALG. Analyzed the data: ALG. Contributed reagents/materials/analysis tools: ALG NHE. Wrote the paper: ALG NHE.

References

1. Euliss NH Jr, Smith LM, Wilcox DA, Browne BA (2008) Linking ecosystem processes with wetland management goals: Charting a course for a sustainable future. Wetlands 28: 553–562.
2. Euliss NH Jr, Smith LM, Liu S, Feng M, Mushet DM, et al. (2010) The need for simultaneous evaluation of ecosystem services and land use change. Environ Sci Technol 44: 7761–7763.
3. Millennium Ecosystem Assessment (2005) Ecosystems and human well-being: Synthesis. Washington DC: Island Press. 137 p.
4. National Agricultural Statistics Service (2009) 2007 Census of agriculture – Summary and state data. U.S. Department of Agriculture, Volume 1 Geographic Area Series, Part 51, AC-07-A-51. 739 p.
5. Batt BDJ, Anderson MG, Anderson CD, Caswell FD (1989) The use of prairie potholes by North American ducks. In: van der Valk AG, editor. Northern prairie wetlands. Ames: Iowa State University Press. pp. 204–227.
6. Smith AG, Stoudt JH, Gallop JB (1964) Prairie potholes and marshes. In: Lindiska JP, editor. Waterfowl tomorrow. Washington DC: U.S. Fish and Wildlife Service. pp 39–50.
7. Farm Service Agency (2008) Conservation Reserve Program (CRP) benefits: water quality, soil productivity and wildlife estimates. U.S. Department of Agriculture Fact Sheet. Available: http://www.fsa.usda.gov/Internet/FSA_File/factsheet_crp_bennies.pdf. Accessed 2012 July 20.
8. Euliss NH Jr, Gleason RA, Olness A, McDougal RL, Murkin HR, et al. (2006) North American prairie wetlands are important nonforested land-based carbon storage sites. Sci Total Environ 36: 179–188.
9. Gleason RA, Laubhan MK, Euliss NH Jr (2008) Ecosystem services derived from wetland conservation practices in the United States Prairie Pothole Region with an emphasis on the USDA Conservation Reserve and Wetland Reserve Programs. U.S. Geological Survey Professional Paper 1745. 58 p.
10. Haufler JB (2005) Fish and wildlife benefits of Farm Bill conservation programs: 2000–2005 update. Wildl Soc Tech Rev 05–02.
11. Auch RF, Sayler KL, Napton DE, Taylor JL, Brooks MS (2011) Ecoregional differences in late-20th-century land-use and land-cover change in the U.S. Northern Great Plains. Great Plains Res 21: 231–243.
12. Claassen R, Carriazo F, Cooper JC, Hellerstein D, Ueda K (2011) Grassland to cropland conversion in the Northern Plains – the role of crop insurance, commodity, and disaster programs. U.S. Department of Agriculture, Economic Research Report EER-120. 77 p.
13. Gutmann MP, Parton WJ, Cunfer G, Burke IC (2005) Population and environment in the U.S. Great Plains. In: Entwisle B, Stern PC, editors. Population, land use, and environment: research directions: National Academies Press. pp. 84–105.
14. Hartman MD, Merchant ER, Parton WJ, Gutmann MP, Lutz SM, et al. (2011) Impact of historical land-use changes on greenhouse gas exchange in the U.S. Great Plains, 1883–2003. Ecol. Appl. 21: 1105–1119.
15. Sylvester KM, Brown DG, Deane GD, Kornak RN (2013) Land transitions in the American plains: multilevel modeling of drivers of grassland conversion (1956–2006). Agric Ecosyst Environ 168: 7–15.
16. Wu JJ, Lin H (2010) The effect of the Conservation Reserve Program on land values. Land Econ 86: 1–21.
17. Hellerstein D, Malcolm S (2011) The influence of rising commodity prices on the Conservation Reserve Program. U.S. Department of Agriculture, Economic Research Service ERR-110.
18. Stubbs M (2007) Land conversion in the Northern Plains. Washington, D.C.: Congressional Research Service Report for Congress RL33950. 13 p.
19. Farm Security Act of 2002 (U.S. Public Law 107-171). Available: http://www.gpo.gov/fdsys/pkg/PLAW-107publ171/html/PLAW-107publ171.htm. Accessed 2014 March 19.
20. Food, Conservation, and Energy Act of 2008 (U.S. Public Law 110-246). Available: http://www.gpo.gov/fdsys/pkg/PLAW-110publ246/html/PLAW-110publ246.htm. Accessed 2014 March 19.
21. Agricultural Act of 2014 (U.S. Public Law 113-79). Available: http://www.gpo.gov/fdsys/pkg/BILLS-113hr2642enr/pdf/BILLS-113hr2642enr.pdf. Accessed 2014 March 19.
22. Energy Independence Security Act of 2007. Available: http://www.gpo.gov/fdsys/pkg/PLAW-110publ140/html/PLAW-110publ140.htm. Accessed 2014 March 19.
23. Fernandez-Cornejo J (2012) Biotechnology and seed use for major U.S. crops. In: Osteen C, Gottlieb J, Vasavada U, editors. Agricultural resources and environmental indicators, 2012 Edition. U.S. Department of Agriculture, Economic Research Service, Economic Information Bulletin 98. pp. 18–20.
24. Balas CJ, Euliss NH Jr, Mushet DM (2012) Influence of conservation programs on amphibians in the prairie pothole region. Wetlands 32: 333–345.
25. Calderone NW (2012) Insect pollinated crops, insect pollinators and US agriculture: Trend analysis of aggregate data for the period 1992–2009. PLoS One 7(5): e37235. doi:10.1371/journal.pone.0037235.
26. National Research Council (2007) Status of pollinators in North America. Washington DC: The National Academies Press. 307 p.
27. Johnson R (2007) Recent honey bee colony declines. Congressional Research Service Report for Congress, RL33938.
28. Skokstad E (2007) The case of the missing hives. Science 316: 970–972.
29. Pettis JS, Delaplane KS (2010) Coordinated responses to honey bee decline in the USA. Apidologie DOI: 10.1051/apido/2010013.
30. Spivak M, Mader E, Vaughan M, Euliss NH Jr (2011). The plight of the bees. Environ Sci Technol 46: 34–38.
31. Morse RA, Calderone NW (2000) The value of honey bees as pollinators of U.S. crops in 2000. Bee Cult 128: 1–15.
32. Rucker RR, Thurman WN, Burgett M (2012) Honey bee pollination markets and the internalization of reciprocal benefits. Am J Agric Econ 94: 956–977.
33. Aizen MA, Harder LD (2009) The global stock of domesticated honey bees is growing slower than agricultural demand for pollination. Curr Biol 19: 1–4.
34. vanEngelsdorp D, Caron D, Hayes J, Underwood R, Henson M, et al. (2012) A national survey of managed honey bee 2010–2011 winter colony losses in the USA: results from the Bee Informed Partnership. J Apic Res 51: 115–124.
35. vanEngelsdorp D, Jayes J Jr, Underwood RM, Pettis JS (2010) A survey of honey bee colony losses in the United States, Fall 2008 to spring 2009. J Apic Res 49: 7–14.
36. Johnson %, Corn ML (2013) Bee health: background and issues for Congress. Congressional Research Service Report, R43191.
37. U.S. Department of Agriculture, National Agricultural Statistics Service. Honey: final estimates for 1986–1992. Statistical Bulletin Number 912. Available: http://usda.mannlib.cornell.edu/MannUsda/viewDocumentInfo.do?documentID = 1520. Accessed 2014 March 17.
38. U.S. Department of Agriculture, National Agricultural Statistics Service. Honey: final estimates 1993–1997. Statistical Bulletin Number 956. Available:

http://usda.mannlib.cornell.edu/MannUsda/viewDocumentInfo.do?documentID = 1520. Accessed 2014 March 17.
39. U.S. Department of Agriculture, National Agricultural Statistics Service. Honey: final estimates 1998–2002. Statistical Bulletin Number 992. Available: http://usda.mannlib.cornell.edu/MannUsda/viewDocumentInfo.do?documentID = 1520. Accessed 2014 March 17.
40. U.S. Department of Agriculture, National Agricultural Statistics Service. Honey: final estimates 2003–2007. Statistical Bulletin Number 1025. Available: http://usda.mannlib.cornell.edu/MannUsda/viewDocumentInfo.do?documentID = 1520. Accessed 2014 March 17.
41. U.S. Department of Agriculture, National Agricultural Statistics Service. Honey report 2009. Released 27 February 2009. Available: http://usda.mannlib.cornell.edu/MannUsda/viewDocumentInfo.do?documentID = 1191. Accessed 2014 March 17.
42. U.S. Department of Agriculture, National Agricultural Statistics Service. Honey report 2010. Released 26 February 2010. Available: http://usda.mannlib.cornell.edu/MannUsda/viewDocumentInfo.do?documentID = 1191. Accessed 2014 March 17.
43. U.S. Department of Agriculture, National Agricultural Statistics Service. Honey report 2011. Released 25 February 2011. Available: http://usda.mannlib.cornell.edu/MannUsda/viewDocumentInfo.do?documentID = 1191. Accessed 2014 March 17.
44. U.S. Department of Agriculture, National Agricultural Statistics Service. Honey report 2012. Released 30 March 2012. Available: http://usda.mannlib.cornell.edu/MannUsda/viewDocumentInfo.do?documentID = 1191. Accessed 2014 March 17.
45. U.S. Department of Agriculture, National Agricultural Statistics Service. Honey report 2013. Released 18 March 2013. Available: http://usda.mannlib.cornell.edu/MannUsda/viewDocumentInfo.do?documentID = 1191. Accessed 2014 March 17.
46. Naug D (2009) Nutritional stress due to habitat loss may explain recent honeybee colony collapses. Biol Conserv 142: 2369–2372.
47. Di Pasquale G, Salignon M, Le Conte Y, Belzunces LP, Decourtye A, et al. (2013) Influence of pollen nutrition on honey bee health: do pollen quality and diversity matter? PLoS One 88(8): e72016. DOI: 10.1371/journal.pone.0072016.
48. Gallant AL, Klaver RW, Casper GS, Lannoo MJ (2007) Global rates of habitat loss and implications for amphibian conservation. Copeia 2007: 967–979.
49. National Agricultural Statistics Service (2012) Honey Report ISSN:1949–1492.
50. Alaux A, Ducloz F, Crauser D, Le Conte Y (2010) Diet effects on honeybee immunocompetence. Biol Lett doi:10.1098/rsbl.2009.0986.
51. Auch RF, Drummond MA, Sayler KL, Gallant AL, Acevedo W (2012) An approach to assess land-cover trends in the conterminous United States (1973–2000). In: Giri C, editor. Remote sensing of land use and land cover. Boca Raton: CRC Press. pp. 351–368.
52. Tuvendal M, Elmqvist T (2011) Ecosystem services linking social and ecological systems: River brownification and response of downstream stakeholders. Ecol Soc 16(4): 21. Available: http://dx.doi.org/10.5751/ES-04456-160421. Accessed 2013 November 2.
53. U.S. Department of Agriculture (1980) Beekeeping in the United States. Washington DC: Agriculture Handbook 335. 193 p.
54. Euliss NH Jr, Smith LM, Liu S, Duffy WG, Faulkner SP, et al. (2011) Integrating estimates of ecosystem services from conservation programs and practices into models for decision makers. Ecol Appl 21: S128–S134.
55. Strong LL, Sklebar TH, Kermes KE (2005) A GAP analysis of North Dakota, final report. Jamestown: U.S. Geological Survey. 118 p.
56. Broome FR, Godwin LS (2003) Partnering for the people: improving the U.S. Census Bureau's MAR/TIGER database. Photogramm Eng Remote Sens 69: 1119–1123.
57. Stewart LO (1935) Public land surveys. Reprinted 1976. Minneapolis: The Meyers Printing Co. 202 p.
58. Watts RD (2005) Distance to nearest road in the conterminous United States. U.S. Geological Survey: Fact Sheet 2005–3011.
59. Watts RD, Compton RW, McCammon JH, Rich CL, Wright SM, et al. (2007) Roadless space of the conterminous United States. Science 316: 736–738.
60. Beekman M, Ratnieks FLW (2000) Long-range foraging by the honey-bee, *Apis mellifera* L. Funct Ecol 14: 490–496.
61. Hagler JR, Mueller S, Teuber LR, Machtley SA, Van Deynze A (2011) Foraging range of honey bees, *Apis mellifera*, in alfalfa seed production fields. J Insect Sci 11: 1–12.
62. Steffan-Dewenter I, Kuhn A (2003) Honeybee foraging in differentially structured landscapes. Proc R Soc Lond B Biol Sci 270: 569–575
63. Dadant MG (1946) The apiary. In: Grout RA, editor. The hive and the honeybee: a new book on beekeeping to succeed the book Langstroth on the hive and the honeybee. Hamilton: Dadant & Sons. pp. 290–299.
64. Boryan C, Yang Z, Mueller R, Craig M (2011). Monitoring US agriculture: the US Department of Agriculture, National Agricultural Statistics Service, Cropland Data Layer Program. Geocarto Int 2011: 1–18.
65. Wilen BO, Bates MK (1995) The US Fish and Wildlife Service's National Wetlands Inventory project. Vegetatio 118: 153–169.
66. Gallant AL (2009) What you should know about land-cover data. J Wildl Manage 73: 796–805.
67. Multi-Resolution Land Characteristics Consortium (MRLC): National Land Cover Database, Frequently asked questions. Available http://www.mrlc.gov/faq_dau.php. Accessed 2012 July 20.
68. Cowan T (2010) Conservation Reserve Program: status and current issues. Washington DC: Congressional Research Service Report for Congress 7-5700, RS21613. 11 p.
69. U.S. Government Accountability Office (2009) Biofuels – potential effects and challenges of required increases in production and use. Washington DC: GAO report GAO-09-446. 175 p.
70. Manuel J (2007) Battle of the biofuels. Environ Health Perspect 115(2): A92–A95.
71. Stubbs M (2009) Agricultural conservation issues in the 111th Congress. Washington DC: Congressional Research Service Report for Congress 7-5700, R40692. 25 p.
72. Thompson W, Meyer S, Green T (2010) The U.S. biodiesel use mandate and biodiesel feedstock markets. Biomass Bioenergy 34: 883–889.
73. National Agricultural Statistics Service (2011) Agricultural Prices. Washington DC: Report ISSN:1937–4216.
74. Homer C, Fry J (2012) The National Land Cover Database. U.S. Geological Survey Fact Sheet 2012–3020.
75. Wickham JD, Stehman SV, Fry JA, Smith JH, Homer CG (2010) Thematic accuracy of the NLCD 2001 land cover for the conterminous United States. Remote Sens Environ 114: 1286–1296.
76. National Agricultural Statistics Service: Quick Stats. Available: http://quickstats.nass.usda.gov. Accessed 2013 January 30.
77. U.S. Geological Survey: WELD: Web-Enabled Landsat Data. Available: http://weld.cr.usgs.gov. Accessed 2013 January 30.
78. Roy DP, Ju J, Kline K, Scaramuzza PL, Kovalsky V, et al. (2010) Web-enabled Landsat data (WELD): Landsat ETM+ composited mosaics of the conterminous United States. Remote Sens Environ 114: 35–49.
79. Pettorelli N, Vik JO, Mysterud A, Gaillard J-M, Tucker CJ, et al. (2005) Using the satellite-derived NDVI to assess ecological responses to environmental change. Trends Ecol Evol 20: 503–510.
80. Undersander D, Becker R, Cosgrove D, Cullan E, Doll J, et al. (2004) Alfalfa management guide. North Central Region Extension Publication NCR547. 51 p.
81. U.S. Department of Agriculture, National Agricultural Statistics Service: Cropland Data Layer metadata. Available: http://www.nass.usda.gov/research/Cropland/metadata/meta.htm. Accessed 2012 August 20.
82. U.S. Department of Agriculture, National Agricultural Statistics Service: CropScape - Cropland Data Layer. Available: http://nassgeodata.gmu.edu/CropScape. Accessed 2012 August 17.
83. Food Security Act of 1985 (U.S. Public Law 99-198). Available: http://history.nih.gov/research/downloads/PL99-198.pdf. Accessed 2014 March 19.
84. CRP enrollment and rental payments by county, 1986-2013. U.S. Department of Agriculture, Farm Service Agency. Available: http://www.fsa.usda.gov/FSA/webapp?area = home&subject = copr&topic = crp-st. Accessed 2014 March 11.
85. U.S. Department of Commerce, Bureau of the Census (1985) 1982 census of agriculture - Volume 2 Subject Series. U.S. Department of Commerce Graphic Summary 189 p.
86. U.S. Department of Commerce, Bureau of the Census (1990) 1987 census of agriculture - Volume 2 Subject Series, Part 1, Agricultural Atlas of the United States. 223 p.
87. U.S. Department of Agriculture, National Agricultural Statistics Service. 1992 Census of Agriculture, Agricultural Atlas of the United States. Available: http://www.agcensus.usda.gov/Publications/1992/Agricultural_Atlas/Maps/index.asp. Accessed 2014 March 19.
88. U.S. Department of Agriculture, National Agricultural Statistics Service (2005) 2002 Agricultural atlas of the United States - Volume 2 Subject Series, Part 1.
89. U.S. Department of Agriculture, Census of Agriculture. 2007 Census Ag Atlas Maps. Available: http://www.agcensus.usda.gov/Publications/2007/Online_Highlights/Ag_Atlas_Maps/Crops_and_Plants. Accessed 2014 March 19.
90. Stehman SV, Wickham JD, Smith JH, Yang L (2003) Thematic accuracy of the 1992 National Land-Cover Data for the eastern United States: statistical methodology and regional results. Remote Sens Environ 86: 500–516.
91. Wickham JD, Stehman SV, Smith JH, Yang L (2004) Thematic accuracy of the 1992 National Land-Cover Data for the western United States. Remote Sens Environ 91: 452–468.
92. U.S. Geological Survey (2008) Imagery for everyone. U.S. Geological Survey Technical Announcement, 21 April 2008. Available: http://landsat.usgs.gov/documents/USGS_Landsat_Imagery_Release.pdf. Accessed 2012 July 20.
93. Thogmartin WE, Gallant AL, Knutson MG, Fox TJ, Suarez MJ (2004) Commentary: a cautionary tale regarding use of the National Land Cover Dataset 1992. Wildl Soc Bull 32: 970–978.
94. Sohl TL, Gallant AL, Loveland TR (2004) The characteristics and interpretability of land surface change and implications for project design. Photogramm Eng Remote Sens 70: 439–448.
95. U.S. Department of Agriculture, National Agricultural Statistics Service (2009) 2006 North Dakota Cropland Data Layer metadata. Available: http://www.nass.usda.gov/research/Cropland/metadata/metadata_nd06.htm#7. Accessed 2012 August 20.
96. Sohl TL, Sleeter BM, Sayler KL, Bouchard MA, Reker RR, et al. (2012) Spatially explicit land-use and land-cover scenarios for the Great Plains of the United States. Agric Ecosyst Environ 153: 1–15.

97. U.S. Department of Agriculture, Farm Service Agency. Conservation programs. Available: http://www.fsa.usda.gov/FSA/webapp?area=home&subject=copr&topic=crp-st. Accessed 2013 January 30.
98. Schnepf R (2010) Agriculture-based biofuels: overview and emerging issues. Congressional Research Service Report 7-5700, R41282. 33 p.
99. U.S. Department of Agriculture, National Agricultural Statistics Service (2002) Acreage. Report ISSN1949-1522. 41 p.
100. U.S. Department of Agriculture, National Agricultural Statistics Service (2012) Acreage. Report ISSN 1949-1522. 40 p.
101. Zhu Z, Woodcock CE, Olofsson P (2012) Continuous monitoring of forest disturbance using all available Landsat imagery. Remote Sens Environ 122: 75–91.
102. Zhu Z, Woodcock CE (2014) Continuous change detection and classification of land cover using all available Landsat data. Remote Sens Environ 144: 152–171.

3

The Social Explanatory Styles Questionnaire: Assessing Moderators of Basic Social-Cognitive Phenomena Including Spontaneous Trait Inference, the Fundamental Attribution Error, and Moral Blame

Michael J. Gill[1]*, Michael R. Andreychik[2]

1 Department of Psychology, Lehigh University, Bethlehem, Pennsylvania, United States of America, **2** Department of Psychology, Fairfield University, Fairfield, Connecticut, United States of America

Abstract

Why is he poor? Why is she failing academically? Why is he so generous? Why is she so conscientious? Answers to such everyday questions—*social explanations*—have powerful effects on relationships at the interpersonal and societal levels. How do people select an explanation in particular cases? We suggest that, often, explanations are selected based on the individual's pre-existing general theories of social causality. More specifically, we suggest that over time individuals develop general beliefs regarding the causes of social events. We refer to these beliefs as *social explanatory styles*. Our goal in the present article is to offer and validate a measure of individual differences in social explanatory styles. Accordingly, we offer the Social Explanatory Styles Questionnaire (SESQ), which measures three independent dimensions of social explanatory style: Dispositionism, historicism, and controllability. Studies 1–3 examine basic psychometric properties of the SESQ and provide positive evidence regarding internal consistency, factor structure, and both convergent and divergent validity. Studies 4–6 examine predictive validity for each subscale: Does each explanatory dimension moderate an important phenomenon of social cognition? Results suggest that they do. In Study 4, we show that SESQ dispositionism moderates the tendency to make spontaneous trait inferences. In Study 5, we show that SESQ historicism moderates the tendency to commit the Fundamental Attribution Error. Finally, in Study 6 we show that SESQ controllability predicts polarization of moral blame judgments: Heightened blaming toward controllable stigmas (assimilation), and attenuated blaming toward uncontrollable stigmas (contrast). Decades of research suggest that explanatory style regarding the self is a powerful predictor of self-functioning. We think it is likely that social explanatory styles—perhaps comprising interactive combinations of the basic dimensions tapped by the SESQ—will be similarly potent predictors of social functioning. We hope the SESQ will be a useful tool for exploring that possibility.

Editor: Brock Bastian, University of New South Wales, Australia

Funding: This work was supported by a Grant-in-Aid award to Michael Gill from the Society for the Psychological Study of Social Issues. The funders had no role in study design, data collection and analysis, decision to publish, or preparation of the manuscript.

Competing Interests: The authors have declared that no competing interests exist.

* Email: m.gill@lehigh.edu

Introduction

Constructing explanations is vital for the human comprehension of reality. Furthermore, as social beings our explanatory abilities are often aimed at understanding other people. *Social explanations* are the product of this social sense-making activity. *Why is he helpful to strangers? Why is she so successful?* Our answers to such everyday questions have powerful effects on interpersonal relationships [1], [2], moral emotions [3–8], reactions to success and failure [9], [10], intergroup relations [11–14], and marital quality [15–17]. It seems that all major domains of social life are shaped by patterns of social explanation.

Here, we are interested in the possibility that individuals have enduring, characteristic styles of social explanation, which we call *social explanatory styles* [18], [19]. Given the centrality of explanation to social life, social explanatory styles should have broad implications for the social life of the individual, pervasively shaping her cognitive, emotional, and behavioral responses to others. Indeed, a large body of work suggests that characteristic styles of explaining one's *own* acts and outcomes have profound effects on individual adaptation [20–22]. We expect that social explanatory styles have similarly potent implications for social functioning.

Below, we offer a measure of individual differences in social explanatory styles: The *Social Explanatory Styles Questionnaire* (*SESQ*). The measure taps three basic explanatory dimensions (described below). To validate the measure, we will provide evidence that each of these basic dimensions moderates an important phenomenon of social cognition: Spontaneous trait inferences [23], the fundamental attribution error [24], and blaming of those with stigmatizing conditions [7]. Although we focus here on the preliminary task of separately validating each dimension of the SESQ, we encourage researchers to consider interactions among these basic dimensions as they try to illuminate particular social judgment phenomena. Prior to presenting evidence regarding the reliability and validity of the SESQ, we will situate the construct of social explanatory styles it in the literature in two ways. First, we will show how our conception of social explanatory styles grows out of classic work regarding the conceptual structure of social explanations. Second, we will elaborate on how our approach is rooted in a particular view of the social explanatory process.

The Conceptual Structure of Social Explanations

Heider [1] pioneered the image of everyday social life as suffused by causal analysis. He also offered seminal ideas about the conceptual structure of lay thinking about social causality. In particular, Heider noted that lay perceivers view others as both "*affected* by their personal and impersonal environment" and as able to "*cause* changes in the environment" (p. 17; italics in original). This distinction between being "affected by" versus "causing" is seen in the longstanding theoretical distinction between *external* (or *situational*) *causes*, which involve personal and impersonal forces that surround an actor and shape her acts or outcomes, and *internal* (or *dispositional*) *causes*, which involve personal abilities, motives, or traits that reside within the actor. This distinction takes center stage in the majority of empirical work on social explanation [25]; but see [26] for an argument that this distinction should not take center stage. Although early work assumed that internal and external causes are mutually exclusive causal choices, research has undermined this assumption [27]; for in-depth discussion see also [28]. Perhaps the most powerful argument against an internal/external dichotomy is that external forces can be seen as creating internal dispositions [e.g., *He lacks confidence* (internal) *because his parents were very critical* (external).]. Thus, our conception of social explanatory styles treats internal and external causes as independent dimensions.

Weiner [7–10] played a major role in pushing psychologists to think beyond internal and external causes. Most famously, Weiner highlights the causal property of *controllability*. For example, according to Weiner and Kukla [9], evaluations of others' achievements are shaped by the perceived causal role of internal-controllable (*effort*) versus internal-uncontrollable (*intelligence*) causes. Controllable failures evoke blame and anger, whereas uncontrollable failures evoke compassion. Broadly speaking, controllability perceptions are high when the perceiver thinks that volitional activity by the actor could have made things turn out otherwise and low when the actor is seen as having little volitional control over how things turned out. Weiner [10] also highlighted the notion of causal *stability*: Some causes are constant (traits), whereas others fluctuate (moods). We included the stability dimension in our research for quite some time, but found no evidence that it mattered for the phenomena we studied. Thus, we will not discuss it further.

The Process of Social Explanation

From Naïve Scientist to Cognitive Miser

In addition to focusing on conceptual structure, classic work also attempted to describe how perceivers select an explanation [29], [30]. Classic models focused on how perceivers choose between internal and external causes, and portray perceivers as engaged in logical analysis like a *naïve scientist*. Furthermore, classic models portray the explanatory process as largely "bottom up," assuming that explanations are selected based on case-specific observations regarding the particular actor and act being explained [25]. For example, Jones and Davis [29] proposed that perceivers select an internal explanation if they answer affirmatively to the question: *Did the actor intentionally bring about effects that most people would try to avoid?* Kelley [30] proposed that internal explanations are selected when the perceiver answers affirmatively to three questions: *Has the actor previously acted like this in similar contexts? Does the actor act like this in many contexts? Is the act different from what others would do?*

Although these models contain some truth [31], research has also uncovered important shortcomings. Most famously, Jones and Harris [24] found that perceivers select internal causes even when classic models suggest it is logically inappropriate to do so (i.e., when there is an obvious external cause present). This pervasive bias has been dubbed the *Fundamental Attribution Error* [32] or the *Correspondence Bias* [27]. Gilbert, Pelham, and Krull [33] illuminated a major cause of the FAE. They presented evidence that perceivers automatically generate internal explanations for acts, and only consider external causes if they are both motivated and able to do so [34], [35]. This work frames the perceiver as an unscientific *cognitive miser* who prefers to exert as little cognitive effort as possible. The miser "prefers" internal explanations because they are easy to generate [23], [36].

The Lay Theories Perspective: Perceiver as *Meaning-Maker*

An alternative perspective—reflected in our concept of social explanatory styles along with other work to be discussed below—is that explanation selection is guided by the perceiver's preexisting theories. This *lay theories perspective* assumes that perceivers vary in their general beliefs and expectations regarding social causality. The starting point for the lay theories perspective is the overwhelming complexity of the social world, the vast array of social events one must explain daily and the vast array of causes that might potentially have given rise to each of those events. In the face of such complexity, pre-existing theories—general beliefs and expectations about "how things typically work"—are indispensable for making sense of it all. Although theories do render the world easier to manage cognitively, the lay theories perspective asserts that needs for *understanding* and *meaning*—not miserliness—are the primary motives underlying theory development [1], [37], [38], [39], [40]. After building a theory, perceivers are not open-minded but rather tend to automatically see the world in terms of their theories. Our major prediction, rooted in this lay theories perspective, is that several well-documented social-cognitive phenomena will be moderated by individual differences in theories of social causality [39–42].

The existing literature contains two major lines of work reflecting a lay theories perspective. The first examines cultural differences. For example, Miller [43] found that Americans show a preference for internal explanations, whereas Indians show a preference for external explanations. Similar results have been reported by Morris and Peng [44]. Various challenges have been offered to the simplistic idea that Westerners prefer internal whereas Easterners prefer external causes. For example, some work has suggested that cultural differences emerge only when external causal information is highly salient, in which case Easterners use it and Westerners continue to ignore it [45], [46]. More subtly, Menon, Morris, Chui, and Hong [47] suggest that Westerners and Easterners both emphasize internal causes, but Easterners are more likely to see dispositions residing in groups (*the organization* is corrupt) whereas Westerners are more likely to see dispositions as residing in individuals (*he* or *she* is corrupt). In spite of these nuances, the literature is clear that there are cultural differences in general theories of social causality, which guide explanation selection in specific cases.

Beyond this work on culture, the best-known approach to lay theories comes from Dweck and her colleagues' work on implicit person theories [39], [40], [48], [49]; see also [50] for a distinct, more recent approach. They take an individual differences (rather than cultural) approach and suggest that lay perceivers can be classified either as *entity theorists*, who believe that the characteristics of human beings are highly stable ("Everyone is a certain kind of person and there is not much that can be done to change that"), or *incremental theorists*, who believe that human characteristics are malleable and unstable ("All people can change even their most basic qualities"). One of the clearest demonstrations of the effects of implicit person theories comes from Chiu, Hong, and Dweck [51]. They found that entity theorists were more likely than incremental theorists to believe that an actor's behavior in one context would predict his behavior in a different context and that even a single instance of behavior is indicative of an enduring behavioral tendency. Other work [Hong, 1994, unpublished] has suggested, in contrast, that incremental theorists favor explanations that point to dynamic processes in the actor's mind (e.g., momentary needs, goals, or strategies), which create expectations of less behavioral stability.

More recently, Church and his colleagues [50] proposed an alternative conceptualization of lay theories. First, they offer the concept of *implicit trait beliefs*, which are a person's beliefs about the stability of traits over time, the consistency of trait-relevant behavior across situations, the ease of predicting behavior from traits, the ease of inferring traits from scant behavioral observations, and the adequacy of traits for understanding a person. They contrast implicit trait beliefs with *implicit contextual beliefs*, which are a person's beliefs about the instability of traits over time, the inconsistency of trait-relevant behavior across situations, the inability to predict specific behaviors from traits, the difficulty of inferring traits from scant behavioral observations, and the importance of context (e.g., roles, statuses) for predicting behavior. Church et al. developed the *Personal Beliefs Inventory* (*PBI*) to measure these two dimensions of lay theories. They found that the PBI comprised two underlying latent factors, which corresponded to implicit trait and implicit contextual theories. This, of course, provides additional evidence regarding the orthogonality of internal and external casual explanations noted above. Furthermore, Church et al. presented evidence that implicit trait beliefs were only weakly related to Dweck et al.'s implicit person theories, and implicit contextual beliefs were not related to them at all.

Our concept of social explanatory styles has much in common with this prior work. How will we contribute beyond it? First, our focus on individual differences distinguishes our approach from work on culture. Second, although Dweck et al. and Church et al. focus on individual differences, we conceive of social explanatory styles in terms of three independent dimensions, only one of which seems likely *a priori* to be empirically related to their constructs (and which we will show below is only moderately related to Church's implicit trait beliefs and is unrelated to Dweck et al.'s theories). To elaborate, unlike the SESQ, Dweck et al. do not directly measure belief in the efficacy of external causes. This is important given the arguments above that such belief is orthogonal to belief in the efficacy of internal causes (which Dweck et al. do measure). Relatedly, unlike the SESQ, Church et al. do not measure belief in the efficacy of actor volition/control. Finally, whereas Church et al. do measure belief in the efficacy of external causes, they conceive of external causes as *contextual* influences that cause an actor to behave differently on different occasions. In contrast, as will be elaborated below, we conceive of external causes as *historical* and *formative* influences that have caused an actor to *become a particular kind of person*. Our conception grows out of our research on moral psychology, which suggests that moral emotions such as blame and compassion are linked to beliefs about the role of historical, formative influences in shaping potentially blameworthy agents [4], [11]. To maintain clarity, we will use more descriptive labels such as *historicism* and *historical causes* when discussing the types of external causes assessed by the Social Explanatory Styles Questionnaire. The upshot here is that, in relation to existing lay theories measures, the SESQ provides predominantly novel information. We will provide evidence below regarding the relation between the SESQ, Dweck et al.'s implicit person theories measure, and Church et al.'s PBI.

Social Explanatory Styles

What are social explanatory styles and where do they come from? We propose that, over time, cultural influences, individual learning experiences, and individual cognitive and motivational influences combine to create individual differences in general beliefs about the causes of action. We propose that important individual differences exist in general beliefs about the causal importance of internal dispositions, historical, formative influences in an agent's life, and agent volition/control. Thus, we conceptualize social explanatory styles in terms of three independent dimensions: *Dispositionism*, *historicism*, and *controllability*. Although we suspect that these different dimensions likely interact to predict certain social judgments, in the present paper we focus on the preliminary task of separately validating our measure of each independent dimension.

Individual differences in social explanatory styles are likely shaped by a wide array of factors. At the broadest level, cultures vary in terms of beliefs about social causality (see above). There is also evidence for ethnic group differences in causal perceptions within the United States [52]. At a more specific level, educational experiences likely shape social explanatory styles. For example, higher education can reduce internal explanations [53] and increase reliance on more sophisticated "interactionist" explanations [52]. Higher education in the social sciences strengthens belief in historicism, at least for understanding group-level outcomes [54], [55]. Finally, at an intrapsychic level, those who are contemplative are relatively likely to adopt a belief in historicism [18]. Surely, much future work is needed to understand the full array of factors that create variability in social explanatory styles.

Understanding the causes and consequences of diversity in social explanatory styles will be greatly facilitated by the availability of a reliable and valid measure. Thus, below we present six studies that examine the convergent and divergent validity of the Social Explanatory Styles Questionnaire. As noted above, given the central role of explanation in social life, individual differences in social explanatory styles—likely involving interactive relations among the independent dimensions tapped by the SESQ—should have broad implications for the individual's social life. That assumption provides the motivation for the present work.

Measuring Social Explanatory Styles

Beyond the work of Dweck et al. and Church et al., other scholars have developed instruments that are similar in some ways to what we are attempting. For example, Fincham and Bradbury [16] developed the Relationship Attribution Measure (RAM). Research using the RAM shows that explanatory styles in the marital context plays a role in shaping marital quality. But, the RAM does not tap broader explanatory tendencies that generalize beyond one's marriage. Relatedly, Peterson, Semmel, von Baeyer, Abramson, Metalsky, and Seligman [21] developed the Attributional Style Questionnaire (ASQ). The ASQ taps *explanatory style*, or one's characteristic style of explaining one's own acts and outcomes [56]. Work with the ASQ has suggested the existence of a *depressive attributional style*: Those who attribute negative personal events to their own stable, global dispositions (i.e., an interactive combination of belief in internality, stability, and globality) are at increased risk of depression. The notion of explanatory styles is quite similar to our notion of social explanatory styles, and its role in predicting depression speaks to the importance of general explanatory theories. The major difference, of course, is that explanatory styles concern the self, whereas social explanatory styles concern others.

To measure our construct, over a period of years we have developed the SESQ, which can be seen in Appendix S1. Respondents are presented with descriptions of the action patterns of eight different individuals. Each of the eight scenarios was designed to describe the general character of a target. That is, the SESQ taps explanations regarding the enduring character of a person rather than explanations for single, isolated acts. Half the targets show positive character and half show negative character. For each target individual, respondents are asked: *Why has [this target] become [this way]?* They provide ratings of the extent to which the cause is the target's traits (*dispositionism*), the target's external circumstances/life experiences (*historicism*), and factors over which the actor can exert control (*controllability*). Scoring of the SESQ involves calculation of mean dispositionism, historicism, and controllability scores.

The Present Studies

Ethics Statement

All studies were approved by Lehigh University's Institutional Review Board (IRB). For each study, participants provided written consent. The consent forms were approved by Lehigh University's IRB.

Overview of Studies

Below, we present six studies. Studies 1, 2 and 3 will examine basic psychometric properties of the SESQ. We will present evidence regarding the internal consistency of responses to each dimension of the SESQ, factor structure of the SESQ, relation to personality traits and political ideologies, and relation to the lay theories measures of Dweck et al. and Church et al.

Studies 4, 5, and 6 address predictive validity. The approach in each study is to validate a particular subscale of the SESQ. As noted above, however, we encourage users to examine interactions among SESQ dimensions for predicting social judgments and behaviors. Such interactions will be more meaningful to the extent that the contributing dimensions from the SESQ have been separately validated. Thus, such preliminary validation is the task of the present studies. Study 4 will test whether SESQ dispositionism moderates the tendency to make spontaneous trait inferences from behaviors [23]. Study 5 will test whether SESQ historicism moderates the tendency to commit the FAE in the classic Jones and Harris [24] attitude attribution paradigm. Study 6 will examine whether SESQ controllability moderates blaming of those from stigmatized categories [7]. Taken together, these studies will show that social explanatory styles play an important role in moderating several basic phenomena of social cognition and thus that each separate subscale of the SESQ has an important degree of predictive validity.

Study 1: Internal Consistency and Factor Structure of the SESQ

Method

Participants. Three-hundred and ten participants (184 males, 126 females) participated on-line via the Mechanical Turk interface created by Amazon. They ranged in age from 18 to 68 ($M = 29.5$). Many participants had completed a 4-year college degree (35%) and some had also completed an advanced professional or graduate degree (8%). Other participants had completed a 2-year degree (11%), less than two years of college (30%), or a high school degree (15%). A few participants (1%) had not completed high school. The sample was predominately White (87%), but also included individuals who identified as East Asian, African-American, and Hispanic.

Procedure. After clicking the "agree" box on an on-line consent form, participants completed the SESQ along with some unrelated measures.

Results and Discussion

We began by examining internal consistency for each scale dimension. Cronbach's alpha suggested strong internal consistency for dispositionism ($\alpha = .89$), historicism ($\alpha = .85$), and controllability ($\alpha = .88$). These support the idea that people have coherent social explanatory styles. Next, we submitted mean ratings on each dimension to a repeated-measures ANOVA. This revealed a strong effect of causal dimension, $F(2, 308) = 113.11$, $p < .001$. The pattern was such that controllability ratings were the highest ($M = 4.37$, $SD = .68$), dispositionism ratings were next ($M = 3.98$, $SD = .64$), and historicism ratings were lowest ($M = 3.51$, $SD = .66$). Controllability ratings were significantly higher than both dispositionism and historicism ratings ($Fs > 46.96$, $ps < .001$, $ds > .78$), and dispositionism ratings were significantly higher than historicism ratings ($F = 67.47$, $p < .001$, $d = .94$). This pattern fits the notion that those in Western cultures tend to view actions as highly controllable [57] and to emphasize internal over external causes [43], [44]. Of course, these mean differences should be interpreted cautiously given that we did not obtain data from a comparison culture to see if the pattern of means would change. Finally, we examined correlations among SESQ dimensions. Supporting our decision to measure them separately, dispositionism and historicism were unrelated, $r(308) = .08$, *ns*. In contrast, dispositionism and controllability showed a modest positive relation, $r(308) = .19$, $p < .001$, and historicism and controllability showed a weak negative relation, $r(308) = -.11$, $p < .05$.

Finally, we computed a principal components factor analysis with varimax rotation. Looking at the scree plot, it was clear that a three factor solution described the data quite well. The eigenvalues of these three factors were 5.77, 4.45, and 3.18, and together they accounted for 56% of the variance. There were two additional factors with eigenvalues between 1.0 and 1.2 but these factors had just one or two items with factor loadings over $|.50|$. Thus, the structure of the SESQ is dominated by three factors. These three factors are displayed in Table 1. Clearly, each causal dimension tapped by the SESQ—dispositionism, historicism, controllability—represents a separate underlying latent factor. Thus, the SESQ reliably measures three independent facets of people's social explanatory styles.

Study 2: Relation of the SESQ to Cognitive Style, Personality Traits, and Political Ideology

Study 2 sought evidence regarding the relation of social explanatory styles to cognitive processing style, personality traits,

Table 1. Factor Analysis of the SESQ (Study 1).

Item	Factor 1	Factor 2	Factor 3
Dispositionism: Susan's Love	.78		
Dispositionism: Bill's Helpfulness	.78		
Dispositionism: Steven's Disagreeableness	.75		
Dispositionism: Robert's Crimes	.74		
Dispositionism: James's Community Service	.74		
Dispositionism: Sarah's Verbal Abuse of Children	.73		
Dispositionism: Janet's Volunteering	.72		
Dispositionism: Beth's Infidelities	.71		
Control: Janet's Volunteering	.33	.85	
Control: James's Community Service		.84	
Control: Bill's Helpfulness		.80	
Control: Susan's Love		.79	
Control: Beth's Infidelities		.56	
Control: Steven's Disagreeableness		.48	
Control: Robert's Crimes		.42	
Control: Sarah's Verbal Abuse of Children		.35	
Historicism: Bill's Helpfulness			.81
Historicism: James's Community Service			.81
Historicism: Janet's Volunteering			.79
Historicism: Susan's Love			.78
Historicism: Robert's Crimes			.57
Historicism: Sarah's Verbal Abuse of Children			.50
Historicism: Steven's Disagreeableness			.36
Historicism: Beth's Infidelities			.26

Note. Factor loadings (including cross-loadings) less than |.25| are deleted.

and political ideology. We propose that social explanatory styles are specific social cognitive orientations and thus they should relate, at most, only modestly to broad personality traits. Beyond this, we expected that individuals prone to thorough cognitive processing would be more historicist and less dispositional in their social explanatory styles [18], [33]. Finally, we expected that social explanatory style would *not* be closely aligned with political ideology. With regard to this latter issue, there is evidence that liberals and conservative do show some differences in their thinking about social causality [58–61]. However, as we have argued elsewhere [18], these differences are specific to thinking about socio-economic inequality and do not reflect the type of broad explanatory theories we are trying to tap with the SESQ; see [60] for a similar perspective.

Method

Participants. Two-hundred eighty undergraduate participants (145 female) participated for credit in their introductory psychology classes.

Procedure. After signing a written consent form, all participants completed the SESQ. In addition, a subset of sixty-seven completed the Need for Cognitive Closure scale (NFCC) [62], a separate subset of ninety-seven completed the Big Five Inventory (BFI) [63] and the Difficulties in Emotion Regulation Scale (DERS) [64], and another subset of one-hundred sixteen completed the Right-Wing Authoritarianism (RWA) [65] and Social Dominance Orientation scales (SDO) [66]. As per standard scoring methods, participants received a single score for NFCC [$M = 3.49$ (scale: 1 to 6), $SD = .42$, $\alpha = .83$], DERS [$M = 2.30$ (scale: 1 to 5), $SD = .64$, $\alpha = .88$], RWA [$M = -1.09$ (scale: -4 to 4), $SD = 1.24$, $\alpha = .92$], and SDO [$M = 3.00$ (scale: 1 to 7), $SD = 1.19$, $\alpha = .94$]. Also as per standard scoring methods, the BFI yielded five scores (scale: 1 to 5), with each score representing one of the Big Five Personality Factors: Extroversion ($M = 3.25$, $SD = .85$, $\alpha = .88$), Agreeableness ($M = 3.67$, $SD = .53$, $\alpha = .66$), Conscientiousness ($M = 3.52$, $SD = .63$, $\alpha = .79$), Neuroticism ($M = 2.90$, $SD = .72$, $\alpha = .79$), and Openness ($M = 3.38$, $SD = .64$, $\alpha = .77$).

Results and Discussion

Correlations were computed between the SESQ dimensions and the other constructs (see Table 2). We also computed multiple regression analyses. For all regression analyses presented in this paper, predictor variables were centered on their means prior to being multiplied to create interaction terms [67]. In the present case, we tested main effects and all 2- and 3-way interactions involving the SESQ dimensions. We found only one significant interaction effect out of 32 possible interactions, so we will treat that effect as spurious (it was not a highly sensible pattern).

Table 2. Correlations of SESQ dimensions with cognitive style, personality traits, and political ideology (Study 2).

	NFCC	DERS	Extroversion	Agreeableness	Conscientiousness	Neuroticism	Openness	RWA	SDO
	(*N*=67)	(*N*=97)	(*N*=97)	(*N*=97)	(*N*=97)	(*N*=97)	(*N*=97)	(*N*=116)	(*N*=116)
Dispositionism	.40**	−.02	.13	.17	.04	−.05	.06	−.07	−.05
Historicism	−.27*	−.04	.14	.21*	.10	.05	.02	−.03	.06
Controllability	.23†	−.24*	−.09	.13	.29**	−.24*	−.25*	−.08	−.13

Note: $^{\dagger}p=.06$; *$p<.05$; **$p<.01$.

As can be seen in Table 2, the strongest correlations were between the SESQ dimensions and NFCC. Specifically, among those high in NFCC social explanatory styles tended to be more dispositional, less historicist, and marginally more likely to emphasize controllability. This is consistent with the notion that careful and thorough thinking increases one's focus on external forces such as agent history, whereas shallow thinking leaves one focused on internal factors such as dispositions and volition. Dispositionism was unrelated to all the other variables measured. In contrast, beyond its relation to NFCC, historicism was also modestly related to Agreeableness. This fits with the idea that historicism is associated with prosocial responding [18], [61]. Finally, controllability was associated with several variables beyond NFCC. In particular, controllability was negatively related to DERS and Neuroticism. It seems likely that these relations involve extrapolation from the self—*my emotions are strong and I have difficulty controlling them*—to a general belief about humanity—*people are not in control.* Also, those high in Openness were similarly likely to reject the idea that people are in control of their actions. This relation likely stems from an influence similar to that of NFCC: Contemplation tends to undermine belief in "free will." Finally, in contrast, those high in Conscientiousness were more likely to score high on controllability. This, as with DERS and Neuroticism, seems likely to reflect extrapolation from the self—*I am consistently able to exercise self-control and enact appropriate behaviors*—to humanity—*people are in control of their actions.* None of the SESQ dimensions were related to political ideology.

Study 3: Social Explanatory Styles, Implicit Person Theories, and Implicit Trait and Contextual Beliefs

In Study 3, we will examine the relation between the SESQ dimensions, Church et al.'s implicit trait and implicit contextual beliefs, and Dweck et al.'s implicit person theories.

Method

Participants. One-hundred thirty-nine participants (76 female) participated for credit in their introductory psychology course. An additional one-hundred nineteen participants (87 males, 32 females) participated on-line via Amazon's Mechanical Turk interface. They ranged in age from 18 to 66 ($M=35$). Many of the on-line participants had completed a 4-year college degree (51%) and some had also completed an advanced professional or graduate degree (10%). Other participants had completed a 2-year degree (10%), less than two years of college (17%), or a high school degree (12%). The sample was predominately White (81%), but also included individuals who identified as East Asian, African-American, and Hispanic.

Procedure. After providing consent, participants completed the SESQ. In addition, the introductory psychology sample completed Levy and Dweck's [unpublished] 8-item IPT measure (e.g., *Everyone is a certain kind of person, and there is not much they can really do to change that*). After appropriate reverse coding, items were averaged such that high scores reflected an entity theory ($M=4.0$ of 7; $SD=1.3$; $\alpha=.93$). In scoring, we followed the procedure of Chiu et al. [51] by deleting those who scored around the midpoint (4) of the scale (who lack a clear theory). Specifically, we categorized those scoring over 4.5 as entity theorists and those scoring below 3.5 as incremental theorists. This resulted in the deletion of roughly 33% of cases, which is comparable to Chui et al. The on-line sample completed Church et al.'s [50] PBI measure, which taps implicit trait ($M=3.83$ of 5; $SD=.34$; $\alpha=.88$) and implicit contextual beliefs ($M=3.22$; $SD=.36$; $\alpha=.86$).

Results and Discussion

We computed correlations between the three SESQ dimensions, IPT, and the two dimensions of the PBI. As can be seen in Table 3, there were no significant relations between the SESQ dimensions and Dweck et al.'s IPT measure. Indeed, there were only two significant correlations among the nine we computed. One of these—a positive relation between SESQ controllability and PBI implicit trait theories—was quite small. There was a somewhat larger relation between SESQ dispositionism and PBI implicit trait theories, although this correlation hardly suggests that the measures are redundant. Taken together, these correlations suggest that the SESQ is providing predominately novel information—not tapped by alternative measures—regarding lay theories of social causality. One task for the future will be to more precisely understand the differences among the constructs being assessed by these measures, a task that will become more achievable as more data are collected involving the newer measures (i.e., PBI, SESQ). Indeed, Church and colleagues [50] showed that the PBI was only weakly related to Dweck et al.'s IPT measure. In particular, then, further investigation is needed to more fully understand why the IPT measure, PBI implicit traits beliefs, and SESQ dispositionism are only weakly to moderately correlated, given their shared emphasis on traits/internal factors.

Study 4: Dispositionism and the Tendency to Make Spontaneous Trait Inferences

Studies 1–3 provided strong evidence regarding the internal consistency, factor structure, and divergent validity of the SESQ. None of the evidence, however, demonstrates the predictive validity of each SESQ dimension. Thus, the purpose of the next three studies is to show that each dimension of the SESQ enables prediction of a relevant social psychological phenomenon. Study 4 will provide evidence that SESQ dispositionism moderates the tendency to make spontaneous trait inferences from behavior. Study 5 will provide evidence that SESQ historicism moderates the tendency to commit the Fundamental Attribution Error. Finally, Study 6 will show that SESQ controllability moderates blaming of those in stigmatized categories. As noted above, here we focus on the preliminary task of separately demonstrating the validity of each SESQ dimension. Future research will, we hope, consider whether interactions among particular social explanatory dimensions might be relevant for understanding a target phenomenon (e.g., as with depressive attributional style).

In Study 4, we utilize a probe recognition paradigm [68] to examine whether the tendency to make *spontaneous trait inferences* (*STIs*) is moderated by the dispositionism facet of social explanatory styles. Such a result takes us outside the realm of self-reports and would provide compelling evidence that dispositionism (as tapped by the SESQ) guides presumably automatic, uncontrollable social cognitive processes.

In the STI paradigm, participants read a series of one-sentence behavior descriptions which are followed by a probe word. Their task is to indicate as quickly and accurately as possible whether the probe word actually appeared in the behavior description. In reality, the probe word did not appear. On critical trials, however, the probe word is a trait (or situation) *implied* by the behavior description. On control trials the probe word is not implied by the behavior description. The logic behind this paradigm [69], [70, [71] is that if participants make a STI, then they should have difficulty correctly reporting that an implied probe word did not actually appear. Indeed, evidence for the occurrence of STIs comes when participants take longer to respond that a probe word (*smart*) did not appear on a critical trial (*John got an A on the test*) than on a control trial (*Ben jumped over the fence*). Such slow responding suggests that participants spontaneously inferred the probe word, an inference that interferes with correctly reporting that the word was not actually in the sentence. Ham and Vonk [70] expanded the STI paradigm to also measure *spontaneous situation inferences* (*SSIs*). The logic is identical to that just described. For example, evidence for an SSI happens if, after reading *Eric lifted the boulder*, participants are slower to report that *light* was not in the sentence than after reading a control behavior description (*Steven swam the lake*). We use the stimuli from Ham and Vonk for our study below.

Our major prediction is that SESQ dispositionism scores will be positively related to the tendency to make STIs. Indeed, because lay theories presumably structure one's understanding of social events on a daily basis, those with strong dispositionist theories should be well-practiced at generating relevant trait concepts from behavioral observations. Thus, such inferences should be highly automatized and hence likely to be detectable in a STI paradigm. If our prediction is confirmed, it will suggest that the dispositionist lay theory tapped by the SESQ is evident even on implicit measures.

One might expect that SESQ historicism scores should predict SSIs, but we were not so sure. The reason has to do with the specific content of the situational explanations used by Ham and Vonk (2003), whose stimuli we use here. Specifically, the SSI stimuli from Ham and Vonk (2003) refer primarily to properties of objects with which an actor has a momentary interaction (e.g., *the fence was low*; *the boulder was light*). In contrast, historicism on the SESQ concerns "nurture" beliefs (e.g., *parents and community have shaped the type of person she is*). It seems to us that these two notions of "external causes" are so different that historicism scores might well be unrelated to SSIs.

Method

Participants. One-hundred fifteen participants (59 female) participated for course credit.

Table 3. Correlations of SESQ dimensions with Dweck et al.'s Implicit Person Theories and Church et al.'s Implicit Trait and Implicit Contextual Theories (Study 3).

	Dweck et al.: Implicit Person Theories	Church et al.: Implicit Trait Theories	Church et al. Implicit Contextual Theories
	(N=93)	(N=119)	(N=119)
Dispositionism	.17	.40***	−.11
Historicism	−.01	.04	.07
Controllability	−.15	.20*	.09

Note: *$p<.05$; ***$p<.001$.

Procedure. After signing a written consent form, participants completed the SESQ at a pretest. A few weeks later, they returned individually to take part in an ostensibly unrelated study. Participants were randomly assigned to either the *STI condition* or *SSI condition* and were seated at a computer terminal. After signing a written consent form, participants received instructions indicating that their task would consist of reading behavior descriptions displayed on the screen and then indicating as quickly and accurately as possible whether or not a word displayed immediately afterward had actually appeared in the behavior description. To motivate participants, a reward of $20 was promised to the participant whose responses were the fastest and most accurate. Participants were instructed to press the "a" key if the probe word had actually appeared in the behavior description and to press the "6" key on the number pad if the probe word had not actually appeared in the behavior description. They were also instructed to keep their left and right index fingers on the keys during the entire task. Participants completed 12 practice trials to familiarize them with the task.

Next, they began the actual task. On each trial, a row of X's was presented in the center of the screen for 1000 ms. Then, a behavior description was displayed for 3000 ms followed by a blank screen which lasted for 500 ms. A row of X's then appeared for 500 ms, followed by a probe word. The probe word remained on the screen until participants indicated "Yes" or "No" (*Was this word actually in the sentence you just read?*). Once an answer was provided, a blank screen was displayed for 1000 ms. Then the next trial began. There were 10 critical trials on which the probe word was implied by the preceding behavior description. There were also 10 control trials on which the probe word was not implied by the preceding behavior description. The critical and control trials consisted of the same behavior descriptions and probe words, but in the control trials the probes were rearranged to be irrelevant to the behavior descriptions. Although the 10 behavior descriptions were always the same, in the STI condition the probe words were traits whereas in the SSI condition probe words were features of the situation. Forty filler trials were also included and these served to add trials on which "yes" was the correct response and on which participants needed to attend to the verb in the behavior description; see Ham & Vonk [69] for rationale. The 60 combinations of behavior descriptions and probes were presented in random order. Response times (RT) and correctness were recorded by the computer.

Results and Discussion

Reaction times. Overall, error rates were very low (M = 1.01%, SD = .02, Range = 0 to 5%). RTs were analyzed only if the response had been correct. Because analyses of RTs can be very sensitive to outliers, we analyzed our response time data using two methods. First, we employed an absolute cutoff criterion of <200 ms and >2000 ms. Using this cutoff criterion resulted in the deletion of only .28% of responses. Second, because the RT data were positively skewed, we performed a natural log transformation. Results using either approach were virtually identical. For ease of interpretation, the analyses presented below are based on the cutoff criterion.

Prior to testing our primary hypotheses, we computed a 2(Trial Type: control, critical) X 2(Probe Type: trait, situation) between-within ANOVA. This revealed a main effect of Trial Type, $F(113) = 9.77$, $p = .002$, which reflected that fact that RTs were slower on critical trials (M = 657) than on control trials (M = 637). Neither the main effect of Probe Type nor the interaction was significant, $Fs < 1.83$. This replicates the findings of Ham and Vonk and suggests that participants were making both STIs and SSIs in our study.

Next, to test our hypotheses regarding dispositionism, we followed the recommendations of Judd, Kenny, and McClelland [72] for testing moderation in a within-subjects design. First, we transformed the within-subjects variable of trial type (critical vs. control) into a difference score that represented the difference between RTs on critical versus control trials. This was done such that higher scores indicated slower RT on critical as compared to control, suggesting the presence of a spontaneous inference. Thus, we will hereafter call this variable *spontaneous inferences.*

We regressed the spontaneous inference variable on condition (STI vs. SSI), SESQ dispositionism, SESQ historicism, and all their 2- and 3-way interactions (the version of the SESQ used in this study omitted the controllability dimension). This analysis revealed only the predicted condition by SESQ dispositionism interaction, $t(107) = 2.93$, $p = .004$ (all other $ts < |1.19|$, $ps > .24$). Follow-up simple slope analyses—plotting the relation between dispositionism and spontaneous inferences separately for the STI and SSI conditions—were computed. See Figure 1. In the STI condition, we found a significant positive relation between SESQ dispositionism and spontaneous inferences, $t(111) = 2.33$, $p = .02$ ($d = .44$). In the SSI condition, there was a slight reversal of this pattern which did not attain statistical significance, $t(111) = -1.47$, $p = .15$ ($d = .28$). Thus, SESQ dispositionism scores predicted an increased tendency to make spontaneous trait inferences, and were weakly predictive of a reduced tendency to make spontaneous situation inferences. As noted earlier, we questioned whether SESQ historicism would predict SSIs, and the evidence suggests that they did not. Validity evidence for SESQ historicism comes next.

Study 5: SESQ Historicism and the Fundamental Attribution Error

In Study 5, we examine the predictive validity of the historicism dimension of the SESQ. To do so, we examine whether historicism moderates one of the most "fundamental" phenomena of social cognition: The *Fundamental Attribution Error* (*FAE*), which is the tendency to neglect or underweight external causes when

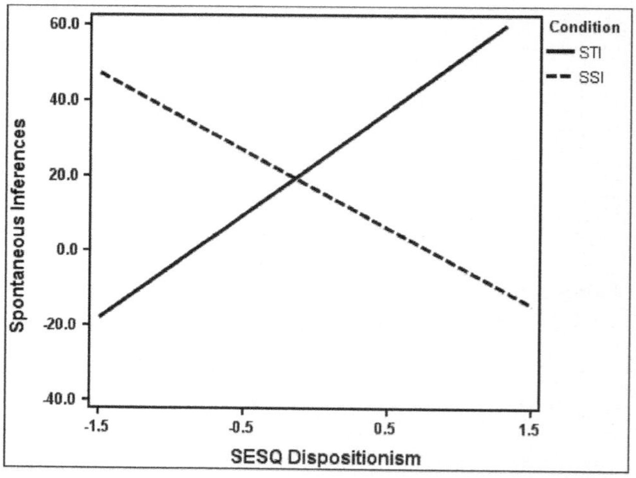

Figure 1. SESQ dispositionism and spontaneous inferences. SESQ dispositionism strongly predicts increased levels of spontaneous trait inference (STI) and weakly predicts decreased levels of spontaneous situation inference (SSI).

making social judgments [24], [27], [73]. To test this, we performed a conceptual replication of Jones and Harris's [24] classic study.

We predicted that SESQ dispositionism would not moderate the tendency to commit the FAE. Given that lay dispositionism is a frequently given explanation for the FAE [27], our prediction deserves some comment. A careful reading of Gilbert and Malone's analysis [27] (see especially pp. 22–24) shows that it is not belief in dispositions *per se* that fosters the FAE. Rather, it is either blindness about or explicit dismissal of the "power of the situation" in shaping actions and dispositions. As noted above, dispositionism is independent of belief in the power of the situation [27] (see also Study 1 regarding the lack of correlation between dispositionism and historicism). Thus, we expect that dispositionism will not moderate the FAE, but rather it will be those who *explicitly affirm the power of external social forces to mold the individual* (i.e., high historicism) who will be less prone to committing the FAE.

Method

Participants. Eighty-nine participants (43 female) participated for credit in their introductory psychology course.

Procedure. After signing a written consent form, participants completed the SESQ at a pretest. A few weeks later, they returned to a different location in small groups, met a different experimenter, signed a written consent form, and completed an experiment modeled after Jones and Harris. Specifically, they learned that they would be reading an essay about Affirmative Action (AA) written by a college student, Pat O'Malley, for a journalism class. Participants were randomly assigned to either the *no choice condition* or the *choice condition* and to the *anti-AA condition* or the *pro-AA condition.*

Participants in the no choice condition learned that "the professor told each student which position to defend. Thus, Pat did not choose which position to argue." Participants in the choice condition learned that "the professor allowed each student to choose which position to defend. Thus, Pat chose to argue the position in the essay you'll read." Next, participants in the anti-AA condition read an essay ostensibly written by Pat that provided several arguments against Affirmative Action, whereas participants in the pro-AA condition read an essay ostensibly written by Pat that provided several arguments in favor of Affirmative Action. Finally, participants were asked to diagnose Pat's "true, personal attitude" on two 9-point scales with endpoints labeled *Definitely Opposes Affirmative Action* and *Definitely Supports Affirmative Action* or *Definitely Against Affirmative Action* and *Definitely In Favor of Affirmative Action.* These two items were highly correlated ($r = .92$), and thus were averaged to form an index of the extent to which Pat was perceived as favorable toward AA ($M = 4.57$, $SD = 2.39$).

Results and Discussion

Ratings of Pat's attitude were regressed on the choice manipulation, the position manipulation (anti or pro), SESQ historicism, SESQ dispositionism, and all their 2-, 3-, and 4-way interactions (again, the controllability dimension was omitted on the version of the SESQ used in this study). The analysis revealed a main effect of position, $t(73) = 8.83$, $p < .001$ ($d = 2.1$), with those in the pro-AA condition perceiving Pat as more favorable to Affirmative Action than those in the anti-AA condition. There was a marginal and not particularly intelligible main effect of dispositionism, $t(73) = 1.67$, $p = .10$, suggesting that those who scored high in dispositionism tended to rate Pat as more favorable toward Affirmative Action. More importantly, replicating Jones and Harris, there was a position by choice interaction, $t(73) = 4.00$, $p < .001$. The nature of this was such that the effect of position on ratings of Pat's attitude was stronger in the choice condition, $t(84) = 9.29$, $p < .001$ ($d = 2.0$), than in the no choice condition, $t(84) = 3.83$, $p < .001$ ($d = .84$). Notably, the fact that there remained a significant difference between the anti- and pro-AA conditions *even in the no choice condition* replicates the evidence for the FAE found by Jones and Harris.

Going beyond Jones and Harris, however, our analysis also revealed that this two-way interaction was moderated by SESQ historicism, creating a three-way interaction, $t(73) = 2.33$, $p = .023$. As can be seen in Figure 2, this interaction was driven by the fact that, as predicted, those high in SESQ historicism were more strongly affected by the choice manipulation than were those low in historicism. Indeed, in the anti-AA condition, those high (+1 SD) in historicism rated Pat as more opposed to Affirmative Action when Pat had choice than when Pat had no choice, $t(41) = -2.27$, $p = .028$ ($d = .71$), whereas the choice manipulation made no difference to those low (−1 SD) in historicism, $t < 1$. Similarly, in the pro-AA condition, those high (+1 SD) in historicism rated Pat as more in favor of Affirmative Action when Pat had choice than when Pat had no choice, $t(39) = 3.31$, p = .002 ($d = 1.06$), whereas the choice manipulation made no difference to those low (−1 SD) in historicism, $t = 1.12$, $p = .27$.

Another way of parsing these data is to look specifically at judgments within the no choice condition, in which, logically, the pro- and anti-AA essay writers should receive similar ratings because of the professor's strong influence on their attitude expressions. Examining that condition reveals that those high in historicism came quite close to avoiding the FAE altogether. Specifically, in the no choice condition those high in historicism (+ 1 SD) showed only a marginal tendency to rate Pat's attitude differently in the anti-AA ($M = 3.8$) as compared to the pro-AA condition ($M = 5.0$), $t(39) = 1.77$, $p = .08$ ($d = .57$). In contrast, this same difference was twice as large among those low (−1 SD) in historicism (Ms = 3.3 and 5.9, respectively; $t(39) = 3.57$, $p = .001$; $d = 1.14$).

Study 6: SESQ Controllability and the Polarization of Moral Judgments

In Study 6, we focus on the controllability dimension of the SESQ. The study is based on Weiner's [8] insight that controllability perceptions play a crucial role in moral blame. In particular, Weiner et al. [7] showed that when a stigmatizing condition is seen as controllable by its possessor, blame is amplified. In contrast, when a stigmatizing condition is seen as uncontrollable by its possessor, blame is inhibited.

Study 6 will examine whether those with a strong general belief in controllability (according to the SESQ) tend to perceive relatively controllable stigmas as *highly* controllable, and thus to show heightened blame compared to those with a weak general belief in controllability. We will also include a condition in which participants respond to relatively uncontrollable stigmas. We are interested in the possibility of a contrast effect: When a stigma is uncontrollable, will those with strong general belief in controllability perceive that stigma as *highly* *un*controllable because the stigma contrasts so markedly with their generally high control expectations? Such a contrast effect would ironically produce attenuated blame responses among those with strong general belief in controllability. In effect, then, Study 6 explores whether the controllability dimension of social explanatory style predicts polarization—both amplification and attenuation—of blame responses.

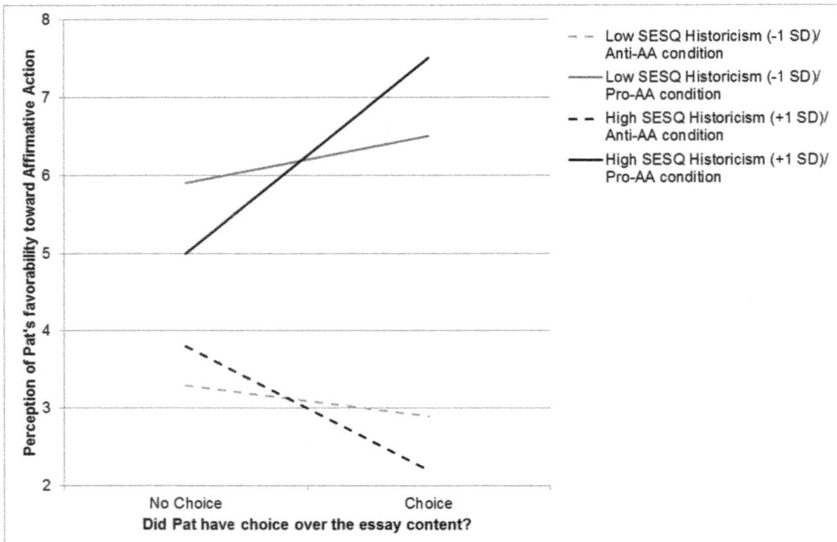

Figure 2. SESQ historicism and the Fundamental Attribution Error. SESQ historicism predicts increased sensitivity to the choice manipulation of the classic Jones and Harris (1967) paradigm, and thus a reduced tendency to commit the FAE.

Method

Participants. Sixty-seven participants (44 female) participated for credit in their introductory psychology course.

Procedure. After signing a written consent form, participants completed the SESQ at a pretest. A few weeks later, they returned to a different location and met a different experimenter. At this follow-up session, after signing a written consent form, they rated four stigmatized categories taken from Weiner et al. [7]. Based on pilot testing, we chose the two categories that were rated highest in controllability (*controllable stigmas*: *Child Abusers, The Obese*) and the two categories that were rated lowest in controllability (*uncontrollable stigmas*: *People with Alzheimer's, The Blind*). Participants in the present study rated the two controllable and the two uncontrollable stigmas in terms of controllability (e.g., *Did a child abuser have control over whether he/she became a child abuser?*). Responses were made on a 9-point scale with endpoints labeled *No Control At All* (1) and *Total Control* (9). Participants also rated how much blame they assigned to each stigma group (e.g., *To what extent do you blame a child abuser?*). Responses were made on a 9-point scale with endpoints labeled *No Blame* (1) and *Total Blame* (9). The order in which these ratings were made was counter-balanced across participants. There were no order effects. To prepare these ratings for analysis, we averaged the controllability ratings for the two controllable stigmas ($M = 7.45$, $SD = 1.24$) and for the two uncontrollable stigmas ($M = 1.75$, $SD = .84$). Next, we averaged the blame ratings for the two controllable stigmas ($M = 7.03$, $SD = 1.22$) and for the two uncontrollable stigmas ($M = 1.28$, $SD = .47$).

Results and Discussion

Our primary hypotheses were that SESQ controllability scores would predict heightened perceptions of control over controllable stigmas (an assimilation effect) and perhaps also attenuated perceptions of control over uncontrollable stigmas (a contrast effect). These alterations in perceived control should, in turn, translate into heightened blame for controllable stigmas and attenuated blame for uncontrollable stigmas.

To test these possibilities, we first looked at perceived control ratings. Specifically, we computed a repeated-measures ANCOVA (repeated measure: controllability ratings for controllable stigmas, controllability ratings for uncontrollable stigmas) with SESQ controllability as a continuous covariate. This analysis revealed a significant interaction, $F(1, 65) = 23.54$, $p < .001$. We calculated predicted means for high and low levels of SESQ controllability and the pattern of means fit our predictions. Specifically, perceived control over controllable stigmas was higher among those with strong general belief in controllability ($M_{controllable} = 8.0$ at +1 SD of SESQ controllability) than among those with weak general belief in controllability ($M_{controllable} = 6.84$ at -1 SD of SESQ controllability). And, in contrast, perceived control over uncontrollable stigmas was *lower* among those with strong general belief in controllability ($M_{uncontrollable} = 1.50$ at -1 SD of SESQ controllability) than among those with weak general belief in controllability ($M_{uncontrollable} = 1.99$).

Next, we examined blame ratings in the same repeated-measures ANCOVA. Once again, the interaction with SESQ controllability was significant, $F(1, 65) = 32.47$, $p < .001$. Once again, we calculated predicted means at high and low levels of SESQ controllability and the pattern of means fit our predictions. Specifically, blame for controllable stigmas was higher among those with strong general belief in controllability ($M_{controllable} = 7.58$ at +1 SD of SESQ controllability) than among those with weak general belief in controllability ($M_{controllable} = 6.39$ at -1 SD of SESQ controllability). And, in contrast, blame for uncontrollable stigmas was *lower* among those with strong general belief in controllability ($M_{uncontrollable} = 1.04$ at -1 SD of SESQ controllability) than among those with weak general belief in controllability ($M_{uncontrollable} = 1.53$ at -1 SD of SESQ controllability).

To capture this blame polarization process in a single analysis, we computed the path model depicted in Figure 3. The model assumes that general belief in controllability (from the SESQ) affects perceived control over both controllable and uncontrollable stigmas, and these controllability perceptions, in turn, contribute to blame. Because they are correlational, of course, the present data cannot rule in any pattern of causal relations. We note, however, that prior literature provides overwhelming evidence for a causal effect of lay theories on perceptions of specific instances [51], [74], [75], [76], [77] and also for a causal effect of perceived

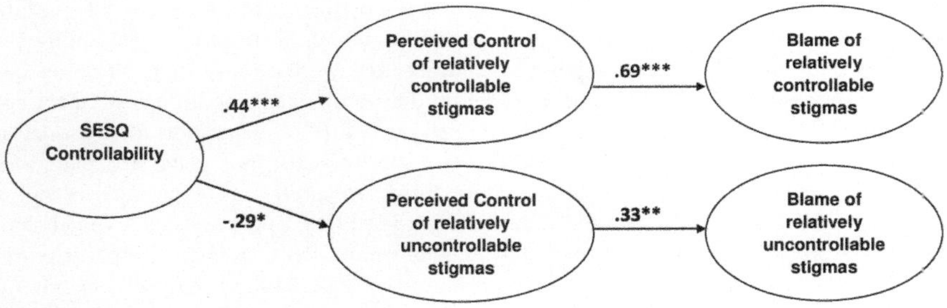

Figure 3. SESQ controllability and blame. SESQ controllability predicts polarization of moral judgments. Among those scoring high on SESQ controllability, perceived control and blame are intensified for relatively controllable stigmas, but attenuated for relatively uncontrollable stigmas. *p<.05, **p<.01, ***p<.001.

control on blame [8]. As can be seen in Figure 3, for controllable stigmas, SESQ controllability scores significantly predicted heightened perceptions of control and these heightened perceptions of control, in turn, significantly predicted heightened blame. In contrast, for uncontrollable stigmas, SESQ controllability scores significantly predicted attenuated perceptions of control and these attenuated perceptions of control, in turn, significantly predicted attenuated blame.

Elsewhere [4] we suggest that historicism can foster compassionate, non-blaming responses. Thus, we examined the relation of SESQ historicism to blaming of the stigma categories. In regression analyses that also included SESQ controllability scores as a predictor, we found that SESQ historicism predicted less blaming of controllable stigmas, $t(64) = -2.90$, $p = .005$ ($\beta = -.31$). In contrast, SESQ historicism was unrelated to blaming of uncontrollable stigmas, $t<1$.

The key finding here is that general belief in controllability—as tapped by the SESQ—is associated with polarized moral blame: Intensifying perceived control and blame for relatively controllable stigmas, and attenuating perceived control and blame for relatively uncontrollable stigmas. Also worthy of note is that SESQ historicism—independent of SESQ controllability—predicts less blame of controllable stigmas.

General Discussion

Explanation pervades social life. Furthermore, the explanations people generate powerfully shape their social emotions and social interactions. How do people select an explanation for an observed social event? Early work suggested that they rely on a logical reasoning process [29], [30], and subsequent work suggested that they do whatever is cognitively easiest [33]. More recent work focuses on the perceiver's pre-existing general theories [40], [43], [44]. Our work grows out of this latter tradition. We suggest that—based on cultural, educational, and personal experiences, filtered through one's cognitive and motivational style—individuals develop various general beliefs regarding the causes of social events. We refer to these beliefs as social explanatory styles. Our main goal in the present article was to offer a measure of individual differences in three dimensions of social explanatory styles, along with separate validity evidence for each of these dimensions.

Accordingly, we have offered the Social Explanatory Styles Questionnaire (SESQ). Rooted in classic theorizing, the SESQ measures three independent dimensions of social explanatory styles: Dispositionism, historicism, and controllability. Studies 1–3 examined basic psychometric properties of the SESQ along with its relations to other relevant constructs (to establish divergent validity). Study 1 revealed that each dimension of the SESQ shows strong internal consistency. Also, based on both factor analysis and correlational analyses, Study 1 suggested that the three SESQ dimensions are largely unrelated to each other. Study 2 provided evidence that the SESQ dimensions are independent of political ideology (RWA, SDO) and only modestly related (in sensible ways) to the Big Five traits and to emotion regulation. Study 2 also suggested that those high in Need for Cognitive Closure are more dispositional and less historicist in their social explanatory styles. Finally, Study 3 looked at relations between the SESQ and other lay theories constructs: Implicit person theories, implicit trait beliefs, and implicit context beliefs. Results indicated that SESQ historicism and SESQ controllability are essentially unrelated to any of these other lay theories measures. Thus, the majority of information provided by the SESQ is not provided by other measures. In contrast, SESQ dispositionism is moderately (not highly) related to the implicit trait beliefs construct offered by Church, Ortiz, and their colleagues [50]. Future work is needed to more precisely understand the differences in what is being assessed by the SESQ dispositionism subscale and the implicit trait beliefs measure.

Do the three dimensions of the SESQ have predictive validity in relation to important social cognitive phenomena? Yes, they do. This was the focus of Studies 4–6. In Study 4, we examined whether SESQ dispositionism moderates the tendency to make spontaneous trait inferences (STIs). Given that STIs can affect downstream consequences such as impression formation and approach/avoidance tendencies, it is important to understand when they will be made. Study 4 presented evidence that STIs are especially likely to be made by perceivers with a strong belief in dispositionism. In Study 5, we examined whether SESQ historicism moderates the tendency to commit the Fundamental Attribution Error. We found that it did, with high scorers on the SESQ historicism dimension being significantly less likely to commit the FAE than were low scorers. Finally, in Study 6, we examined whether general controllability beliefs would moderate blame judgments. Study 6 revealed that, interestingly, SESQ controllability predicted polarization of blame judgments: Heightened perceptions of control and blameworthiness for controllable stigmas, and attenuated perceptions of control and blameworthiness for uncontrollable stigmas. Thus, general controllability beliefs might paradoxically contribute to both condemnation and compassion toward others, a possibility surely worthy of further exploration. Indeed, existing work tends to emphasize the negative, condemnatory side of controllability beliefs [7], [57]. SESQ historicism also predicted reduced blame of those with controllable stigmas, independent of SESQ controllability scores.

In sum, Studies 4–6 provide predictive validity evidence regarding the three fundamental dimensions of social explanatory styles tapped by the SESQ. It is worth noting that SESQ scores in Studies 4–6 were always obtained several weeks prior to the main dependent variables, suggesting that social explanatory styles are robust and stable dimensions of people's thinking.

Where do we go from here? First, as noted above, we expect that social explanatory styles develop from a variety of influences including culture, socialization experiences, extrapolation from the self, general cognitive styles, and so on. Future work is needed to examine the contributions of these various factors to the development and modification of the three social explanatory dimensions tapped by the SESQ. Such work will be especially valuable if social explanatory styles are eventually shown to have the types of pervasive effects on social responding that we expect they will have.

Furthermore, we anticipate that, as with the Attributional Style Questionnaire [21], future research will suggest that certain configurations of explanatory beliefs—interactive combinations of the three basic explanatory dimensions—are particularly important. Researchers should therefore think in terms of interactions among the SESQ dimensions when attempting to understand social phenomena. Indeed, the fact that we independently validated each subscale of the SESQ should not be taken to mean that those subscales should always be treated separately in future theorizing and research. In fact, unpublished data from our lab already highlight the importance of interactions among social explanatory style dimensions for predicting implicit blame. In one study, we had participants learn about a violent criminal. Immediately afterwards, we assessed the extent to which blame-relevant constructs were automatically activated by priming with the criminal's name. The theoretical question was whether implicit blame is impacted by social explanatory styles in the same manner as explicit blame (as in Study 6 above), or whether, alternatively, implicit blame shows a different pattern than explicit blame [e.g., everyone experiences blame at the implicit level, but certain people—based on their general beliefs in controllability and historicism (see Study 6)—adjust their explicit judgments towards reduced blame]. We found an interaction between historicism and controllability beliefs (the same dimensions relevant for predicting explicit blame; see Study 6) for predicting implicit blame: Those who score both high on historicism *and* low on controllability show especially low levels of implicit blame. In addition to showing interactive effects of social explanatory style dimensions, this study also highlights how social explanatory styles shape immediate, uncontrollable responses to social stimuli (see also Study 4 above).

What other types of effects on social responding should be explored? We have an enduring interest in moral emotions, especially prosocial moral emotions that reflect concern for others (e.g., compunction regarding mistreatment of others and compassion for the plight of others; [4] [11], [18], [78]). Thus, an ongoing program of research in our labs involves connecting social explanatory styles to enduring moral emotional tendencies. To date, we have shown that the SESQ historicism predicts dispositional compassion-proneness and that historicism has a causal impact on compassionate responding [18]. One issue that remains to be investigated is why historicism has these effects. Gill et al. [4] offer a model in which historicist explanations for negative aspects of a target increase the sense that the target has suffered, and perceived suffering mediates the impact of historicist explanations on compassion. Gill et al. examined their model in the context of intergroup attitudes and not general explanatory styles. Thus, a task for future research is to examine whether a general belief that suffering lies behind people's negative acts and outcomes mediates the connection between SESQ historicism and dispositional compassion-proneness. More broadly, research on social explanatory styles needs to move beyond predicting personality self-reports (e.g., compassion-proneness) and responses to verbal stimuli in the lab (as in Studies 4–6 above). Researchers should examine whether social explanatory styles predict patterns of responding in face-to-face interactions with novel social partners, emotional responding within enduring relationships, patterns of blame vs. compassion reflected in social policy positions, and so on. We are examining all these domains of social life in our labs. Also, more work is needed regarding causal effects of social explanatory styles, although, of course, it is no easy task to manipulate *general* beliefs in social causality.

We will conclude by noting the massive body of work supporting the importance of self-oriented explanatory style in shaping self-relevant cognitive, emotional, and behavioral outcomes [20]. Explanatory style—an interactive combination internality, globality, and stability beliefs—is most famously linked to the development of depression [22], [79]. Beyond this, however, it has also been linked to performance in law school [80], productivity in the workplace [81], athletic performance [82], tendency toward risky aggression [83], and even physical health [84]. If explanatory style regarding the self is such a potent predictor of diverse areas of self-functioning, then it is plausible that social explanatory styles—perhaps including particular, interactive configurations of basic social explanatory dimensions—will be a similarly potent predictor of diverse areas of social functioning. We believe that this is a possibility worthy of exploration and we hope the SESQ will be a useful tool in that endeavor.

Supporting Information

Appendix S1 The Social Explanatory Styles Questionnaire (SESQ).
(DOCX)

Acknowledgments

Sincere thanks are extended to Dorian Arbelaez, Derek DeBellis, Shaundra Gallogly, Melissa Knapp, Jessica Lubitz, Syreeta McCutcheon, Tim Palumbo, Dheera Reddy, Kurt Schmenger, and Melissa Yates for their assistance with data collection and management.

Author Contributions

Conceived and designed the experiments: MJG MRA. Performed the experiments: MRA. Analyzed the data: MJG MRA. Wrote the paper: MJG MRA.

References

1. Heider F (1958). The psychology of interpersonal relations. Hoboken, NJ, USA: John Wiley & Sons Inc. doi: 10.1037/10628-000
2. Krieglmeyer R, Wittstadt D, Strack F (2009). How attribution influences aggression: Answers to an old question by using an implicit measure of anger. J Exp Soc Psychol 45(2): 379–385.
3. Alicke MD (2000). Culpable control and the psychology of blame. Psychol Bull 126(4): 556–574. doi: 10.1037/0033-2909.126.4.556
4. Gill MJ, Andreychik MR, Getty PD (2013). More than a lack of control: External explanations evoke compassion for outgroups by increasing perceptions of suffering (independent of perceived control). Pers Soc Psychol Bull 39(1): 73–87.
5. Pizarro D, Uhlmann E, Salovey P (2003). Asymmetry in judgments of moral blame and praise. Psychol Sci 14(3): 267–272. doi: 10.1111/1467-9280.03433

6. Tetlock PE, Visser PS, Singh R, Polifroni M, Scott A, et al. (2007). People as intuitive prosecutors: The impact of social-control goals on attributions of responsibility. J Exp Soc Psychol 43(2): 195–209. doi: 10.1016/j.jesp.2006.02.009
7. Weiner B, Perry RP, Magnusson J (1988). An attributional analysis of reactions to stigmas. J Pers Soc Psychol 55(5): 738–748. doi: 10.1037/0022-3514.55.5.738
8. Weiner B (2006). Social motivation, justice, and the moral emotions: An attributional approach Mahwah, NJ, US: Lawrence Erlbaum Associates Publishers.
9. Weiner B, Kukla A (1970). An attributional analysis of achievement motivation. J Pers Soc Psychol 15(1): 1–20. doi: 10.1037/h0029211
10. Weiner B (1985). An attributional theory of achievement motivation and emotion. Psychol Rev 92(4): 548–573. doi: 10.1037/0033-295X.92.4.548
11. Gill MJ, Andreychik MR (2007). Explanation and intergroup emotion: Social explanations as a foundation of prejudice-related compunction. Group Process Intergroup Relat 10(1): 87–106. doi: 10.1177/1368430207071343
12. Jayaratne TE, Ybarra O, Sheldon JP, Brown TN, Feldbaum M, et al. (2006). White Americans' genetic lay theories of race differences and sexual orientation: Their relationship with prejudice toward blacks, and gay men and lesbians. Group Process Intergroup Relat 9(1): 77–94.
13. Yzerbyt V, Rogier A (2001). Blame it on the group: Entitativity, subjective essentialism, and social attribution. In, The psychology of legitimacy: Emerging perspectives on ideology, justice, and intergroup relations. New York, NY, US: Cambridge University Press.
14. Hewstone M (1990). The ultimate attribution error? A review of the literature on intergroup causal attribution. Eur J Soc Psychol 20(4): 311–335.
15. Bradbury TN, Fincham FD (1990). Attributions in marriage: Review and critique. Psychol Bull 107(1): 3–33. doi: 10.1037/0033-2909.107.1.3
16. Fincham FD, Bradbury TN (1992). Assessing attributions in marriage: The relationship attribution measure. J Pers Soc Psychol 62(3): 457–468. doi: 10.1037/0022-3514.62.3.457
17. Fincham FD (2007). Attributions in close relationships: From balkanization to integration. In Fletcher GJO, Clark MS (Eds), Blackwell Handbook of Social Psychology: Interpersonal Processes. Malden: Blackwell Publishing.
18. Gill MJ, Andreychik MR (2009). Getting emotional about explanations: Social explanations and social explanatory styles as bases of prosocial emotions and intergroup attitudes. Soc Personal Psychol Compass 3(6): 1038–1054.
19. Moskowitz GB, Gill MJ (2013). Person perception: From snap judgments to the regulation of enduring relationships. In Reisberg D (Ed), Oxford handbook of cognitive psychology. Oxford, UK: Oxford University Press.
20. Buchanan GMCE, Seligman MEP (1995). Explanatory style. Hillsdale, NJ, USA: Lawrence Erlbaum Associates, Inc.
21. Peterson C, Semmel A, von Baeyer C, Abramson LY, Metalsky GI, et al. (1982). The attributional style questionnaire. Cognit Ther Res 6(3): 287–299.
22. Sweeney PD, Anderson K, Bailey S (1986). Attributional style in depression: A meta-analytic review. J Pers Soc Psychol 50(5): 974–991.
23. Winter L, Uleman JS (1984). When are social judgments made? Evidence for the spontaneousness of trait inferences. J Pers Soc Psychol 47(2): 237–252.
24. Jones EE, Harris VA (1967). The attribution of attitudes. J Exp Soc Psychol 3(1): 1–24.
25. Gilbert DT (1998). Ordinary personology. In Gilbert DT, Fiske ST, Lindzey G (Eds), The handbook of social psychology (4th ed). New York, NY, US: McGraw-Hill.
26. Malle BF (2004). How the mind explains behavior: Folk explanations, meaning, and social interaction. MIT Press.
27. Gilbert DT, Malone PS (1995). The correspondence bias. Psychol Bull 117(1): 21–38.
28. Rangel U, Keller J (2011). Essentialism goes social: Belief in social determinism as a component of psychological essentialism. J Pers Soc Psychol 100(6): 1056–1078. doi: 10.1037/a0022401
29. Jones EE, Davis KE (1965). A theory of correspondent inferences: From acts to dispositions. Adv Exp Soc Psychol 2: 219–266.
30. Kelley HH (1973). The process of causal attribution. Am Psychol 28(2): 107–128.
31. McArthur LA (1972). The how and what of why: Some determinants and consequences of causal attribution. J Pers Soc Psychol 22(2): 171–193.
32. Ross L (1977). The intuitive psychologist and his shortcomings: Distortions in the attribution process. Adv Exp Soc Psychol 10: 173–220.
33. Gilbert DT, Pelham BW, Krull DS (1988). On cognitive busyness: When person perceivers meet persons perceived. J Pers Soc Psychol 54(5): 733–740.
34. Quattrone GA (1982). Overattribution and unit formation: When behavior engulfs the person. J Pers Soc Psychol 42(4): 593–607.
35. Trope Y (1986). Identification and inferential processes in dispositional attribution. Psychol Rev, 93(3), 239–257.
36. Uleman JS, Saribay A, Gonzalez CM (2008). Spontaneous inferences, implicit impressions, and implicit theories. Annu Rev Psychol, 59, 329–360.
37. Bruner J (1990). Acts of meaning: Four lectures on mind and culture. Harvard University Press.
38. Kelly G (1955). The psychology of personal constructs New York: Norton.
39. Molden DC, Dweck CS (2006). Finding "meaning" in psychology: A lay theories approach to self-regulation, social perception, and social development. Am Psychol 61(3): 192–203.
40. Plaks JE, Levy SR, Dweck CS (2009). Lay theories of personality: Cornerstones of meaning in social cognition. Soc Personal Psychol Compass 3(6): 1069–1081.
41. Hong Y, Levy SR, Chiu C (2001). The contribution of the lay theories approach to the study of groups. Pers Soc Psychol Rev 5(2): 98–106.
42. Levy SR, Chiu C, Hong Y (2006). Lay theories and intergroup relations. Group Process Intergroup Relat 9(1): 5–24.
43. Miller JG (1984). Culture and the development of everyday social explanation. J Pers Soc Psychol 46(5): 961–978.
44. Morris MW, Peng K (1994). Culture and cause: American and Chinese attributions for social and physical events. J Pers Soc Psychol 67(6): 949–971.
45. Choi I, Nisbett RE (1998). Situational salience and cultural differences in the correspondence bias and actor-observer bias. Pers Soc Psychol Bull 24(9): 949–960. doi: 10.1177/0146167298249003
46. Norenzayan A, Choi I, Nisbett RE (2002). Cultural similarities and differences in social inference: Evidence from behavioral predictions and lay theories of behavior. Pers Soc Psychol Bull 28(1): 109–120.
47. Menon T, Morris MW, Chiu C, Hong Y (1999). Culture and the construal of agency: Attribution to individual versus group dispositions. J Pers Soc Psychol 76(5): 701–717.
48. Dweck CS (1999). Self-theories: Their role in motivation, personality, and development. Psychology Press.
49. Levy S, Plaks J, Dweck C (1999). Modes of social thought. Dual-Process Theories in Social Psychology.
50. Church AT, Ortiz FA, Katigbak MS, Avdeyeva TV, Emerson AM, et al. (2003). Measuring individual and cultural differences in implicit trait theories. J Pers Soc Psychol 85(2): 332–347.
51. Chiu C, Hong Y, Dweck CS (1997). Lay dispositionism and implicit theories of personality. J Pers Soc Psychol 73(1): 19–30.
52. Bauman CW, Skitka LJ (2006). Ethnic group differences in lay philosophies of behavior in the United States. J Cross Cult Psychol 37(4): 438–445. doi: 10.1177/0022022106288479
53. Kluegel JR, Bobo L (1993). Dimensions of whites' beliefs about the black-white socioeconomic gap. In Sniderman PM, Tetlock P, Carmines EG (Eds), Prejudice, politics, and the American dilemma. Stanford, CA, USA: Stanford University Press.
54. Guimond S, Begin G, Palmer DL (1989). Education and causal attributions: The development of "person-blame" and "system-blame" ideology. Soc Psychol Q 52(2): 126–140.
55. Lopez GE, Gurin P, Nagda BA (2002). Education and understanding structural causes for group inequalities. Polit Psychol 19(2): 305–329.
56. Peterson C, Buchanan GM (1995). Explanatory style: History and evolution of the field. In, Explanatory style. Hillsdale, NJ, England: Lawrence Erlbaum Associates, Inc.
57. Savani K, Stephens NM, Markus HR (2011). The unanticipated interpersonal and societal consequences of choice. Psychol Sci 22(6): 795–802. doi: 10.1177/0956797611407928
58. Skitka LJ (1999). Ideological and attributional boundaries on public compassion: Reactions to individuals and communities affected by a natural disaster. Pers Soc Psychol Bull 25(7): 793–808. doi: 10.1177/0146167299025007003
59. Skitka LJ, Tetlock PE (1993). Providing public assistance: Cognitive and motivational processes underlying liberal and conservative policy preferences. J Pers Soc Psychol 65(6): 1205–1223. doi: 10.1037/0022-3514.65.6.1205
60. Skitka LJ, Mullen E, Griffin T, Hutchinson S, Chamberlin B (2002). Dispositions, scripts, or motivated correction? Understanding ideological differences in explanations for social problems. J Pers Soc Psychol 83(2): 470–487. doi: 10.1037/0022-3514.83.2.470
61. Zucker GS, Weiner B (1993). Conservatism and perceptions of poverty: An attributional analysis. J Appl Soc Psychol 23(12): 925–943. doi: 10.1111/j.1559-1816.1993.tb01014.x
62. Webster DM, Kruglanski AW (1994). Individual differences in need for cognitive closure. J Pers Soc Psychol 67(6): 1049–1062.
63. John O, Donahue E, Kentle R (1991). The Big Five Inventory: Versions 4a and 54. Institute of Personality and Social Research. University of California, Berkeley, CA.
64. Gratz KL, Roemer L (2004). Multidimensional assessment of emotion regulation and dysregulation: Development, factor structure, and initial validation of the difficulties in emotion regulation scale. J Psychopathol Behav Assess 26(1): 41–54.
65. Altemeyer B (1988). Enemies of freedom: Understanding right-wing authoritarianism San Francisco, CA, US: Jossey-Bass.
66. Sidanius J, Pratto F (2001). Social dominance: An intergroup theory of social hierarchy and oppression. Cambridge University Press.
67. Cohen J, Cohen P (1983). Applied multiple regression/correlation analysis for the behavioral sciences. Hillsdale, NJ: Erlbaum.
68. McKoon G, Ratcliff R (1986). Inferences about predictable events. J Exp Psychol Learn Mem Cogn 12(1): 82–91.
69. Uleman JS, Newman LS, Moskowitz GB (1996). People as flexible interpreters: Evidence and issues from spontaneous trait inference. Adv Exp Soc Psychol 28: 211–279.
70. Ham J, Vonk R (2003). Smart and easy: Co-occurring activation of spontaneous trait inferences and spontaneous situational inferences. J Exp Soc Psychol 39(5): 434–447.
71. Wigboldus DH, Dijksterhuis A, Van Knippenberg A (2003). When stereotypes get in the way: Stereotypes obstruct stereotype-inconsistent trait inferences. J Pers Soc Psychol 84(3): 470–484.

72. Judd CM, Kenny DA, McClelland GH (2001). Estimating and testing mediation and moderation in within-subject designs. Psychol Methods 6(2): 115–134.
73. Ross LD, Amabile TM, Steinmetz JL (1977). Social roles, social control, and biases in social-perception processes. J Pers Soc Psychol 35(7): 485–494.
74. Levy SR, Stroessner SJ, Dweck CS (1998). Stereotype formation and endorsement: The role of implicit theories. J Pers Soc Psychol 74(6): 1421–1436.
75. McConnell AR (2001). Implicit theories: Consequences for social judgments of individuals. J Exp Soc Psychol 37(3): 215–227.
76. Plaks JE, Stecher K (2007). Unexpected improvement, decline, and stasis: A prediction confidence perspective on achievement success and failure. J Pers Soc Psychol 93(4): 667–684.
77. Poon CS, Koehler DJ (2006). Lay personality knowledge and dispositionist thinking: A knowledge-activation framework. J Exp Soc Psychol 42(2): 177–191.
78. Andreychik MR, Gill MJ (2009). Ingroup identity moderates the impact of social explanations on intergroup attitudes: External explanations are not inherently prosocial. Pers Soc Psychol Bull 39: 73–87.
79. Joiner TE, Wagner KD (1995). Attributional style and depression in children and adolescents: A meta-analytic review. Clin Psychol Rev 15(8): 777–798.
80. Satterfield JM, Monahan J, Seligman ME (1997). Law school performance predicted by explanatory style. Behav Sci Law 15(1): 95–105.
81. Seligman ME, Schulman P (1986). Explanatory style as a predictor of productivity and quitting among life insurance sales agents. J Pers Soc Psychol 50(4): 832–838.
82. Seligman ME, Nolen-Hoeksema S, Thornton N, Thornton KM (1990). Explanatory style as a mechanism of disappointing athletic performance. Psychol Sci 1(2): 143–146.
83. Satterfield JM, Seligman ME (1994). Military aggression and risk predicted by explanatory style. Psychol Sci 5(2): 77–82.
84. Kamen LP, Seligman ME (1987). Explanatory style and health. Curr Psychol 6(3): 207–218.

4

Self-Reported Parental Exposure to Pesticide during Pregnancy and Birth Outcomes: The MecoExpo Cohort Study

Flora Mayhoub[1,6], Thierry Berton[1,2], Véronique Bach[1], Karine Tack[2], Caroline Deguines[1,3], Adeline Floch-Barneaud[1,4], Sophie Desmots[1,5], Erwan Stéphan-Blanchard[1], Karen Chardon[1]*

1 Laboratoire PériTox, Unité mixte Université – INERIS (EA 4285-UMI 01), Université de Picardie Jules Verne, Amiens, France, **2** Unité NOVA, Institut National de l'Environnement Industriel et des Risques, Verneuil en Halatte, France, **3** Médecine Néonatale, Pôle Femme-Couple-Enfant, Centre Hospitalier Universitaire d'Amiens, Amiens, France, **4** Unité ISAE, Institut National de l'Environnement Industriel et des Risques, Verneuil en Halatte, France, **5** Unité TOXI, Institut National de l'Environnement Industriel et des Risques, Verneuil en Halatte, France, **6** Faculty of Medicine, Tishreen University, Latakia, Syria

Abstract

The MecoExpo study was performed in the Picardy region of northern France, in order to investigate the putative relationship between parental exposures to pesticides (as reported by the mother) on one hand and neonatal parameters on the other. The cohort comprised 993 mother-newborn pairs. Each mother completed a questionnaire that probed occupational, domestic, environmental and dietary sources of parental exposure to pesticides during her pregnancy. Multivariate regression analyses were then used to test for associations between the characteristics of parental pesticide exposure during pregnancy and the corresponding birth outcomes. Maternal occupational exposure was associated with an elevated risk of low birth weight (odds ratio (OR) [95% confidence interval]: 4.2 [1.2, 15.4]). Paternal occupational exposure to pesticides was associated with a lower than average gestational age at birth (−0.7 weeks; p = 0.0002) and an elevated risk of prematurity (OR: 3.7 [1.4, 9.7]). Levels of domestic exposure to veterinary antiparasitics and to pesticides for indoor plants were both associated with a low birth weight (−70 g; p = 0.02 and −160 g; p = 0.005, respectively). Babies born to women living in urban areas had a lower birth length and a higher risk of low birth length (−0.4 cm, p = 0.006 and OR: 2.9 [1.5, 5.5], respectively). The present study results mainly demonstrate a negative correlation between fetal development on one hand and parental occupational and domestic exposure to pesticides on the other. Our study highlights the need to perform a global and detailed screening of all potential physiological effects when assessing in utero exposure to pesticides.

Editor: Olga Y. Gorlova, Geisel School of Medicine at Dartmouth College, United States of America

Funding: This work was funded by the Picardy Regional Council. F. Mayhoub was funded by Tishreen University (Latakia, Syria) and T. Berton was funded by the European Regional Development Fund. The funders had no role in study design, data collection and analysis, decision to publish, or preparation of the manuscript.

Competing Interests: The authors have declared that no competing interests exist.

* Email: karen.chardon@u-picardie.fr

Introduction

Human exposure to pesticides is a very complex phenomenon, since it involves many different compounds, sources of exposure and exposure pathways (i.e. respiratory, cutaneous and intestinal pathways). Once pesticides have been applied, the primary compounds and their degradation products are dispersed into the air, water and soil. Human exposure to pesticides can be occupational (through agriculture, floristry, municipal maintenance, etc.), dietary (through the consumption of food contaminated by pesticide residues), domestic (through the spraying of houseplants or garden plants, the eradication of domestic insect pests (such as mosquitoes, flies, etc.) and the use of antiparasitics in humans or in domestic pets) or environmental (i.e. the inhalation of volatilized pesticides of agricultural or non-agricultural origin) [1–2]. Although occupational exposure has been extensively investigated, there are few studies of domestic exposure [2].

Pesticide exposure during pregnancy is becoming an increasingly important public health issue because it may affect the development of the exposed fetus. The association between pesticide exposure in pregnant women and fetal growth has [11,14]. However, this topic is still subject to debate because the various studies did not reach consistent conclusions - probably because of differences in location, exposure assessment methods and the type and number of compounds investigated [3–12]. Furthermore, most of these epidemiological studies focused on a very specific population, such as farmers or other populations with high levels of pesticide exposure (e.g. those living near to crop-farming areas or other areas with intensive pesticide use). To the best of our knowledge, very few studies [9,10,13,14] have studied the relationship between "routine" domestic/dietary parental exposure on one hand and birth outcomes on the other. There are few data on the need for prevention of these types of exposure, and these data can only be gathered in general population cohorts.

The primary objective of the present MecoExpo study was to assess the different types of prenatal exposure to pesticides in the Picardy region of northern France (a region which is characterized by a high birth rate (13.1‰, according to the French National Institute of Statistics and Economic Studies (*Institut National de la*

Statistique et des Études Économiques), relative to the national average. A secondary objective was to investigate the relationship between the different modes of exposure on one hand and birth outcomes on the other. Prenatal exposure to pesticides was assessed via a self-questionnaire filled out by the mother; this is the only method that can simultaneously gather information on all the various sources of intrauterine exposure to pesticides (i.e. occupational, domestic, environmental and dietary exposure) in a sample of the general population.

Methods

2.1 Study participants

The MecoExpo cohort (comprising 993 mother-newborn pairs) was recruited between January 2011 and January 2012. Eleven of Picardy's 16 maternity clinics agreed to participate in the study. Unfortunately, the region's neonatal intensive care units (which treat newborns suffering from a severe neonatal disease or with a gestational age <32 weeks at birth) did not participate.

To be included in the MecoExpo cohort, the mother had to be had to be (i) 18 years of age or older and (ii) fluent enough in French to understand the study's objectives and procedures. Mothers aged under 18 and mothers who did not have full parental authority over their child (such as incarcerated persons) were excluded from the study. Multiple births were also excluded from the present study.

The study and both maternal and neonatal data collection (questionnaire, medical records) were approved by the local investigational review board (*Comité de Protection des Personnes dans la Recherche Biomédicale de Picardie*). Potential participants were given a verbal presentation of the study by their attending pediatrician in the maternity clinic. All mothers signed an informed consent giving us permission to enroll them and their infants in the study. A study information sheet was given to the women prior to their completion of the study questionnaire. During completion of the self-administred questionnaire, an investigating physician was always on hand to provide explanations but did not influence the answers. In view of the many different aspects of possible exposure probed by the questionnaire and in order to shorten and facilitate the questionnaire's completion, the respondee was instructed not to answer a given question if in any doubt. Most of the questions were "yes"/"no" or multiple choice questions. Open questions were used to gather additional information, when necessary. None of the data collected during the study enabled the direct identification of participants.

2.2 Characteristics of intrauterine exposure to pesticides in a questionnaire-based survey

Mothers from the cohort completed the questionnaire during their stay in the maternity clinic (4 to 5 days after giving birth). The questionnaire addressed occupational, domestic, environmental and dietary sources of pesticide exposure. Prior to use in the study, the questionnaire was validated in a sample of 25 women (aged between 25 and 45 and from various socio-professional categories). It was then modified by taking account of the women's answers, comments and questions. The final questionnaire comprised 44 items and took respondees about 15 minutes to read and complete.

2.2.1 Occupational exposure to pesticides. The mother was asked to state (i) whether she had ever worked during the pregnancy (and, if so, the duration), (ii) whether her occupation and/or that of the father involved exposure to pesticides (e.g. in agriculture, animal husbandry, gardening, etc.) and (iii) the modalities of maternal exposure to pesticides (the duration and location of exposure, the type of compound and the use or not of protective equipment).

2.2.2 Domestic exposure to pesticides. The questionnaire probed possible uses of pesticides in the mother's home during her pregnancy (whether applied directly by the mother or indirectly by another person). The mother was asked to report use of (i) antiparasitics for human administration (to treat lice, scabies, ticks, etc.), (ii) antiparasitics for domestic pets (to treat fleas, ticks, etc.) and the number and type of treated animals, (iii) insecticides, herbicides, fungicides and plant growth regulators for treating houseplants or garden plants and (iv) pesticides for eradicating domestic insect pests (such as flies, mosquitoes, etc.).

2.2.3 Environmental exposure to pesticides. The mother was asked to state whether she lived within 1 km of (i) green areas (a park, a sports field, etc.), (ii) a crop field, (iii) a highway, a railway or an airport. The mother was also asked to state the locality in which she had lived during her pregnancy. We then queried a database (produced by the French National Institute of Statistics and Economic Studies) to obtain the population density for each locality. The localities were then arbitrarily divided into rural localities (<2 000 inhabitants/km^2) and urban localities (≥2 000 inhabitants/km^2).

2.2.4 Questions on dietary exposure. The mother was asked to state (i) her total dietary intake of the main food categories (fruits and vegetables, cereals, milk products and meat) during pregnancy (possible answers were "never or almost never", "not every day", "every day", "several times a day") and (ii) the frequency with which the consumed fruits and vegetables, milk products and meat were organic foods (with possible answers of "never", "sometimes", "most of the time ").

2.3 Birth outcomes

Neonatal data - gestational age (weeks of amenorrhea), birth weight (g), birth length (cm) and head circumference at birth (cm) - were extracted from medical records by the maternity clinic's pediatrician. Prematurity was defined as birth before 37 weeks of amenorrhea. Low birth weight or length was defined as a birth weight or length (adjusted for the mother's age, weight, and height, the rank of pregnancy, the gestational age and the baby's gender) below the 5th percentile (relative to normative data for France) [15–16]. Small head circumference was defined as a measurement (adjusted for gestational age and the baby's gender) below the 5th percentile (relative to normative data for France) [15]. Infants with missing neonatal or maternal data on adverse birth outcomes were not considered in these analyses.

2.4 Confounding factors

Factors known or suspected (on the basis of the scientific literature) to have an effect on fetal development were considered as confounding factors, i.e. the mother's age and body mass index (BMI), parity, diabetes, hypertension, tobacco use, alcohol use, drug abuse, socioprofessional category (educational level and type of work), and the baby's gender.

2.5 Data processing

The study data (questionnaire data, birth outcomes and covariates) were recorded using Sphinx plus^2 software (version 5.1.0.6, Le Sphinx Développement, Chavanod, France). Some questionnaire answers were combined, in order to obtain new, composite variables that were more relevant than those obtained from single questions. Thus, the composite variables used in the assessment of intrauterine exposure to pesticides included maternal or paternal occupational exposure, maternal domestic exposure to human antiparasitics, veterinary antiparasitics, and

Table 1. Maternal characteristics in the MecoExpo cohort (n = 993).

Variables	
Age (year)	Mean (SD)
	29 (5.2)
Parity:	n(%)
Primiparous	409 (41.7)
Multiparous	573 (58.3)
Missing data	*11*
Maternal diabetes during pregnancy:	n(%)
Yes	62 (6.2)
No	931 (93.8)
Maternal hypertension during pregnancy:	n(%)
Yes	47 (4.7)
No	946 (95.3)
Maternal smoking during pregnancy:	n(%)
Yes	293 (29.5)
No	700 (70.5)
Maternal educational level:	n(%)
≤High school completed	504 (53.7)
>High school completed	434 (46.3)
Missing data	*55*
Working during pregnancy:	n(%)
Yes	671 (67.6)
No	322 (32.4)
Place of residence during pregnancy:	n(%)
Rural locality	774 (85.9)
Urban locality	127 (14.1)
Missing data	*92*

Table 2. Newborn characteristics in the MecoExpo cohort (n = 993).

Variables	Mean (SD)	n (%)
Gestational age (weeks)	39.3 (1.3)	924 (93.1)
Missing data		*69 (6.9)*
Birth weight (g)	3340 (492)	932 (93.9)
Missing data		*61 (6.1)*
Birth length (cm)	49.5 (2.1)	922 (92.8)
Missing data		*71 (7.2)*
Head circumference at birth (cm)	34.4 (1.4)	911 (91.7)
Missing data		*82 (8.3)*
Gender:		
male		508 (51.2)
female		485 (48.8)
Prematurity:		
Yes		24 (2.6)
No		900 (97.4)
Missing data		*69*
Low birth weight:		
Yes		788 (94.9)
No		42 (5.1)
Missing data		*163*
Low birth length:		
Yes		56 (6.8)
No		764 (93.2)
Missing data		*173*
Small head circumference:		
Yes		34 (4.0)
No		822 (96.0)
Missing data		*137*

domestic pesticides for houseplants or garden plants, environmental exposure (the home's proximity to a crop fields, green areas, highways, railways or airports) and dietary exposure (consumption of fruits and vegetables, cereals, milk products and meat; consumption of organic fruits and vegetables, etc.).

2.6 Statistical analyses

The MecoExpo cohort's demographics and intrauterine exposure to pesticides were first characterized in a descriptive analysis. Quantitative parameters (gestational age, birth weight, etc.) were expressed as the mean and the standard deviation (SD). Qualitative parameters (prematurity, low birth weight, maternal occupational exposure to pesticides, etc.) were expressed as the number and the percentage of the study population.

Multivariate linear regression and logistic regression analyses were used to study the putative associations between birth outcomes and the characteristics of *in utero* exposure to pesticides. Using forward selection, covariates with a $p\text{-value}<0.20$ in a univariate analysis were fed into in the multivariate analyses. The risk of an adverse birth outcome (prematurity, small head circumference, and low birth weight and low birth length) was expressed as an odds ratio (OR) [95% confidence interval (CI)]. The 95% CI was calculated according to Woolf's method, with an alpha risk of 0.05. All statistical analyses were performed with SPSS software (V.20.0, Chicago, IL, USA).

Results

3.1 Characteristics of the study population

A total of 993 mother-newborn pairs were included in the MecoExpo cohort. Given that some questionnaire answers or clinical values were missing, the total n for some variables was below 993 and so the corresponding missing data rates are also reported.

The characteristics of the MecoExpo study population are summarized in Table 1 and Table 2. The mean (SD) maternal age was 29 (5.2) and the mean pre-pregnancy BMI was 24.4 (5.5) kg/m^2. Six percent of the mothers were diabetic and less than 5% had arterial hypertension during pregnancy. Forty-two percent of the women were primiparous, 46% had completed high school and 68% had been working during their pregnancy. About 30% of the mothers stated smoking during pregnancy; the corresponding values for drinking alcohol and illicit drug use were 3% and 1%, respectively. Overall, 86% of the women lived in rural localities (<2 000 inhabitants/km^2).

Table 3. Characteristics of prenatal exposure to pesticides (n = 993).

Variables	n (%)
Occupational exposure to pesticides	
Mother:	
Yes	43 (4.3)
No	950 (95.7)
Father:	
Yes	86 (8.7)
No	907 (91.3)
Maternal domestic exposure to pesticides	
Human antiparasitics:	
Yes	328 (33.0)
No	665 (67.0)
Veterinary antiparasitics:	
Yes	215 (21.7)
No	776 (78.3)
Missing data	*2*
Pesticides against insects:	
Yes	127 (13.0)
No	850 (87.0)
Missing data	*16*
Pesticides for indoor plants:	
Yes	37 (3.7)
No	956 (96.3)
Pesticides for outdoor plants:	
Yes	166 (17.0)
No	813 (83.0)
Missing data	*14*
Maternal environmental exposure to pesticides	
Proximity to a crop field (<1 km):	
Yes	527 (58.2)
No	378 (41.8)
Missing data	*88*
Proximity to a green area:	
Yes	707 (72.7)
No	266 (27.3)
Missing data	*20*
Proximity to a highway, railway or airport:	
Yes	366 (37.4)
No	612 (62.6)
Missing data	*15*

Table 4. Characteristics of prenatal exposure to pesticides (n = 993) (continued).

Variables	n (%)
Maternal dietary exposure to pesticides (total food intake)	
Fruits and vegetables:	
Never or almost never	18 (1.8)
Not every day	319 (32.3)
Every day	362 (36.6)
Several times a day	289 (29.3)
Missing data	*5*
Cereals:	
Never or almost never	4 (0.4)
Not every day	173 (17.6)
Every day	532 (54.1)
Several times a day	274 (27.9)
Missing data	10
Dairy products:	
Never or almost never	8 (0.8)
Not every day	111 (11.3)
Every day	430 (43.7)
Several times a day	436 (44.3)
Missing data	*8*
Meat:	
Never or almost never	23 (2.4)
Not every day	365 (37.5)
Every day	489 (50.2)
Several times a day	97 (10.0)
Missing data	*19*
Maternal dietary exposure to pesticides (organic food intake)	
Fruits and vegetables:	
Never	518 (52.4)
Sometimes	375 (38.0)
Most of the time	95 (9.6)
Missing data	*5*
Dairy products:	
Never	654 (66.3)
Sometimes	265 (26.9)
Most of the time	68 (6.9)
Missing data	*6*
Meat:	
Never	827 (84.0)
Sometimes	137 (13.9)
Most of the time	20 (2.0)
Missing data	*9*

3.2 Characteristics of in utero exposure to pesticides

The main characteristics of prenatal exposure to pesticides (as assessed by the mothers' questionnaire data) are summarized in Table 3 and 4.

3.2.1 Occupational exposure to pesticides. 43 mothers and 86 fathers (4.3% and 8.7% of the total sample, respectively) worked in an occupation in which there was potential for exposure to pesticides. Fifteen mothers and 42 fathers (1.5% and 4.2% of the total sample, respectively) had agricultural occupations.

3.2.2 Domestic exposure to pesticides. 33% of the mothers were exposed to human antiparasitics, with 22% exposed to veterinary antiparasitics, 13% exposed to domestic insecticides, 4% exposed to pesticides for houseplants and 17% exposed to pesticides for garden plants.

Table 5. Multivariate associations between factors related to *in utero* exposure to pesticides and gestational age and prematurity.

Variable	Gestational age (weeks)		Prematurity	
	n	Mean (SD)	Cases/ controls	OR [95% CI]
Total sample	924	-	24/900	-
Occupational exposure				
Mother:				
Yes	21	39.2 (1.4)	1/20	NA
No	903	39.5 (1.3)	23/880	Reference
Father:				
Yes	80	38.8 (1.7)**	6/74	3.7 [1.4, 9.7]*
No	844	39.5 (1.3)	18/826	Reference
Maternal domestic exposure				
Human antiparasitics:				
Yes	307	39.6 (1.2)	7/300	0.8 [0.3, 2.0]
No	617	39.4 (1.4)	17/600	Reference
Veterinary antiparasitics:				
Yes	201	39.4 (1.4)	6/195	1.2 [0.5, 3.1]
Non	721	39.5 (1.3)	18/703	Reference
Missing data	*2*		*0/2*	-
Pesticides against insects:				
Yes	115	39.6 (1.2)	3/112	1.0 [0.3, 3.4]
No	794	39.4 (1.3)	20/774	Reference
Missing data	*15*	-	*1/14*	-
Pesticides for indoor plants:				
Yes	35	39.4 (1.2)	1/34	NA
No	889	39.5 (1.3)	23/866	Reference
Pesticides for outdoor plants:				
Yes	156	39.5 (1.2)	2/154	NA
No	754	39.5 (1.3)	21/733	Reference
Missing	*14*	-	*1/13*	-
Maternal environmental exposure				
Proximity to a crop field:				
Yes	490	39.4 (1.4)	17/473	2.1 [0.8, 5.4]
No	356	39.6 (1.3)	6/350	Reference
Missing data	*78*	-	*1/77*	-
Proximity to a green area:				
Yes	660	39.5 (1.3)	19/641	1.8 [0.6, 5.3]
No	244	39.5 (1.3)	4/240	Reference
Missing data	*20*	-	*1/19*	-
Proximity to a highway, railway or airport:				
Yes	339	39.5 (1.3)	8/331	0.9 [0.4, 2.2]
No	571	39.5 (1.3)	15/556	Reference
Missing data	*14*	-	*1/13*	-

3.2.3 Environmental exposure to pesticides. 58% of the mothers lived near to a crop field crop, 73% lived near to a green area and 37% lived near to a highway, railroad line or airport.

3.2.4 Dietary exposure to pesticides. 29% of mothers consumed fruits and vegetables "several times" a day and 44% consumed milk products "several times a day". Fifty percent consumed cereals "every day" and 50% consumed meat "every day".

Only 10% of the mothers consumed organic fruits and vegetables "most of the time", whereas the corresponding proportions organic milk products and organic meat were 7% and 2%, respectively.

3.3 Multivariate associations between fetal growth and estimated in utero exposure to pesticides

3.3.1 Gestational age and prematurity (Table 5, 6). Estimated paternal occupational exposure to pesticides was significantly associated with lower gestational age (−0.7 weeks, relative to infants whose parents were not occupationally exposed to pesticides; $p = 0.006$) and a higher risk of prematurity (OR [95% CI]: 3.7 [1.4, 9.7]; $p = 0.02$). Maternal exposure (whether occupational, domestic, environmental or dietary) was not significantly associated with either gestational age or the risk of prematurity.

3.3.2 Birth weight (as a continuous variable) and low birth (Table 7, 8). Estimated maternal occupational exposure was associated with higher risk of low birth weight (OR [95% CI]: 4.2 [1.2, 15.4]; $p = 0.01$). Exposure to human and veterinary antiparasitics were both significantly associated with a lower birth weight (−70 g; $p = 0.02$ and −85 g; $p = 0.04$, respectively). Exposure to pesticides for houseplants was also associated with lower birth weight (−160 g; $p = 0.03$). No association with dietary exposure was observed.

3.3.3 Birth length (as a continuous variable) and low birth length (Table 9, 10). The risk of low of low birth length was significantly associated with the mother's residence in an urban area (OR [95% CI]: 2.9 [1.5, 5.5]; $p = 0.01$]. No associations with parental occupational exposure or dietary exposure were observed.

3.3.4 Birth head circumference at birth (as a continuous variable) and small head circumference (Table 11, 12). In multivariate statistical models, no significant association was found between head circumference at birth or small head circumference on one hand and the variables describing the *in utero* exposure to pesticides on the other.

Discussion

To the best of our knowledge, this study is the first one to simultaneously examine the association between all sources of *in utero* exposure to pesticides (i.e. occupational, domestic, environmental and dietary sources) and four common descriptors of fetal development (gestational age, birth weight, birth length and head circumference at birth). The prevalence of fetal growth restriction with respect to these parameters (i.e. prematurity, low birth weight, low birth length and small head circumference) was also considered.

Fetal growth is conditioned by many different environmental, genetic, metabolic, nutritional and placental factors. It is well known that adverse fetal growth is a good predictor of neonatal mortality and morbidity [17–19]. Fetal growth restriction may therefore be a determining factor for some diseases of childhood (since infants with poor head growth appear to run an increased risk of cerebral palsy, cognitive impairment and behavioral disorders) [20,21] (ii) diseases of adolescence (since extremely low birth weight may be associated with a higher prevalence of developmental delay, neurosensory impairments (seizures, visual

Table 6. Multivariate associations between factors related to *in utero* exposure to pesticides and gestational age and prematurity (continued).

Place of residence during pregnancy:				
Rural locality	714	39.4 (1.4)	21/693	Reference
Urban locality	123	39.6 (1.3)	1/122	NA
Missing data	*87*	-	*2/85*	-
Maternal dietary exposure (total food intake)				
Fruits and vegetables:				
Never or almost never	16	39.3(1.4)	0/16	NA
Not every day	298	39.5(1.3)	8/290	Reference
Every day	333	39.4(1.3)	10/323	1.1 [0.4, 2.9]
Several times a day	272	39.6(1.3)	6/266	0.8 [0.3, 2.4]
Missing data	*5*	-	*0/5*	-
Cereals:				
Never or almost never	4	39.7 (0.5)	0/3	NA
Not every day	162	39.4 (1.2)	3/159	Reference
Every day	488	39.5 (1.4)	15/473	1.7 [0.5, 5.9]
Several times a day	260	39.5(1.3)	6/254	1.3 [0.3, 5.1]
Missing data	79	-	0/79	-
Dairy products:				
Never or almost never	7	39.6 (0.7)	0/7	NA
Not every day	105	39.4 (1.1)	2/103	Reference
Every day	399	39.4 (1.3)	10/389	1.3 [0.3, 6.1]
Several times a day	405	39.5 (1.4)	12/393	1.6 [0.4, 7.1]
Missing data	*8*	-	*0/8*	-
Meat:				
Never or almost never	22	39.5 (2.0)	1/21	NA
Not every day	338	39.5 (1.2)	4/334	Reference
Every day	458	39.4 (1.4)	16/442	3.0 [1.0, 9.1]
Several times a day	88	39.5 (1.6)	3/85	3.0 [0.7, 13.4]
Missing	*87*	-	*0/87*	-
Maternal dietary exposure (organic food intake)				
Fruits and vegetables:				
Never	481	39.4 (1.4)	13/468	0.6 [0.2, 1.9]
Sometimes	347	39.6 (1.2)	7/340	0.5 [0.1, 1.6]
Most of the time	91	39.3 (1.5)	4/87	Reference
Missing data	*5*	-	*0/5*	-
Dairy products:				
Never	607	39.5 (1.3)	17/590	1.8 [0.2, 13.9]
Sometimes	247	39.5 (1.3)	6/241	1.6 [0.2, 13.3]
Most of the time	64	39.5 (1.3)	1/63	Reference
Missing data	*6*	-	*0/6*	
Meat:				
Never	773	39.5 (1.3)	21/752	Reference
Sometimes	124	39.5 (1.3)	2/122	NA
Most of the time	18	39.2 (1.4)	1/17	NA
Missing data	*78*	-	*0/78*	-

*p = 0.05;
**p = 0.01;
***p = 0.001.
NA: an odds ratio was not available because too few cases were observed (n<3).

Table 7. Multivariate associations between (i) variables related to *in utero* exposure to pesticides, (ii) birth weight (BW, in g) and low birth weight (LBW).

Variables	BW (g)		LBW	
	n	Mean (SD)	Cases/controls	OR [95% CI]
Total sample	932		42/786	
Occupational exposure				
Mother:				
Yes	19	3177 (521)	3/14	4.2 [1.2, 15.4]**
No	913	3343 (491)	39/772	Reference
Father:				
Yes	83	3213 (517)	1/96	NA
No	849	3353 (488)	41/690	Reference
Domestic exposure				
Humans antiparasitic:				
Yes	309	3397 (477)*	11/241	0.8 [0.4, 1.6]
No	623	3312 (497)	31/545	Reference
Veterinary antiparasitic:				
Yes	206	3286 (520)*	10/177	1.1 [0.5, 2.3]
No	724	3358 (482)	31/608	Reference
Missing data	*2*	-	*1/1*	-
Pesticides against insects:				
Yes	120	3373 (472)	4/95	0.8 [0.3, 2.2]
No	796	3338 (493)	37/680	Reference
Missing data	*16*	-	*1/11*	-
Pesticides for indoor plants:				
Yes	33	3186 (464)**	2/26	NA
No	899	3346 (492)	40/760	Reference
Pesticides for outdoor plants:				
Yes	156	3369 (479)	2/136	NA
No	762	3337 (492)	40/638	Reference
Missing data	14	-	0/12	-
Environmental exposure				
Proximity to a crop field:				
Yes	490	3328 (491)	25/411	1.2 [0.6, 2.4]
No	359	3352 (486)	15/304	Reference
Missing data	83	-	2/71	-
Proximity to a green area:				
Yes	663	3365 (498)	26/564	0.6 [0.3, 1.1]
No	250	3275 (470)	16/204	Reference
Missing data	*19*	-	*0/18*	-
Proximity to a highway, railway or airport:				
Yes	344	3380 (523)	15/259	0.9 [0.5, 1.8]
No	573	3317 (470)	27/484	Reference
Missing data	15	-	0/13	-

problems), learning disabilities and hyperactivity) and diseases of adulthood (hypertension, diabetes and hyperlipidemia) [20,21]. Unfortunately, these factors are only seldom analyzed in the literature.

The inconsistency of the literature results may be explained (at least in part) by the fact that studies evaluating the association between pesticide exposure and fetal growth have used several different definitions of low birth weight. In fact, studies considering the proportion of small-for-gestational-age infants generally consider the 10th percentile and include only the gestational age (plus, in some cases, the baby's gender) as an adjustment parameter. In contrast, our study low birth weight or length as being below the 5th percentile after adjustment for various maternal and neonatal characteristics (the mother's age, weight,

Table 8. Multivariate associations between (i) variables related to *in utero* exposure to pesticides, (ii) birth weight (BW, in g) and low birth weight (LBW) (continued).

Dietary exposure (Total food intake)				
Fruits and vegetables:				
Never or almost never	17	3152 (501)	2/13	Reference
Not every day	298	3316 (481)	16/250	0.4 [0.1, 2.0]
Every day	342	3329 (483)	11/289	0.3 [0.1, 1.3]
Several times a day	270	3388 (511)	13/230	0.4 [0.1, 1.8]
Missing data	5	-	0/4	-
Cereals:				
Never or almost never	4	3525 (527)	0/4	NA
Not every day	164	3360 (466)	7/141	Reference
Every day	495	3321 (489)	22/409	0.6 [0.3, 1.5]
Several times a day	259	3360 (508)	12/227	1.1 [0.4, 2.8]
Missing data	*71*	-	*1/5*	-
Dairy products:				
Never or almost never	8	3098 (431)	1/5	NA
Not every day	103	3251 (473)	8/86	Reference
Every day	408	3345 (475)	17/341	0.5 [0.1, 4.5]
Several times a day	405	3357 (510)	16/348	0.3 [0.0, 2.3]
Missing data	*8*		*0/6*	
Meat:				
Never or almost never	22	3275 (520)	1/20	NA
Not every day	340	3329 (465)	19/288	Reference
Every day	458	3332 (494)	19/388	0.7 [0.4, 1.4]
Several times a day	93	3393 (557)	3/78	0.6 [0.2, 2.0]
Missing data	*80*	-	*0/12*	-
Dietary exposure (organic food intake)				
Fruits and vegetables:				
Never	483	3304 (509)	23/399	1.6 [0.5, 5.4]
Sometimes	354	3399 (472)	16/300	1.5 [0.4, 5.2]
Most of the time	90	3283 (453)	3/83	Reference
Missing data	5	-	0/5	-
Dairy products:				
Never	617	3327 (505)	32/508	1.4 [0.7, 2.8]
Sometimes	245	3367 (469)	10/216	Reference
Most of the time	64	3346 (439)	0/4	NA
Missing data	6	-	0/6	-
Meat:				
Never	777	3329 (490)	39/657	Reference
Sometimes	126	3422 (492)	2/108	NA
Most of the time	20	3238 (518)	1/16	NA
Missing data	70	-	0/5	-

*P<0.05;
**P<0.01.
BW: birth weight; LBW: Low birth weight; NA: an odds ratio was not available because too few cases were observed (n<3).

and height, the rank of birth, the gestational age and the baby's gender), as recommended by the AUDIPOG study [15–16].

In the present study, we considered almost all the confounding factors known or suspected in the literature to have an effect on fetal development. However, some of these factors (such as the consumption of alcohol and/or illicit drugs during pregnancy) could not be analyzed further because of the low number of affirmative replies. For ethical reasons, we chose not to probe a number of other factors (such as the parent's financial situation and ethnic origin); this might constitute a source of study bias. Moreover, the fact that pesticide levels were not measured in this study might constitute another source of bias; however, data

Table 9. Multivariate associations between (i) variables related to *in utero* exposure to pesticides, (ii) birth length (BL, in cm) and low birth length).

Variable	BL (cm)		LBL	
	n	Mean (SD)	Cases/controls	OR [95% CI]
Total sample	922		56/764	
Occupational exposure				
Mother:				
Yes	19	49.5 (1.9)	2/15	NA
No	903	49.5 (2.1)	54/749	Reference
Father:				
Yes	79	49.3 (2.0)	1/67	NA
No	843	49.5 (2.1)	55/697	Reference
Domestic exposure				
Humans antiparasitics:				
Yes	309	49.8 (2.0)	19/252	1.0 [0.6, 1.9]
No	613	49.3 (2.1)	37/512	Reference
Veterinary antiparasitics:				
Yes	201	49.3 (2.1)	9/173	0.7 [0.3, 1.4]
No	719	49.5 (2.1)	46/590	Reference
Missing data	*2*	-	*1/1*	-
Pesticides against insects:				
Yes	115	49.5 (1.9)	8/88	1.3 [0.6, 2.9]
No	793	49.5 (2.1)	46/666	Reference
Missing data	*14*	-	*2/10*	-
Pesticides for indoor plants:				
Yes	35	49.2 (2.0)	4/26	2.2 [0.7, 6.5]
No	887	49.5 (2.1)	52/738	Reference
Pesticides for outdoor plants:				
Yes	157	49.7 (2.2)	9/130	0.9 [0.4, 1.9]
No	752	49.4 (2.1)	47/623	Reference
Missing data	*13*	-	*0/11*	-
Environmental exposure to pesticides				
Proximity to a crop field (<1 km):				
Yes	491	49.6 (2.1)	32/404	1.0 [0.6, 1.8]
No	350	49.3 (2.0)	22/289	Reference
Missing data	*81*	-	*2/71*	-
Proximity to a green area:				
Yes	655	49.6 (2.2)	42/541	1.1 [0.6, 2.1]
No	249	49.2 (1.9)	14/206	Reference
Missing data	*18*	-	*0/17*	-
Proximity to a highway, railway or airport:				
Yes	339	49.6 (2.1)	23/276	1.2 [0.7, 2.9]
No	570	49.4 (2.1)	33/477	Reference
Missing data	*13*	-	*0/11*	-
Level of urbanization:				
Rural	726	49.5 (2.1)	34/606	Reference
Urban	119	49.1 (2.0)	15/93	2.9 [1.5, 5.5]*
Missing data	*77*	-	*7/65*	-

Table 10. Multivariate associations between (i) variables related to *in utero* exposure to pesticides, (ii) birth length (BL, in cm) and low birth length) (continued).

Dietary exposure (total food intake)				
Fruits and vegetables:				
Never or almost never	18	49.3 (2.2)	1/15	Reference
Not every day	301	49.4 (2.0)	19/253	1.1 [0.1, 9.0]
Every day	329	49.4 (2.2)	19/268	1.1 [0.1, 8.5]
Several times a day	269	49.7 (2.1)	17/224	1.1 [0.1, 9.2]
Missing data	*5*	-	*0/4*	-
Cereals:				
Never or almost never	4	50.2 (1.7)	0/4	NA
Not every day	159	49.4 (2.1)	11/132	Reference
Every day	493	49.4 (2.1)	27/402	0.8 [0.4, 1.7]
Several times a day	256	49.6 (2.2)	18/218	1.0 [0.5, 2.2]
Missing data	*81*	-	*0/8*	-
Dairy products:				
Never or almost never	7	48.1 (1.2)	0/5	NA
Not every day	105	49.3 (2.1)	8/87	Reference
Every day	396	49.4 (2.0)	21/328	0.7 [0.3, 1.6]
Several times a day	407	49.6 (2.2)	27/339	0.9 [0.4, 2.0]
Missing data	*7*	-	*0/5*	-
Meat:				
Never or almost never	22	49.3 (2.2)	0/20	NA
Not every day	338	49.4 (2.1)	25/279	Reference
Every day	457	49.5 (2.1)	24/382	0.7 [0.4, 1.3]
Several times a day	87	49.6 (2.3)	6/71	0.9 [0.4, 2.4]
Missing data	*89*	-	*1/12*	-
Dietary exposure (organic food intake)				
Fruits and vegetables:				
Never	484	49.3 (2.2)	36/388	1.5 [0.6, 4.0]
Sometimes	345	49.7 (1.9)	15/330	0.6 [0.3, 2.1]
Most of the time	88	49.4 (2.1)	5/83	Reference
Missing data	*5*	-	*0/4*	-
Dairy products:				
Never	611	49.4 (2.1)	39/498	1.1 [0.6, 2.0]
Sometimes	242	49.6 (2.0)	15/207	2.0 [0.4, 9.0]
Most of the time	62	49.8 (2.0)	2/55	Reference
Missing data	*3*	-	*0/4*	-
Meat:				
Never	769	49.4 (2.1)	47/642	Reference
Sometimes	126	49.6 (1.9)	7/102	0.9 [0.4, 2.1]
Most of the time	18	49.0 (2.1)	1/14	NA
Missing data	*80*	-	*1/6*	-

*P<0.05;
**P<0.01.
BL: birth length, LBL: low birth length. NA: an odds ratio was not available because too few cases were observed (n<3).

obtained from maternal questionnaires were used as a proxy for pesticide exposure.

4.1 Occupational exposure to pesticides

Our results revealed that 4.3% of the mothers and 8.7% of the fathers had an occupation that potentially involved pesticide exposure. We found that 1.5% of the mothers and 4.2% of the fathers worked in agriculture (i.e. 2.9% of all parents). The literature studies differ in terms of their locations, study populations, exposure assessment methods and fetal parameters - making it difficult to compare the respective results. Our results highlighted an association between self-reported maternal occu-

Table 11. Multivariate associations between (i) variables related to *in utero* exposure to pesticides, (ii) head circumference at birth (HCB, in cm) and (iii) small head circumference at birth.

Variable	HCB (cm)		SHCB	
	N	Mean (SD)	Cases/controls	OR [95% CI]
Total sample	911		34/822	
Occupational exposure				
Mother:				
Yes	21	34.5 (1.7)	2/36	NA
No	890	34.4 (1.4)	32/786	Reference
Father:				
Yes	79	34.2 (1.6)	4/70	1.3 [0.5, 4.2]
No	832	34.4 (1.4)	30/752	Reference
Domestic exposure				
Human antiparasitics:				
Yes	305	34.5 (1.4)	9/276	0.7 [0.3, 1.5]
No	606	34.3 (1.4)	25/546	Reference
Veterinary antiparasitics:				
Yes	193	34.3 (1.5)	8/175	1.1 [0.5, 2.6]
No	717	34.4 (1.4)	26/646	Reference
Missing data	*1*	-	*0/1*	-
Pesticides against insects:				
Yes	115	34.4 (1.3)	7/99	1.9 [0.8, 4.4]
Non	781	34.4 (1.4)	27/709	Reference
Missing data	*15*	-	*0/14*	-
Pesticides for indoor plants:				
Yes	33	34.2 (1.4)	2/29	NA
No	878	34.4 (1.4)	32/793	Reference
Pesticides for outdoor plants:				
Yes	149	34.6 (1.4)	8/135	1.5 [0.7, 3.5]
No	748	34.4 (1.4)	26/674	Reference
Missing data	*14*	-	*0/13*	-
Environmental exposure				
Proximity to a crop field:				
Yes	487	34.4 (1.4)	20/437	1.3 [0.6, 2.8]
No	345	34.4 (1.4)	11/314	Reference
Missing data	*79*	-	*3/71*	-
Proximity to a green area:				
Yes	644	34.5 (1.4)	21/586	0.7 [0.3, 1.3]
No	249	34.2 (1.4)	12/219	Reference
Missing data	*18*	-	*1/17*	-
Proximity to a highway, railway or airport:				
Yes	332	34.4 (1.4)	12/301	0.9 [0.5, 1.9]
No	565	34.5 (1.4)	22/508	Reference
Missing data	*14*	-	*0/13*	-

pational exposure to pesticides during pregnancy and the risk of low birth weight. We also found an association between estimated paternal occupational exposure to pesticides on one hand and low gestational age and the risk of the prematurity on the other. However, it is important to note that our cohort was recruited from the general population, in which only some of the parents were occupationally exposed to pesticides. This situation contrasts with literature studies of specifically exposed cohorts of farmers or other agricultural workers. The retrospective study of the general population performed in the USA by Savitz et al. [3] found an association between small-for-gestational-age status and self-reported occupational parental exposure to pesticides. In Colombia, the study by Restrepo et al. [5] revealed a moderately strong relationship between an increased risk of prematurity and reported

Table 12. Multivariate associations between (i) variables related to *in utero* exposure to pesticides, (ii) head circumference at birth (HCB, in cm) and (iii) small head circumference at birth (continued).

Place of residence during pregnancy:				
Rural locality	722	34.4 (1.4)	24/649	Reference
Urban locality	114	34.4 (1.5)	9/102	2.4 [1.1, 5.3]
Missing data	*75*	-	*1/71*	-
Dietary exposure (total food intake)				
Fruits and vegetables:				]
Never or almost never	18	34.0 (1.3)	0/16	NA
Not every day	292	34.4 (1.4)	16/263	Reference
Every day	334	34.4 (1.4)	11/297	0.6 [0.3, 1.3]
Several times a day	262	34.5 (1.5)	7/241	0.5 [0.2, 1.2
Missing data	*5*	-	*0/5*	-
Cereals:				
Never or almost never	4	34.7 (2.2)	0/4	NA
Not every day	162	34.4 (1.4)	5/148	Reference
Every day	488	34.4 (1.4)	24/428	2.6 [1.0, 6.9]
Several times a day	247	34.5 (1.4)	5/232	0.6 [0.2, 2.3]
Missing data	*92*	-	*0/10*	-
Dairy products:				
Never or almost never	7	33.1 (1.1)	2/4	Reference
Not every day	104	34.3 (1.3)	5/94	0.1 [0.0, 0.8]
Every day	395	34.4 (1.4)	14/356	0.1 [0.0, 0.5]
Several times a day	397	34.4 (1.5)	13/360	0.1 [0.0, 0.4]
Missing data	*8*	-	*0/8*	-
Meat:				
Never or almost never	22	34.0 (1.4)	1/20	NA
Not every day	336	34.5 (1.4)	11/302	Reference
Every day	449	34.4 (1.4)	16/409	1.1 [0.5, 2.3]
Several times a day	85	34.4 (1.6)	6/73	2.3 [0.8, 6.3]
Missing	*101*	-	*0/18*	-
Dietary exposure (organic food intake)				
Fruits and vegetables:				
Never	481	34.2 (1.4)	25/425	2.6 [1.1, 6.1]
Sometimes	340	34.6 (1.4)	7/312	Reference
Most of the time	85	34.4 (1.3)	2/80	NA
Missing data	*5*	-	*0/5*	-
Dairy products:				
Never	612	34.3 (1.4)	25/549	1.3 [0.3, 5.6]
Sometimes	231	34.6 (1.5)	7/210	1.0 [0.2, 4.7]
Most of the time	62	34.5 (1.3)	2/57	Reference
Missing data	*2*	-	*0/6*	-
Meat:				
Never	762	34.4 (1.4)	31/688	Reference
Sometimes	123	34.7 (1.5)	3/110	0.6 [0.2, 2.0]
Most of the time	17	34.1 (1.2)	0/15	NA
Missing data	*91*	-	*0/9*	-

HCB: head circumference at birth. SHCB: small head circumference at birth. NA: an odds ratio was not available because too few cases were observed (n<3).

occupational exposure to pesticides among female workers and the wives of male workers in floriculture. In contrast, the study in agricultural areas in Norway by Kristensen et al. [4] found that the rates of prematurity and small-for-gestational-age status were lower for farmers than for non-farmers. In the latter study, pesticide exposure was assessed by means of national census data on indicators such as farm size, the number and types of livestock, and so on.

Despite some small discrepancies between the above-mentioned results, there appears to be a general consensus in which maternal and/or paternal occupational exposure to pesticides is associated with adverse effects on fetal development and adverse birth outcomes.

4.2 Domestic exposure to pesticides

Our study also considered domestic pesticides but did not focus on any one substance or group of substances in particular (in contrast to several literature studies). We found that self-reported maternal exposure to pesticides for houseplants was correlated with lower birth weight. In contrast, we did not find any association between maternal exposure to pesticides for outdoor plants and poor fetal growth. Our findings are consistent with Petit et al.'s [14] results on insecticide use on indoor plants in the Brittany region of western France but not with their data on use on garden plants. In fact, Petit et al.'s retrospective study found that higher self-reported *in utero* exposure to household insecticides for use on plants (and especially outdoor plants) was related to lower birth weight and head circumference [14].

We did not find any association between fetal growth and maternal exposure to domestic insecticides. Our findings are consistent with those of Petit et al. [14] regarding the association between residential use of insect control on one hand and birth weight and head circumference at birth on the other hand. Similarly, our results are in line with the reports by Berkowitz et al. [8] and Whyatt et al. [9] in the USA, which did not find any association between self-reported use of domestic pesticides, prenatal personal ambient air or umbilical cord blood levels of some domestic insecticides on one hand and birth weight, birth length or head circumference at birth on the other. The questionnaire used in these two studies of the same cohort probed domestic use of pesticides against three groups of pests only (cockroaches, rodents and others). In the retrospective study performed by Savitz et al. [3] in the USA, self-reported exposure to household pesticides was associated with the risk of small-for-gestational-age status but not with prematurity. The questionnaire used in Savitz et al.'s study [1] probed exposure very generally via a single question on whether or not the mother and/or the father had been exposed to household pesticides.

In the present study, we found that maternal exposure to veterinary antiparasitics was associated with a lower birth weight. To the best of our knowledge, our study is the first to have assessed the relationship between maternal exposure to veterinary anti-parasitics and fetal growth. In contrast, we did not find any association between fetal growth and maternal exposure to human antiparasitics.

4.3 Environmental exposure to pesticides

In our questionnaire, environmental exposure was assessed as self-reported proximity (within 1 km) of the mother's home during pregnancy to areas in which pesticides are usually widely applied (crop fields, green areas and transportation networks (highways, railroads and airports)). We did not observed any association between fetal growth and this proximity, in agreement with the results of the study by Petit et al. [14] in France; the latter researchers did not find any association between agricultural activities in the mother's place of residence during early pregnancy (based on data on agricultural activities from the national census) and birth weight (as a continuous variable) or the risk of low birth weight. In contrast, Xiang et al.'s [6] study in the USA (based on remote sensing and a geographic information system (GIS)) found an association between low birth weight and total crop production area within a 300 m buffer zone around the mother's residence. However, Xiang et al. [6] did not examine fetal growth parameters other than low birth weight. However, it is possible that the mothers in the present MecoExpo study (especially those living on the outskirts of cities) may have over-estimated the distance between their residence and crop fields.

4.4 Dietary exposure to pesticides

We did not find a significant association between fetal growth on one hand and overall or organic food intake on the other. Our questionnaire asked the mother about her eating behavior during a period (pregnancy) in which the diet is very likely to change. We cannot rule out the presence of recall bias, since the questionnaire was completed after delivery.

In conclusion, our present results demonstrate that both maternal and paternal occupational exposure to pesticides during pregnancy is associated with low gestational age and a greater risk of prematurity and low birth weight. Maternal domestic exposure to pesticides for houseplants and to veterinary antiparasitics was associated with low birth weight. Our questionnaire served as a wide-ranging tool for characterizing all the possible sources of prenatal exposure to pesticides. In the future, we could better characterize the exposure pathways and the nature of the compounds involved by complementing our questionnaire-based data with data generated by tools such as GISs and environmental or biological assays of pesticide residues.

Acknowledgments

We thank the parents who participated in this study, the staff at the maternity clinics and the staff from Picardy's perinatal networks. We also wish to thank the *Biobanque de Picardie* for technical assistance. Lastly, we thank Dr. David Fraser for advice on the manuscript's English.

This work was funded by the Picardy Regional Council and the Grenelle Environment. F. Mayhoub was funded by Tishreen University (Latakia, Syria) and T. Berton was funded by the European Regional Development Fund.

Author Contributions

Conceived and designed the experiments: FM VB KT AFB SD ESB KC. Performed the experiments: FM TB CD KC. Contributed reagents/materials/analysis tools: TB KT AFB. Wrote the paper: FM VB ESB KC.

References

1. Bedos C, Cellier P, Calvet R, Barriuso E, Gabrielle B (2002) Mass transfer of pesticides into the atmosphere by volatilization from soils and plants: overview. Agronomie 22 21–33
2. Whyatt RM, Barr DB, Camann DE, Kinney PL, Barr JR, et al. (2003) Contemporary-use pesticides in personal air samples during pregnancy and blood samples at delivery among urban minority mothers and newborns. Environ Health Perspect 111(5):749–56.
3. Savitz DA, Whelan EA, Kleckner RC (1989) Self-reported exposure to pesticides and radiation related to pregnancy outcome-results from National Natality and Fetal Mortality Surveys. Public Health Rep 104(5): 473–477.
4. Kristensen P, Irgens LM, Andersen A, Bye AS, Sundheim L (1997) Gestational age, birth weight, and perinatal death among births to Norwegian farmers, 1967–1991. Am J of Epidemiol 146(4): 329–338.
5. Restrepo M, Munoz N, Day NE, Parra JE, de Romero L, et al. (1990) Prevalence of adverse reproductive outcomes in a population occupationally exposed to pesticides in Colombia. Scand J Work Environ Health 16(4): 232–238.
6. Xiang H, Nuckols JR, Stallones L (2000) A geographic information assessment of birth weight and crop production patterns around mother's residence. Environ Res 82(2): 160–167.

7. Eskenazi B, Harley K, Bradman A, Weltzien E, Jewell NP, et al. (2004) Association of in utero organophosphate pesticide exposure and fetal growth and length of gestation in an agricultural population. Environ Health Perspect 112(10): 1116–1124.
8. Berkowitz GS, Wetmur JG, Birman-Deych E, Obel J, Lapinski RH, et al. (2004) In utero pesticide exposure, maternal paraoxonase activity, and head circumference. Environ Health Perspect 112(3): 388–391.
9. Whyatt RM, Camann D, Perera FP, Rauh VA, Tang D, et al. (2005) Biomarkers in assessing residential insecticide exposures during pregnancy and effects on fetal growth. Toxicol Appl Pharmacol 206(2): 246–254.
10. Sathyanarayana S, Basso O, Karr CJ, Lozano P, Alavanja M, et al. (2010) Maternal pesticide use and birth weight in the agricultural health study. J Agromedicine 15(2): 127–136.
11. Petit C, Chevrier C, Durand G, Monfort C, Rouget F, et al. (2010) Impact on fetal growth of prenatal exposure to pesticides due to agricultural activities: a prospective cohort study in Brittany, France. Environ Health 9: 71.
12. Brucker-Davis F, Wagner-Mahler K, Bornebusch L, Delattre I, Ferrari P, et al. (2010) Exposure to selected endocrine disruptors and neonatal outcome of 86 healthy boys from Nice area (France). Chemosphere 81(2): 169–176.
13. Wohlfahrt-Veje C, Main KM, Schmidt IM, Boas M, Jensen TK, et al. (2011) Lower birth weight and increased body fat at school age in children prenatally exposed to modern pesticides: a prospective study. Environ Health 10: 79.
14. Petit C, Blangiardo M, Richardson S, Coquet F, Chevrier C, et al. (2012) Association of environmental insecticide exposure and fetal growth with a Bayesian model including multiple exposure sources: the PELAGIE mother-child cohort. Am J Epidemiol 175(11): 1182–1190.
15. Association des Utilisateurs de Dossiers Informatisés en Pédiatrie, Obstétrique et Gynécologie. Étude sur la croissance fœtale et infantile. www.audipog.net.
16. Mamelle N, Boniol M, Rivière O, Joly MO, Mellier G, et al. (2006) Identification of newborns with Fetal Growth Restriction (FGR) in weight and/or length based on constitutional growth potential. Eur J Pediatr 165: 717–725.
17. McCormick MC (1985) The contribution of low birth weight to infant mortality and childhood morbidity. N Engl J Med 312(2): 82–90.
18. Kramer MS, Olivier M, McLean FH, Willis DM, Usher RH (1990) Impact of intrauterine growth retardation and body proportionality on fetal and neonatal outcome. Pediatrics 86(5): 707–713.
19. McIntire DD, Bloom SL, Casey BM, Leveno KJ (1999) Birth weight in relation to morbidity and mortality among newborn infants. N Engl J Med 340(16): 1234–1238.
20. Yanney M, Marlow N (2004) Paediatric consequences of fetal growth restriction. Semin Fetal Neonatal Med 9(5): 411–418.
21. Strauss RS, Dietz WH (1997) Effects of intrauterine growth retardation in premature infants on early childhood growth. J Pediat 130(1): 95–102.

5

Balancing Energy Budget in a Central-Place Forager: Which Habitat to Select in a Heterogeneous Environment?

Martin Patenaude-Monette[1], Marc Bélisle[2], Jean-François Giroux[1]*

1 Groupe de recherche en écologie comportementale et animale, Département des sciences biologiques, Université du Québec à Montréal, Montréal, Québec, Canada,
2 Département de biologie, Université de Sherbrooke, Sherbrooke, Québec, Canada

Abstract

Foraging animals are influenced by the distribution of food resources and predation risk that both vary in space and time. These constraints likely shape trade-offs involving time, energy, nutrition, and predator avoidance leading to a sequence of locations visited by individuals. According to the marginal-value theorem (MVT), a central-place forager must either increase load size or energy content when foraging farther from their central place. Although such a decision rule has the potential to shape movement and habitat selection patterns, few studies have addressed the mechanisms underlying habitat use at the landscape scale. Our objective was therefore to determine how Ring-billed gulls (*Larus delawarensis)* select their foraging habitats while nesting in a colony located in a heterogeneous landscape. Based on locations obtained by fine-scale GPS tracking, we used resource selection functions (RSFs) and residence time analyses to identify habitats selected by gulls for foraging during the incubation and brood rearing periods. We then combined this information to gull survey data, feeding rates, stomach contents, and calorimetric analyses to assess potential trade-offs. Throughout the breeding season, gulls selected landfills and transhipment sites that provided higher mean energy intake than agricultural lands or riparian habitats. They used landfills located farther from the colony where no deterrence program had been implemented but avoided those located closer where deterrence measures took place. On the other hand, gulls selected intensively cultured lands located relatively close to the colony during incubation. The number of gulls was then greater in fields covered by bare soil and peaked during soil preparation and seed sowing, which greatly increase food availability. Breeding Ring-billed gulls thus select habitats according to both their foraging profitability and distance from their nest while accounting for predation risk. This supports the predictions of the MVT for central-place foraging over large spatial scales.

Editor: Michael Sears, Clemson University, United States of America

Funding: The research was supported by grants to JFG and MB from the Natural Sciences and Engineering Research Council of Canada, the Canadian Wildlife Service, ICI Environnement, Falcon Environmental Services, Chamard et Associés, Waste Management, and BFI Canada. MPM was supported by a scholarship from the Natural Sciences and Engineering Research Council of Canada. The funders had no role in study design, data collection and analysis, decision to publish, or preparation of the manuscript.

Competing Interests: ICI Environnement, Falcon Environmental Services, Chamard et Associés, Waste Management, and BFI Canada provided funding towards this study. There are no patents, products in development or marketed products to declare. This does not alter the authors' adherence to all the PLOS ONE policies on sharing data and materials.

* Email: giroux.jean-francois@uqam.ca

Introduction

Animals face time and energy constraints leading to trade-offs in their activity budget, which can also be modulated by factors such as the spatio-temporal distribution of food resources, conspecifics, predation risk, and phenology. How animals respond to these constraints in order to maximize their fitness through foraging behaviour has been the main focus of optimal foraging theory [1], [2]. For instance, the marginal-value theorem (MVT) has been used to predict which resource patch an animal should exploit and how long it should stay before moving to another patch or return to its nest or shelter [3], [4]. Assuming that animals maximize their net energy gain, this model has provided relevant qualitative predictions [5]. However, it has been developed and used for small-scale systems in which animals are assumed to incur few or no travel costs and to be highly informed about their environment [1], [2].

This model may therefore be difficult to apply at the landscape level because of information uncertainty about the environment, which influences learning ability and because of the limited motion and navigation capacity of animals [6], [7], [8]. For example, classical central-place foraging models based on the MVT predict that prey load size should increase with the distance traveled by a forager from its central place [4], [9]. However, a forager moving across the landscape with a large load can incur increased travel costs due to greater energy expenditures or can encounter higher predation risks through increased exposure and reduced manoeuvrability [5]. Therefore, the impact of carrying a heavy load can influence the time and energy budget of a central-place forager in different ways, sometime far from the conclusions of the classical models [10].

The MVT predicts that a foraging path is the outcome of balancing trade-offs between energy expenditures and gains, especially within landscapes where resources are heterogeneously distributed. Although it is difficult to use the MVT to make precise predictions under relaxed assumptions, classical central-place foraging models nevertheless allow to predict that distant patches must provide higher energy "prey" than those found in nearby patches [9]. Hence, the profitability of a given load size may vary for a generalist forager traveling through a heterogeneous landscape. Also, habitats providing low energy food should only be used close to the central place whereas habitats with high-energy food may be exploited near or far from the central place. It remains that travel costs may increase the use of poor quality habitats when individuals must sample and learn the quality of their environment [11], [12]. Moreover, temporal variation in habitat availability and forager condition may alter the pattern of habitat use along a distance gradient [13].

Although assessing the costs and benefits of large spatio-temporal scale movements is difficult, analytical methods based on accurate location data (e.g., GPS) are now available to study movement behaviour. Combining these analytical methods with *in situ* observations of individual foraging strategies, patch quality, and environmental conditions while considering the individuals' characteristics has the capacity to provide insights into the cost-benefit trade-offs associated with foraging movements underlying habitat selection [13], [14]. For instance, resource selection functions (RSF) have been widely used to assess habitat selection. They are based on the comparison of relative habitat use (defined by presence-only data) and availability or on the presence/absence of individuals in habitat patches [15]. RSF are particularly informative if a distinction can be made between actively selected locations, such as foraging patches, and the incidentally selected locations visited during inter-patch movements [16], [17]. Bastille-Rousseau *et al.* [18] have advocated the use of a combination of RSF, residence time analysis, and ground surveys to study resource selection and foraging strategies at the landscape level. Considering the hierarchical aspect of the selection process, the difficulty of defining available habitats with presence-only data can be avoided by building RSF based on the habitats actually visited for foraging vs. those crossed when moving to a patch [19], [20]. Measuring the time spent by an animal within the surroundings of recorded locations (residence time) should allow discriminating between locations occurring within foraging patches and those found along movement paths [16], [21].

We used RSF and residence time analyses from GPS-tracking data, as well as survey data, diet characterization and calorimetric analyses to study the processes that determine habitat use by breeding Ring-billed gulls (*Larus delawarensis*). This species is a colonial central-place forager that feeds opportunistically upon a wide variety of prey items found in both aquatic and terrestrial habitats [22], [23]. We expected that gulls should be more likely to forage in a patch where the amount of habitats providing high-energy food increases and that such a relationship should be more pronounced far from the colony so that gulls reach a threshold of profitability. We also hypothesized that gulls should select habitats with a temporally variable food availability only when those habitats provide high food returns. For instance, agricultural lands and lawns should be selected on rainy days when annelids (earthworms) are more available to gulls [24]. By testing these predictions, our study sheds light on the process of habitat selection by animals from an energy trade-off perspective.

Materials and Methods

Ethics statement

Field methods to capture, mark, and collect Ring-billed gulls were approved by the Institutional Animal Protection Committee of the Université du Québec à Montréal (No. 646). The capture and marking of gulls was conducted under Environment Canada scientific permit to capture and band migratory birds (No. 10546) while the collection of specimens was carried out under Environment Canada scientific research permit (No. SC-23)

Study area

We tracked the movements of Ring-billed gulls breeding on Deslauriers Island located in the St. Lawrence River 3 km downstream from Montreal, QC, Canada (45.717°N, 73.433°W). This colony covered 11.4 ha and supported 48,000 pairs at the time of the study. The surrounding foraging area encompassed approximately 6,000 km^2 and consisted of a mosaic of high and low density urban areas, agricultural lands of intensive (soybean, maize, and small cereals) and extensive cultures (hayfields and pastures), as well as riparian habitats along the River and its tributaries (Fig. 1). Four landfills and two waste material transhipment sites were located in the vicinity of the colony. Landfills attract gulls because of the anthropogenic food they supply but the implementation of deterrence programs may reduce their accessibility [25], [26]. During our study, the St-Thomas (41 km) and Lachute (63 km) landfills, as well as the two transhipment sites (12 and 27 km), had no deterrence program. On the other hand, the Ste-Sophie landfill (37 km) initiated a deterrence program in 2009 that combined pyrotechnics and selective culling. However, the program was limited to weekdays from 07:00 to 15:00 thereby leaving some feeding opportunities for gulls [26]. Lastly, the Terrebonne landfill (8 km) conducted a deterrence program since 1995 that included falconry, distress calls, and pyrotechnics. This program was in operation every day from sunrise to sunset, preventing all but few gulls to use the landfill (Thiériot, E., unpublished data).

Telemetry

Breeding Ring-billed gulls were fitted with 10–16-g GiPSy-2 data loggers (TechnoSmart, Italy) between April and June 2009–2010. The loggers represented (mean ± SD) 2.8±0.5% of the birds' body mass (485±49 g). Most gulls were captured and recaptured with nest traps or dip nets but some had to be recaptured by rifle shooting; carcasses were then kept for further analyses (see *Diet and calorimetric analyses*). Data loggers were attached on the two median rectrices with white TESA tape (no. 4651) and programmed to acquire locations at 4-min intervals. Tracking lasted 1 to 3 days depending on battery life. Half of the birds included in the analyses returned to their nest within 15 min after being released and 81% of them returned within 60 min. Birds that spent more than 1 h away from their nest took on average 4.5±3.9 h to return. Breeding stage upon capture was categorized as incubating or brood rearing. Gulls were sexed with genomic DNA isolation from chest feathers [27].

We recaptured 109 Ring-billed gulls (41 females, 68 males) with loggers that provided reliable data (Table S1). After removing locations within a 300-m buffer zone around the colony (see *Data analyses*), there were only 28 missing locations on a potential of 15,948. The remaining 15,920 locations had a low dilution of precision metric (DOP ≤6) and an estimated precision of ±5 m [28]. A total of 67 gulls were followed during incubation (164 foraging trips) and 42 during the brood rearing period (239 foraging trips).

Gull Surveys

We conducted weekly surveys from April to June alternating between three periods (05:00–10:00, 10:00–15:00, and 15:00–20:00) to determine the proportion of time Ring-billed gulls spent

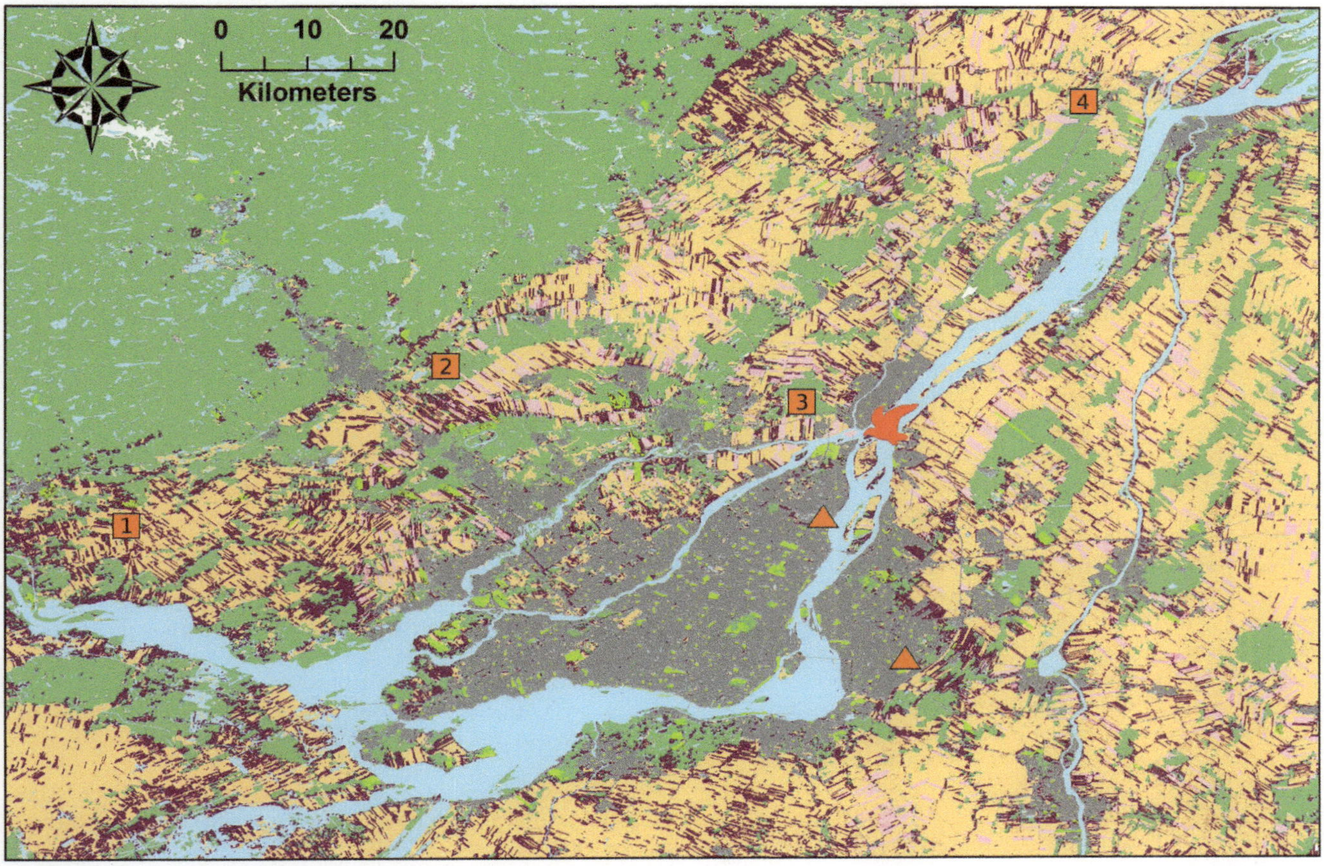

Figure 1. Map of the study area. Land cover types include water (blue), urban areas (gray), intensive cultures (mango), extensive cultures (purple), unidentified cultures (rose), lawns (olive green), and woodlots (dark green). Numbers in squares indicate landfill locations (1- Lachute, 2- Ste-Sophie, 3- Terrebonne, 4- St-Thomas), red triangles indicate transhipment site locations, and the bird pictogram indicates the location of the Deslauriers Island Ring-billed gull colony.

foraging in their main feeding habitats. In agricultural habitats, we surveyed a 50-km roadside transect on each shore of the St. Lawrence River ($N = 13$ and 21 surveys in 2009 and 2010, respectively). We tallied the number of birds in each flock and performed an instantaneous scan sampling to determine the proportion of birds foraging (head down below the horizontal or

Table 1. Cover percentage of eight habitat types available in the foraging range of 109 Ring-billed gulls breeding on Deslauriers Island established as the minimum convex polygon calculated with all gull locations and mean cover percentage (±1 SD) in movement (residence time <100 s) and foraging (residence time ≥100 s) patches (200-m radius), 2009–2010.

Habitat type	% cover Foraging range (5,565 km²)	Movement patches ($N = 2,599$)	Foraging patches ($N = 4,490$)
Lawns (parks, golf courses, etc.)	1.2	1.8±8.3	2.1±9.4
Woodlots	20.6	13.7±28.8	4.8±16.0
Urban areas	16.8	27.8±38.5	23.1±36.6
Water bodies	5.3	18.7±34.8	22.4±37.9
Intensive cultures	39.5	24.3±34.1	31.4±38.7
Extensive cultures	11.7	8.4±16.2	8.0±15.6
Unidentified cultures	4.1	3.4±12.3	4.2±14.3
Landfills/Transhipment sites	0.1	1.3±11.3[a]	4.2±20.0[a]

[a]Percent occurrence.

probing into the soil) that we considered as the proportion of time spent foraging [29]. A flock was defined as a group of gulls using the same field type and not separated by more than 200 m from each other. Birds using different field types but closer than 200 m from each other were considered as different flocks. The total number of tractors and their activity (ploughing, harrowing or sowing) was also noted over the entire transect during each survey.

Observations in other habitats were conducted weekly in 2010 at fixed points located in urban (N= 25 points), suburban (N= 53 points), and riparian (N= 10 points) areas on the Montreal Island (N= 16 surveys) and along the North (N= 18 surveys) and the South shores (N= 22 surveys) of the St. Lawrence River. These sites were selected because they were susceptible to be visited by gulls while insuring that observers driving vehicles could stop safely. At each point, gulls using different habitat types (lawns, shores, water, grounds covered with concrete, asphalt or gravel, building roofs, and post lights) were counted and scanned to determine the proportion of birds foraging (erratic flight in emergent insect clouds above waterbodies, feeding on garbage, head down below the horizontal or probing into the soil or water).

Finally, we estimated the proportion of time gulls spent foraging at landfills by conducting 5-h observation periods once a week in 2009 (N= 7) and five days a week in 2010 (N= 59) at the Ste-Sophie landfill, again alternating among the three daily periods including periods with and without deterrence. Total bird counts and instantaneous scan sampling were conducted every half hour. The mean daily abundance of gulls was computed for each day as well as the proportion of birds that were actually foraging (flying less than 5 m above the active tipping area, head down below the horizontal or probing into refuse).

Diet and calorimetric analyses

We collected 496 boli from chicks of both sexes during weekly visits to the Deslauriers colony during the rearing period of 2009 and 2010. We selected chicks haphazardly and slightly pressed their proventriculus to make them regurgitate recently swallowed food. Spontaneous regurgitations of adults (N= 13) captured during banding operations throughout the breeding period were also collected. Samples were frozen until they were analysed. We also kept frozen the carcasses (N= 51) of adults fitted with data loggers and recaptured by shooting until the content of their oesophagus and proventriculus could be analysed. Similarly, we analysed stomach contents of birds collected by rifle shooting in agricultural lands (N= 69), riparian areas (N= 54), and at the Ste-Sophie landfill (N= 85). We made sure that birds were actively feeding in these habitats before collecting them. For safety reasons, gulls could not be collected in urban areas. Each food item of a bolus or stomach was separated, identified, dried to constant weight and weighted (±0.01 g). Food items were grouped into broad categories (e.g., arthropods, annelids, vertebrates, refuse, vegetation, other).

Food availability could not be assessed throughout the 6,000 km^2 of the foraging area to estimate the benefits obtained by gulls when feeding in different habitats. Instead, we relied on the relative area of each habitat and the food quality in these habitats based on energy content of the various food items. We therefore performed duplicate or triplicate calorimetric analyses of each food category using a bomb calorimeter (Parr, model 1108P).

Data analyses

We first created a 300-m buffer zone around Deslauriers Island (colony) to discriminate between foraging trips and short movements to the shore or surrounding shallow water where gulls rest and preen [30]. Our analyses were limited to locations outside this zone. The mean number of foraging trips per day, the mean direct (Euclidean) distance between the colony and the farthest location reached during a foraging trip (whether a stopover or not), the mean distance traveled on a foraging trip and the mean sinuosity of movement paths (traveled distance divided by round trip direct distance, [31]) were compared between breeding stages and sexes using linear mixed models with gull ID as a random factor.

For each foraging trip, we calculated the total amount of time spent at different locations on the landscape by estimating residence time without rediscretization [16]. Residence time was defined as the time spent in a circle of radius r centred on a given location along the foraging path. The circle, with its specific habitat composition and features, could then be viewed as a potential foraging patch. In the absence of precise information regarding the spatio-temporal distribution of resources, the hierarchy of spatial scales at which animals are likely to respond to landscape heterogeneity (i.e., patches, [32]) can only be identified through behaviour [16], [33]. For each trip, we thus computed the coefficient of variation (CV) of residence times for radii ranging between 200 and 2,000 m with 100-m increments. We averaged the CV across paths and plotted them against the circle radii (Fig. S1). The mean CVs of residence time across paths showed a plateau for radii of 200 to 400 m instead of a clear peak.

Table 2. Summary of *a priori* models based on resource selection functions that predict the probability that a breeding Ring-billed gull will forage in a patch (200-m radius) for a 100-s residence time threshold.

Model	Deviance	K	ΔAICc	w_i
H+D+B	7,891	26	0.00	0.813
H+D+R+B	7,886	30	2.94	0.187
H+D	7,940	19	35.06	0.000
H+D+R	7,936	23	38.63	0.000
H+B	8,466	18	558.98	0.000
H+R+B	8,459	22	560.26	0.000
H	8,533	11	611.33	0.000
H+R	8,527	15	613.67	0.000

H: habitat types; D: distance between a location and the colony; R: mean daily rainfall; B: breeding stage (egg incubation vs. chick rearing); K: number of parameters; w_i: Akaike weight.

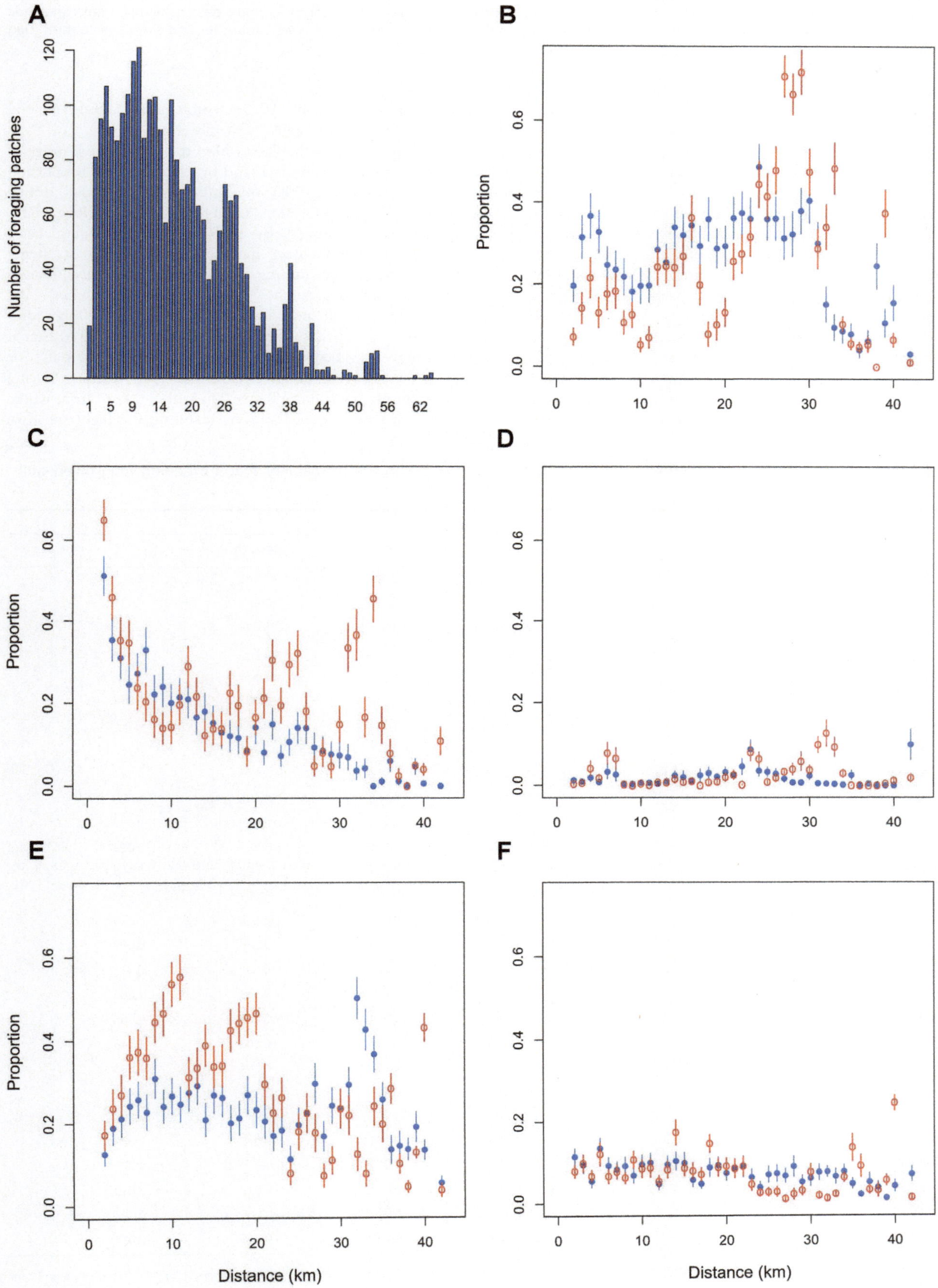
A
B
C
D
E
F
Number of foraging patches
Proportion
Distance (km)
1 5 9 14 20 26 32 38 44 50 56 62
0 20 40 60 80 100 120
0 10 20 30 40
0.0 0.2 0.4 0.6

Figure 2. The effect of distance on habitat selection by foraging Ring-billed gulls. Number of foraging patches within 1-km concentric bands from the colony (a). Mean (±1 SD) proportion of urban areas (b), waterbodies (c), lawns (d), intensive cultures (e), and extensive cultures (f) in foraging (blue) and movement patches (red) in relation with the distance from the colony.

There was no significant difference in CVs distribution between males and females. We thus chose a 200-m radius to get a stronger contrast in habitat composition between foraging and movement patches. We finally retained locations distanced by at least two radii to limit spatial autocorrelation.

We calculated the landscape composition within each circle in which residence time was estimated based on a land cover map created in ArcGIS 9.3.1 [34] using both agricultural and topographic data ([35], [36], [37]; planimetric precision <30 m). Landscape composition was defined as the proportion of different habitats including lawns, woodlots, urban areas, and water as well as intensive, extensive and unidentified cultures. Because of their relatively small size, landfills and transhipment centres were noted as presence/absence in each circle. We also measured the distance between each location where a residence time was computed and the nest of the tracked gull. Finally, we calculated the mean daily rainfall using data from 10 meteorological stations located throughout the entire foraging area [38].

We first described the habitats within the global home range of gulls breeding on Deslauriers Island by estimating the proportion of habitats within the 100% minimum convex polygon drawn using the foraging trip locations of all birds. Next, we built a RSF based on patches visited by gulls on their foraging trips. Considering that a foraging individual must reduce its flying speed and increase its turning rate, we used residence time to discriminate "foraging patches" from "movement patches". We assumed that if a gull spent more than 100 s in a 200-m radius circle, it was actively foraging. Otherwise, we considered that it was moving either between the colony and a foraging patch or between two foraging patches. Gulls observed foraging during surveys typically spent more than 100 s within 200 m from where they were first detected. Moreover, based on the flight speed of

Table 3. Mixed-effects averaged logit resource selection functions quantifying the probability that a breeding Ring-billed gull forage in a patch.

Variable	*β*	SE	95% CI	
Intercept	−0.612	0.491	−1.575	0.351
Distance*	0.089	0.013	0.063	0.115
Woodlots*	−2.963	0.448	−3.840	−2.086
Lawns	−0.212	0.834	−1.846	1.422
Urban areas*	−2.550	0.521	−3.570	−1.529
Landfills	0.992	0.510	−0.007	1.992
Water*	−1.130	0.516	−2.142	−0.118
Extensive cultures	−1.037	0.619	−2.251	0.177
Intensive cultures	−0.901	0.516	−1.913	0.111
Unidentified cultures	−0.319	0.688	−1.666	1.029
Lawns × Distance	0.017	0.033	−0.049	0.083
Urban areas × Distance*	0.067	0.016	0.036	0.098
Landfill × Distance	0.001	0.017	−0.033	0.035
Water × Distance	0.031	0.016	−0.001	0.063
Extensive cultures × Distance	−0.005	0.021	−0.045	0.035
Intensive cultures × Distance	−0.026	0.015	−0.056	0.004
Unidentified cultures × Distance	−0.036	0.026	−0.087	0.015
Lawns × Incubation	−0.050	0.671	−1.365	1.266
Urban areas × Incubation	0.210	0.244	−0.267	0.688
Landfill × Incubation	0.271	0.446	−0.603	1.145
Water × Incubation	0.205	0.254	−0.294	0.703
Extensive cultures × Incubation	−0.349	0.418	−1.168	0.469
Intensive cultures × Incubation*	1.429	0.237	0.965	1.893
Unidentified cultures × Incubation	0.911	0.474	−0.018	1.839
Lawns × Rainfall*	0.038	0.019	0.001	0.075
Extensive cultures × Rainfall	0.000	0.007	−0.013	0.013
Intensive cultures × Rainfall	−0.002	0.004	−0.009	0.005
Unidentified cultures × Rainfall	−0.003	0.008	−0.019	0.012

Model-averaged coefficients (*β*), unconditional standard errors (SE), and 95% confidence intervals (CI) are presented. Variables followed by an asterisk are significant (95% CI excluding 0).

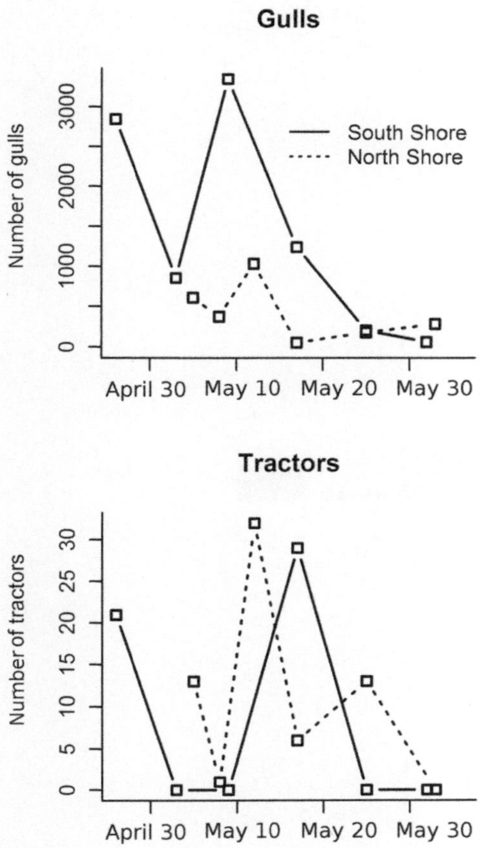

Figure 3. Use of agricultural lands by breeding Ring-billed gulls. Number of gulls and of tractors observed during surveys on the North and South shores of the St. Lawrence River, 2010.

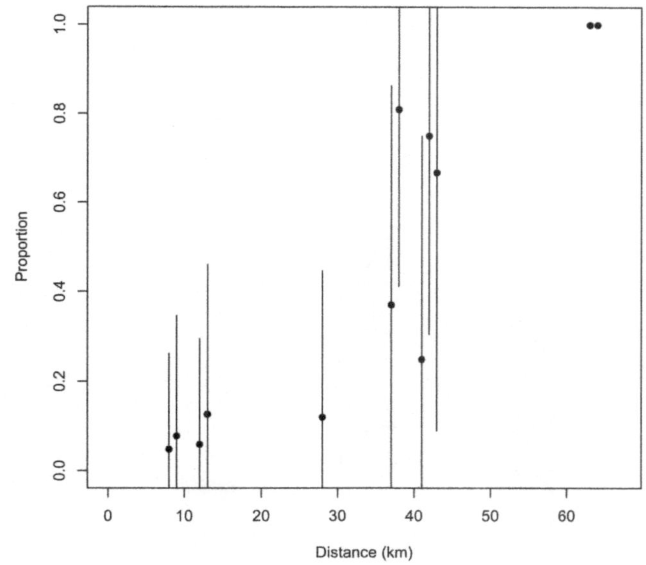

Figure 4. Use of landfills and transhipment sites by Ring-billed gulls. Mean (±1 SD) proportion of Ring-billed gull locations at landfills and transhipment sites in foraging patches within 1-km concentric bands located at different distances from the colony. All landfills and open transhipment sites were visited by at least one tagged individual. Some sites encompassed more than one band.

Black-headed gulls (*Chroicocephalus ridibundus*) and Lesser Black-backed gulls (*Larus fuscus*), which are respectively slightly smaller and larger than Ring-billed gulls (14.7–15.5 m/s, respectively; [39]), at least 26 s is required for a gull to cross a circle of 200-m radius. The remaining 74 s appears insufficient for a gull to forage significantly in such a circular patch. Although our tracking device did not allow to determine the precise activity of the birds while not moving, we consider justified to assume that gulls were actually foraging in patches where they spend more than 100 s. Indeed, during the breeding period, gulls must brood their eggs or feed their young and must therefore spend as much time as possible on the colony allowing the rest of their time to foraging.

We used mixed effects logistic regressions to quantify the influence of landscape composition on the probability that a gull foraged in a patch along its movement path. Gull ID and foraging trip ID (nested within gull ID) were treated as random factors. The addition of these terms dealt with the hierarchical structure of the data and allowed the estimation of the variability across individuals and foraging trips. Eight different models were built and compared based on the second-order Akaike information criterion (AIC_c, [40]). We included the proportion of each habitat type and the occurrence of landfills and transhipment sites in all eight models. We considered the interaction of rainfall with lawns as well as with each type of agricultural cover because annelids are more prevalent under wet conditions [24]. We also included the distance between the location of a gull while foraging and its nest as a proxy for foraging costs and accessibility [41]. We considered distance both as a main effect and in interaction with the relative amount of each habitat type (except woodlots) as well as with the occurrence of landfills or transhipment sites. We used this approach because we do not know which fitness currency gulls may be maximizing and because the profitability of the different habitats may not scale linearly with distance. Although woodlots are accessible, gulls avoid being under canopy and should thus avoid forest habitats whatever the distance from the colony. We included breeding stage in interactions with each habitat type to take into consideration the gulls' breeding phenology and their associated requirements as well as habitat phenology, particularly for agricultural cover types where farming practices and field conditions vary throughout the season. Finally, we built a second set of eight models, adding the sex of the birds in interaction with each habitat type and the distance of the patch from the colony as males and females differ in size (affecting travel costs and dominance on food patches) and provide different levels of parental care [23]. We fitted mixed effects logistic regressions using the Laplace approximation using the lme4 package (version 0.999375-39; [42]) run in the R statistical environment (version 2.12.2; [43]). AIC_c were computed based on maximum log-likelihoods. Multi-model inference was performed following Burnham and Anderson [41] after testing that there was no problem of collinearity.

The effect of distance on habitat selection may be non-linear partly because central-place foragers often avoid habitats near their central-place by moving further away [44], [45]. Moreover, the relative abundance of different habitats varied with distance from the colony. To overcome this problem, we first draw 1-km wide circular bands up to 67 km from the colony, which corresponds to a few kilometers further than the farthest gull location (see *Results*). For each band with at least five foraging patches, we calculated the mean area covered by each habitat type within patches to estimate habitat use. We also calculated the mean area covered by the different habitats in movement patches

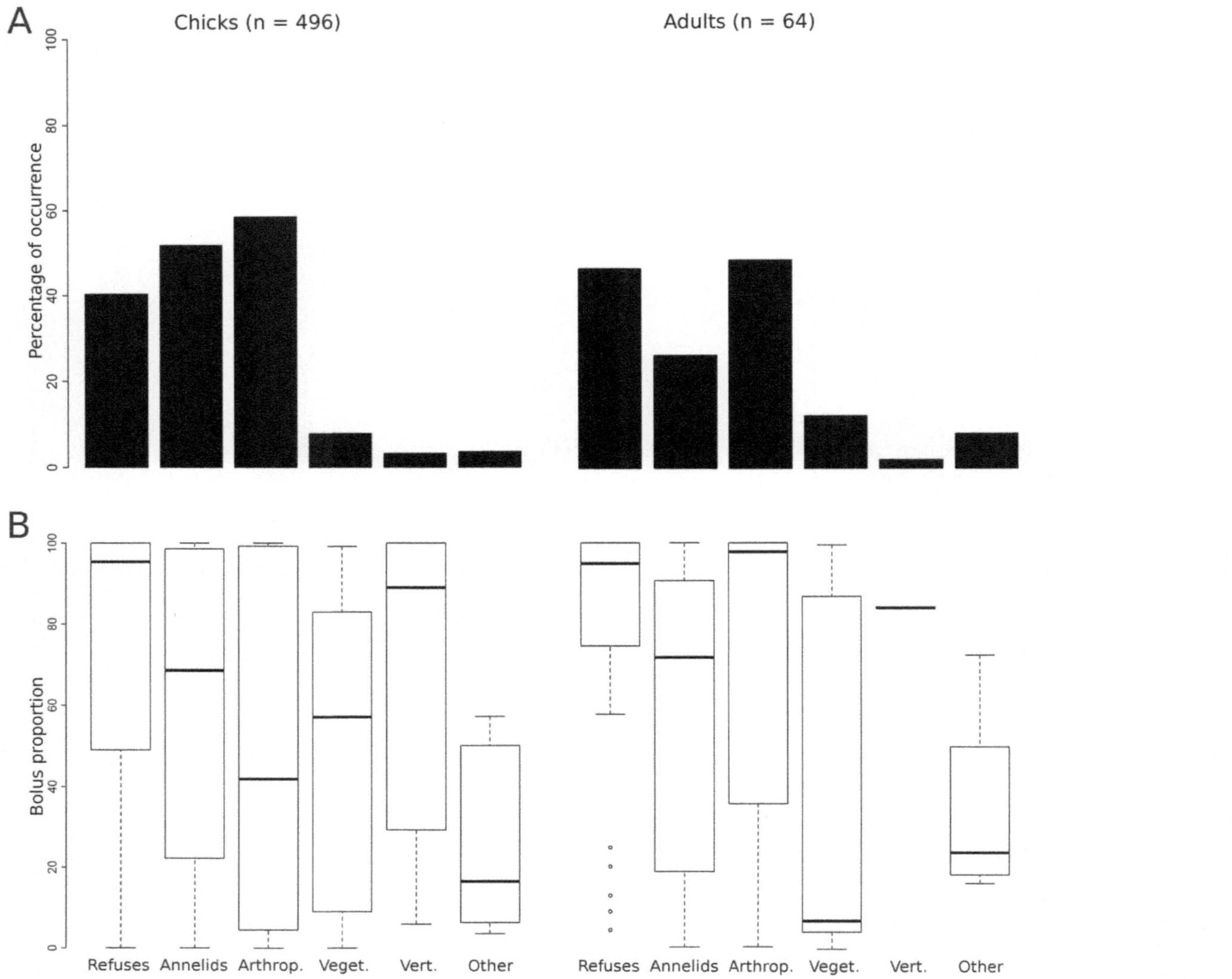

Figure 5. Diet of chicks and breeding adults of Ring-billed gulls. Diet of Ring-billed gull chicks (boli) and breeding adults (boli and stomach contents) at the Deslauriers Island colony, 2009–2010, expressed as the percentage of occurrence of each food category (a) and the proportion based on dry mass of each food category when present (b). Boxplots provide the first (bottom line), second (black midline) and third (top line) quartiles; whiskers extend to observations found up to 1.5 times the interquartile range; observations outside this range are indicated by empty dots.

(≥5 patches) within each circular band. We then plotted these two values for each band and each habitat to explore habitat selection as a function of distance.

The proportion of gulls observed foraging in a flock was considered as the time spent foraging in a given habitat [29]. This proportion was modeled as a two-column matrix, with the first column giving the number of gulls foraging and the second column giving the number of gulls involved in other activities for each flock, using a GLM with a binomial error distribution and logit link function (i.e., a logistic regression) using the stats package run in R. We also assessed whether the abundance of gulls in agricultural lands was related to the total number of tractors encountered along transects, which was considered an index of agricultural field work. This was done using a GLM with a Poisson error distribution and log link function (i.e., a Poisson regression) in R. This model included tractor number, transect location (South or North shore) and their interaction as explanatory variables.

Finally, we computed the proportion of boli containing at least one item of each food category for both chicks and adults. We then calculated the mean relative amount of each food item category when present in a bolus based on dry mass. The energy value of boli (kJ) was calculated for each gull collected at the Ste-Sophie landfill, in agricultural lands and at riparian sites by combining the dry mass of each item found in the stomach and their energy value. We compared the mean energy value of boli across habitats using an ANOVA.

Results

Characteristics of foraging trips

The mean number of foraging trips per day was greater during the rearing period (3.1±1.0 trips/day, ±SD) than during incubation (1.9±0.8 trips/day; $t_{107} = -7.01$, $P<0.001$). The mean direct distance between the colony and the furthest location reached during a foraging trip (whether a stopover or not) was also greater during brood rearing (16.6±12.4 km, maxi-

Table 4. Mean dry mass (g ± SD) and mean energy value (kJ) of nine food items gathered by sub-adult and adult Ring-billed Gulls in three habitat types (*N* = number of birds with food items present in their stomach).

Food items	Mean dry mass (g) Landfills (*N* = 81)	Agricultural lands (*N* = 54)	Riparian habitats (*N* = 22)	Energy (kJ)
Meat	1.84±4.71	-	0.87±2.81	30.1
Bread/rice	1.27±2.62	-	0.47±1.05	19.9
Potatoes/French fries	0.15±0.79	-	0.32±0.89	21.8
Miscellaneous refuse	0.79±2.69	-	-	22.6
Annelids	0.10±0.32	1.99±2.80	-	13.8
Arthropods	0.06±0.24	0.03±0.08	0.09±0.24	22.8
Corn/soybean grains	-	1.44±3.36	-	18.1
Vertebrates	0.01±0.11	-	0.46±0.61	19.4
Miscellaneous	0.10±0.32	0.08±0.35	-	21.3
TOTAL	4.47±6.37	3.55±3.68	2.36±3.39	-

mum = 63.5 km vs. 12.5±9.9 km, maximum = 42.4 km; $t_{107} = -2.22$, $P = 0.03$). Furthermore, the mean foraging distance traveled was greater during the rearing period compared to incubation (38.6±29.0 km, maximum = 156 km vs. 30.2±23.8 km, maximum 105 km; $t_{107} = -2.55$, $P = 0.01$). However, there was no difference in path sinuosity during the two periods (incubation: 1.2±0.2, maximum = 2.5; rearing: 1.2±0.2, maximum = 2.9; $t_{107} = 1.38$, $P = 0.17$). Finally, the mean trip duration was similar throughout the breeding period (incubation: 2.5±2.0 h, maximum = 9.6 h; rearing: 2.3±1.7 h, maximum = 12.4 h; $t_{107} = 0.91$, $P = 0.36$) but the trips lasted longer when a landfill was visited (3.5±1.8 h vs. 2.2±1.8 h; $t_{107} = 5.95$, $P < 0.0001$). No significant effect of sex was found for the trip characteristics (all $P > 0.21$).

Habitat selection

The composition of foraging and movement patches was highly variable (Table 1). Nevertheless, both movement and foraging patches were on average composed of smaller percentages of woodlots and of intensive and extensive cultures than what was found over the whole foraging range. An opposite trend was found for urban areas, waterbodies, landfills, and transhipment sites. While woodlots and urban areas covered a smaller proportion of foraging patches than movement patches, intensive cultures were relatively more important in foraging patches. Landfills and transhipment sites also occurred more often in foraging than movement patches. The distribution of residence time was strongly skewed to the right, with a peak under 100 s and a maximum reaching 19,377 s or 5.4 h (Fig. S2).

Model ranking based on AIC_c remained similar when considering the sex of individuals and its interaction with habitat types or patch distance. Yet, we only show results for models without sex as they performed better with much less parameters ($\Delta AICc = 3.04$). The best model ($w_i = 0.813$) included habitat types as well as the distance separating the foraging patch from the colony, the breeding stage and their two-way interactions with habitat types (Table 2). The model that also included rainfall and its interaction with habitat types scored as the second best model ($w_i = 0.187$), leaving barely any support from the data for the remaining models. Note that the same two models were selected with similar, strong levels of evidence for other residence time thresholds (60, 80, 120, and 140 s) and with patch radii of 200 and 400 m, underlining the robustness of our results with respect to these two assumptions.

Ring-billed gulls had a greater probability of foraging in patches located farther from the colony (Table 3). The distribution of these patches with respect to their distance from the colony was skewed to the right and showed a noticeable mode at ~10 km notwithstanding habitat types (Fig. 2a). Not surprisingly, gulls strongly avoided foraging in patches that included large amounts of woodlots (Table 3). Patches containing urban areas were significantly avoided close to the colony but increasingly selected further away. In fact, gulls tended to forage in patches with more urban cover compared to movement patches when the birds were between 25 and 35 km from their nest site (Fig. 2b). Because the colony was surrounded by water and gulls foraged little near the colony, there was a significant overall avoidance of this habitat (Table 3). Nevertheless, there was nearly a significant positive interaction between waterbodies and distance. In fact, waterbodies were relatively more important in foraging patches compared to movement patches when the birds were at 12 km or more from the colony (Fig. 2c). As expected, Ring-billed gulls foraged to a greater extent in patches containing lawns on rainy days (Table 3). We observed a greater proportion of lawns in foraging than in movement patches at around 5 km and again between 27 and 35 km (Fig. 2d).

The probability that a gull foraged in a patch increased with the proportion of intensive cultures (i.e., cereal fields) during incubation but tended to decrease during chick rearing (Table 3). More specifically, there were more intensive cultures in foraging than in movement patches up to 23 km from the colony (Fig. 2e). Similarly, the likelihood that gulls foraged in patches with extensive cultures (i.e., hayfields and pastures) tended to decrease with increasing amounts of this habitat (Table 3). The effect of distance on the use of extensive cultures by foraging gulls was not important (Fig. 2f). Gull surveys conducted in agricultural landscapes support the above patterns as the presence of gulls in intensive agricultural lands was related to the occurrence of ploughing, harrowing, and sowing, which all took place during the incubation period (mid-April to mid-May; Fig. 3). Indeed, the number of gulls observed along transects in agricultural lands increased with cultivation activities as indexed by the number of operating tractors seen in the fields (Poisson regression: β ±

SE = 0.064±0.001, z = 53.9, P<0.01). Of 20,900 gulls counted along transects, 52% were observed on bare soil fields (ploughed or recently sown), 34% on cereal fields with short vegetation (< 10 cm), 8% on stubble cereal fields and the remaining 6% on recently mowed hayfields. Finally, Ring-billed gulls had a greater tendency to forage in patches where a landfill or transhipment site was present (Table 3) and this was especially true as distance from the colony increased (Fig. 4).

Foraging behaviour, diet, and energy

The mean proportion of time that Ring-billed gulls spent foraging varied among habitats (deviance = -1.5×10^4; df = 1351, P<0.01). It was higher in agricultural lands (0.54±0.40) than in landfills and transhipment sites (0.17±0.20; z = −76.9, P<0.01), riparian habitats (0.12±0.25; z = −78.4, P<0.01), urban areas (0.15±0.32; z = −53.4, P<0.01) and on lawns (0.43±0.41; z = −3.1, P<0.01).

The four main food items (i.e., refuse, annelids, arthropods, and vegetation) were found in 40–60% of the boli collected from chicks reared on Deslauriers Island (Fig. 5a). The same items were found in the stomachs and boli of breeding adults, but in lower proportions (25–30%); it was compensated by a greater frequency of vertebrates and miscellaneous items. Yet, vertebrates occurred in less than 10% of the boli/stomachs in both chicks and adults. When refuse items were present, they contributed to a large proportion of the contents based on dry mass, unlike vegetation and miscellaneous items that usually represented a small proportion (Fig. 5b). The importance of annelids and arthropods was much more variable when present. Vertebrates were also quite variable in chick boli, whereas they clearly contributed to a very large proportion of the adult diet when they occurred.

Stomach contents from gulls collected in landfills were largely composed of fat meat typically found in refuse (Table 4). In agricultural lands, stomach contents were composed more or less equally of annelids and grains (soybean and corn). Stomach contents from riparian areas contained edible refuse, wild fishes, and arthropods. By pooling data on the relative importance of each food item and their respective energy content, we found that the mean energy value of stomach contents differed significantly among habitats ($F_{2,144}$ = 3.51, P = 0.03). It was significantly higher in landfills (112.8±169.8 kJ) than in agricultural lands (55.8±63.6 kJ) and riparian areas (56.5±97.5 kJ), which were not significantly different.

Discussion

By combining analyses of GPS-tracking data and information on the gulls' abundance, diet, and proportion of time spent foraging in different habitats, we found that the distance from the colony and habitat phenology had strong effects on the process of habitat selection by breeding Ring-billed gulls foraging in a heterogeneous environment. For instance, they positively selected areas managed intensively for agriculture at a distance up to about 23 km from the colony but only when fields were being ploughed, harrowed, or sown. Gulls also selected areas where landfills and transhipment sites were present, especially as the distance from the colony increased. The mean energy intake being significantly greater in landfills than in agricultural lands, these results clearly suggest a trade-off by Ring-billed gulls to balance their energy budget. The St. Lawrence River and its tributaries are often used as passageways when flying to and from the insular colony, which resulted in a general avoidance of this habitat as feeding site. Over 12 km, however, gulls may stop along the shores of the rivers and the lakes or feed on emergent insects over water resulting in a selection of this habitat.

Energy trade-offs in selected habitats

The spatial and temporal variation in food availability could not be measured across the 6,000-km^2 study area. Nevertheless, we believe that using energy as an index of food quality and the relative area covered by each habitat allowed us to assess the relative benefits of different habitats. The strong selection for intensive cultures during incubation corresponded to the period when fields were being cultivated and the new cereal shoots were still at a height that allowed the birds to feed without visual obstruction. This seems to be associated with the occurrence of short periods of high food availability. Although it is difficult to differentiate the confounding effects of the breeding stage from the timing of field work and food availability, the positive effect of soil preparation and seed sowing on the abundance of gulls in agricultural lands during the incubation period (vs. brood-rearing) supports the hypothesis that selection for a specific habitat is higher during the peak of food availability. During our surveys, most gulls foraged in bare soil fields as observed for Black-headed gulls [46]. Moreover, half of the gulls' diet in agricultural lands was made of annelids, which are more accessible when tractors are ploughing and harrowing. Sibly and McCleery [24] have shown a positive relationship between the abundance of Herring gulls (*Larus argentatus*) in agricultural lands and the biomass of earthworms near the ground surface. Yet, the averaged RSFs did not detect an effect of rainfall on the use of agricultural lands despite the positive effect of ground wetness on the availability of annelids and their use by gulls [24]. In agricultural fields, gulls rely on the presence of heavy machinery that cannot work on wet soils. This contrasts with the use of lawns by gulls that was strongly associated with rainfall. Although we could not sample birds using urban areas, the greater availability of annelids on rainy days on lawns and their use by gulls is well established [22]. The other half of the gulls' diet in agricultural lands was made of soybeans and corn, which availability increases when sowing takes place (e.g., seeds accidentally dropped along road and field edges when farmers fill their seeders and seeds sown in superficial ground; M. Patenaude-Monette, pers. obs.). Annelids, soybeans and corn composed a less energy-rich diet than the food gathered by gulls at landfills. Considering that gulls selected the intensive agricultural lands no further than 23 km, we suggest that the profitability of this habitat was limited by the travel costs associated with the distance from the colony and the relatively low energy value of the food.

Gulls selected areas comprising landfills or transhipment sites throughout the breeding season, a period during which food availability at these sites does not vary with time. Although the accessibility (distance from the colony and deterrence program effectiveness) and volume of refuse differed among sites, we could only account for variation in distance from the colony. The selection of landfills was stronger, but also more variable, as the distance increased. Thus, the selection of landfills was probably not constrained by their distance from the colony as was the selection of agricultural lands at the scale of the study area. Nevertheless, its high variability suggests that not all gulls used landfills and transhipment sites. Indeed, landfills and transhipment sites were present in less than 5% of foraging patches of all individuals. Moreover, when refuse food items occurred in boli, they accounted for a much larger proportion of the bolus than any other food items. Furthermore, both the mean bolus mass and the mean energy content of food were much higher in landfills than in any other habitats.

We can hypothesize that gulls incur higher travel costs when foraging in landfills, which are located farther from the colony than agricultural lands [47]. Habitat accessibility is indeed likely to be negatively correlated with the distance separating the foraging site from the nest as travel costs (time, energy) increase with distance [41], [48]. Accordingly, intensively managed agricultural lands may thus provide a profitable net energy gain to foraging gulls despite food items of lower energy value, at least during the incubation period. On the other hand, landfills with their more energy rich food may be valuable foraging sites despite their remoteness and are thereby selected by gulls. The stronger selection observed with increasing distance to the colony (up to 63 km) may result from the fact that the closest sites (<30 km from the colony) included two transhipment sites where refuse is less available than at landfills. Moreover, the Terrebonne landfill that received the largest tonnage of refuse and which is located the closest to the colony has a very effective deterrence program (É. Thiériot, unpublished data).

Time constraints in urban areas

Gulls are known to feed on refuse in commercial and residential areas and on handouts offered by citizens [49]. Nevertheless, we found that breeding Ring-billed Gulls avoided foraging in urban areas located <10 km from the colony, but showed the opposite trend at greater distances. This pattern may result from the profitability of urban areas as foraging sites, which likely depends on the type of development (e.g., residential, commercial, or industrial) and population density. The proportion of time foraging was indeed very low in urban areas where gulls adopted a sit-and-wait strategy to exploit spatially and temporally scattered feeding opportunities (e.g., people handouts and overfilled garbage bins). While the proportion of time foraging was comparable in urban areas and in landfills, foraging opportunities are probably much less predictable in the former habitat. Furthermore, commercial and residential areas of high population densities (i.e., with greater foraging opportunities) were located about 20 km from the colony, which is much further than the closest landfill or agricultural lands. Although urban refuse food may present high energy contents, the time to gather enough refuse is likely too long to make foraging trips to urban areas profitable, particularly during the rearing period when chicks are waiting to be fed at the colony [50], [51]. The situation may nevertheless be different during the post-breeding period when gulls are then actively using urban areas ([52], C. Girault and J.-F. Giroux, unpublished data).

Conclusion

Combining RSF to survey data, diet characterization, and calorimetric analyses allowed us to characterize habitat selection processes of a central-place forager from an energy trade-off perspective. It also shows that other factors such as predation risk associated to deterrence programs at landfills can also play a role in the process of habitat selection at large spatial scales as suggested through the concept of landscape of fear [53]. This approach was applied to a species that had to move over a large area to find food in a heterogeneous environment where habitat profitability also varied in time. Despite the complexity brought up by travel costs and habitat sampling issues, we were able to show that classical optimal foraging theory can make qualitative predictions applicable at the landscape level. This adds to the few evidences that optimal foraging theory has the potential to be scaled-up to the landscape level as predicted by Lima and Zollner [6]. Moreover, once classical models will have been modified such that their constraints are adapted to large spatio-temporal scales (e.g., [11], [54], [55]), GPS data loggers will allow us to test these models by linking the foraging behaviour of individuals to their breeding performance [14]. Such progress would make significant strides toward understanding the links between movement behaviour, habitat selection, fitness, and population dynamics within heterogeneous landscapes. For instance, this approach could be applied to many gull populations around the world to link their dynamics to food availability through landfill, agriculture, and fishery management.

Supporting Information

Figure S1 Residence times of breeding Ring-billed gulls in relation with patch size. Mean coefficient of variation (CV) of residence times within circular patches of different radii centred on locations obtained by GPS data loggers (*N* = 109 birds).
(TIF)

Figure S2 Frequency distribution of residence times of breeding Ring-billed gulls. Residence times were established for 200-m radius circular patches centred on locations obtained by GPS data loggers (*N* = 109 birds).
(TIF)

Table S1 Characteristics of individual Ring-billed gulls tracked during the study.
(PDF)

Acknowledgments

This research was conducted in partnership with the municipalities of Terrebonne, Repentigny, Laval, Charlemagne, Mascouche, Saint-Hippolyte, Sainte-Sophie, Sainte-Anne-des-Plaines, and Saint-Lin-Laurentides. We thank F. St-Pierre and M. Tremblay for field and laboratory assistance and R. Zamojska for diet and calorimetric analyses. S. Benhamou provided valuable advice about residence time computation while A. Desrochers, P. Peres-Neto, and G. Bastille-Rousseau commented an earlier draft of this manuscript.

Author Contributions

Conceived and designed the experiments: MPM JFG MB. Performed the experiments: MPM JFG. Analyzed the data: MPM MB. Contributed reagents/materials/analysis tools: JFG MB. Wrote the paper: MPM. Provided methodological and editorial comments: JFG MB. Supervised the overall field study: JFG.

References

1. Stephen DW, Krebs JR (1986) Foraging theory. Princeton: Princeton University Press. 247 p.
2. Giraldeau L-A, Caraco T (2000) Social foraging theory. Princeton: Princeton University Press. 376 p.
3. Charnov EL (1976) Optimal foraging, the marginal-value theorem. Theor Popul Biol 9: 129–136.
4. Orians GH, Pearson NE (1979) On the theory of central place foraging. In: Horn DJ, Stairs GR, Mitchell DR, editors. Analysis of ecological systems. Columbus: Ohio State University Press. 155–177.
5. Nonacs P (2001) State dependent behavior and the marginal value theorem. Behav Ecol 12: 71–83.
6. Lima SL, Zollner PA (1996) Towards a behavioral ecology of ecological landscapes. Trends Ecol Evol 11: 131–135.
7. Zollner PA, Lima SL (1999) Search strategies for landscape-level interpatch movements. Ecology 80: 1019–1030.
8. Nathan R, Getz WM, Revilla E, Holyoak M, Kadmon R, et al. (2008) A movement ecology paradigm for unifying organismal movement research. P Natl Acad Sci-Biol 105: 19052–19059.

9. Schoener TW (1979) Generality of the size-distance relation in models of optimal feeding. Am Nat 114: 902–914.
10. Olsson O, Brown JS, Helf KL (2008) A guide to central place effects in foraging. Theor Popul Biol 74: 22–33.
11. Bernstein C, Kacelnik A, Krebs JR (1991) Individual decisions and the distribution of predators in a patchy environment. II. The influence of travel costs and structure of the environment. J Anim Ecol 60: 205–225.
12. Beauchamp G, Bélisle M, Giraldeau L-A (1997) Influence of conspecific attraction on the spatial distribution of learning foragers in a patchy habitat. J Anim Ecol 66: 671–682.
13. Owen-Smith N, Fryxell JM, Merrill EH (2010) Foraging theory upscaled: the behavioural ecology of herbivore movement. Philos T Roy Soc B 365: 2267–2278.
14. Gaillard J-M, Hebblewhite M, Loison A, Fuller M, Powell R, et al. (2010) Habitat-performance relationships: finding the right metric at a given spatial scale. Philos T Roy Soc B 365: 2255–2265.
15. Manly BFJ, McDonald LL, Thomas DL, McDonald TL, Erickson WP (2002) Resource Selection by Animals: Statistical Design and Analysis for Field Studies. Second Edition, London: Kluwer Academic, 221 p.
16. Barraquand F, Benhamou S (2008) Animal movements in heterogeneous landscapes: identifying profitable places and homogeneous movement bouts. Ecology 89: 3336–3348.
17. Beyer HL, Haydon DT, Morales JM, Frair JL, Hebblewhite M, et al. (2010) The interpretation of habitat preference metrics under use-availability designs. Philos T Roy Soc B 365: 2245–2254.
18. Bastille-Rousseau G, Fortin D, Dussault C (2010) Inference from habitat-selection analysis depends on foraging strategies. J Anim Ecol 79: 1157–1163.
19. Fauchald P, Tveraa T (2006) Hierarchical patch dynamics and animal movement pattern. Oecologia 149: 383–395.
20. Freitas C, Kovacs KM, Lydersen C, Ims RA (2008) A novel method for quantifying habitat selection and predicting habitat use. J Appl Ecol 45: 1213–1220.
21. Fauchald P, Tveraa T (2003) Using first-passage time in the analysis of area-restricted search and habitat selection. Ecology 84: 282–288.
22. Brousseau P, Lefebvre J, Giroux J-F (1996) Diet of ring-billed gull chicks in urban and non-urban colonies in Quebec. Colon Waterbird 19: 22–30.
23. Pollet IL, Shutler D, Chardine J, Ryder JP (2012) Ring-billed Gulls (*Larus delawarensis*). The Birds of North America Online. Ithaca: Cornell Lab of Ornithology. Available: http://bna.birds.cornell.edu.bnaproxy.birds.cornell.edu/bna/species/033doi:10.2173/bna.33. Accessed 5 July 2013.
24. Sibly RM, McCleery RH (1983) The distribution between feeding sites of herring gulls breeding at Walney island, U.K. J Anim Ecol 52: 51–68.
25. Belant JL, Ickes SK, Seamans TW (1998) Importance of landfills to urban-nesting herring and ring-billed gulls. Landscape Urban Plan 43: 11–19.
26. Thiériot E, Molina P, Giroux J-F (2012) Rubber shots not as effective as selective culling in deterring gulls from landfill sites. Appl Anim Behav Sci 142: 109–115.
27. Fridolfsson AK, Ellegren H (1999) A simple and universal method for molecular sexing of non-ratite birds. J Avian Biol 30: 116–121.
28. Frair JL, Fieberg J, Hebblewhite M, Cagnacci F, DeCesare NJ, et al. (2010) Resolving issues of imprecise and habitat-biased locations in ecological analyses using GPS telemetry data. Philos T Roy Soc B 365: 2187–2200.
29. Altmann J (1974) Observational study of behavior: Sampling methods. Behaviour 49: 227–267.
30. Racine F, Giraldeau L-A, Patenaude-Monette M, Giroux J-F (2012). Evidence of social information on food location in a ring-billed gull colony, but the birds do not use it. Anim Behav 84: 175–182.
31. Batschelet E (1981) Circular statistics in biology. London: Academic Press. 371p.
32. Kotliar NB, Wiens JA (1990) Multiple scale of patchiness and patch structure: a hierarchical framework for the study of heterogeneity. Oikos 59: 253–260.
33. Bellier E, Certain G, Planque B, Monestiez P, Bretagnolle V (2010) Modelling habitat selection at multiple scales with multivariate geostatistics: an application to seabirds in open sea. Oikos 119: 988–999.
34. ESRI (2009) ArcGIS version 9.3.1. Redlands, California.
35. FADQ (2010) Bases de données des cultures assurées 2009 et 2010. Direction des ressources informationnelles, la Financière agricole du Québec, Saint-Romuald, Canada. Available: http://www.fadq.qc.ca/geomatique/professionnels_en_geomatique/base_de_donnees_de_cultures_assurees.html. Accessed 5 December 2011.
36. Natural Resources Canada (2009) Land Cover, Circa 2000, Vector. NRCan, Earth Sciences Sector, Centre for Topographic Information, Sherbrooke, Canada. Available: http://geobase.ca/geobase/en/find.do?produit=csc2000v. Accessed 12 January 2012.
37. Natural Resources Canada (2010) CanVec version 1.1. NRCan, Earth Sciences Sector, Centre for Topographic Information, Sherbrooke, Canada. Available: ftp://ftp2.cits.rncan.gc.ca/pub/canvec/. Accessed 12 January 2012.
38. Environment Canada (2010) National Climate Data and Information Archive. Government of Canada website. Available: http://climate.weather.gc.ca. Accessed 10 January 2011.
39. Shamoun-Baranes J, van Loon E (2006) Energetic influence on gull flight strategy selection. J Exp Biol 209: 3489–3498.
40. Burnham KP, Anderson DR (2002) Model selection and multimodel Inference: a practical information-theoretic approach. Second Edition, New-York: Springer-Verlag. 448 p.
41. Matthiopoulos J (2003) The use of space by animals as a function of accessibility and preference. Ecol Model 159: 239–268.
42. Bates D, Maechler M, Bolker B (2011) Lme4: Linear mixed-effects models using S4 classes. R package version 0.999375-39. Available: http://CRAN.R-project.org/package=lme4. Accessed 20 June 2011.
43. R Development Core Team (2011) R: a language and environment for statistical computing. Version 2.12.2, Vienna. http://www.r-project.org/.
44. Gaston AJ, Ydenberg RC, Smith GEJ (2007) Ashmole's halo and population regulation in seabirds. Mar Ornithol 35: 119–126.
45. Elliot KE, Woo KJ, Gaston AJ, Benvenuti S, Dall'Antonia L, et al. (2009) Central-place foraging in an arctic seabird provides evidence for Storer-Ashmole's halo. Auk 126: 613–625.
46. Schwemmer P, Garthe S, Mundry R (2008) Area utilization of gulls in a coastal farmland landscape: habitat mosaic supports niche segregation of opportunistic species. Landscape Ecol 23: 355–367.
47. Wilson RP, Quintana F, Hobson VJ (2012). Construction of energy landscapes can clarify the movement and distribution of foraging animals. P Roy Soc Lond B Bio 279: 975–980.
48. Rosenberg DK, McKelvey KS (1999) Estimation of habitat selection for central place foraging animals. J Wildl Manage 63: 1028–1038.
49. Belant JL (1997) Gulls in urban environments: landscape-level management to reduce conflict. Landscape Urban Plan 38: 245–258.
50. Bukacinska M, Bukacinski D, Spaans AL (1996) Attendance and diet in relation to breeding success in Herring gulls (*Larus argentatus*). Auk 113: 300–309.
51. Shaffer SA, Costa DP, Weimerskirch H (2003) Foraging effort in relation to the constraints of reproduction in free-ranging albatrosses. Funct Ecol 17: 66–74.
52. Maciusik B, Lenda M, Skorka P (2010) Corridors, local food resources, and climatic conditions affect the utilization of the urban environment by the Black-headed Gull *Larus ridibundus* in winter. Ecol Res 25: 263–272.
53. Searle KR, Stokes CJ, Gordon IJ (2008) When foraging and fear meet: using foraging hierarchies to inform assessments of landscapes of fear. Behav Ecol 19: 475–482.
54. Amano T, Ushiyama K, Moriguchi S, Fujita G, Higuchi H (2006) Decision-making in group foragers with incomplete information: Test of individual-based model in Geese. Ecol Monogr 76: 601–616.
55. Mueller T, Fagan WF (2008) Search and navigation in dynamic environments – from individual behaviors to population distributions. Oikos 117: 654–664.

6

Honey Pollen: Using Melissopalynology to Understand Foraging Preferences of Bees in Tropical South India

Raja Ponnuchamy[1,2], Vincent Bonhomme[1¤a¤b], Srinivasan Prasad[1], Lipi Das[3], Prakash Patel[3], Cédric Gaucherel[1], Arunachalam Pragasam[2], Krishnamurthy Anupama[1*]

1 Department of Ecology, French Institute of Pondicherry, UMIFRE 21 CNRS-MAEE/USR 3330, Pondicherry, India, 2 Department of Botany, Kanchi Mamunivar Centre for Post-Graduate Studies, Pondicherry, India, 3 Sri Aurobindo International Centre of Education, Pondicherry, India

Abstract

The aim of the study was to use melissopalynology to delineate the foraging preferences of bees in tropical environs. This was done by comparing pollen spectra obtained from the same hives every three months for three years at four sampling locations (in two sites) within a confined landscape mosaic. If melissopalynology is highly replicable, the spatial variation of the pollen spectrum from the honey samples would be much more than the temporal (inter-annual) variations. In other words, given the three factors, Month, Year and Location, honey pollen from different Locations, in a given Year and Month, would be much less similar than samples from different Years, in a given Location and Month. We then determined how the factors, Month, Year and Location, influenced the pollen influx of honey. The pollen analyses of the 42 honey samples collected during the three years yielded 80 pollen taxa/types: 72 dicotyledonous and 8 monocotyledonous, encompassing 41 botanical families spread into seven life forms namely, trees, shrubs, epiphytes, herbs, climbers, grasses, and sedges. Our results showed that pollen spectra were equally comparable between Locations and between Months and Years; the importance of this result is that it helped to demonstrate the complexity of ecological/environmental phenomena involved in the process of foraging by bees in a heterogeneous and complex landscape.

Editor: Fabio S. Nascimento, Universidade de São Paulo, Faculdade de Filosofia Ciências e Letras de Ribeirão Preto, Brazil

Funding: Ms. Sieglind D'Arcy provided financial support through a donation that helped provide a Doctoral fellowship to the first author (RP). She had no role in study design, data collection and analysis, decision to publish, or preparation of the manuscript. No other funding is available for this project. Publication fee has been provided by The French Institute of Pondicherry.

Competing Interests: The authors have declared that no competing interests exist.

* Email: anupama.k@ifpindia.org

¤a Current address: School of Mathematics and Statistics, The University of Sheffield, Sheffield, United Kingdom
¤b Current address: Centre de Bio-Archéologie et d'Ecologie, UMR 5059 Université de Montpellier II/CNRS/EPHE, Montpellier, France

Introduction

Bees, the primary pollinators of the world, play a crucial role for wild and cultivated plants, especially in the tropics where insect pollination is vital [1–2]. Melissopalynology is the study of the pollen they collect, intentionally and accidentally, which gets into honey. Melissopalynology has been extensively used [3–10] to determine the purity, geographical and floral origins of honey. It is also used to assess correlations with *in situ* climatic parameters such as rainfall and temperature [11–12] important in the context of external factors influencing pollinators and pollination networks [13–19]. Statistical analyses, mainly ordination, have been carried out on melissopalynological data in quantitative studies to obtain more robust characterization of the honeys in terms of their geographic and botanic origins [20–22].

The many variables that come into play in the production of honey, including the ability of honeybees to remove certain types and certain amounts of pollen from the nectar they collect prior to returning to the hive, have been summarized [23]. Though acknowledged that the complexity introduced by these different variables implies a substantial variation from year to year or season to season in terms of the pollen contents of honey produced in the same hive [23], to our knowledge, this replicability, *i.e.*, stability in time and space, has not been tested statistically. This study attempts to fill the gap using the primary data generated in the course of a pluri-annual melissopalynological survey near Puducherry, South India.

The aim of the study was to use melissopalynology to delineate the foraging preferences of bees in tropical environs. There are several methods, including direct observations and video monitoring (11,14,18–19) to understand the foraging preferences of bees. Analyzing pollen in honey provides a complementary, robust, rapid and quantitative method to do this. This was done by comparing pollen spectra obtained from the same hives every three months for three years at four sampling locations (in two sites) within a confined landscape mosaic. Our hypothesis is that if melissopalynology is highly replicable, the spatial variation of the pollen spectrum from the honey samples would be statistically much more than the temporal (inter-annual) variations. In other words, given the three factors, Month, Year and Location, honey pollen from different Locations, in a given Year and Month, would be much less similar than samples from different Years, in a given Location and Month. We then determined how the factors, Month, Year and Location, influenced the pollen influx into honey.

Here, we test the replicability of melissopalynology for the first time in the tropics and delineate the foraging preferences of bees and provide methodological recommendations for further melissopalynological experimental designs.

Materials and Methods

Ethics statement

The study was conducted in privately owned areas where prior permission was obtained: site 1 to which two of the authors (LD and PP) are affiliated, and site 2 managed by Bernard Declercq and Deepika Kundaji, Auroville. The study did not include any human subjects or vertebrate animals, and honey was collected with minimal disturbance to the honeybees.

Study site

The study was conducted in four locations in two sites that are 6 km apart. The first three locations were in site 1, spread over 160 ha at 40–50 m a.s.l. (11°57′8.3″ N, 79°45′57.2″ E). Location 4 was in site 2 (11°59′20.4″ N, 79°47′4.2″ E and 50 m a.s.l.), spread over 10 ha (Figure 1).

In the Puducherry region, rainfall is distributed over a part of the summer and a part of the (tropical) winter, *i.e.*, from July to January. Much of the rain occurs during the northeast monsoon between October and December (records from Puducherry weather station). Mean temperature in December was 25°C for the years from 1911 to 1961 [24]. In the last three decades (1980–2009), the pattern remained similar.

Bee species, beehive locations, and surrounding vegetation

As part of an ongoing eco-restoration project, particular effort was made to rear the Asiatic honeybee *Apis cerana* Fabricius, one of the native honeybees of India [25]. The bees were reared in wooden beehives placed in four locations. The locations were chosen to reflect the complex mosaic of vegetation (Figure 1; [26]). One beehive per location was considered in this study.

The four locations are Garden and Tropical Dry Evergreen Forest (GT), Coconut Grove (CG), Agricultural Field (AF), and Scrub Jungle (SJ). GT contains ornamental plants, several introduced drought-tolerant *Acacia* spp., *Casuarina junghuhniana* Miq., small patches of restored Tropical Dry Evergreen Forest (TDEF) with characteristic species like *Memecylon umbellatum* Burm. f. and *Allophylus serratus* (Roxb.) Kurz and scrub thicket elements like *Benkara malabarica* (Lam.) Tirveng. and *Ziziphus oenoplia* L. (Mill.). CG comprises a mixed plantation of *Cocos nucifera* L., *Casuarina junghuhniana* Miq. and *Manilkara zapota* (L.) P. Royen, where cereals are intercropped during the monsoon. AF comprises cereals, vegetables, pulses, and tubers, cultivated by usual crop rotation practices, and surrounding plantations of *Citrus* spp., *Cocos nucifera* L., *Mangifera indica* L., *Musa paradisiaca* L., and *Psidium guajava* L. Local herbaceous plants like *Trianthema portulacastrum* L. and *Waltheria indica* L. are common in the CG and AF. The dominant species in SJ are characteristic of scrub jungles: *Benkara malabarica* (Lam.) Tirveng, *Catunaregum spinosa* (Thunb.) Tirveng., *Dodonaea viscosa* (L.) Jacq., *Glycosmis mauritiana* (Lam.) Tanaka, *Flacourtia indica* (Burm. f.) Merr., *Securinega leucopyrus* (Willd.) Muell. -Arg., *Toddalia asiatica (L.)* Lam. var. *gracilis* Gamble, and *Ziziphus oenoplia* L.

Sampling of honey and identification of pollen content

Samples were collected seasonally in the fourth week of February, May, August, and November during 2007, 2008, and 2009 in the four locations, later referred to as the independent variables Month, Year, and Location. A contiguous 10 cm×10 cm area containing pollen cells as well as honey cells from a brood comb was chosen for (pseudo-random) collection. Each sample was collected by squeezing out honey along with pollen without harm to the bees. The honey and pollen samples were collected in sterile containers by two of the authors (LD, RP) exclusively for the melissopalynological studies. We retrieved 42 honey samples; six samples could not be retrieved due to hive abandonment.

Honey was dissolved in warm, distilled water to remove sugars and water soluble components and centrifuged. The supernatant was discarded with care to check for loss of pollen during this procedure. The residue was then processed for pollen studies using standard acetolysis method [27], mounted in glycerine medium and observed under ×500 magnification using a Light optical microscope (Wild M20). Pollen morphological features, as revealed by the qualitative and quantitative features of the outer wall [28–30], formed the basis for the identification and enumeration of pollen types [31–32]. They were identified and enumerated using the reference pollen slides of the French Institute of Pondicherry as well as pollen floras [33–36]. High pollen counts, averaging 6933±3097 were obtained, keeping in mind both tropical diversity and the under- and over- representation of pollen in honey [23]. Pollen frequency classes were assigned using standard procedures [37]. The primary data generated in the course of this study is represented as a pollen diagram (Figure 2) drawn using TILIA [38] and a plate of pollen photomicrographs (Figure 3).

Statistical analysis

All statistical analyses were done using the statistical environment R 2.15.1 [39]. Similarities between pollen spectra were computed using two indices: binary Bray-Curtis' index (bBC) and Bray-Curtis' index (BC). These two indices compare pollen presence/absence and pollen frequencies between samples, respectively, and are calculated as follows [39]:

$$bBC_{jk} = bBC_{kj} = \frac{A+B-2J}{A+B}$$

and

$$BC_{jk} = BC_{kj} = \frac{\sum_i^n |x_{ij} - x_{ik}|}{\sum_i^n (x_{ij} + x_{ik})}$$

For the bBC index, A and B are the numbers of species in samples j and k, and J is the number of species found in the two samples. The BC index uses the absolute distance between x_{ij} and x_{ik}, which are pollen frequencies for the ith over n species in samples j and k.

Multivariate analyses of variance (MANOVA) were performed to test the effects of the independent variables Month, Year and Location on the pollen spectra, the latter being the dependent variable since we aimed at testing if the pollen spectra vary between Months between Years, and between the Locations and if any interaction between these factors exists in our dataset.

We nested Month and Year factors within the Location factor since their repetitions are meaningful only within the same location. For model selection, as no information-based criterion (e.g. Akaike information criterion) is available for MANOVA performed on distances matrices, we used the vegan package [39] and 10^5 permutations to estimate the distribution of the statistics. Then all interactions starting from the full model have been tested; backward procedures were adopted for model selection, with the successive removal of the interactions of the highest order with an

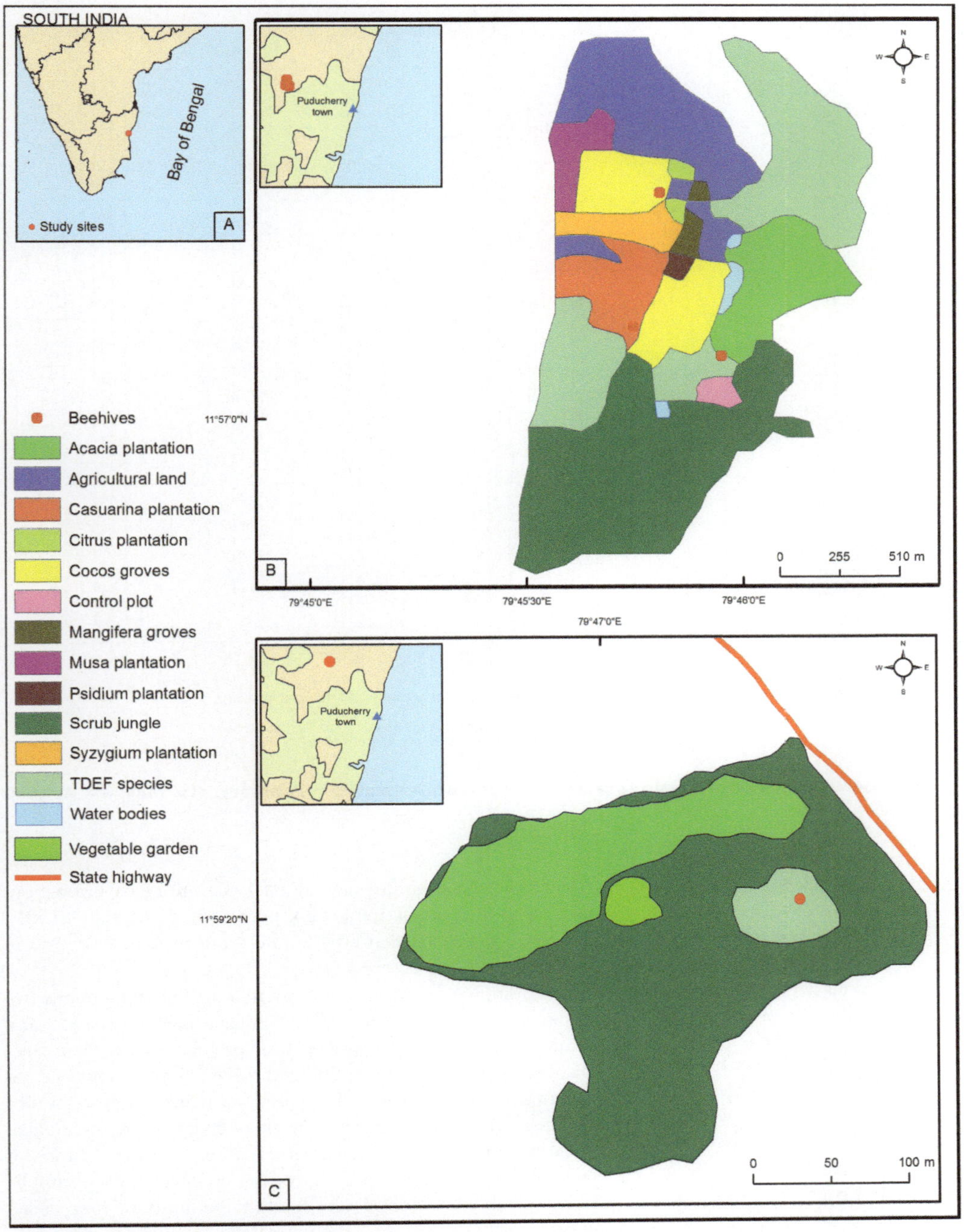

Figure 1. Location detail and mosaic vegetation of study areas. A. South India with state boundaries, B. First three locations in site 1 with surrounding vegetation C. Fourth location in site 2 with surrounding vegetation.

arbitrary threshold $\alpha = 0.05$. Forward selection led to the same final models. Distance matrices and their graphical representation as heatmaps were built using the pair-wise distances for the two indices and between samples.

Principal Component Analyses (PCA) explored how the structure of our experimental design (Month, Year, Location) interplay in the total variance of our dataset as summarized by the principal components. In other words, if the replicability is high among sites, we expect samples of each site to cluster together, no matter which Year or Month they were collected. Then, Linear Discriminant Analyses (LDA) with and without cross-validation (leave-one-out) determined the classification error, i.e., the value of previous knowledge. In other words, if for every sample, we use the grouping structure of all the samples collected but one, and then introduced the left out sample, do we classify it correctly? PCA was performed and illustrated using the ade4 package [40] to explore how pollen taxa and different Months, Years, and Locations are distributed. Confidence ellipses (± 1.5SD on every PC), corresponding to the categories of every factor and drawn a posteriori on the factorial map, help graphically to understand the patterns observed. Scatter correlation circles were then used to explore and attribute the influences of each pollen taxon. Percentages of the

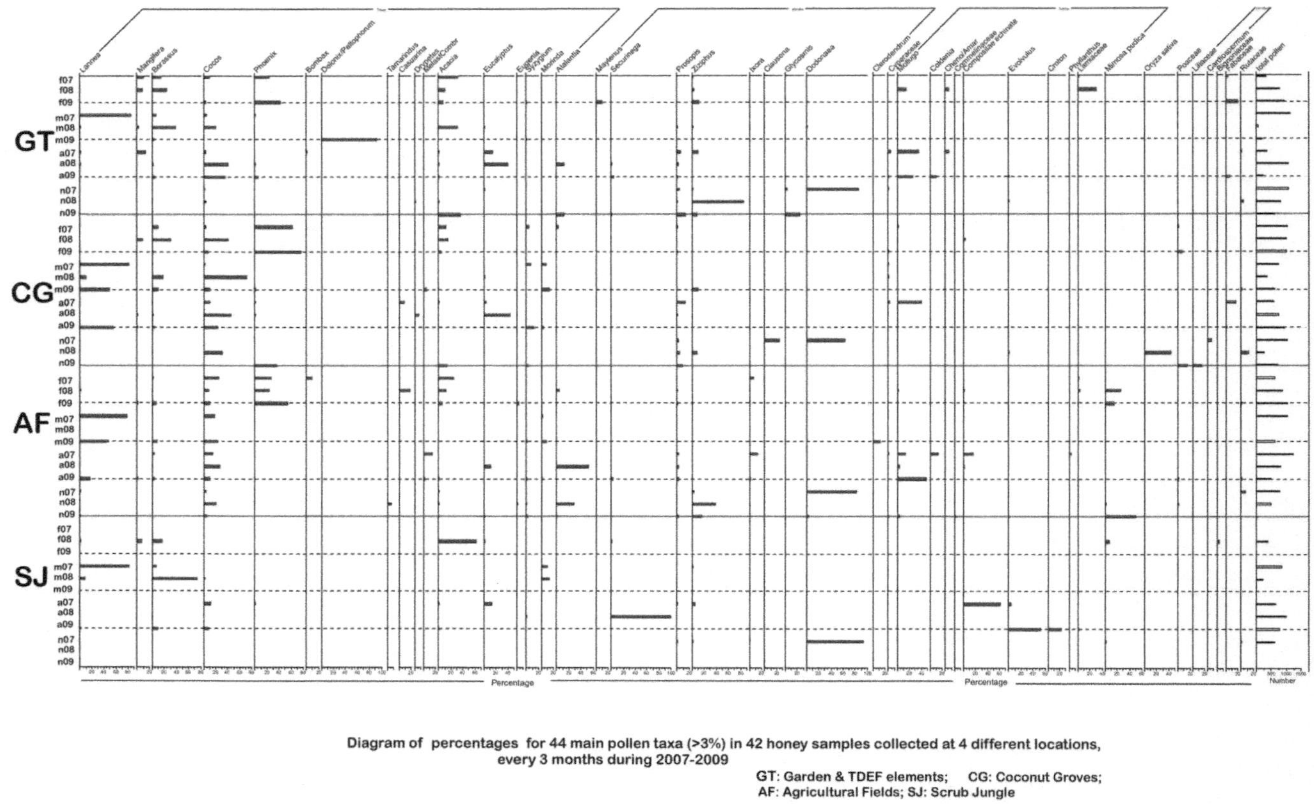

Figure 2. Pollen diagram showing the percentages of the main taxa and the total pollen sum (f = February; m = May; a = August; n = November; 07 = 2007; 08 = 2008; 09 = 2009).

variance explained by the successive PC axes were calculated using the Eigen values of the variance/covariance matrix. LDA was performed using the package MASS [41] to test whether the discriminant linear combinations of pollen taxa were able to discriminate between groups. The standardized discriminant coefficients were used to compare the relative importance of the pollen taxa in order to discriminate within/between groups of samples. Three LD axes were obtained for Month and Location (4 levels each) and two LD axes were obtained for the factor Year (3 levels each).

The LD axes that brought the maximum between-groups differences were considered for each of the factors. LDA was first performed on the complete dataset of 80 taxa. We then tested if LDA can also be used in our case as a tool to classify additional pollen spectra based on this discriminant function, using the leave-one-out cross-validation implemented in the MASS package [41]. The idea behind this validation is simple: every pollen spectrum is successively removed from the dataset and an LDA is performed and then used to classify the pollen spectrum removed. For the final analyses, we retained only the 51 taxa that occurred at least 3 times in our dataset of 42 samples.

Results

Honey pollen content

The pollen analyses of the 42 honey samples collected during the three years yielded 80 pollen taxa/types: 72 dicotyledonous and 8 monocotyledonous, encompassing 41 botanical families spread into seven life forms namely, trees, shrubs, epiphytes, herbs, climbers, grasses, epiphytes and sedges (Table S1). On average, 6933±3097 pollen grains (average ±1 SD are given throughout the text) were counted (min = 283, max = 12356, median = 7591), and 18±7 pollen types (min = 5, max = 30, median = 18.5) were identified per sample.

Three families accounted for more than half the total number of pollen grains: Arecaceae (29%), Anacardiaceae (14%), and Mimosaceae (11%). Arecaceae was present in all, but one, samples. The three most abundant life forms, expressed as percentages of the total pollen count, were trees (39%), shrubs (24%), and herbs (20%). Forty-four out of 80 taxa were recorded at ≥3% of the total (Figure 2). The graph at the extreme right in this figure shows the total number of pollen counted in each sample. Twenty-six honey samples were found to be uni-floral (one pollen taxon occurring at ≥45% of the total pollen count per sample), represented by 14 predominant pollen taxa (Figure 3). As expected, pollen spectra and predominant pollen taxa varied in space and time, a few examples being *Lannea, Dodonaea, Phoenix, Borassus*, and *Cocos* (Figure 2).

Statistical analyses

We performed MANOVAs on the distance matrices calculated using the two similarity indices (Table 1 & Table 2). All the tested factors were highly significant and hence the pollen spectra were not highly replicable.

The average Bray-Curtis (BC) index was 0.3 and the average binary Bray-Curtis (bBC) index was 0.4, graphically shown as heatmaps (Figure 4). Taken individually, each factor was highly significant ($P<10^{-4}$) and retained in the final model. Only the two interactions Year × Location ($P<10^{-3}$) and Year × Month

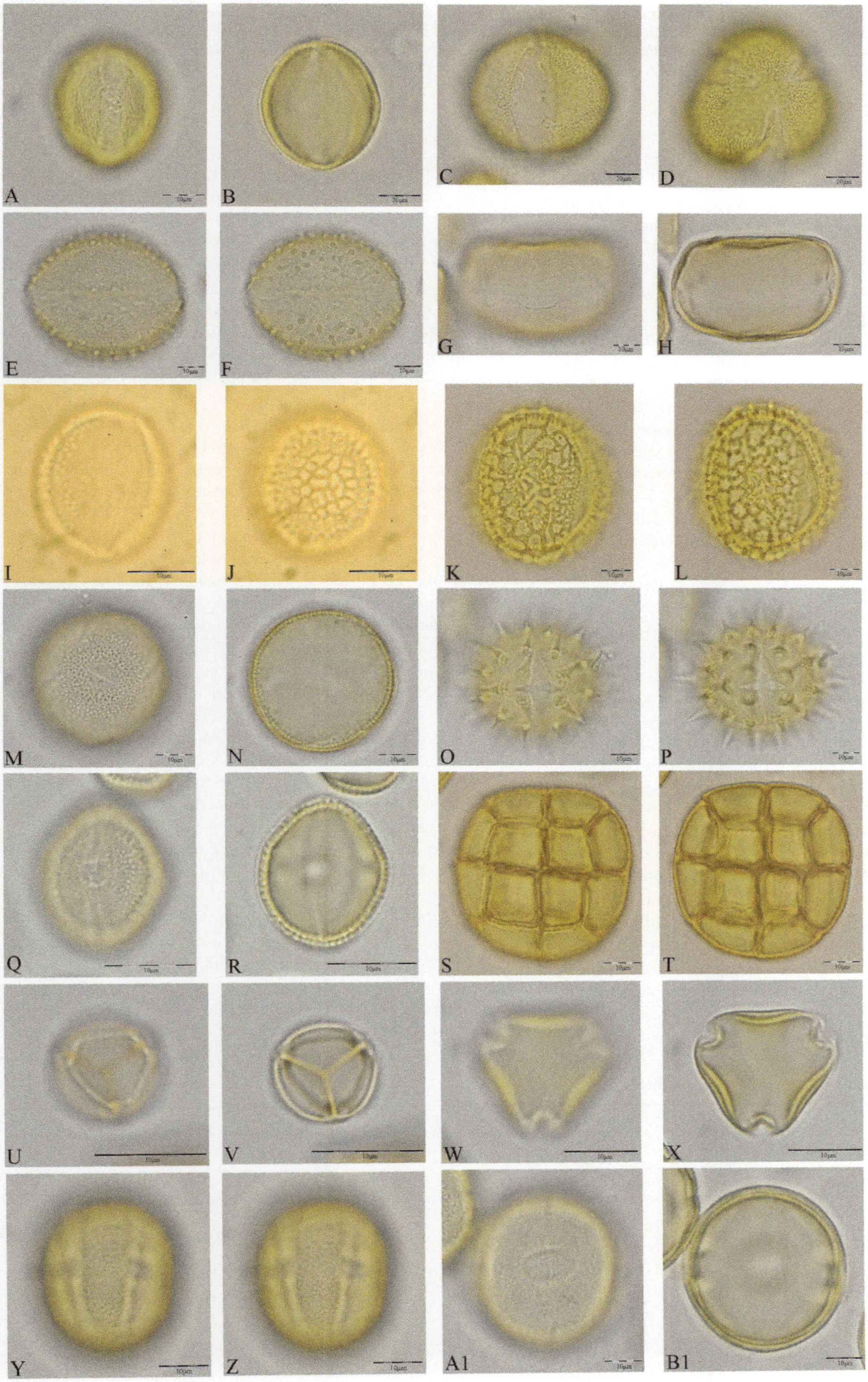
A
B
C
D
E
F
G
H
I
J
K
L
M
N
O
P
Q
R
S
T
U
V
W
X
Y
Z
A1
B1

Figure 3. Photomicrographs showing the 14 predominant pollen types *i.e.*, uni-floral origin (a single pollen type represented >45% of total observed pollen types in a sample) in the 42 honey samples arranged ascending order of family: A–B *Lannea*; C–D *Mollugo*; E–F *Borassus*; G–H *Cocos*; I–J *Phoenix*; K–L *Delonix/Peltophorum*; M–N *Evolvulus*; O–P Compositae-echinate; Q–R *Securinega*; S–T *Acacia*; U–V *Mimosa pudica*; W–X Rhamnaceae; Y–Z *Atalantia*; A1–B1 *Dodonaea*.

($P<10^{-4}$) were significant in the bBC model; only Year × Month ($P<10^{-2}$) was retained in the final BC model (Tables 1a & 1b). The heatmaps showed accordingly no well-defined patterns: when samples were arranged location-wise, there were no higher similarity values along the matrix diagonal (Figure 4), as expected. The only "structure" was that the least similar sample pairs (blue and shades of blue) correspond to samples in different locations in a given year and month (Figure 4, BC model). Similar heatmaps were obtained when arranged month-wise and year-wise.

Only a few highly abundant taxa (*Dodonaea*, *Lannea*, *Phoenix*, and *Acacia*) appeared distinctive in the plots on the first two PC axes. The first two PC axes captured 38% (PC1 = 21%; PC2 = 17%) of the total variance (Figure 5D). The graphical relative distribution of the pollen taxa showed two trends on the plot using PC1 and PC2 as principal axes (Figure 5A–D). Moreover, *Dodonaea* and *Lannea* were pronounced on the two directions along two PC axes. First, a clear Month effect was identified (Figure 4A). Then, in the factors Year (Figure 5B) and Location (Figure 5C), such grouping was not as pronounced. In addition, most multi-floral honey samples overlapped.

In the final LDA, retaining only 51 taxa, samples were well classified with reference to all three factors (Figure 6). The discriminant coefficient values were high for 15 taxa with reference to one or more factors (Figure 6). *Madhuca* was identified as the most discriminant taxa for Month and Year and, overall, the taxa with the highest discriminant value. Other taxa with high discriminant values for all factors were *Cassia*, *Grewia*, Commelinaceae, and Malvaceae. Most of the taxa with high discriminant power were "low abundance" taxa. The discriminant coefficient values were low (<0.01) for the remaining 35 taxa (Figure 6). Several of the set of taxa with coefficient values closer to zero corresponded to "high abundance" taxa (*e.g.*, *Dodonaea*, *Lannea*, *Phoenix*, *Acacia*, and *Cocos*), of which many were pronounced along the first two PC axes. Results of leave-one-out cross validation also indicated that only one sample was misclassified for each of the tested factors: Month ("CGn08"), Year ("GTn09"), and Location ("SJa09"). Two out of 3 misclassified samples were designated as multi-floral origin. The analysis helped delineate the pollen taxa of importance *vis-à-vis* the considered factors, found in both high and low proportions in the honey samples.

Discussion

Our results showed that pollen spectra were equally comparable between Locations and also between Months and Years; the importance of this result, is that it helped to demonstrate the complexity of ecological/environmental phenomena involved in the process of foraging by bees in a heterogeneous and complex landscape. This shows that single, random samples of honey are not likely to provide reliable replicates of the pollen spectra. Furthermore, samples and taxa groups were well delineated based on the three factors considered; the importance of this result is that we now have a tool to classify additional pollen spectra, even when there is a low overall replicability.

The honey pollen content reflected the vegetation characterized by Tropical Dry Evergreen Forest (TDEF) species typical of Coromandel Coast [42–44]; markers were both predominant (*e.g.*, *Lannea*, *Dodonaea*, and *Mollugo*) and less-represented (*e.g.*, Melastomataceae/Combretaceae, *Drypetes* and *Glycosmis*). Taxa such as *Lannea*, *Dodonaea*, *Cocos* and *Borassus* have been reported to be foraged by the same bee species in other parts of south India [8,45]. Some taxa such as Poaceae and Cyperaceae, generally reported in very low proportions, were frequently found in our samples, sometimes in considerable proportions. The present study, one of the first comprehensive melissopalynological contributions to the TDEF in the context of plant-pollinator interaction, is unique in that it documents, over time and space, differences in the pollen contents of honey, even within the confined landscape mosaic. At larger spatial sampling scales, this method is likely to throw up even more differences. As floral availability in the immediate vicinity of the beehive was ensured at all sites during most seasons, we assumed that the bees did not go into neighbouring sites to forage.

Bees are considered to be predominant pollen vectors in tropical forests [46–49], yet studies limited to bees in Southeast Asia are rare [48], thus there is an urgent need for forest bee community level data [50] for natural regeneration and restoration.

We found 80 pollen taxa from 42 samples. In a compilation of honey collected across a few hundred kilometers of Andhra Pradesh in south India, 104 taxa were reported from 164 samples [8]. In general, melissopalynological studies used random sampling because the main concern was determining the broad geographic

Table 1. MANOVA table for binary Bray-Curtis' distance.

MANOVA on binary Bray-Curtis' distances						
Response variable: Bray-Curtis' distances	**df**	**SSQ**	**MSQ**	**F**	**R^2**	**Pr(>F)**
Year	2	1.3910	0.6955	4.3182	0.0906	**<0.0001**
Location	3	1.1849	0.3950	2.4522	0.0772	**<0.0001**
Month	3	4.5184	1.5061	9.3511	0.2944	**<0.0001**
Year × Location	6	1.5822	0.2637	1.6373	0.1031	**0.0021**
Year × Month	6	3.2889	0.5482	3.4033	0.2143	**<0.0001**
Residuals	21	3.3823	0.1610		0.2204	
Total	41	15.3477			1	

Table 2. MANOVA table for Bray-Curtis' distances. df, SSQ, MSQ stand for degrees of freedom, sum of squares, mean squares.

MANOVA on Bray-Curtis' distances						
Response variable: Binary Bray-Curtis' distances	**df**	**SSQ**	**MSQ**	**F**	**R^2**	**Pr(>F)**
Year	2	0.7887	0.39435	3.4524	0.1091	**0.0002**
Location	3	0.7635	0.25450	2.2281	0.1056	**<0.0001**
Month	3	1.6813	0.56044	4.9065	0.2326	**<0.0001**
Year × Month	6	0.9098	0.15163	1.3275	0.1259	0.0637
Residuals	27	3.0840	0.11422		0.4267	
Total	41	7.2273			1	

Only the final models are shown.

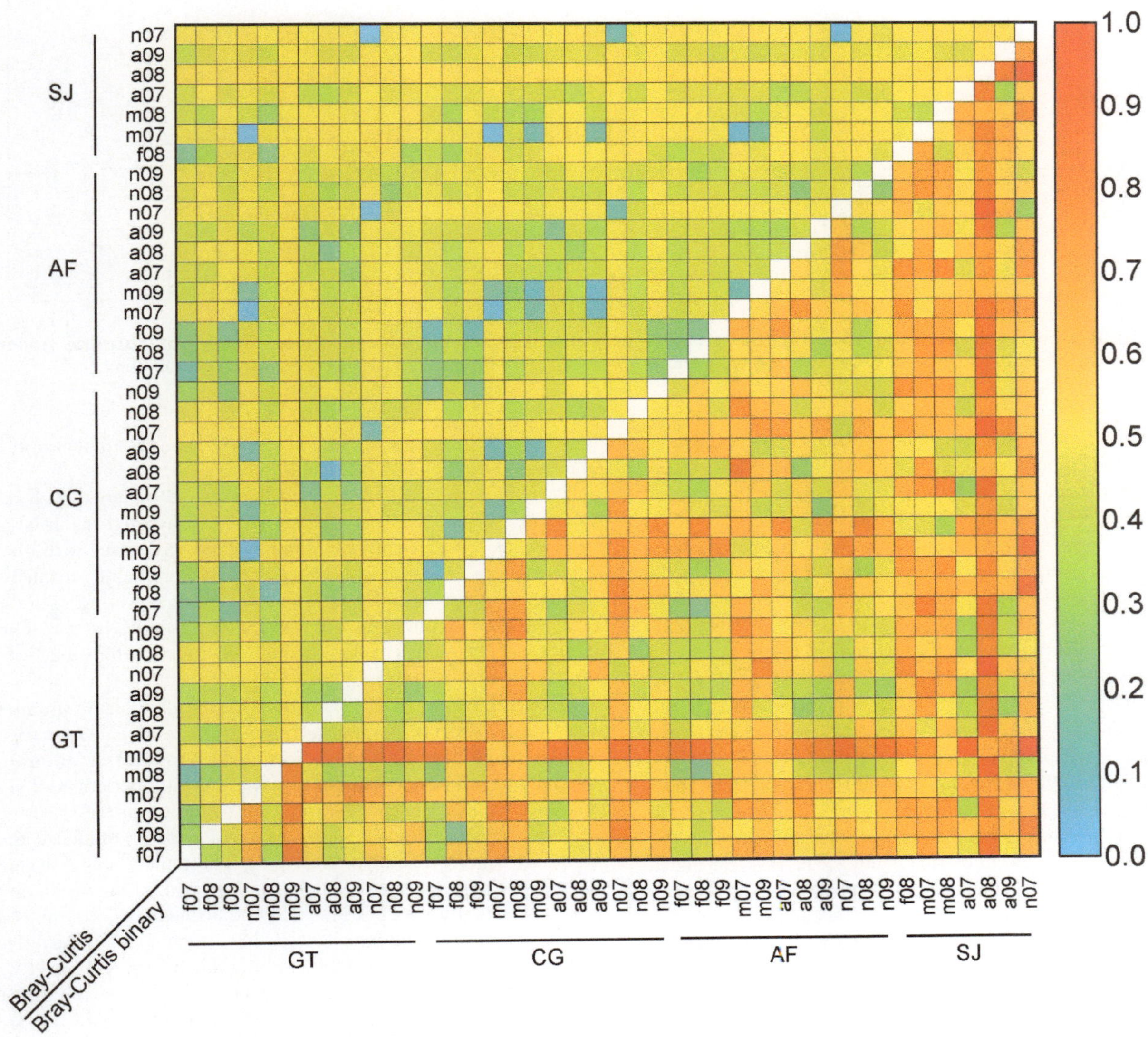

Figure 4. Pair-wise comparison of qualitative and quantitative melissopalynology for pollen similarity studies.

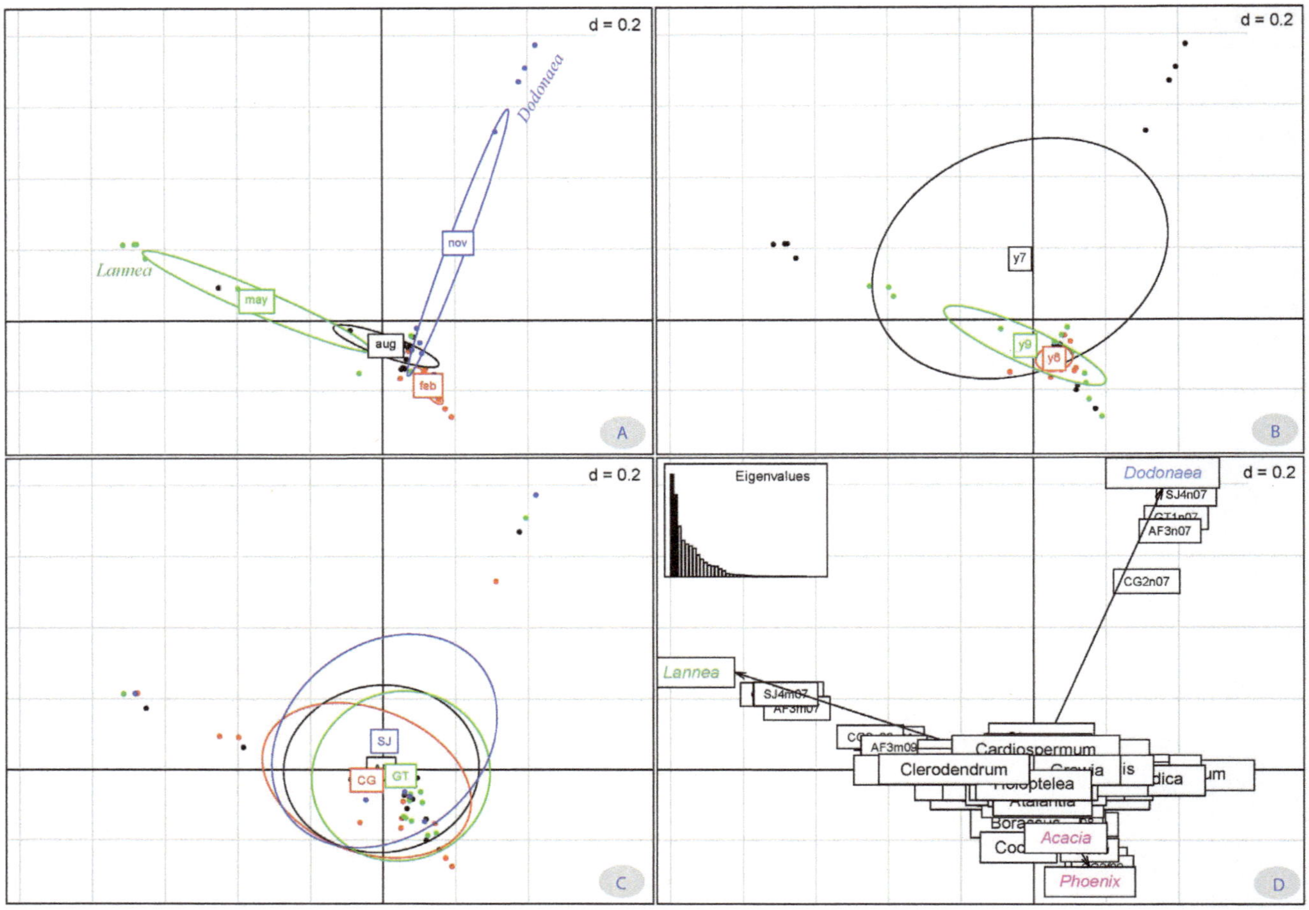

Figure 5. Multivariate analyses (PCA) showing the structure of pollen spectra in reduced dimensionality of absolute pollen frequency. A = Month-wise, B = Year-wise, C = Location-wise, and D = Percentage of Eigen value and overall variance distribution.

origins of honey, which did not require long term monitoring. Thanks to our methodology of achieving high pollen counts, we report here, in a smaller geographic space, a comparable number of taxa, allowing us to exploit other statistical analyses.

We found a higher degree of similarity with qualitative index (bBC) and no structure with quantitative index (BC), probably due to the complex web of factors influencing the pollen content of honey. Apart from phenology and such other "external" ecological/environmental factors, factors related to bee behaviour such as the individual ability of some bees to remove more or less pollen from the nectar they collect [23] also come into play in this complexity. Similarity indices and ordination analyses were used to classify honey samples based on their spatial location over two provinces in Spain [20]. They found similar trends, the focus being botanical and again broad geographic origins. However, the temporal variations were not taken into account in that study. To our knowledge, in India only one study [51] has calculated qualitative indices on 6 samples collected in the same season; quantitative indices have not been reported for India.

Recent studies have effectively used similarity indices as well as ordination techniques such as PCA and LDA [21,52–53] to classify the honey samples in terms of their botanical and geographic origins. Because of the temporal dimension in our study adding MANOVA was useful. Combining multivariate techniques (MANOVA, PCA, and LDA) with the pollen counts helped us to classify the samples in terms of factorial influences and understand the dynamics of bee foraging preferences.

Ordination analyses helped delineate pollen taxa such as *Dodonaea*, *Lannea*, *Phoenix* and *Acacia* collected by the bees in large proportions. Species corresponding to these taxa have a distinct flowering season in contrast with *Cocos*, which remained available through most seasons. Even during the peak flowering of these taxa, the bees continued to visit and gather pollen from *Cocos*. This finding supports the results of others [8,45] regarding the bees' preference of *Cocos* pollen.

Lannea and *Dodonaea* were consistently recorded during summer and winter seasons, respectively, but their abundances varied inter-annually due to variations in rainfall. Seasonal variations in rainfall and soil water availability drive flowering periodicity [54–56]. In a tropical context, the physical condition of the sites, the neighboring vegetation, and the effect of animals influence the variation of individual phenology [57]. These may have reflected spatial differences in the pollen assemblages within the vegetation mosaic of our study area, which however seemed less pronounced than the other (temporal) factors like phenology. Thus, this method can be used for tracing floral phenology across years (scarce versus good flowering) and its effect on bees as the major pollinator in the community.

Discriminant analysis helped to highlight taxa found in small proportions in the honey, such as *Madhuca*, *Cassia*, *Grewia*, Commelinaceae and Malvaceae. Our direct observations [Pon-

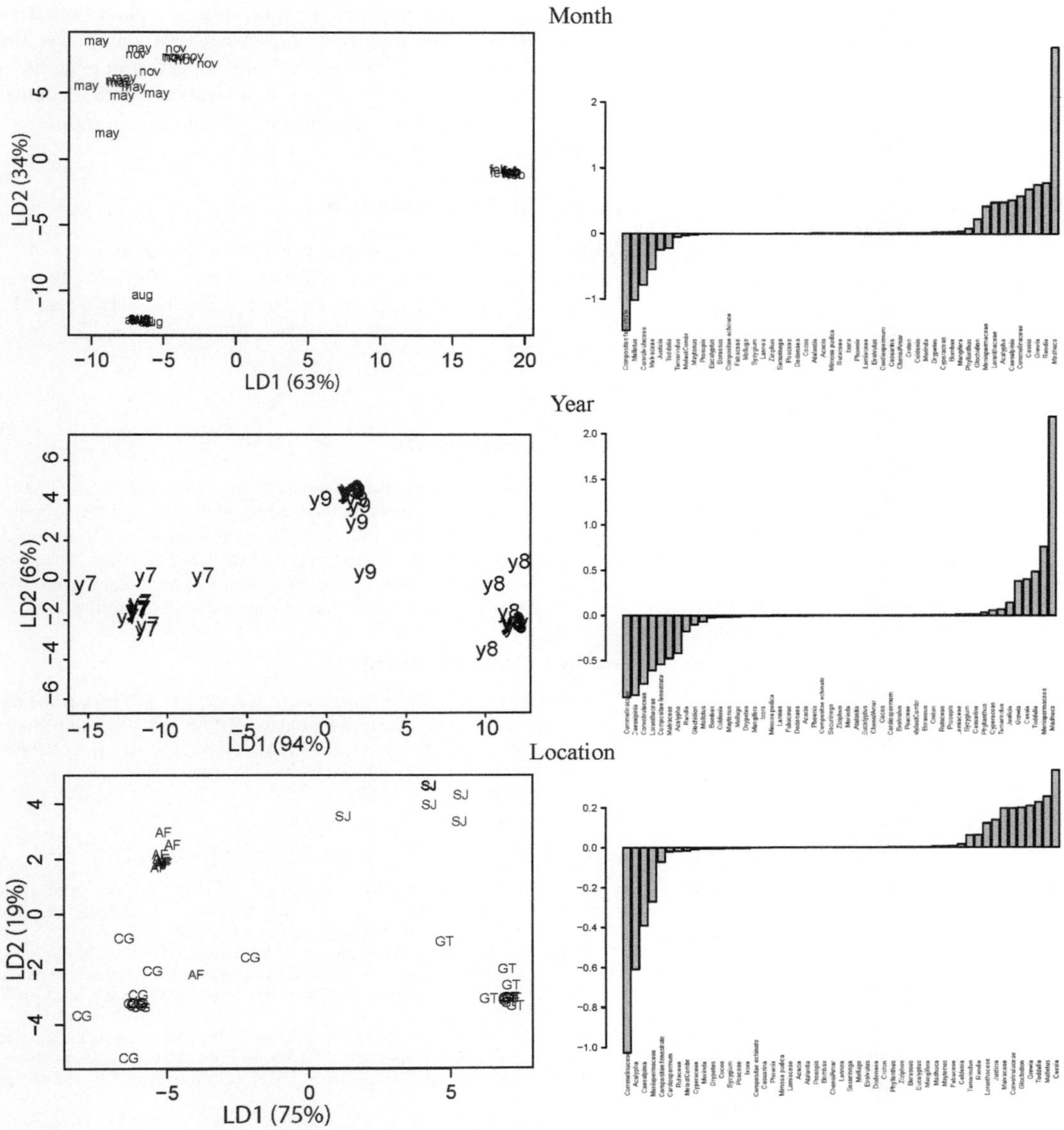

Figure 6. Multivariate analyses (LDA) showing the group membership of honey with reference to spatio-temporal factor and discriminant coefficient value of individual pollen type. For Month and Location, the third LD axis did not bring major between-groups differences; therefore only the first two axes have been retained.

nuchamy (2014), PhD Thesis, Pondicherry University, India] corroborate that they frequently visit the species corresponding to these taxa. Though frequently in low abundances, the consistent presence of these taxa in the honey suggests that, rather than serving as the bees' reward, they may actually be getting the benefit of pollination (by the bees). Some other studies [21–22,53] also used discriminant analyses to highlight low abundance taxa. Though not in the purview of the present study, this highlights the need to quantify the pollen present in the nectar [58], for the tropical plant taxa, documented here as potential bee-plants (Table S1).

Though our analyses highlighted only a few outliers or misclassified samples, it seems likely that this may be a result of source scarcity or bees' preference. Some additional taxa with low discriminant power such as *Atalantia, Phoenix* and *Ziziphus* are among the broad geographic indicators of the Coromandel Coastal environment.

Part of the reason for the apparent wide variation in the pollen data results may be directly attributed to sampling a combination of both pollen cells and honey cells. We accept that such sampling could account for much of the differences found in the samples collected during different seasons as well as years. In other words, our results reflect not only the primary nectar sources of the bees but also the primary pollen collecting plant sources. Studies in other geographic areas [9,46] have shown that the primary nectar and primary pollen foraging plants are usually different. It is true that sometimes in a hive a minor amount of pollen might be collected from a primary nectar source, as the bees eliminate much, but not all, of the pollen they collected with the nectar; the reverse is sometimes also true when the bee has no time to remove large quantities of pollen from the nectar, but rarely are the same plants used primarily for both aspects [7,59]. However, our field observations in south India have shown that bees can source a) nectar alone from some plants (e.g., *Lawsonia inermis* L., *Neolamarckia cadamba* (Roxb.) Bosser and *Pongamia pinnata* (L.) Pierre) b) pollen alone from some plants (e.g., *Cocos nucifera* L., *Oryza sativa* L. and *Peltophorum pterocarpum* (DC.) K. Heyne) and c) pollen and nectar from some plants (e.g., *Haematoxylum campechianum* L., *Derris ovalifolia* (Wight & Arn.) Benth. and *Dodonaea viscosa* (L.) Jacq.,). The other aspect is that bees are opportunists that often gather pollen from plants that are easily accessed from their hives and as opportunists, choose plants that can provide them both nectar and pollen. This aspect could easily explain how the honey examined from our study area in South India contained ample amounts of anemophilous pollen from plants that are not used for nectar sources. Those pollen undoubtedly came from the pollen storage cells that were incorporated into honey samples that were studied.

A potential future experimental design is a small tweak to the methodology: to separately collect and process 1) only the pollen cells from the brood comb 2) only the capped honey cells from the brood comb and c) only capped honey cells from the super, with the hypothesis of a higher overall replicability.

Spatial and temporal factors as well as bees' preferences can play a vital role in honey pollen influx, which ultimately affects replicability. Results show that melissopalynological sampling in conjunction with multivariate statistics is a powerful tool to help classify honeys and understand the foraging preferences of bees in space and time. Our methodology also allowed us to assess replicability, which underlined the need for systematic studies incorporating both the spatial and temporal dimensions, especially in tropical conditions. With an appropriate experimental design taking into account all the complexities of plant-pollinator interactions at a community level, melissopalynology has the potential to provide a holistic ecological perspective in generating data from several landscapes or within a landscape in the context of climate change or effects on the pollinator community or ecosystem functions and services.

Supporting Information

Table S1 List of pollen taxa recorded during the analyses of 42 honey samples collected over a 3 year period (2007–2009) near Puducherry South India. Note: Herbs (H); Shrubs (SH); Trees (T); Climbers (C); Sedges (SE); Grasses (G); Epiphytes (E); Non-Classified (NC).
(DOC)

Acknowledgments

We are thankful to the team members of Project Ecolake for facilitating and helping with the fieldwork and colleagues at the Ecology Department, French Institute of Pondicherry for useful discussions during this project. We thank Dr. Nina Sengupta, Auroville and Dr. Gary Burkhart, School of Medicine, Marseille for reading earlier versions of this manuscript. We thank the two reviewers for their suggestions on our manuscript.

Author Contributions

Conceived and designed the experiments: KA PP LD SP. Performed the experiments: RP LD SP. Analyzed the data: RP SP KA VB. Contributed reagents/materials/analysis tools: LD PP AP VB. Wrote the paper: RP KA VB SP. Research design of statistics: VB RP. Critical review and suggestions: CG.

References

1. Winfree R (2010) The conservation and restoration of wild bees. Annals of the New York Academy of Sciences 1195: 169–197.
2. Ollerton J, Winfree R, Tarrant S (2011) How many flowering plants are pollinated by animals? Oikos 120: 321–326.
3. Waters R (1915) Pollen grains as source-indicators of honey. The Journal of Agriculture 11: 213–215.
4. Nair PKK (1964) A pollen analytical study of Indian honeys. The Journal of the Indian Botanical Society 43(2): 171–191.
5. Maurizio A (1975) Microscopy of honey. In: Crane E (ed.) Honey, a comprehensive survey; Crane, Russak & Co., New York. 240–257.
6. Moar NT (1985) Pollen analysis of New Zealand honey. New Zealand Journal of Agricultural Research 28: 39–70.
7. Jones GD, Bryant VM (1992) Melissopalynology in the United States: a review and critique. Palynology 16: 63–71.
8. Ramanujam CGK, Kalpana TP, Fatima K (1992) Melittopalynology and recognition of major nectar and pollen sources for honey bees in some districts of Andhra pradesh. In: Venkatachala BS, Jain KP, Awasthi N (eds)- Proc. Birbal Sahni Birth Centenary Palaeobotanical Conference. Geophytology 22: 261–271.
9. Sajwani A, Farooq SA, Patzelt A, Eltayeb EA, Bryant VM (2007) Melissopalynological studies from Oman. Palynology 31: 63–79.
10. Song XY, Yao Y-F, Yang W-D (2012) Pollen analysis of natural honeys from the central region of Shanxi, North China. Plos One 7(11): e49545. doi:10.1371/journal.pone.0049545.
11. Jato MV, Iglesias MI, Rodriguez-Gracia VR (1994) A contribution to the environmental relationship of the pollen spectra of honeys from Ourense (NW Spain). Grana 33: 260–267.
12. Bilisik A, Cakmak I, Blcakci A, Malyer H (2008) Seasonal variation of collected pollen loads of honeybees (*Apis mellifera* L. anatoliaca). Grana 47: 70–77.
13. Herrera CM (1995) Floral biology, Microclimate, and Pollination by Ectothermic bees in an early-blooming herb. Ecology 76(1): 218–228.
14. Jens MO, Bascompte J, Elberling H, Jordano P (2008) Temporal dynamics in a pollination network. Ecology 89:1573–1582. http://dx.doi.org/10.1890/07-0451.1.
15. Rands SA, Whitney HM, (2008) Floral temperature and optimal foraging: Is heat a feasible floral reward for pollinators? Plos One 3(4): e2007. doi:10.1371/journal.pone.0002007.
16. Thomas SG, Rehel SM, Varghese A, Davidar P, Potts SG (2009). Social bees and food plant associations in the Nilgiri Biosphere Reserve, India. Tropical Ecology 50(1): 79–88.
17. Baldock KCR, Memmott J, Ruiz-Guajardo JC, Roze D, Stone GN (2011) Daily temporal structure in African Savanna flower visitation networks and consequences for network sampling. Ecology 92(3): 687–698.
18. Selva Singh Richard P, Muthukumar S, Malleshappa H (2011) Relationship between Floral Characters and Floral Visitors of Selected Angiospermic Taxa from Kalakad Mundanthurai Tiger Reserve, Southern Western Ghats, India. Indian Forester 137(8): 962–975.
19. Nascimento DL, Nascimento FS (2012) Extreme effects of season on the foraging activities and colony productivity of a stingless bee (Melipona asilvai Moure, 1971) in Northeast Brazil. 2012: Article ID 267361, 6 pages. doi:10.1155/2012/267361.
20. Herrero B, Valencia-Barrera RM, Martin RS, Pando V (2002) Characterization of honeys by melisssopalynology and statistical analysis. Canadian Journal of Plant Science 82: 75–82.
21. Corbella E, Cozzolino D (2008) Combining multivariate analysis and pollen count to classify honey samples accordingly to different botanical origins. Chilean Journal of Agricultural Research 68(1): 102–107.
22. Aronne G, De micco V (2010) Traditional melissopalynology integrated by multivariate analysis and sampling methods to improve botanical and geographical characterization of honeys. Plant Biosystems 144(4): 833–840.
23. Bryant VM, Jones GD (2001) The R-values of honey: Pollen coefficients. Palynology 25: 11–18.
24. Meher-Homji VM (1966) The climate of Pondicherry. The Indian Geographical Journal 41(1&2): 9–17.
25. Oldroyd BP, Nanork P (2009). Conservation of Asian bees. Apidologie 40: 296–312.
26. Ponnuchamy R, Pragasam A, Aravajy S, Patel P, Das L, et al. (2013) A floristic study on herbs and climbing plants at Puducherry, South India - an approach to biodiversity conservation and regeneration through eco-restoration. Check List: 9(3): 555–600.
27. Erdtman G (1960) The acetolysis method a revised description. Svensk Botanisk Tidskrift 54: 561–564.
28. Wodehouse RP (1959) Pollen Grains Their structure, identification and significance in science and medicine. Hafner Publishing Co. New York, 574pp.
29. Erdtman G (1969) Pollen morphology and Plant taxonomy. Hafner publishing company, 553pp.
30. Punt W, Hoen PP, Blackmore S, Nilsson S, Le Thomas A (2007) Glossary of pollen and spore terminology. Review of Palaeobotany and Palynology 143: 1–81.
31. Faegri K, Iversen J, Kaland PE, Krzywinski K (1989) Text Book of Pollen Analysis. 4th Edition, John Wiley & Sons Ltd, 328pp.

32. Moore PD, Webb JA, Collinson ME (1991) Pollen analysis. 2nd edition, Blackwell Scientific Publications, 216pp & 271 plates.
33. Huang T-C. (1972) Pollen Flora of Taiwan. National Taiwan University Botany Department Press, 297pp & 177 plates.
34. Vasanthy G (1976) Pollen of the South Indian Hills. Institut Francais de Pondichery, 74pp & 34 plates.
35. Nayar TS (1990) Pollen flora of Maharashtra State, India. Today & Tomorrow's printers & publishers, New Delhi, 157pp & 67 plates.
36. Tissot C, Chikhi H, Nayar TS (1994) Pollen of wet evergreen forests of the Western Ghats, India. Publications du departement d'écologie, Institut Francais de Pondichéry, 55pp & 78plates.
37. Louveaux J, Maurizio A, Vorwohl G (1978) Methods of melissopalynology. Bee World 59: 139–157.
38. Grim EC (1987) TILIA and TILIA * Graph. Illinois state Museum, Springfield, IL, USA (http://wwwncdcnoaagov/paleo/tiliahtml).
39. Oksanen FJ, Blanchet G, Kindt R, Legendre P, Minchin PR, et al. (2011) vegan: Community Ecology Package. R package version 2.0-2. http://CRAN.R-project.org/package = vegan.
40. Dray S, Dufour AB (2007) The ade4 package: implementing the duality diagram for ecologists. Journal of Statistical Software 22: 1–20.
41. Venables WN, Ripley BD (2002) Modern Applied Statistics with S. Fourth Edition. Springer, New York.
42. Champion HG, Seth SK (1968) A revised survey of the Forest Types of India. Government of India Press, New Delhi, 404pp.
43. Meher-Homji VM (1974) On the origin of the Tropical Dry Evergreen Forest of South India. Journal of Ecology and Environmental Sciences 1: 19–39.
44. Parthasarathy N, Selwyn MA, Udayakumar M (2008) Tropical Dry Evergreen forests of Peninsular India: ecology and conservation significance. Tropical Conservation Science 1(2): 89–110.
45. Bhargava HR, Jyothi JVA, Bhushanam M, Surendra NS (2009) Pollen analysis of Apis honey, Karnataka, India. Apiacta 44: 14–19.
46. Sharma M (1970) An analysis of pollen loads of Honeybees from Kangra, India. Grana 10: 35–42.
47. Bawa KS (1990) Plant-pollinator interactions in tropical rain forests. Annual Review of Ecology and Systematics 21: 399–422.
48. Corlett RT (2004) Flower visitors and pollination in the oriental (Indo-Malayan) region. Biological Review 79: 497–532.
49. Schemske DW, Mittelbach GH, Cornell HV, Sobel JM, Roy K (2009) Is there a latitudinal gradient in the importance of biotic interactions? Annual Review of Ecology and Systematics 40: 245–269.
50. Liow LH, Sodhi NS, Elmqvist T (2001) Bee diversity along a disturbance gradient in tropical lowland forests of Southeast Asia. Journal of Applied Ecology 38: 180–192.
51. Jhansi P, Kalpana TP, Ramanujam CGK (1994) Pollen analysis of some Apis cerana Fabr honeys from Andhra Pradesh, India. Apidologie 25: 289–296.
52. Bogdanov S, Haldimann M, Luginbuhl W, Gallmann P (2007) Minerals in honey: environmental, geographical and botanical aspects. Journal of Agricultural Research and Bee World 46(4): 269–275.
53. Montenegro G, Pena RC, Pizarro R (2010) Multivariate analysis of pollen frequency of the native species *Escallonia pulverulenta* (Saxifragaceae) in Chilean honeys. Rivista Brasilian Botany 33(4): 615–630.
54. Sivaraj N, Krishnamurthy VK (1989) Flowering phenology in the vegetation of Shervaroys, South India. Vegetatio 79: 85–88.
55. Rivera G, Borchert R (2001) Induction of flowering in tropical trees by a 30-min reduction in photoperiod: evidence from field observations and herbarium specimens. Tree Physiology 21: 201–212.
56. Borchert R, Meyer SA, Felger RS, Porter-Bolland L (2004) Environmental control of flowering periodicity in Costa Rican and Mexican tropical dry forests. Global Ecology and Biogeography 13: 409–425.
57. Bawa KS, Kang H, Grayum MH (2003) Relationship among time, frequency, and duration of flowering in tropical rain forest trees. American Journal of Botany 90(6): 877–887.
58. Todd FE, Vansell GH (1942). Pollen grains in nectar and honey. Journal of Economic Entomology 35: 728–731.
59. Sajwani A, Farooq SA, Bryant VM (2014). Studies of bee foraging plants and analysis of pollen pellets from hives in Oman. Palynology. doi:10.1080/01916122.2013.871652.

Green Manure Addition to Soil Increases Grain Zinc Concentration in Bread Wheat

Forough Aghili[1]*, Hannes A. Gamper[1], Jost Eikenberg[2], Amir H. Khoshgoftarmanesh[3], Majid Afyuni[3], Rainer Schulin[4], Jan Jansa[5], Emmanuel Frossard[1]

1 Institute of Agricultural Sciences, Department of Environmental Systems Science, Swiss Federal Institute of Technology (ETH) Zürich, Switzerland, **2** Paul Scherrer Institute (PSI), Radioanalytics Laboratory, Villigen, Switzerland, **3** College of Agriculture, Department of Soil Sciences, Isfahan University of Technology, Isfahan, Iran, **4** Institute of Terrestrial Ecosystems, Department of Environmental Systems Science, Swiss Federal Institute of Technology (ETH) Zürich, Switzerland, **5** Institute of Microbiology, Academy of Sciences of the Czech Republic, Prague, Czech Republic

Abstract

Zinc (Zn) deficiency is a major problem for many people living on wheat-based diets. Here, we explored whether addition of green manure of red clover and sunflower to a calcareous soil or inoculating a non-indigenous arbuscular mycorrhizal fungal (AMF) strain may increase grain Zn concentration in bread wheat. For this purpose we performed a multifactorial pot experiment, in which the effects of two green manures (red clover, sunflower), $ZnSO_4$ application, soil γ-irradiation (elimination of naturally occurring AMF), and AMF inoculation were tested. Both green manures were labeled with ^{65}Zn radiotracer to record the Zn recoveries in the aboveground plant biomass. Application of $ZnSO_4$ fertilizer increased grain Zn concentration from 20 to 39 mg Zn kg^{-1} and sole addition of green manure of sunflower to soil raised grain Zn concentration to 31 mg Zn kg^{-1}. Adding the two together to soil increased grain Zn concentration even further to 54 mg Zn kg^{-1}. Mixing green manure of sunflower to soil mobilized additional 48 μg Zn (kg soil)$^{-1}$ for transfer to the aboveground plant biomass, compared to the total of 132 μg Zn (kg soil)$^{-1}$ taken up from plain soil when neither green manure nor $ZnSO_4$ were applied. Green manure amendments to soil also raised the DTPA-extractable Zn in soil. Inoculating a non-indigenous AMF did not increase plant Zn uptake. The study thus showed that organic matter amendments to soil can contribute to a better utilization of naturally stocked soil micronutrients, and thereby reduce any need for major external inputs.

Editor: Raffaella Balestrini, Institute for Sustainable Plant Protection - C.N.R., Italy

Funding: This study was supported by the grant 123920 of the Swiss National Science Foundation (SNF) and the Swiss Agency for Development and Cooperation (SDC) in the framework of Research Partnerships with Developing Countries. The funding body and host institutions had no role in study-design, data collection, analysis, and manuscript preparation. JJ was further supported by the J.E. Purkyně Fellowship and the long-term development program RVO61388971.

Competing Interests: The authors have declared that no competing interests exist.

* Email: forough.aghili@usys.ethz.ch

Introduction

Wheat is the third most-grown cereal after maize and rice, draws on the largest cropping area, and ranks first in global cereal trade [1]. It is the crop contributing most calories to large segments of the global human population. Yet, wheat-based diets do not provide sufficient zinc (Zn), which is a leading cause of widespread Zn deficiency [2]. Low grain Zn concentration is cause of low plant-availability of Zn in many soils on which wheat is produced [3,4]. Efforts have been made to breed wheat cultivars efficient in acquiring Zn from soil and effective in (re-) translocating Zn to grains [5,6]. Zinc supply from soil has, however, to be increased for such elite crop cultivars to become fully effective, which can be achieved via appropriate soil fertility management, such as application of mineral Zn fertilizer [7], addition of green manure [8], and/or a strengthening of nutrient acquisition traits, including symbioses of roots with naturally occurring and newly introduced arbuscular mycorrhizal fungi (AMF) [9–12].

Plants and probably also AMF take up Zn from the soil solution in form of free Zn^{2+} and $ZnOH^{+}$ ions, or as Zn-organic ligand complexes [13,14]. The depleted soil solution is replenished with Zn via desorption or dissolution from the soil matrix, followed by dispersion by diffusion [15]. Desorption from the soil matrix is controlled by soil pH, salinity, and clay, carbonate, and organic matter contents [15]. To promote Zn dissolution plants and microorganisms exude soil-acidifying protons and Zn-chelating low-molecular-weight organic compounds [16,17]. These Zn mobilizing activities of roots and microorganisms are promoted under iron (Fe), Zn, and other nutrient deficiencies [18]. The most well known classes of exuded organic Zn ligands are carboxylates, amides, and non-proteinaceous amino acids (= siderophores) [19,20]. A recent study on Zn uptake by wheat in the field [8] suggests that residues from the previous crop in crop rotations and thus possibly also addition of green manure to soil can raise the plant-available Zn in soil and promote Zn uptake in crop plants, mainly by contributing Zn-chelating dissolved organic carbon and amino acids.

Arbuscular mycorrhizal fungi, phylum Glomeromycota), because of their ubiquity and crucial involvement in plant nutrient acquisition and health, are a plant production-relevant group of root symbionts [21,22]. Their hyphae form effective, large-distance conduits for the transport of temporarily and spatially heterogeneously available nutrients of low mobility in soil, such as phosphate (P) and Zn [23]. Crop residue or green manure addition to soil and sporadic rain and irrigation may create nutrient flushes that crop plants with root systems extended by extraradical AMF hyphae may much more effectively utilize [24]. Arbuscular mycorrhizal fungi, whether indigenous or deliberately introduced as inoculants, were repeatedly reported to benefit Zn uptake in crop plants [9,10]. While the phenomenon of increased plant Zn uptake of mycorrhized as opposed to non-mycorrhized plants has already often been demonstrated [10], we still lack information about controlling factors [8] and the possible reinforcing effect of combined enrichment of soils with organic matter and mineral Zn fertilizer.

Here we report findings of a cross-factorial pot experiment on Zn nutrition of bread wheat involving the enrichment of calcareous soil with green manure of red clover and sunflower and inoculating plants with a non-indigenous AMF strain. For comparison and to study its interactions with the other experimental factors also a water-soluble mineral Zn fertilizer ($ZnSO_4$) was applied. To compare the effect of all naturally occurring AMF and possibly associated other soil microorganisms, the soil of half of the experimental units was γ-irradiated and re-inoculated with an AMF-free microbial filtrate of a water suspension of non-sterilized soil. An AMF inoculation treatment was further included in an attempt to assess the potential of this rapidly growing technology and for controlling against non-AMF mediated biotic effects by the soil γ-irradiation and microbial re-inoculation procedure. We predicted that 1) green manure addition to soil improves Zn uptake by wheat, 2) green manure addition improves Zn uptake from mineral Zn fertilizer and 3) inoculation of wheat plants with a foreign AMF strain improves Zn uptake, particularly from soil whose indigenous AMF had been killed by γ-irradiation.

Materials and methods

Experimental design

A complete cross-factorial experiment with the factors green manure (3 levels: none, red clover, sunflower), mineral Zn fertilization (2 levels: none, $ZnSO_4$), γ-irradiation (2 levels: non-irradiated; γ-irradiated and re-inoculated with soil microbes, except AMF), and AMF inoculation (2 levels: none, inoculated) was set up with each treatment replicated five times. The 120 experimental pots were arranged randomly on a glasshouse bench.

Soil origin and physicochemical soil analyses

The soil was collected in September 2009 to a depth of 30 cm from an arable field at the Rudasht research station (32, 29/N, 52, 10/E, 1560 m above sea level), located 65 km south-east of Isfahan in central Iran [permission for soil sampling was given by the Isfahan Agricultural and Natural Resource Research Center and for its import to Switzerland by the Swiss Federal Department of Agriculture]. The soil was air-dried and passed through a 5 mm sieve, before being shipped to Switzerland, where 5 kg were further passed through a 2 mm sieve for physicochemical analyses.

This experimental soil was a Typic Haplocambid, according to the USDA soil taxonomy [25]. The field where the soil was sampled had been under agricultural use with periodical irrigation from a nearby river. The crop rotation prior to soil sampling comprised barley, wheat, sugar beet, and wheat, interrupted by dry fallow periods. The climate in central Iran is semi-arid with a long-term mean annual temperature of 16.8°C, a mean annual rainfall lower than 100 mm, and a potential annual evaporation higher than 2000 mm [26].

The soil texture was a silty clay loam based on the measurements by the hydrometer method [27] and according to the USDA soil classification scheme [6]. The pH was 7.9 and the electrical conductivity (EC) 23 dSm^{-1}, as determined by the procedure of Rhoades [28], using an ISE pH meter 720A (Mettler Toledo LLC, Columbus, OH, USA) and an E- 518 conductometer (Metrohm Herisau, Switzerland), respectively. The soil was low in organic carbon [5 g (kg soil) $^{-1}$] and nitrogen [0.6 g (kg soil) $^{-1}$], as estimated by the methods of Walkley and Black [29] and on a Carlo Erba flash combustion CN-analyzer (NA1500, Carlo Erba, Milano, Italy), respectively. The soil contained 300 mg $CaCO_3$ (kg soil)$^{-1}$ as determined after neutralization with hydrochloric acid and back titration with sodium hydroxide [30].

The total Zn concentration of the soil was 80.2 mg Zn (kg soil)$^{-1}$, according to energy dispersive X-ray fluorescence spectrometry (XRF) measurements on a Spectra X-Lab 2000 instrument (SPECTRO Analytical Instruments GmbH, Kleve, Germany). Potentially plant-available Zn was extracted from 25 g of soil, using 50 ml of 0.05 M diethylene triamine-penta-acetic acid (DTPA), adjusted to pH 7.2 [31], and measured on an Agilent 7500 C inductively coupled plasma mass spectrometer (ICP-MS, Agilent Technologies, Santa Clara, California, USA). The amount of DTPA-extractable Zn was 0.45 mg Zn (kg soil)$^{-1}$.

Partial soil desalination, γ-irradiation and fertilization

Preliminary tests showed that wheat growth on the untreated soil was severely impaired by salinity stress (Forough Aghili et al., unpubl. data). Therefore, we flushed the soil in five rounds, with a volume ratio of 1:1 soil:deionized water each prior to the experiment. This treatment can be considered comparable to repeated flood irrigation, used by farmers at the field site prior to sowing. Soil washing lowered the EC from 23 to 6.7 dS m^{-1}, which is close to the threshold value of 5.9 dS m^{-1} for salinity-induced growth depression in wheat [32]. Flushing with water also slightly decreased the soil pH from 7.9 to 7.7. Analyses of the leachate indicated that large amounts of sodium, chlorine and sulfur had been removed, but virtually none of the total soil Zn (data not shown). The DTPA-extractable concentration of Zn in the soil even increased slightly from 0.45 to 0.47 mg Zn (kg soil)$^{-1}$. No spores of AMF could be retrieved from the leachate. The partially desalinated soil was again air-dried and sieved to a particle size of ≤5 mm.

Half of the soil was γ-irradiated with a dose of 25–75 kGy using a ^{60}Co source (Studer-Hard, Däniken, Switzerland, http://www.leoni-irradiation-services.com) in order to kill the indigenous soil microbes. To reintroduce soil microbes, but not AMF, 50 ml of a filtrate of a 2.5% (w:v) soil water suspension was added per kilogram soil. This microbial filtrate was prepared by passing the soil suspension twice through Whatman No 1 filter papers, which size-excluded AMF propagules. This procedure was recommended by Thompson [33] for studying the effect of AMF on Zn nutrition and is also utilized in many comparable studies to analyze the relative effect of different soil microorganisms on plant nutrition [34,35]. Indeed, soil γ-irradiation is currently the only way to create a control treatment, free of naturally occurring AMF, since mycorrhiza-defective mutants of wheat are not available [36].

The flushed soils (non-irradiated and γ-irradiated) received 400 mg K, 200 mg P, and 80 mg Fe per kilogram soil in the form of finely ground K_2SO_4, $CaHPO_4$ and $FeSO_4$ $7H_2O$ salts.

Preparation and application of ^{65}Zn-labeled green manure

We chose red clover (*Trifolium pratense L.*) and sunflower (*Helianthus annuus* L.) for the production of experimental green manures, because they are also often grown before wheat in the region of Isfahan [8]. Furthermore, Soltani et al. [8] found that compared to other possible green manure plants, red clover and sunflower introduced significant amounts of dissolved organic carbon into the soil solution, which was probably important for Zn solubilization.

Seeds of clover and sunflower were surface sterilized in 15% H_2O_2 for 15 min, rinsed with distilled water and germinated on moistened filter papers for two days. The most vigorously growing seedlings were transferred to a combined sand bed-hydroponics system, which consisted of compartmented seedling trays filled with silica sand of a particle size of 0.7–1.2 mm, partially immersed in a full-strength Hoagland nutrient solution [37]. After 28 days, the nutrient solution was exchanged for one that contained radioactive ^{65}Zn for an additional 26 days of vegetative plant development. While 30 liters of Hoagland nutrient solution were labeled with 5.55 MBq of ^{65}Zn for about 400 red clover plantlets, 40 l of Hoagland nutrient solution were labeled with 9.25 MBq of ^{65}Zn for about 140 sunflower plantlets. The ^{65}Zn radiotracer was added as carrier-free $ZnCl_2$, dissolved in weak HCl (Amersham plc, GE Healthcare, Little Chalfont, UK). The photoperiod in the glasshouse was set to 14 h, the minimal light intensity to 12 kLux, the temperature to 22°C during the day and 16°C at night, and the relative air humidity was allowed to vary between 30 and 40%.

At harvest, the entire shoots of red clover and only the leaf blades of sunflower, without petioles and stems, were collected, air-dried and finely ground to powder. The total tissue C and N concentrations were determined in 4 mg tissue samples using the above-mentioned CN-analyzer. The total P and Zn concentrations were measured in 100 mg subsamples of each of the green manures, using the above-mentioned ICP-MS after incineration at 550°C for 6 h and extracted with 3 ml of hot 14.4 M nitric acid (HNO_3). The concentration of radioactive ^{65}Zn in the green manures was measured by γ-spectrometry in 300 mg subsamples using IGC2 high purity germanium detectors (ORTEC Advanced Measurements Technologies Inc, Oak Ridge, Tennessee, USA). Selected characteristics of both green manures are presented in Table 1.

The green manures (Table 1) were homogenously mixed into the soils at a dosage of 4 g dry matter per kilogram of dry soil. This dosage corresponds approximately to an addition of 18 tons of dry matter per hectare considering a soil bulk density of 1.5 t m^{-3} and incorporation to a soil depth of 30 cm.

Mineral Zn fertilization

Half of the soil in each green manure × irradiation treatment combination was fertilized with water soluble Zn in the form of $ZnSO_4$ at a dosage of 4.7 mg Zn (kg soil)$^{-1}$, corresponding approximately to 19 kg Zn ha^{-1}.

AMF inoculation

Finally, half of all pots in each combination of the above treatments were inoculated with approximately 250 spores of a pot culture of the Swiss isolate BEG155 of the AMF species *Claroideoglomus claroideum* [38]. The spores of the inoculum were extracted by wet-sieving and decanting [39] and directly pipetted onto the roots of the transplanted wheat seedlings. This careful spore isolation and inoculation procedure prevented co-inoculation of many other microbes and introduction of organic matter in the form of root pieces, which would have been the case with so-called whole inoculum {= growth substrate, containing fungal spores, hyphae and colonized root fragments [40]}.

Data on AMF root colonization were not systematically collected in this experiment, since microscopic and molecular genetic quantification in a previous experiment with the same wheat cultivar and soil clearly showed a high infection pressure by the naturally occurring AMF (Forough Aghili et al., unpublished data). However, successful colonization of the roots by the AMF isolate BEG155 and by naturally occurring AMF were confirmed in a subset of all experimental treatments by quantitative polymerase chain reaction as in the previous study and additionally by phylogenetic sequence analysis of a 1.6 kb-long ribosomal DNA amplicon of the AMF colonizing the roots of a subset of all experimental units (Anouk Guyer et al., unpublished data).

Planting, growth conditions, harvest and mineral nutrient analyses

Wheat kernels {*Triticum aestivum* cv. Kavir, a cultivar widely grown in Iran [41]} were surface-sterilized with 15% H_2O_2 for 15 min and pre-germinated on moistened filter paper for three days prior to transplantation. Four seedlings were planted into each pot with 550 g soil and later thinned to the most vigorously growing two individuals. Nitrogen in the form of NH_4NO_3 was applied weekly, six times, amounting to 600 mg N (kg soil)$^{-1}$ until tillering.

Table 1. Mineral nutrient concentrations of the two types of applied green manure prepared from red clover and sunflower.

	Red clover (Mean ± SE)	Sunflower (Mean ± SE)
N mg (g DM*)$^{-1}$	43.3±0.6	58.4±0.4
C/N (mass ratio)	9.1±0.1	6.3±0.1
P mg (g DM)$^{-1}$	5.0±0.1	7.3±0.1
Zn µg (g DM)$^{-1}$	45.6±0.6	104.4±2.4
^{65}Zn kBq¶ (g DM)$^{-1}$	6.9±0.02	15.8±0.1

* DM: dry matter.

¶Radioactivity at the time of harvest of the experiment.

The means and associated standard errors (SE) of three replicate subsamples of the nitrogen (N) concentration, carbon (C) to N mass ratio, phosphorus (P) and zinc (Zn) concentrations, and ^{65}Zn concentration are listed.

The climatic conditions in the glasshouse were set to a photoperiod of 14 h with a minimum light intensity of 10 kLux, a 22/17°C day/night air temperature regime, and 40–45% relative air humidity. Soil moisture was kept at about 70% soil water holding capacity by daily watering to weight.

Harvest took place at grain maturity, 125 days after planting. The total weight of the grains and straw of the two plants in each pot was determined after drying to constant weight at 60°C for 72 h. Subsamples of 200 mg of finely ground wheat straw and grain were incinerated in porcelain crucibles at 550°C for 6 h and the ashes dissolved in 2 ml of boiling 13 M HNO_3. Zinc concentrations were measured using ICP-MS. Measurement accuracy and precision were ensured by regular inclusion of a certified plant reference standard in the analyses (hay powder IAEA-V-10, 24 mg Zn kg^{-1}) and by running blank samples with each sample batch. The concentration of radioactive ^{65}Zn was measured in the grains and straw by γ-spectrometry as described for the green manure above. Zinc uptake into roots could not be determined because it was not possible to recover the roots quantitatively from the clay-rich soil. Soil pH and the concentrations of total N and DTPA-extractable soil Zn were measured at the end of the experiment, using the above-described analytical procedures.

Calculations and data analyses

Plant Zn uptake from green manure, soil and mineral Zn fertilizer. Plant Zn uptake was calculated as the product of Zn concentration and biomass for both the grain and straw fractions and summed to obtain the amount of Zn contained in the entire aboveground biomass. All radioactivity measurements were related to the harvest time, taking the radioactive decay into account (^{65}Zn half-life time: 243.9 d). The percentage of Zn in the aboveground biomass derived from the green manure [Zn_{dgm} (%)] was calculated as:

$$Zn_{dgm}(\%) = 100 \times SA_p \times (SA_{gm})^{-1} \quad (1)$$

where SA_p [Bq (mg Zn^{-1})] is the specific activity (SA) of Zn in the aboveground biomass and SA_{gm} the specific activity of Zn in the added green manure. The specific activity of Zn in the plant was calculated as:

$$SA = [^{65}Zn] \times [Zn]^{-1} \quad (2)$$

where [^{65}Zn] stands for the concentration of radioactivity per kilogram of plant material [Bq (kg $DM)^{-1}$] and [Zn] stands for the concentration of total Zn in the plant [mg Zn (kg $DM)^{-1}$].

Using the equations 1 and 2, the amount of Zn taken up to the aboveground biomass from green manure [Zn_{dgm}, µg Zn (kg $soil)^{-1}$] was calculated as:

$$Zn_{dgm} = (Zn_{dgm} \times Zn_{upt}) \times 10^{-2} \quad (3)$$

where Zn_{upt} is the amount of Zn taken up to the aboveground plant biomass per kilogram of soil [µg Zn (kg $soil)^{-1}$].

Knowing Zn_{dgm}, it is possible to calculate the percentage of Zn recovered by the aboveground plant biomass from the added green manure [Zn_{rec_gm} (%)]:

$$Zn_{rec\_gm} = 100 \times Zn_{dgm} \times Zn_{added\_gm}{}^{-1} \quad (4)$$

where Zn_{added_gm} is the amount of Zn added with the green manure [µg Zn (kg $soil)^{-1}$].

Knowing Zn_{dgm}, it is also possible to calculate the amount of Zn in the plant that is derived from non-labeled Zn sources in soil, i.e. in the non-fertilized soil from the native soil Zn pool and in the mineral Zn-fertilized soil from the native soil Zn pool as well as the applied $ZnSO_4$ [Zn_{dsoil}, µg Zn (kg $soil)^{-1}$]:

$$Zn_{dsoil} = Zn_{upt} - Zn_{dgm} \quad (5)$$

Statistical analyses. The results were analyzed by fixed factor four-way or three-way analyses of variance (ANOVA) with two levels (γ-irradiated and non-irradiated) of 'soil γ-irradiation', three levels (none, red clover and sunflower) of 'green manure addition', two levels [0 and. 4.7 mg Zn (kg $soil)^{-1}$] of 'mineral Zn fertilization', and two levels (with and without inoculation with *C. claroideum*) of 'AMF inoculation'. The interaction terms were sequentially removed from the initially complete ANOVA model when not significant (backward elimination). In addition, a one-way ANOVA was carried out on the saved residuals of a three-way ANOVA with the factors 'soil γ-irradiation', 'mineral Zn fertilization' and 'AMF inoculation' in order to specifically analyze the effect of green manure addition. Compliance of data dispersion with ANOVA model assumptions was verified using Shapiro-Wilcoxon's normality and Levene's equal variance tests. If necessary, data were log_{10} or squareroot transformed. All statistical analyses were carried out using the software package SPSS version 17 (SPSS Inc., Chicago, Ill inois, USA). Means of factor levels were compared by least-significant-difference (LSD) tests at the significance level of $p<0.05$. The figures were prepared in SigmaPlot version 12 [Systat Software Inc. (SSI), San Jose, California, USA].

Results

Plant biomass and grain nitrogen concentration

The grain yield of the experimental wheat plants was not significantly affected by any of the treatments (Figure 1A, Table 2), but the large variance may have concealed a similar γ-irradiation effect as on the total aboveground biomass (Figure 1B). The total aboveground biomass (= straw + grains) was significantly larger for the wheat plants grown in γ-irradiated than non-irradiated soil ($F_{1,96} = 10.45$, $p = 0.002$). Inoculation with *C. claroideum* had no significant effect on aboveground biomass production (Table 2).

Both types of green manure significantly increased grain N concentration ($F_{2,70} = 31.41$, $p<0.001$, Table 2), which ranged between 30 and 45 g N (kg $DM)^{-1}$ in the plants grown on γ-irradiated soil and between 25 and 37 g N (kg $DM)^{-1}$ in the plants grown on non-irradiated soil (Figure 2). Soil γ-irradiation also led to a significant increase in grain N concentrations ($F_{1,70} = 10.04$, $p = 0.003$, Table 2). Inoculation with *C. claroideum* and $ZnSO_4$ addition had no significant effects on grain N concentration (Table 2).

Grain Zn concentration and Zn uptake to grains and aboveground biomass

Grain Zn concentration increased significantly with application of mineral Zn fertilizer ($F_{1,70} = 50.96$, $p<0.001$) and green manure ($F_{2,70} = 13.48$, $p<0.001$), but was not affected by inoculation of *C. claroideum* and soil γ-irradiation (Figure 3A, Table 2). The lowest grain Zn concentration [20±1.64 mg Zn (kg $DM)^{-1}$] was measured in the treatment with neither mineral Zn fertilization, nor addition of green manure, while the highest grain Zn

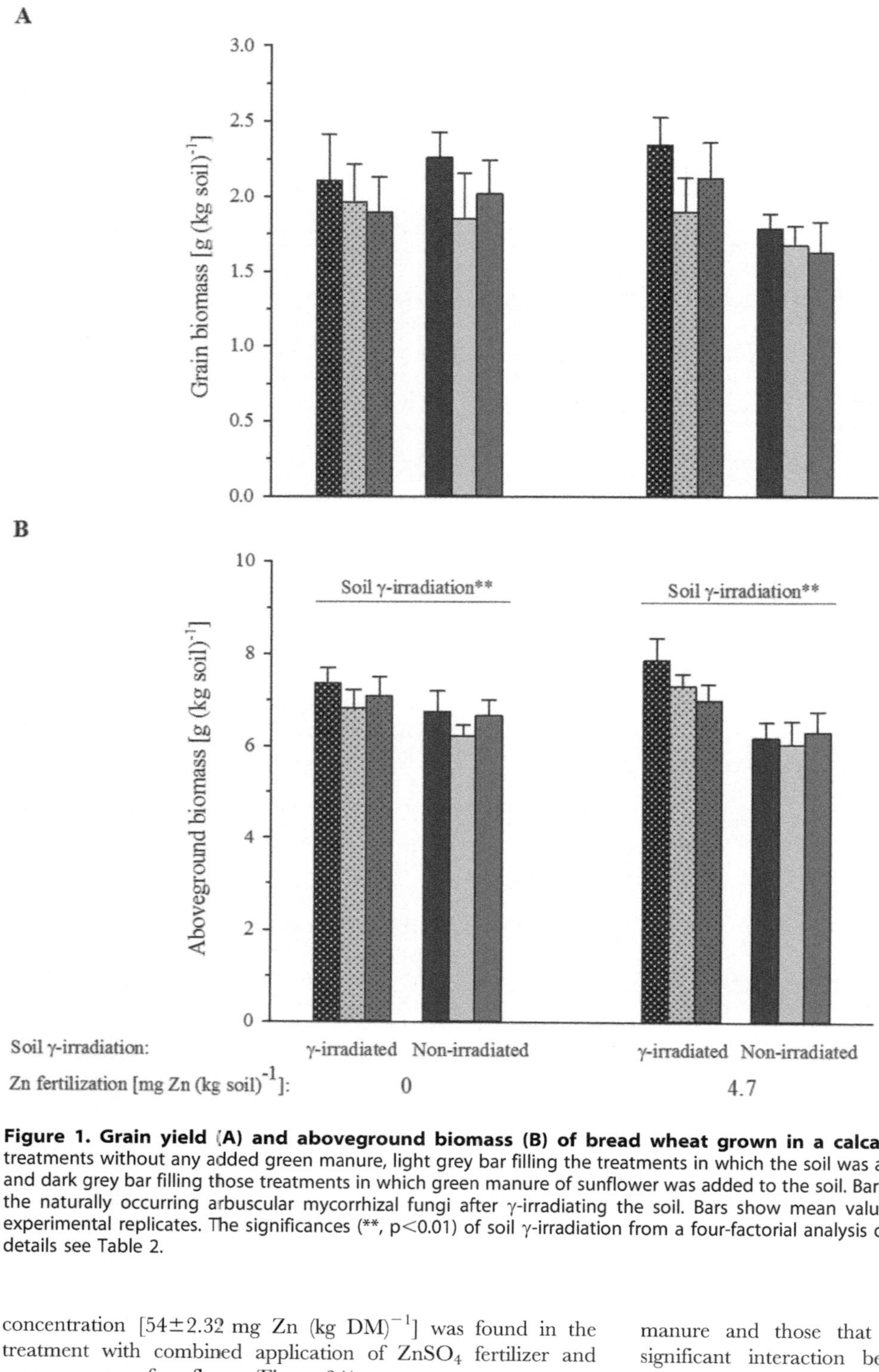

Figure 1. Grain yield (A) and aboveground biomass (B) of bread wheat grown in a calcareous soil. Black bar filling denotes the treatments without any added green manure, light grey bar filling the treatments in which the soil was amended with green manure of red clover, and dark grey bar filling those treatments in which green manure of sunflower was added to the soil. Bar hatching highlights the treatment missing the naturally occurring arbuscular mycorrhizal fungi after γ-irradiating the soil. Bars show mean values and associated standard errors of five experimental replicates. The significances (**, $p<0.01$) of soil γ-irradiation from a four-factorial analysis of variance are indicated. For full statistical details see Table 2.

concentration [54±2.32 mg Zn $(kg\ DM)^{-1}$] was found in the treatment with combined application of $ZnSO_4$ fertilizer and green manure of sunflower (Figure 3A).

The highest Zn concentration in the aboveground biomass [46.1±1.43 mg Zn $(kg\ DM)^{-1}$] was found in plants grown on non-irradiated soil amended with green manure of sunflower in combination with $ZnSO_4$ (Figure 3B). The lowest aboveground Zn concentration was observed in plants grown on γ-irradiated soil that had neither been fertilized with mineral Zn, nor amended with green manure (Figure 3B). Application of mineral Zn fertilizer reduced the differences between the aboveground biomass Zn concentrations of those plants that had received green manure and those that had not, resulting in a statistically significant interaction between green manure addition and mineral Zn fertilization ($F_{2,96}=6.24$, $p<0.01$; Table 2). Inoculation with *C. claroideum* had no significant effect on the concentration of Zn in the aboveground biomass (Table 2).

The amount of Zn taken up from the native soil Zn pool and mineral Zn fertilizer that was allocated to grains ranged between 46 and 88 μg Zn $(kg\ soil)^{-1}$, while the total amount of Zn accumulated in the aboveground biomass ranged between 117 and 367 μg Zn $(kg\ soil)^{-1}$ (Table 3). The lowest values were again observed in the absence of mineral Zn fertilization and green manure addition, while the highest values were observed after

Table 2. Results of fixed factor four-way analyses of variance (ANOVA) on plant and soil parameters.

ANOVA model	Grain biomass		Aboveground biomass		Grain N concentration		Grain Zn concentration		Aboveground Zn concentration		Zn uptake into grains	
Source of variance	**F value**	**df**	**F value**	**df**	**F value**	**df**	**F value**	**df**	**F value**	**df**	**F value**	**df**
Full model	0.29^{ns}	23	2.47*	23	4.45***	23	5.92***	23	8.91***	23	2.78**	23
Green manure (A)	0.33^{ns}	2	0.26^{ns}	2	31.41***	2	13.48***	2	13.71***	2	1.98^{ns}	2
Zn fertilization (B)	0.19^{ns}	1	0.12^{ns}	1	0.09	1	50.96***	1	125.23***	1	40.52***	1
Soil γ-irradiation (C)	0.20^{ns}	1	10.45**	1	10.04	1	2.99^{ns}	1	9.15**	1	0.17^{ns}	1
Inoculation (D)	0.76^{ns}	1	0.13^{ns}	1	2.97	1	1.95^{ns}	1	1.04^{ns}	1	0.95^{ns}	1
A×B	r	2	r	2	R	2	12.71**	2	6.24**	2	12.71***	2
A×C	r	2	0.61^{ns}	2	0.98^{ns}	2	3.36*	2	4.41*	2	1.22^{ns}	2

ANOVA model	Zn uptake into aboveground biomass		Zn_{dgm}		Zn_{rec_gm}		Zn_{dsoil}		DTPA-extractable soil Zn	
Source of variance	**F value**	**df**	**F value**	**df**	**F value**	**df**	**F value**	**df**	**F value**	**df**
Full model	4.26***	23	5.95***	15	8.61***	15	6.15***	23	16.40***	23
Green manure (A)	4.13*	2	39.92***	2	72.25***	2	3.50*	2	85.22***	2
Zn fertilization (B)	53.49***	1	21.23***	1	22.31***	1	77.13***	1	168.84***	1
Soil γ-irradiation (C)	0.01^{ns}	1	5.21*	1	8.85**	1	1.14^{ns}	1	0.64^{ns}	1
Inoculation (D)	2.34^{ns}	1	8.25**	1	4.82*	1	1.26^{ns}	1	2.10^{ns}	1
A×B	0.49^{ns}	2	2.12^{ns}	2	0.13^{ns}	2	2.70^{ns}	2	2.17^{ns}	2
A×C	0.44^{ns}	2	0.63^{ns}	2	4.64*	2	2.95^{ns}	2	0.54^{ns}	2

DTPA: diethylene triamine-penta-acetic acid.

na: not applied, r: removed from the statistical model, ns: not significant, *, $p<0.05$; **, $p<0.01$; ***, $p<0.001$.

The measurements of the plant parameters {grain biomass, total above ground biomass, grain N concentration, grain Zn concentration, aboveground Zn concentration, Zn uptake to grains, Zn uptake to the aboveground biomass, Zn derived from green manure in the aboveground biomass [Zn_{dgm}], proportion of the Zn recovered in the above ground biomass [Zn_{rec_gm}] of the Zn added with the green manure Zn derived from the soil and fertilizer in the aboveground biomass [Zn_{dsoil}]}and soil parameter (DTPA-extractable Zn from soil) were made at grain maturity. Effect sizes of the experimental factors and their significant interactions are indicated as F-values alongside with the statistical significance level. The interactions of the factors A×D, B×C, B×D, C×D, A×B×C, A×B×D, A×D×C, B×C×D, A×B×C×D were not significant in any of the 11 ANOVAs and thus these results are not listed.

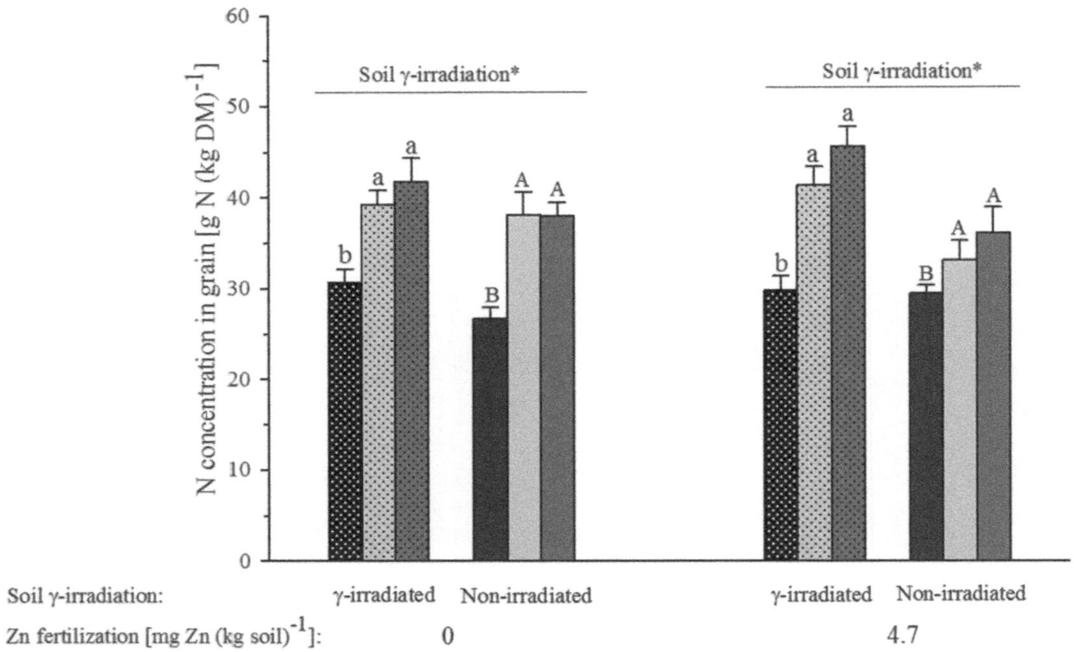

Figure 2. Grain nitrogen (N) concentration of wheat grown in a calcareous soil. Bar filling denoting the different green manure addition treatments is the same as in Figure 1. Bars show mean values and associated standard errors of five experimental replicates. The significances (*, $p<0.05$) of the effect of soil γ-irradiation from a four-factorial analysis of variance are shown. Different letters indicate statistical differences of separate least significant difference tests at $p<0.05$ for the different green manure addition treatments within the combinations of soil γ-irradiation and mineral Zn fertilization. For full statistical details see Table 2.

addition of mineral Zn fertilizer and green manure of sunflower. Adding green manure to the soil tended to increase Zn accumulation in the grains, when no mineral Zn fertilizer had been applied, but this effect was not statistically significant (Table 2). Inoculation with *C. claroideum* had no significant effect on Zn uptake to the grains (Table 2).

Zn derived from green manure and both, soil and mineral Zn fertilizer, in the aboveground biomass

The Zn from the added green manure recovered in the aboveground biomass (Zn_{rec_gm}) ranged between 2.5% and 4.1% for red clover, and between 1.4% and 2.7% for sunflower (Figure 4). These Zn recoveries from the two types of green manures differed significantly across all treatments ($F_{1,79}=72.25$, $p<0.001$). Mineral Zn fertilization lowered Zn_{rec_gm} for both forms of green manure ($F_{1,64}=22.31$, $p<0.001$, Figure 4 & Table 2), as did soil γ-irradiation ($F_{1,64}=8.85$, $p<0.01$). The recovered Zn fraction from sunflower residues was also reduced by the inoculation of *C. claroideum* when also mineral Zn fertilizer was applied ($F_{1,18}=10.84$, $p<0.01$; Figure 4).

The amount of Zn in the aboveground biomass derived from green manure (Zn_{dgm}) ranged between 4.5 μg Zn (kg soil)$^{-1}$ in the treatment of combined soil γ-irradiation, mineral Zn fertilization, and addition of green manure of red clover, and 11 μg Zn (kg soil)$^{-1}$ in the treatment with green manure of sunflower but without mineral Zn fertilization, soil γ-irradiation, and AMF inoculation (Table 3). The amount of plant Zn derived from green manure of sunflower (Zn_{dgm}) was consistently higher than that derived from red clover ($F_{1,64}=39.92$, $p<0.001$; Tables 2 & 3).

The amount of Zn derived from the native soil Zn pool (Zn_{dsoil}) was significantly increased with green manure addition, when no $ZnSO_4$ was applied ($F_{2,96}=3.50$, $p=0.034$, Table 2 & Figure 5). This apparent soil Zn mobilization was more pronounced for green manure produced from sunflower than from red clover (Figure 5). Under conditions of co-application of $ZnSO_4$, the effect of green manure addition was, however, variable and weak and statistically not significant. There was also no significant effect of γ-irradiation, nor any effect by the non-indigenous *C. claroideum* inoculant on the total amount of Zn derived from soil and mineral Zn fertilizer, either (Table 2).

Changes in DTPA-extractable Zn from soil, total N and pH in soil

The concentration of DTPA-extractable Zn from soil measured after plant harvest was significantly higher in the treatments with green manure than without green manure ($F_{1,96}=169$, $p<0.001$). Application of mineral Zn fertilizer also significantly increased DTPA-extractable Zn ($F_{2,96}=85.2$, $p<0.001$; Tables 2 & 3). There was a highly significant correlation between the total Zn taken up into the aboveground biomass (Y) and the DTPA-extractable Zn concentration in the soil (X) according to a double reciprocal regression model [$Y=1/(0.004+2.05/X)$] with $r^2=0.56$ and $p<0.0001$.

Green manure addition slightly decreased soil pH, independently of the soil γ-irradiation treatment ($F_{2,96}=139.4$, $p<0.001$; Table 4). The total soil N content was higher at harvest in the treatments that received green manure than in those that did not ($F_{2,96}=321.7$, $p<0.001$, Table 2 & 4).

Discussion

The results confirmed our first prediction, because green manure addition to soil increased Zn uptake by bread wheat. The findings, however, did not unequivocally support our second

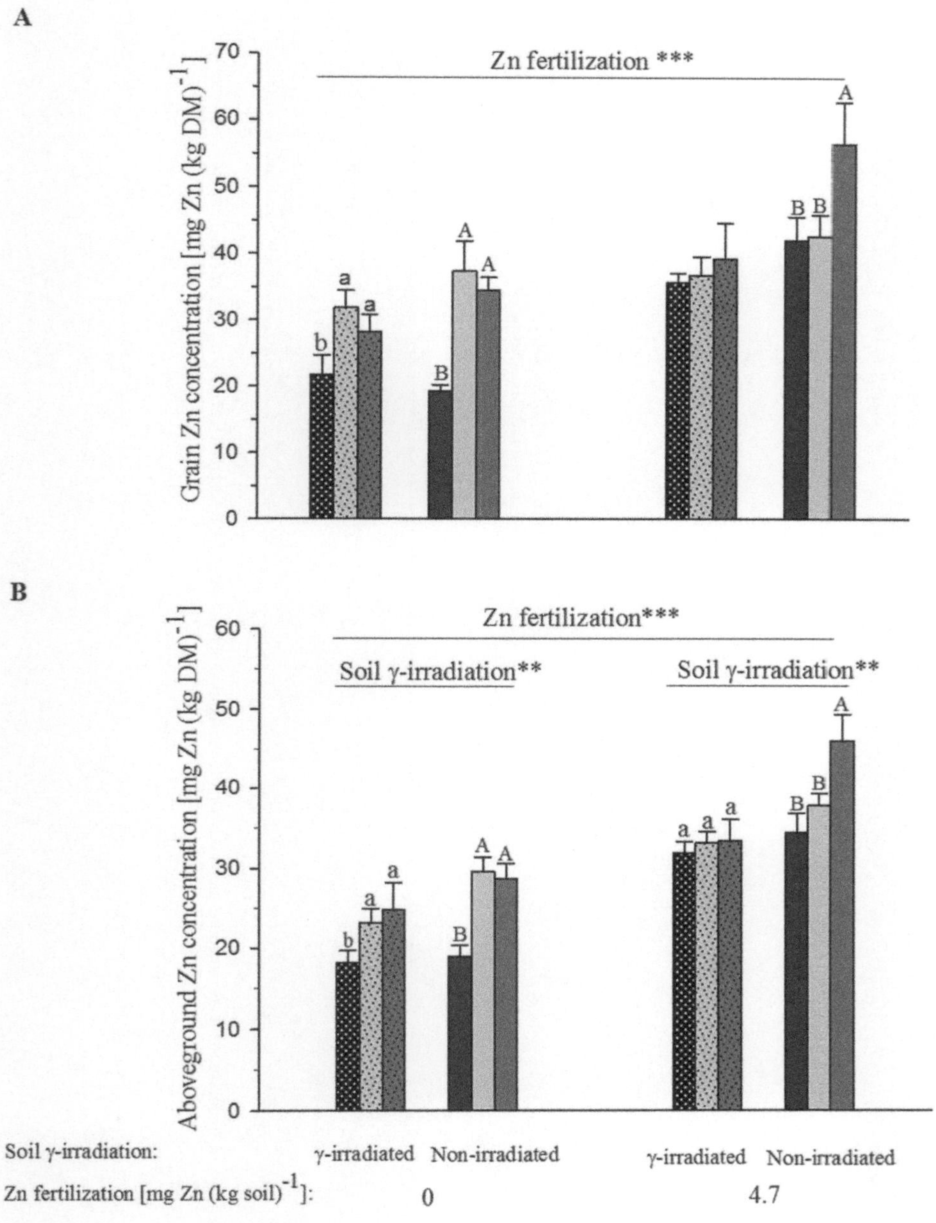

Figure 3. Grain (A) and aboveground (B) zinc (Zn) concentrations of wheat grown in a calcareous soil. Bar filling denoting the different green manure addition treatments is the same as in Figure 1. Bars show mean values and associated standard errors of five experimental replicates. The significances (**, $p<0.01$; ***, $p<0.001$) of the effect of mineral Zn fertilization, soil γ-irradiation of fixed factor four-way analyses of variance are shown. Different letters indicate statistical differences of separate least significant difference tests at $p<0.05$ for the different green manure addition treatments within the combinations of soil γ-irradiation and mineral Zn fertilization. For full statistical details see Table 2.

prediction, since utilization of the applied mineral Zn fertilizer by the plants did not improve in response to green manure addition. Also our last prediction that inoculation of a non-indigenous AMF strain would improve Zn transfer from soil to plants was not confirmed, not even in AMF- and thus competitor-free soil after removal of naturally occurring AMF by soil γ-irradiation. These two later findings appear to be related to the fact that Zn availability in the studied soil was neither limiting plant growth, nor yield.

In agreement with previous studies [43,44], we observed a clear increase in grain Zn concentration after application of mineral Zn fertilizer. However, application of mineral Zn fertilizer did neither translate into increased plant growth, nor higher grain yields, showing that Zn availability was not the primary plant growth-limiting factor in this soil. Sadeghzadeh [42] reports DTPA-extractable Zn levels below 0.6 mg Zn (kg soil)$^{-1}$ to limit wheat growth in calcareous soil. Since our soil contained 0.47 mg Zn (kg soil)$^{-1}$ and application of mineral Zn fertilizer did not promote wheat growth, it appears that the threshold for growth-limitation of soil Zn concentration may even be lower, although Zn uptake can obviously be raised by application of mineral Zn fertilizer.

Table 3. Effects of green manure addition and $ZnSO_4$ application to soil, soil γ-irradiation and inoculation of a non-indigenous arbuscular mycorrhizal fungus (AMF) on plant and soil parameters.

Green manure addition	Soil γ-irradiation	Zn added with $ZnSO_4$	Zn added with green manure	AMF inoculation	Zn uptake into aboveground biomass	Zn_{dgm}	Zn_{dsoil}	DTPA-extractable soil Zn
		μg Zn (kg soil)$^{-1}$			μg Zn (kg soil)$^{-1}$	μg Zn (kg soil)$^{-1}$		μg Zn (kg soil)$^{-1}$
None	**γ-irradiated**	0	0	no	159.3±12.4		159.3±12.4	450± 20
	γ-irradiated	0	0	yes	127.6± 6.9		127.6± 6.9	440± 32
	Non-irradiated	0	0	no	117.4± 13.2		117.4± 13.2	460± 35
	Non-irradiated	0	0	yes	127.2± 10.4		127.2± 10.4	480± 42
	γ-irradiated	4700	0	no	251.6± 16.6		251.6± 16.6	2150± 100
	γ-irradiated	4700	0	yes	227.3± 14.3		227.3± 14.3	1960± 93
	Non-irradiated	4700	0	no	206.6± 13.2		206.6± 13.2	2180± 110
	Non-irradiated	4700	0	yes	228.4± 27.5		228.4± 27.5	1990± 160
Red clover	**γ-irradiated**	0	183	no	152.9± 21.4	5.56± 0.59	147.4± 21.3	1220± 100
	γ-irradiated	0	183	yes	156.9± 25.3	5.86± 1.03	151.1± 19.6	1500± 120
	Non-irradiated	0	183	yes	205.0± 18.6	8.52± 0.35	196.5± 18.4	2010± 70
	Non-irradiated	0	183	yes	176.0± 23.8	6.10± 0.42	169.9± 20.2	2430± 110
	γ-irradiated	4700	183	no	224.0± 34.1	4.51± 0.39	219.5± 34.1	5050± 120
	γ-irradiated	4700	183	yes	243.9± 10.6	4.93± 0.38	239.0± 12.6	3550± 74
	Non-irradiated	4700	183	no	202.9± 25.2	5.32± 0.52	197.6± 23.8	4430± 32
	Non-irradiated	4700	183	yes	226.7± 22.4	6.11± 0.54	220.6± 21.5	3950± 92
Sunflower	**γ-irradiated**	0	418	no	227.9± 39.6	10.32± 1.39	217.6± 31.4	3310± 66
	γ-irradiated	0	418	yes	128.9± 11.4	8.38± 0.96	120.6± 22.6	1750± 120
	Non-irradiated	0	418	no	189.9± 14.3	11.05± 0.87	178.9± 16.4	3230± 86
	Non-irradiated	0	418	yes	174.9± 30.2	9.45± 1.61	165.5± 20.7	1950± 33
	γ-irradiated	4700	418	no	258.9± 25.8	8.44± 0.64	250.5± 41.3	3850± 82
	γ-irradiated	4700	418	yes	205.8± 20.4	5.94± 0.75	200.0± 19.5	4990± 36
	Non-irradiated	4700	418	no	367.0± 40.2	8.5± 0.64	358.5± 37.4	4540± 120
	Non-irradiated	4700	418	yes	227.9± 24.5	5.97± 0.80	222.0± 26.2	4680± 130

DTPA: diethylene-triamine-penta-acetic acid

Mean values and associated standard errors of five experimental replicates of Zn uptake to the aboveground biomass, Zn in the aboveground biomass derived from green manure (Zn_{dgm}), Zn derived from soil and fertilizer (Zn_{dsoil}) and DTPA-extractable Zn from soil at grain maturity are listed.

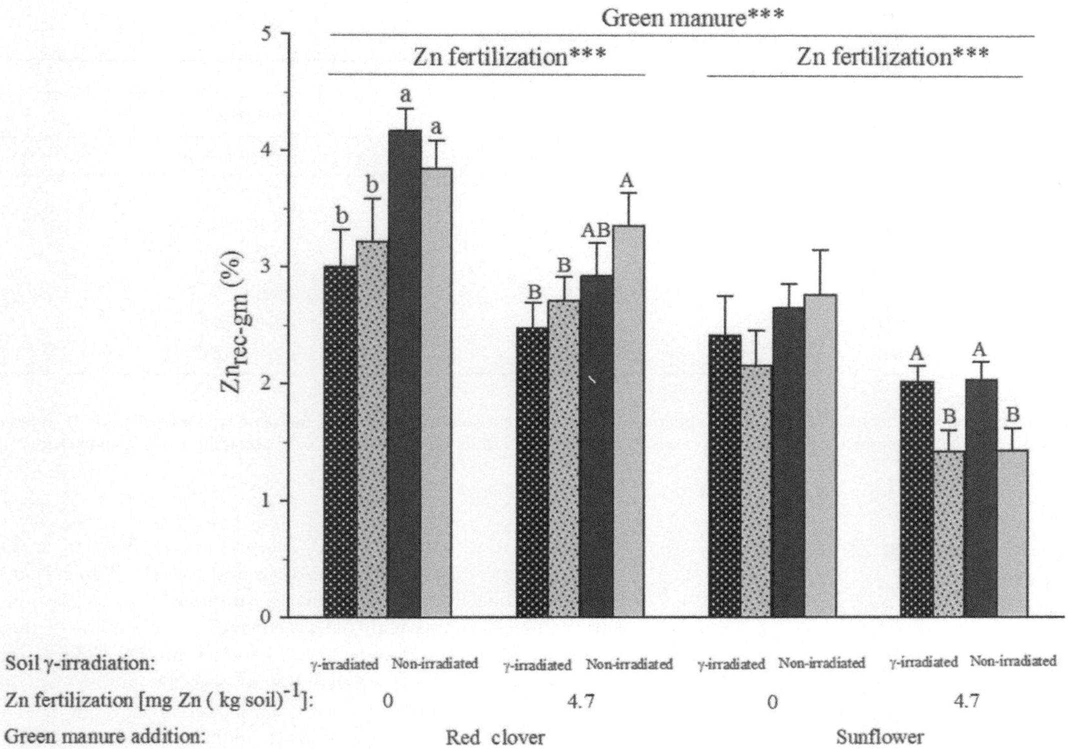

Figure 4. Percentage of zinc (Zn) recovered from green manure (Zn_{rec-gm}) in the aboveground wheat biomass. Black bar filling denotes treatments with arbuscular mycorrhizal fungus (AMF) inoculation and light grey filling treatments without AMF inoculation. Bar hatching highlights treatments in which the naturally occurring AMF were missing after γ-irradiating the soil. Bars show mean values and associated standard errors of five experimental replicates. The significances (***, $p<0.001$) of the effect of green manure addition and mineral Zn fertilization from a fixed factor four-way analysis of variance are indicated above the bars. For full statistical details see Table 2.

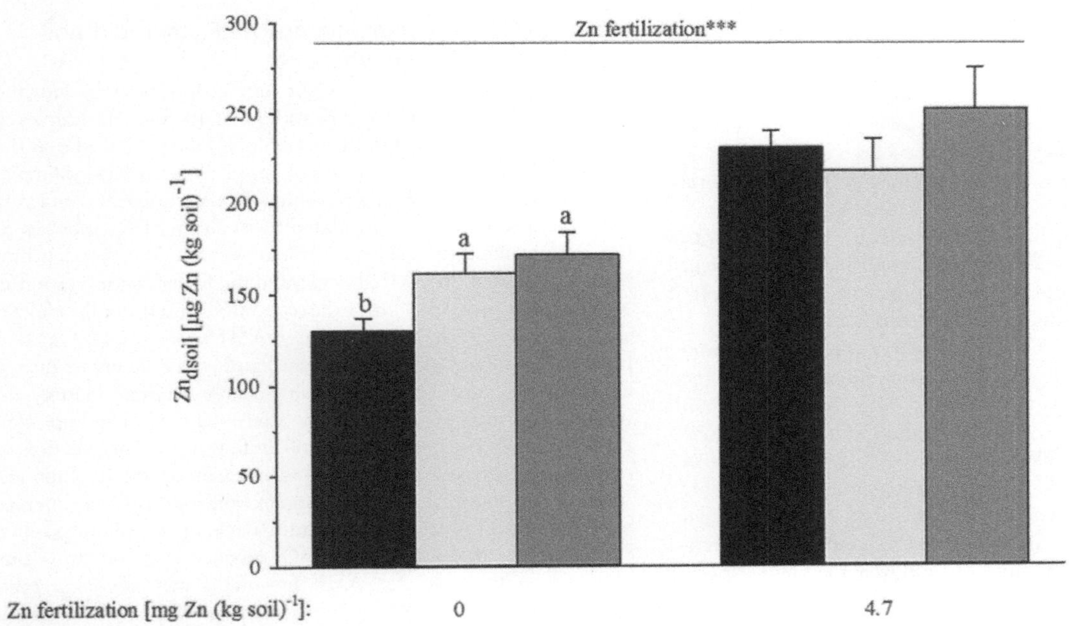

Figure 5. Zinc (Zn) uptake from soil to the aboveground biomass of bread wheat grown in a calcareous soil after addition of two types of green manure. The Zn taken up from soil either originated from the native soil Zn pool or from soil as well as applied $ZnSO_4$ fertilizer. Bar filling denoting the different green manure addition treatments is the same as in Figure 1. Bars show mean values and associated standard errors of five experimental replicates. The significance (***, $p<0.001$) of the effect of mineral Zn fertilization from a fixed factorial four-way analysis of variance is indicated above the bars. Different letters indicate statistical differences of separate least significant difference tests at $p<0.05$ for the different green manure addition treatments within the different Zn fertilization levels. For full statistical details see Table 2.

Table 4. Total soil nitrogen (N) concentration and pH in water at wheat harvest.

Soil	Green manure	Total N (g kg^{-1})	pH (H_2O)
		(Mean ± SE)	(Mean ± SE)
Non-irradiated	None	0.55±0.02[B]	7.75±0.03[A]
	+ Red clover	0.87±0.02[A]	7.50±0.02[B]
	+ Sunflower	0.88±0.02[A]	7.53±0.01[B]
γ-irradiated	None	0.63±0.01[b]	7.64±0.02[a]
	+ Red clover	0.89±0.02[a]	7.46±0.01[b]
	+ Sunflower	0.96±0.02[a]	7.48±0.01[b]

DTPA: diethylene-triamine-penta-acetic acid

The values represent the means and associated standard errors (SE) of 20 experimental units. Different superscript letters of the same type following the SE indicate statistical difference among the means of the three green manure treatments within each soil γ-irradiation treatment at $p<0.05$, according to least significance difference tests.

Mixing green manure to soil increased Zn uptake by wheat via Zn mobilizing effects

The observed increase in Zn uptake from the native soil Zn pool after green manure addition could originate from changes to the soil conditions, root growth, and/or plant physiology. Only addition of green manure to the soil increased the DTPA-extractable Zn from 0.47 to 0.5 or 2 mg Zn (kg soil)$^{-1}$, when green manure of red clover and sunflower were added, respectively. Combining $ZnSO_4$ application with green manure addition to soil increased the DTPA-extractable Zn concentration even further, namely up to 3.8 mg Zn (kg soil)$^{-1}$ when red clover was used and up to 5.0 mg Zn (kg soil)$^{-1}$ when sunflower was used, respectively (Table 3). We thus can conclude that the lack of a plant growth response to application of mineral Zn fertilizer (Figure 1A&B) must be explained by an alternative plant growth-limiting factor and not the >0.6 mg Zn (kg soil)$^{-1}$ of DTPA-extractable Zn [42].

The larger increase in DTPA-extractable soil Zn in response to addition of green manure of sunflower than such of red clover (Table 3) could have been due to the Zn-richer green manure of sunflower than the green manure of red clover. For production of the green manure of sunflower, but not that of red clover, only leaf laminae were used, which could explain the higher mineral nutrient concentrations of it (Table 1). Moreover, the relatively young age (54 day) and bigger sunflower than red clover seeds with own nutrient reserves may have further contributed to nutrient concentration differences of the two types of green manure (Table 1), translating into differences in plant Zn uptake.

There may have been further co-nutritional or root- and microbial growth-mediated Zn uptake stimulation, because the green manure produced of sunflower was also richer in N than that of red clover (Table 1). The green manure of the leaf laminae of the well N-supplied sunflower plants could have released N during its decomposition and stimulated root growth and possibly the synthesis of Zn facilitating N-rich plant and microbial compounds. Elevated root and microbial exudation and necromass in response to green manure of sunflower may also explain the higher DTPA-extractable Zn concentrations of the soil and increased plant Zn uptake. Root- and microbe-derived organic acids, amides and (phyto-) siderophores may have chelated and thereby mobilized Zn for uptake by the wheat plants. More N released from the decomposing green manure of more N-rich sunflower than red clover material (Table1) may have supported the N-demanding biosynthesis of Zn chelating compounds [8,14,45].

Elevated root and microbial activity in response to green manure addition may further have lowered soil pH (Table 4) and thereby mobilized soil Zn. Similarly, stimulation of nitrification upon higher N inputs with the green manure of sunflower than that of red clover and thus release of protons into the soil solution may have raised Zn bioavailability in soil for uptake by the mycorrhized wheat plants.

All in all, the effectiveness of green manure addition to soil to release Zn from the native soil Zn pool for plant uptake was remarkable (Figure 5). This stimulatory effect on plant Zn uptake diminished, however, when additionally $ZnSO_4$ fertilizer was applied. This is probably, because the applied $ZnSO_4$ fertilizer introduced already a high amount of Zn, compared to the amount solubilized by chelating compounds released upon addition of green manure, reducing Zn mobilization form soil.

Inoculation of a non-indigenous AMF strain did not increase Zn uptake in wheat

A previous experiment (Forough Aghili, unpublished) with the same soil and wheat cultivar and additional analyses on samples of this experiment (Anouk Guyer, unpublished data) showed that the roots of the wheat plants were colonized by naturally occurring AMF of this soil. 1.6 kb-long ribosomal DNA sequences confirmed root colonization by the inoculated Swiss strain of *C. claroideum* of the wheat plants raised in γ-irradiated soil. We suspect that maladaptation of the AMF inoculant to the living conditions in the experimental soil [46] must have compromised symbiotic Zn acquisition by wheat. The inoculated AMF was originally isolated from Swiss arable soil, not calcareous, and with a loamy texture, a lower, near neutral pH, and much richer in organic matter and bioavailable nutrients [47] than the study soil here. The improved Zn recovery from green manure of sunflower after application of mineral Zn fertilizer by the plants inoculated with the foreign AMF strain points at possibly complex soil-root-microbe interactions beneficial to mycorrhized plants. Lack, or just minor positive effects by the non-indigenous AMF inoculant should draw our attention to the fact that AMF inoculants can not be *a priori* considered effective in assisting crop plants to take up Zn from soil when introduced to soils of different physicchemical and biological properties.

γ-Irradiation has been shown to modify the physicochemical soil properties to some degree [48,49]. However, we believe that this did not invalidate our results. While the increased biomass (Figure 1) and N uptake (Figure 2) of the wheat plants grown in γ-irradiated soil can probably be related to released N from decomposing microbial necromass [49], the magnitude of this effect was certainly much smaller than that by the N added with the green manures (Figure 2, Table 2). Likewise, the levels of dissolved organic compounds [48] must have risen in response to γ-irradiation, but again this effect must have been considerably smaller than that caused by mixing 0. 4% (w/w) finely ground green manure to soil. Therefore, following Thompson [33], and until a mycorrhiza symbiosis-defective wheat mutant becomes available, we see no better approach than using γ-irradiation for the study of the influence of entire natural AMF assemblages on plant Zn uptake from real arable soil.

The finding of higher grain and aboveground Zn concentrations in plants raised on native than γ-irradiated soil (Figure 3) points at no Zn uptake stimulatory effect by elevated levels of dissolved organic compounds [48] and N after soil γ-irradiation [49]. The generally increased Zn tissue concentration after addition of green manure to soil (Figure 3) and higher Zn recovery from less N- and Zn-rich green manure of red clover than more N- and Zn-rich green manure of sunflower point at considerable influences by C- rather than N-limited saprotrophic soil microbes on Zn uptake of mycorrhized bread wheat plants. Being obligate biotrophs, AMF rely on saprotrophs for remobilization of mineral nutrients from decomposing green manure that they may as soon as available take up and then possibly deliver to their host plants as observed for the Zn from the green manure of sunflower (Figure 4). Much higher Zn recovery from the Zn- and N-poorer green manure of red clover than the Zn-richer and N-poorer green manure of sunflower (Figure 4) points at faster decomposition of the earlier than latter and thus also different speeds in nutrient recycling from different green manures. However, the two types of green manure appear not to have differed in Zn mobilization from soil (Figure 5).

Native as opposed to γ-irradiated soil after back-addition of an AMF propagule-free microbial filtrate of a water suspension of living soil does certainly not only differ in AMF occurrence. Besides the physicochemical changes discussed above [49], largely stochastic epidemic population growth of saprophytic organisms must occur [35]. Therefore, importance of fungi and microbes conferring similar nutritional benefits to plants as AMF [50] may increase in absence of otherwise naturally occurring AMF and much reduced population sizes of most of other just re-introduced soil microbes. Microbial nutrient competition with plants [34] may be particularly harsh when microbial population growth after inoculation coincides with release of nutrients from new microbial necromass and freshly applied mineral fertilizer, as it must have occurred in the γ-irradiated control soil of this experiment. The re-introduced soil microbes in the filtrate of the soil suspension and the newly inoculated foreign AMF inoculant may thus have mainly sequestered Zn and other nutrients in their newly formed biomass in γ-irradiated soil [34]. This would further explain why the inoculated foreign AMF strain did not assist much in plant Zn uptake.

In summary, this study advanced our knowledge on possible agronomic practices to biofortify cereal grains with Zn. i) It showed that addition of readily decomposable N-rich green manure to calcareous soil can raise grain Zn concentration of bread wheat to levels approaching those of only $ZnSO_4$ fertilizer-fed wheat plants; ii) The study showed that combined addition of N-rich green manure and $ZnSO_4$ fertilizer can considerably raise grain Zn concentration; iii) Mixing green manure to the soil showed that the native soil Zn pool can contribute considerably to total Zn accumulation in the aboveground plant biomass even when no additional mineral Zn fertilizer had been applied to the soil; iv) Lastly, the study emphasizes that care should be taken when trying to utilize AMF inoculants for supporting crop plants in their Zn uptake, when the fungi are not adapted to the prevailing soil conditions.

Acknowledgments

The authors would like to thank Dr. Laurie P. Mauclaire Schönholzer, Thomas Flura and Max Ruethi for their assistance in running the analytical equipment and Simon Ineichen for practical help in sample processing. We acknowledge critical comments by two anonymous reviewers that helped to clarify the main message of this study.

Author Contributions

Conceived and designed the experiments: JJ FA EF. Performed the experiments: FA. Analyzed the data: FA EF HAG. Wrote the paper: FA HAG EF RS. Provided the AM fungal inoculant: JJ. Provided the plant seeds and the soil: AHK MA. Enabled gamma-countingL JE. Approved the final manuscript version: JJ FA EF HAG AHK MA JE RS.

References

1. Curtis BC (2002) Wheat in the world. In B. C. . Curtis, S. . Rajaram, H. Gomez Macpherson (eds.), Bread wheat: Improvement and production. Food and Agriculture Organization of the United Nations, Rome, Italy.
2. Black RE, Victora CG, Walker SP, Bhutta ZA, Christian P, et al. (2013) Maternal and child undernutrition and overweight in low-income and middle-income countries. Lancet 382: 427–451.
3. Welch RM, Graham RD (2004) Breeding for micronutrients in staple food crops from a human nutrition perspective. J Exp Bot 55: 353–364.
4. Cakmak I, Kalayci M, Kaya Y, Torun AA, Aydin N, et al. (2010) Biofortification and localization of zinc in wheat grain. J Agr Food Chem 58: 9092–9102.
5. Cakmak I (2008) Enrichment of cereal grains with zinc: Agronomic or genetic biofortification? Plant Soil 302: 1–17.
6. Khoshgoftar AH, Shariatmadari H, Karimian N, Khajehpour MR (2006) Responses of wheat genotypes to zinc fertilization under saline soil conditions. J Plant Nutr 29: 1543–1556.
7. White PJ, Broadley MR (2011) Physiological limits to zinc biofortification of edible crops. Front Plant Sci 2: 80.
8. Soltani S, Khoshgoftarmanesh AH, Afyuni M, Shrivani M, Schulin R (2013) The effect of preceding crop on wheat grain zinc concentration and its relationship to total amino acids and dissolved organic carbon in rhizosphere soil solution. Biol Fert Soils 50: 239–247.
9. Cavagnaro TR (2008) The role of arbuscular mycorrhizas in improving plant zinc nutrition under low soil zinc concentrations: a review. Plant Soil 304: 315–325.
10. Lehmann A, Veresoglou SD, Leifheit EF, Rillig MC (2014) Arbuscular mycorrhizal influence on zinc nutrition in crop plants – A meta-analysis. Soil Biol Biochem 69: 123–131.
11. Ryan MH, Angus JF (2003) Arbuscular mycorrhizae in wheat and field pea crops on a low P soil: increased Zn-uptake but no increase in P-uptake or yield. Plant Soil 250: 225–239.
12. Ryan MH, Derrick JW, Dann PR (2004) Grain mineral concentrations and yield of wheat grown under organic and conventional management. J Sci Food Agr 84: 207–216.
13. Diesing WE, Sinaj S, Sarret G, Manceau A, Flura T, et al. (2008) Zinc speciation and isotopic exchangeability in soils polluted with heavy metals. Eur J Soil Sci 59: 716–729.
14. Gramlich A, Tandy S, Frossard E, Eikenberg J, Schulin R (2013) Availability of zinc and the ligands citrate and histidine to wheat: does uptake of entire complexes play a role? J Agric Food Chem 61: 10409–10417.
15. Alloway BJ (2009) Soil factors associated with zinc deficiency in crops and humans. Environ Geochem Hlth 31: 537–548.
16. Gao X, Zhang F, Hoffland E (2009) Malate exudation by six aerobic rice genotypes varying in zinc uptake efficiency. J Environ Qual 38: 2315–2321.
17. Daneshbakhsh B, Khoshgoftarmanesh AH, Shariatmadari H, Cakmak I (2013) Phytosiderophore release by wheat genotypes differing in zinc deficiency tolerance grown with Zn-free nutrient solution as affected by salinity. J Plant Physiol 170: 41–46.
18. Dakora FD, Phillips DA (2002) Root exudates as mediators of mineral acquisition in low-nutrient environments. Plant Soil 245: 35–47.
19. Hoffland E, Wei CZ, Wissuwa M (2006) Organic anion exudation by lowland rice (*Oryza sativa L.*) at zinc and phosphorus deficiency. Plant Soil 283: 155–162.
20. Ueno D, Rombola AD, Iwashita T, Nomoto K, Ma JF (2007) Identification of two novel phytosiderophores secreted by perennial grasses. New Phytol 174: 304–310.

21. Parniske M (2008) Arbuscular mycorrhiza: the mother of plant root endosymbioses. Nat Rev Microbiol 6: 763–775.
22. Bonfante P, Genre A (2010) Mechanisms underlying beneficial plant-fungus interactions in mycorrhizal symbiosis. Nat Commun 1: 48.
23. Fitter AH (1991) Costs and benefits of mycorrhizas - implications for functioning under natural conditions. Experientia 47: 350–355.
24. Joner EJ, Jakobsen I (1995) Growth and extracellular phosphatase-activity of arbuscular mycorrhizal hyphae as influenced by soil organic-matter. Soil Biol Biochem 27: 1153–1159.
25. Anonymous (2010). Keys to soil taxonomy. Natural Resources Conservation Service, United States Department of Agriculture, Washington, D.C., 338 p.
26. Mostafazadeh-Fard B, Mansouri H, Mousavi SF, Feizi M (2009) Effects of different levels of irrigation water salinity and leaching on yield and yield components of wheat in an arid region. J Irrig Drain E-Asce 135: 32–38.
27. Gee GW, Bauder JW (1986) Particle size analysis. In: A Klute, editor editors. Methods of soil analysis. Madison, Wisconsin, USA: American Society of Agronomy. pp. 383–411.
28. Rhoades JD (1996) Salinity: Electrical conductivity and total dissolved salts. Methods of soil analysis. Madison, Wisconsin, USA: Soil Science Society of America. pp. 417–435.
29. Walkey A, Black IA (1934) An examination of the Degtjareff method for determinig soil organic matter and proposed modification of the chromic acid titration method. Soil Sci 37: 29–38.
30. Burt R (2004) Soil survey laboratory methods manual: soil survey investigations report Nebraska: United States Department of Agriculture. Natural Resources Conservation Servic.
31. Lindsay WL, Norvell WA (1978) Development of a DTPA soil test for zinc, iron, manganese, and copper. Soil Sci Soc Am J 42: 421–428.
32. Maas EV (1986) Salt tolerance of plants. Appl Agric Res 1: 12–25.
33. Thompson JP (1990) Soil sterilization methods to show VA-mycorrhizae aid P and Zn nutrition of wheat in vertisols. Soil Biol Biochem 22: 229–240.
34. Nazeri N, Lambers H, Tibbett M, Ryan M (2013) Do arbuscular mycorrhizas or heterotrophic soil microbes contribute toward plant acquisition of a pulse of mineral phosphate? Plant Soil 373: 699–710.
35. van de Voorde TFJ, van der Putten WH, Bezemer TM (2012) Soil inoculation method determines the strength of plant–soil interactions. Soil Biol Biochem 55: 1–6.
36. Barker SJ, Stummer B, Gao L, Dispain I, O'Connor PJ, et al. (1998) A mutant in *Lycopersicon esculentum* Mill. with highly reduced VA mycorrhizal colonization, isolation and preliminary characterisation. Plant J 15: 791–797.
37. Hogland DR, Arnon OD (1938) The water-culture method of growing plants without soil. University of California college of agriculture, agricultural experiment station Berkeley, California. USA.
38. Schenck NC, Smith GS (1982) Additional new and unreported species of mycorrhizal fungi (Endogonaceae) from Florida. Mycologia 74: 77–92.
39. Gerdemann JW, Nicolson TH (1963) Spores of mycorrhizal *Endogone* species extracted from soil by wet sieving and decanting. T Brit Mycol Soc 46: 235–244.
40. Cavagnaro TR, Smith FA, Hay G, Carne-Cavagnaro VL, Smith SE (2004) Inoculum type does not affect overall resistance of an arbuscular mycorrhiza-defective tomato mutant to colonisation but inoculation does change competitive interactions with wild-type tomato. *New Phytol* 161: 485–494.
41. Karami M, Afyuni M, Khoshgoftarmanesh AH, Papritz A, Schulin R (2009) Grain zinc, iron, and copper concentrations of wheat grown in central Iran and their relationships with soil and climate variables. J Agr Food Chem 57: 10876–10882.
42. Sadeghzadeh B (2013) A review of zinc nutrition and plant breeding. J Soil Sci Plant Nutr 13: 905–927.
43. Kalayci M, Torun B, Eker S, Aydin M, Ozturk L, et al. (1999) Grain yield, zinc efficiency and zinc concentration of wheat cultivars grown in a zinc-deficient calcareous soil in field and greenhouse. Field Crop Res 63: 87–98.
44. Rengel Z (1999) Zinc deficiency in wheat genotypes grown in conventional and chelator-buffered nutrient solutions. Plant Sci 143: 221–230.
45. Neilands JB (1995) Siderophores: Structure and function of microbial iron transport compounds. J. Biol. Chem 270: 26723–26726.
46. Oliveira RS, Vosatka M, Dodd JC, Castro PML (2005) Studies on the diversity of arbuscular mycorrhizal fungi and the efficacy of two native isolates in a highly alkaline anthropogenic sediment. Mycorrhiza 16: 23–31.
47. Jansa J, Mozafar A, Anken T, Ruh R, Sanders IR, et al. (2002) Diversity and structure of AMF communities as affected by tillage in a temperate soil. Mycorrhiza 12: 225–234.
48. Marschner B, Bredow A (2002) Temperature effects on release and ecological properties of dissolved organic matter (DOM) in sterilized and biologically active soil samples. Soil Biol Biochem 34: 459–466.
49. McNamara NP, Black HIJ, Beresford NA, Parekh NR (2003) Effects of acute gamma irradiation on chemical, physical and biological properties of soils. Appl Soil Ecol 24: 117–132.
50. Kariman K, Barker SJ, Jost R, Finnegan PM, Tibbett M (2014) A novel plant–fungus symbiosis benefits the host without forming mycorrhizal structures. New Phytol 201: 1413–1422.

8

Fat Content and Nitrite-Curing Influence the Formation of Oxidation Products and NOC-Specific DNA Adducts during *In Vitro* Digestion of Meat

Thomas Van Hecke[1], Els Vossen[1], Julie Vanden Bussche[2], Katleen Raes[3], Lynn Vanhaecke[2], Stefaan De Smet[1]*

1 Laboratory for Animal Nutrition and Animal Product Quality, Department of Animal Production, Faculty of Bioscience Engineering, Ghent University, Melle, Belgium, 2 Laboratory of Chemical Analysis, Department of Veterinary Public Health and Food Safety, Faculty of Veterinary Medicine, Ghent University, Merelbeke, Belgium, 3 Laboratory for Food Microbiology and Biotechnology, Department of Industrial Biological Sciences, Faculty of Bioscience Engineering, Ghent University - Campus Kortrijk, Kortrijk, Belgium

Abstract

The effects of fat content and nitrite-curing of pork were investigated on the formation of cytotoxic and genotoxic lipid oxidation products (malondialdehyde, 4-hydroxy-2-nonenal, volatile simple aldehydes), protein oxidation products (protein carbonyl compounds) and NOC-specific DNA adducts (O^6-carboxy-methylguanine) during *in vitro* digestion. The formation of these products during digestion is suggested to be responsible for the association between red meat and processed meat consumption and colorectal cancer risk. Digestion of uncured pork to which fat was added (total fat content 5 or 20%), resulted in significantly higher lipid and protein oxidation in the mimicked duodenal and colonic fluids, compared to digestion of pork without added fat (1% fat). A higher fat content also significantly favored the formation of O^6-carboxy-methylguanine in the colon. Nitrite-curing of meat resulted in significantly lower lipid and protein oxidation before and after digestion, while an inconsistent effect on the formation of O^6-carboxy-methylguanine was observed. The presented results demonstrate that haem-Fe is not solely responsible for oxidation and nitrosation reactions throughout an *in vitro* digestion approach but its effect is promoted by a higher fat content in meat.

Editor: Roger A. Coulombe, Utah State University, United States of America

Funding: This study was financed by the Federal Public Service of Health, Food Chain Safety and Environment, Belgium (grant RF-11/625 MEATNOX) (http://www.health.belgium.be/eportal). L. Vanhaecke is supported by a postdoctoral fellowship from the Research Foundation - Flanders (FWO) (http://www.fwo.be/Postdoctorale-mandaten.aspx). The funders had no role in study design, data collection and analysis, decision to publish, or preparation of the manuscript.

Competing Interests: The authors have declared that no competing interests exist.

* Email: stefaan.desmet@ugent.be

Introduction

Several meta-analyses have reported a significant epidemiological association between colorectal cancer (CRC) and high intake of red and processed meat [1,2]. However, the biochemical mechanisms underlying this association have not been completely elucidated yet. To date, the formation of cyto- and genotoxic oxidation products and genotoxic *N*-nitroso-compounds (NOCs) during digestion are considered the most plausible factors contributing to the increased risk of developing CRC when consuming large amounts of red and in particular processed meat [3]. Meat contains proteins, unsaturated lipids, haem-Fe and in case of processed meat also nitrite, which are all compounds involved in oxidation and nitrosation processes.

Major cyto- and genotoxic aldehydes such as malondialdehyde (MDA) and 4-hydroxy-2-nonenal (4-HNE), and less cytotoxic simple aldehydes, e.g. hexanal, are formed by free radical-induced damage to polyunsaturated fatty acids (PUFA). Lipid oxidation products are formed during processing, storage and preparation of meat, as well as during digestion in the gastro-intestinal tract. Next to fat, also proteins can be oxidized, resulting in the formation of protein carbonyl compounds (PCC). Lipid and protein oxidation products may cause oxidative stress and induce DNA damage due to their highly reactive nature. MDA and 4-HNE are prevailing in higher concentrations in colonic mucosae of CRC patients compared to a healthy control group [4]. Also PCC were described to be higher in plasma of CRC patients compared to a control group [5].

Previously, it was shown that volunteers on a high red meat diet had higher endogenous formation of genotoxic NOCs in feces compared to vegetarians, measured as 'apparent total nitroso-compounds' (ATNC) [6]. Furthermore, colonic exfoliated cells in the red meat-eating group of this study displayed higher concentrations of the NOC-specific DNA adduct O^6-carboxy-methylguanine (O^6-C-MeG), which were positively correlated with ATNC concentrations in feces [6]. Measurement of O^6-C-MeG is far more specific than ATNC since the latter also include nitrosothiols and nitrosyl-heme in addition to the genotoxic NOCs.

Haem-Fe in meat has been shown to be the main promoter of the peroxidation and nitrosation pathway [3]. However, when rats were fed a diet rich in haem-Fe, the effect of haem on colonic epithelial proliferation and cytolytic activity of fecal water was lower in a low fat diet (4.2%), compared to diets containing more fat (11.5 and 20.3%) [7]. A lean beef diet (5.0% fat) high in haem-

Fe did not promote colon carcinogenesis in cancer-induced rats [8]. Hence, we hypothesized that the fat content in meat might modulate the effect of haem on peroxidation and nitrosation.

Nitrite salt is widely used as a curing agent in meat products for color formation, to inhibit outgrowth of *Clostridium botulinum*, and to delay oxidative rancidity. However, nitrite-curing has also been suggested to increase NOC formation in meat products. Several studies have reported on the influence of nitrite-cured meats on the promotion of colorectal carcinogenesis. Rats consuming nitrite-cured hot-dogs (4.7% fat) had 3.7 to 5.0 fold higher NOC levels in feces compared to a control group, while consumption of beef (3.6% fat) resulted in a 2.0 to 2.9 fold increase [9]. A nitrite-cured ham diet increased cytotoxicity, lipid peroxidation and amount of 'mucin depleted foci' (MDF) in the colon of rats, compared to a control group [10]. However, fresh meat and processed meats differ in more properties than only nitrite-curing. Variation in haem-Fe content, fat content, and different processing procedures such as mincing and heating do not allow to draw conclusions on the isolated effect of nitrite-curing in previously mentioned studies. In a controlled study, Santarelli *et al.* [11] showed that consumption of nitrite-cured meat and oxidized meat increased ATNC and MDF in the colon of rats compared to consumption of similar non-cured and non-oxidized meat. Moreover, a human intervention study showed increased fecal ATNC when a high proportion of red meat (21.4% fat) or nitrite-cured processed meat (24.0% fat) was consumed, compared to a vegetarian diet, but no significant difference was seen between the red meat and processed meat diets [12].

Therefore, we aimed at elucidating the likely modulating effects of fat content and nitrite-curing of meat on lipid and protein oxidation markers, and the formation of NOC-specific DNA adducts during digestion. For this purpose, we used an *in vitro* digestion protocol adapted from Versantfoort *et al.* [13], followed by a colonic fermentation step according to Van de Wiele *et al.* [14].

Materials and Methods

1. Experimental set-up

Uncured and nitrite-cured heated pork samples differing in fat content (targeted at 1, 5 or 20% fat) were compared before and after mimicked duodenal and colonic digestion. Each incubation run included all treatments in quadruplicate from which 2 duplicates underwent *in vitro* digestion until the duodenum and the remaining 2 until the colon. Each incubation run was performed three times with fecal inoculum originating from three different persons. In total, 2 meat samples before digestion, 6 duodenal digests and 6 colonic digests were obtained for each of the 6 prepared meat products.

2. Preparation of the meat samples

Commercially available lean meat samples from the *m. Longissimus dorsi* of pig were purchased in a local supermarket. The loin was manually chopped into cubes of approximately 1–2 cm^3. Subcutaneous pork fat from one batch was added to the chopped meat to obtain a targeted total fat content of 1 (no fat added), 5 and 20%. Meat samples with added fat were first minced in a grinder equipped with a 10 mm plate, followed by grinding through a 3.5 mm plate. After grinding, nitrite-curing was applied by adding 20 g 0.6% nitrite salt/kg meat, corresponding to an added concentration of 120 mg nitrite/kg meat. All meat samples were heated in a warm water bath for 15 min after the core temperature had reached 65°C. After manufacturing, all meat samples were homogenized in three 5 s bursts using a food processor, vacuum packed and stored at −20°C until the start of the incubation.

3. Digestive simulations

The *in vitro* digestions consisted of an enzymatic digestion simulating the mouth, stomach, and duodenum, followed by a simulation of the colonic fermentation. For the enzymatic digestion, the protocol described by Versantfoort *et al.* [13] was adapted by adding oxidants and antioxidants that are normally present in digestive juices (Table 1). Hence, peroxidase [15] and $NaNO_2$ [16] were added to the saliva juice, and ascorbic acid [17], H_2O_2 [18] and ferrous iron [18] were added to the gastric juice. Meat samples (4.5 g) were sequentially incubated for 5 minutes with 6 ml saliva, 2 hours with 12 ml gastric juice, and 2 hours with 2 ml bicarbonate buffer (1 M, pH 8.0), 12 ml duodenal juice and 6 ml bile. These enzymatic incubations were performed in quadruplicate. After completion, 2 of the 4 replicates were diluted with 44 ml H_2O to obtain the same solid/liquid ratio as in the colon (see below), homogenized with an ultraturrax (9500 rpm) and stored at −20°C and −80°C pending analysis. The 2 remaining replicates underwent the additional colonic fermentation stage according to Van de *Wiele et al.* [14]. SHIME (simulator of the human intestinal microbial ecosystem) medium (22 ml) [19] and a human fecal inoculum (22 ml) (for preparation cfr. 2.4) were added to the digesta. The vessels were continuously flushed with N_2 for 30 minutes to obtain an anaerobic environment. Anaerobic conditions of the flasks containing digesta at the colonic digestion stage were confirmed, using resazurin saturated test strips. Subsequently, the vessels were incubated for 72 hours while stirring at 37°C. To evaluate the rate of bacterial fermentation, total anaerobic bacteria were counted after 72 h of fermentation. One ml digestive fluid was serially diluted (10-fold) using a sterile peptone solution (1 g/l peptone, 0.4 g/l agar, 8.5 g/l NaCl and 0.5 g/l cystein), after which 0.1 ml was added on an RCM-plate (Reinforced Clostridial Medium). After 48 hours of incubation at 37°C, colony forming units (CFU) were counted and expressed as log_{10} CFU/ml digesta. As for the duodenal samples, colonic digestive fluids were homogenized by ultraturrax at 9500 rpm and subdivided in 1.3 ml aliquots while stirring on a magnetic field in dark and stored at −20°C and −80°C till analyses. Undigested control samples were obtained in duplicate by homogenizing 4.5 g meat in 82 ml H_2O, mimicking the liquid/solid ratio in the digested samples.

4. Preparation of human fecal inoculum

Fresh fecal material was collected from 3 volunteers without known gastro-intestinal diseases and without intake of antibiotics for at least 6 months. The 3 human donors of fecal material were recruited among the laboratory personnel through informal announcement and volunteers have given their written informed consent. The research was approved by the Federal Public Service of Health, Food Chain Safety and Environment, Belgium, but was not submitted to an ethical committee for approval, nor a waiver was received. The data and volunteer information were analyzed anonymously and de-identified. All volunteers were male, meat-eaters on a Western diet, and aged 49, 26 and 38 years, respectively. Fresh fecal material was diluted in pre-cooked PBS solution (1/4; w/v), to which sodium thioglycolate (1 g/l) was added as a reducing agent. The fecal slurry was filtered by a 1 mm metal sieve to remove the particulate matter. Afterwards, the inocula were stored at −80°C on glycerol stock (20%) in different aliquots. Before use in the colonic fermentation stage, the bacterial inoculum was cultured during 24 hours at 37°C to obtain the necessary microbiotic culture. For this purpose, fecal inoculum

Table 1. Composition of digestive juices used for the *in vitro* digestion of meat samples.

	DIGESTION[1]				FERMENTATION[7]	
	Mouth	Stomach	Duodenum		Colon	
	Saliva (1 L)	Gastric juice (1 L)	Duodenal juice (1 L)	Bile (1 L)	SHIME medium[8] (1 L)	Cultured bacterial inoculum* (1 L)
Inorganic sol.	0.90 g KCl	2.75 g NaCl	7.01 g NaCl	5.26 g NaCl	6.8 g KH_2PO_4	0.51 g NaCl
	0.20 g KSCN	0.27 g NaH_2PO_4	3.39 g $NaHCO_3$	5.79 g $NaHCO_3$	8.8 g K_2HPO_4	0.01 g KCl
	0.90 g NaH_2PO_4	0.82 g KCl	0.08 g KH_2PO_4	0.38 g KCl		0.23 g $Na_2HPO_4.12H_2O$
	0.57 g $NaSO_4$	0.40 g $CaCl_2$,$2H_2O$	0.56 g KCl	0.15 ml HCl 37%		0.02 g KH_2PO_4
	0.30 g NaCl	0.31 g NH_4Cl	0.05 g $MgCl_2$			
	1.69 g $NaHCO_3$	6.50 ml HCl 37%	0.18 ml HCl 37%			
Organic sol.	0.20 g Urea	0.09 g Urea	0.10 g Urea	0.25 g Urea	1.0 g Arabinogalactan	0.06 g $C_2H_3NaO_2S$
	11.5 mg Uric acid	0.02 g Glucuronic acid	1.00 g BSA	1.80 g BSA	3.0 g Yeast extract	33.3 g Brain heart infusion
	25.0 mg Mucin	0.65 g Glucose	9.00 g Pancreatin	30.0 g Bile	0.4 g Glucose	0.45 g L-Cystein-HCl
	2.50 IU Peroxidase[2]	0.33 g Glucoseamine-HCl	1.50 g Lipase		0.5 g L-Cystein-HCl	16.0 g Fecal matter
		17.6 mg Ascorbic acid[4]			4.0 g Mucin	20.0 ml Glycerol
		1.00 g BSA			2.0 g Pectin	
		2.50 g Pepsin			1.0 g Pepton	
		3.00 g Mucin			1.0 g Xylan	
					4.0 g Potato starch	
Add	6.90 mg $NaNO_2$[3]	10.0 µl H_2O_2 (30%)[5]	0.20 g $CaCl_2.2H_2O$	0.22 g $CaCl_2.2H_2O$		
		11.2 mg $FeSO_4.7H_2O$[6]				

DIGESTION[1]: based on Versantfoort *et al.* (13) unless otherwise indicated; Peroxidase[2]: Güven *et al.* (15), $NaNO_2$[3]: Takahama *et al.* (16), Ascorbic acid[4]: Dabrowska-Ufniarz *et al.* (17), H_2O_2[5]: Nalini *et al.* (18), $FeSO_4$[6]: Nalini *et al.* (18), FERMENTATION[7]: Based on Van de Wielle *et al.* (14), SHIME MEDIUM[8]: Molly *et al.* (19), *Bacterial inoculum was cultured under anaerobic conditions for 24 hours at 37°C and used immediately in the fermentation procedure.

was diluted with BHI broth (37 g/l Brain Heart Infusion and 0.5 g/l cysteine) at a 1/9 ratio. Subsequently, anaerobic conditions in the flask were reached by continuously flushing the headspace with N_2 during 1 hour.

5. Chemical composition of the meat samples

The meat samples were analyzed for dry matter, crude protein and crude fat content according to the ISO 1442–1973, ISO 937–1978 and ISO 1444–1973 methods, respectively. Lipids were extracted using chloroform/methanol (2/1; v/v) [20], whereas fatty acids (FA) were analyzed as described by Raes *et al.* [21]. Briefly, FA were methylated and analyzed by gas chromatography (HP6890, Brussels, Belgium) using a CP-Sil88 column for fatty acid methyl esters (FAME; 100 m×0.25 mm×0.25 µm; Chrompack, the Netherlands). Peaks were identified, based on their retention times corresponding with standards (NuChek Prep. Inc., Sigma, Bornem, Belgium). Nonadecanoic acid (C19:0) was used as an internal standard to quantify the individual and total FA content. The fatty acid profiles were expressed in g/100 g FAME. Residual nitrite concentrations were measured colorimetrically at 538 nm after diazotization with sulfanilamide and N-(1-naphtyl)-ethylenediamine dihydrochloride (ISO 2918–1975). Nitrite concentrations were calculated based on a standard curve obtained with SN and expressed as mg nitrite/kg meat. Hematin was determined colorimetrically by the method of Hornsey *et al.* [22], converted to haem-Fe using the formula haem-Fe = hematin *atomic weight Fe/molecular weight hematin and expressed as mg haem-Fe/100 g meat. Total Fe was determined by ICP-AES (Iris Intrepid II XSP, Thermo Electron corporation) following destruction by Bunsen burner and dry incineration at 550°C for 4 h, followed by dissolving in 3 ml concentrated HNO_3, diluting to 10 ml bidistilled water and filtration. Total Fe was calculated based on a standard curve and expressed as mg Fe/100 g meat.

6. Oxidation products

MDA concentrations in digesta (−20°C) were measured by a modified method in accordance with Grotto *et al.* [23]. TBARS were formed from the reaction of MDA with 2-thiobarbituric acid in an acid environment. After extraction in 1-butanol, the absorbance of the colored complex was measured colorimetrically at 532 nm. A standard curve with 1,1,3,3-tetramethoxypropane was used and the concentration was expressed as nmol MDA/ml solution.

Levels of 4-HNE, pentanal, hexanal, heptanal, octanal and nonanal were analyzed in digesta (−80°C) through HPLC (Agilent 1200 series, provided with a degasser, autosampler, quaternary pump, column oven and fluorescence detector) using an adapted method of Holley *et al.* [24]. All solutions were purified with activated carbon and filtrated. For preparation of the cyclohexanedione (CHD) reagent, 10 g ammonium sulfate and 0.29 ml acetic acid were resolved in 100 ml, adjusted to pH 5, and purified with activated carbon. After filtration, 0.25 g CHD, dissolved in 2 ml activated carbon purified MeOH, was added to the mixture. All glassware was cleaned with ethanol and H_2O and dried in a 100°C oven to remove contaminating aldehydes. One ml digest was mixed with 4 ml $CHCl_3$:MeOH (2:1, v/v) and 0.4 ml NaCl (9%). After 30 s vortex, the mixture was centrifuged (5 min, 1100 g) and the $CHCl_3$ phase was collected. The remaining aqueous solution was mixed again with 2 ml $CHCl_3$:MeOH and the $CHCl_3$ phase was collected as described before. The combined $CHCl_3$ phases were dried under gentle N_2 stream. The dried residue was resolved in 0.1 ml MeOH, 0.4 ml H_2O and 1 ml CHD reagent. After 1 h of heating at 60°C in a warm water bath, samples were filter sterilized (0.2 µm cellulose membrane filter) in dark HPLC vials. The injection volume was 80 µl and flow rate 1 ml/min. Separation was done on a Supelcosil LC-18 column (25 cm×4.6 mm, 5 µm, cat. 58295 Supelco), using stepwise elution (50% tetrahydrofuran from 0–40 min). The derivatized aldehydes were detected by a fluorescence detector at an excitation wavelength of 380 nm and an emission wavelength of 446 nm. Aldehydes were quantified using a standard curve and expressed as pmol aldehyde/ml digest.

The measurement of PCC following their covalent reaction with 2,4-dinitrophenylhydrazine (DNPH) was done according to Ganhão *et al.* [25]. This reaction leads to the formation of a stable 2,4-dinitrophenyl hydrazone product. Total carbonyl content was quantified colorimetrically at 370 nm, using a molar absorption coefficient of 21.0/(mM·cm) and expressed as nmol DNPH/mg protein. Protein concentrations were measured at 280 nm after reaction with 2 M HCl instead of DNPH, quantified using a standard curve with BSA and expressed as mg/ml solution.

7. O^6-Carboxy-methylguanine and O^6- methylguanine

The NOC-specific DNA adduct O^6-C-MeG was quantified using U-HPLC-MS/MS [26]. In brief, 182 µl of filter sterilized sample was incubated for 18 hours at 37°C with 100 µg calf thymus (CT-)DNA. After addition of the internal standard (50 µL, 20 ng/ml O^6-D3-MeG), the mixture was dissolved in 2 ml of 0.1 M formic acid and hydrolyzed by heating (80°C for 30 min). The hydrolysate was cooled on ice and then applied to an Oasis HLB cartridge (SPE) (30 mg, 1 ml), which was conditioned with 2 ml of 100% MeOH and equilibrated with 2 ml deionized water. After loading the hydrolysate, a vacuum suction was applied on the SPE cartridge, followed by the elution step with 2 ml of 100% MeOH. The collected fraction was evaporated to dryness (90 min, 20°C) using a SpeedVac Plus (Savant, Holbrook, NY, USA). Finally, the dried residue was dissolved in a total volume of 100 µl of mobile phase consisting of 95:5 0.05% aqueous acetic acid:H_2O. Chromatographic separation of the DNA-adducts was achieved by reversed phase chromatography and gradient elution. Separation of the DNA-adducts was carried out on a Nucleodur C18 ISIS column (5 µm, 250×4 mm, Machery Nagel, Düren, Germany), kept at 30°C. Analysis was performed on a triple quadrupole mass analyzer (TSQ Vantage, Thermo Electron, San Jose, USA), fitted with a heated electrospray ionization (HESI II) source operating in the positive ion mode. A standard curve of O^6-C-MeG was made by derivatization of O^6-carboxymethyl-deoxyguanosine (O^6-C-MedG) with 0, 1 M formic acid at 70°C for 1 hour [27]. O^6-C-MeG was quantified using the standard curve and the area ratio of internal standard O^6-D3-MeG and expressed as ng O^6-C-MeG/ml digesta.

8. Short chain fatty acids and NH_3

Five ml of 10% formic acid containing internal standard (1 mg 2-ethyl butyric acid) was added to 1 ml digest. After 15 min centrifugation at 4°C and 22.000 *g*, supernatant was filtered and an aliquot was transferred into a 1.5 ml glass vial. Samples were stored at 4°C until analysis using gas chromatography (Shimadzu Corporation, 's-Hertogenbosch, The Netherlands) equipped with a Nukol column (30 m×0.25 mm×0.25 µm, Supelco) with a flame ionization detector. Briefly, 0.5 µl of sample was injected with the carrier gas N_2, the injector temperature was 250°C and the inlet pressure 52.7 kPa. The temperature program was 90°C at the start of the injection, increasing 20°C/min until 160°C (kept for 8.5 min), increasing 10°C/min until 170°C (kept for 2 min). The detection temperature was 250°C. Ammoniac concentrations were measured by a colorimetrical method described by Chaney and Marbach [28].

9. Statistical analysis

Data were analyzed using SAS enterprise guide 5. For the data on the meat samples prior to digestion, a linear model with the fixed effects of fat content, nitrite-curing and fat content × nitrite was used. For the duodenal and colonic digestion samples, a mixed model was used with the same fixed effects and the random effect of incubation run. Data on O^6-C-MeG were analyzed per incubation run separately due to very high variation between runs related to the use of different human fecal inocula. Tukey-adjusted *post hoc* tests were performed for all pairwise comparisons. $P<0.05$ was considered significant.

Results

1. Meat characteristics

The characteristics of the prepared meats prior to digestion are shown in Table 2. Dry matter content and fatty acid concentrations increased, whereas protein content decreased with increasing fat content. There was an unexpected effect of nitrite and fat content × nitrite interaction for the fat content due to a lower than targeted fat content of the 20% fat uncured samples. Addition of subcutaneous pork fat to the lean meat resulted in a significantly lower proportion of LC n-3 and n-6 PUFA and higher ALA, LA and SFA proportions in the fatty acid profile of the prepared meat samples. Residual nitrite levels in the cured meat samples amounted to approximately 41%, 30% and 17% of the added amount (120 mg/kg meat), hence there was a significant effect of fat content on the residual nitrite level. Even though originating from the same pork batch, nitrite-cured meats contained significantly less Fe than the corresponding uncured meats. However, no effect was observed on haem-Fe. The pH was slightly lower in the nitrite-cured meats while no effect of fat content was observed.

2. Total anaerobic bacterial count

Colonic digestive samples counted 7.4 ± 0.6 $\log_{10}$ CFU/ml and was not influenced by fat content ($P=.442$) or nitrite-curing ($P=.241$) (data not shown). However, colonic digestive fluids incubated with fecal inoculum 1 contained significantly less $\log_{10}$ CFU/ml (6.8 ± 0.4) than with inoculum 2 (7.6 ± 0.2) and 3 (7.9 ± 0.2).

3. Lipid oxidation

In the meat samples prior to digestion, MDA, pentanal and hexanal were significantly affected by fat content and nitrite-curing, the interaction term appeared also significant (Table 3). MDA was by far the most abundant aldehyde. Octanal was not detected at all, whereas 4-HNE and heptanal were detected in uncured but not in nitrite-cured meats. The concentration of nonanal was not affected by fat content, but nitrite-curing had a significant effect. MDA and volatile aldehyde concentrations were at least 2-fold up to 20-fold lower in the nitrite-cured versus the uncured meat samples. Aldehyde concentrations generally increased with increasing fat content in the uncured samples, but no clear effect of fat content on the aldehyde concentrations in the nitrite-cured samples was observed.

After digestion, MDA was by far the most abundant aldehyde, followed by hexanal. The effects of fat content, nitrite-curing and their interaction term were significant for most aldehydes. Nitrite-curing had no significant effect on pentanal and heptanal concentrations after colonic digestion. Higher concentrations of MDA were measured in both uncured and nitrite-cured meats compared to undigested meat. In contrast, concentrations of 4-HNE and volatile aldehydes were lower or similar after digestion of uncured meats, but higher for cured meats compared to before digestion. However, nitrite-cured meats had significantly lower concentrations of all measured aldehydes compared to uncured meats after the duodenal digestion and significantly lower MDA and hexanal with trends of lower 4-HNE and nonanal after colonic digestion. After duodenal digestion, nitrite-curing resulted in equal MDA independent of the fat content, while 4-HNE and pentanal were significantly higher in the cured 20% fat meat digest. Compared to their uncured equivalents, 4-HNE formation was only 2.5-fold lower in the 20% fat meat digest, while 12-fold lower concentrations were found in the 5% fat meat digest and no 4-HNE was detected in the 1% fat meat digest.

Because MDA was the only aldehyde that was present in higher concentrations in the colonic as compared to the duodenal digestion, it was hypothesized that MDA might be present in the human fecal inocula. To investigate this, blank incubations were performed without meat for the duodenal and colonic digestive simulation in a separate run. No aldehydes were detected in the blank duodenal digest, while MDA concentrations after 72 h of incubation were 5.1 ± 0.1; 17.0 ± 0.2 and 18.3 ± 1.1 nmol/ml digest for the three fecal inocula respectively, indicating a significant contribution of the fecal inoculum to the MDA levels in the colonic meat digests. One might assume similar effects for the other aldehydes, but these were not measured in the present experimental set up.

4. Protein oxidation

Increasing PCC concentrations were observed in the following order: undigested < duodenal < colonic digests independent of nitrite-curing (Table 4). Fat content did not affect the concentration of PCC before digestion, but nitrite-cured products had lower PCC concentrations than its uncured equivalents before digestion. In the duodenal digests, uncured samples with added fat showed significantly higher PCC concentrations than the ones without added fat. Nitrite-curing led to significantly lower PCC concentrations for the duodenal digests with no significant differences between digests with different fat content. After 72 h of colonic fermentation, a marginal effect of fat content was observed with lower PCC concentrations in the 5% fat meat digests as compared to the other samples.

Due to digestion, lower protein concentrations were measured in the duodenal and colonic digestive fluids compared to the meat before digestion (Table 4). Cured meats had significantly lower protein levels after duodenal and colonic simulation compared to uncured equivalent meats. From the blank incubations, it was estimated that the fecal inocula and SHIME medium contributed for 30–40% of the protein in the colonic fluid. Fecal proteins contained between 5.0 and 8.5 nmol DNPH/mg protein and hence largely contributed to the higher PCC concentrations in the meat colonic digests.

5. O^6-Carboxy-methylguanine and O^6-methylguanine

No O^6-C-MeG was detected in meats prior to digestion or at the end of the duodenal digestive simulation (Table 5). After mimicking colonic digestion, detection was highly dependent on the applied fecal inoculum. Colonic incubation with the inoculum from volunteer 1 did not result in detectable O^6-C-MeG. The fecal inocula from volunteers 2 and 3 resulted however in low and very high levels of O^6-C-MeG, respectively. A significant influence of fat content was observed, with higher concentrations of O^6-C-MeG in both cured and uncured samples containing 20% fat compared to samples lower in fat. The effect of nitrite-curing on the O^6-C-MeG content was not consistent with significantly lower O^6-C-MeG when using inoculum 2 and higher O^6-C-MeG when

Table 2. Composition of the pork model products used in the *in vitro* digestion.

Nitrite-curing		Uncured			Nitrite-cured				P-values		
Fat content (%)		**1**	**5**	**20**	**1**	**5**	**20**	**RMSE**	**F**	**NC**	**F×NC**
Item	**Unit**										
Dry matter	%	29.1^{c}	31.9^{b}	39.0^{a}	29.3^{c}	31.1^{b}	43.6^{a*}	0.41	**<.001**	**.002**	**<.001**
Protein	%	24.5^{a}	21.5	17.8^{b}	22.2	22.2	18.4	1.08	**.001**	.597	.171
Fat	%	1.6^{c}	5.6^{b}	17.7^{a}	1.7^{c}	5.4^{b}	20.6^{a*}	0.38	**<.001**	**.006**	**<.001**
SFA	g/100 g FAME	35.0^{c}	38.0^{b}	39.6^{a}	38.3^{b*}	38.3^{b}	39.6^{a}	0.22	**.026**	**<.001**	**<.001**
MUFA	g/100 g FAME	41.3	42.2	43.1	41.5	42.2	42.9	0.91	.178	.958	.942
PUFA	g/100 g FAME	15.4	16.0	16.4	15.4	15.9	16.1	0.23	.101	**.042**	.348
ALA	g/100 g FAME	0.32^{b}	0.68^{a}	0.79^{a}	0.31^{b}	0.69^{a}	0.75^{a}	0.02	**<.001**	.209	.868
LC n-3 PUFA	g/100 g FAME	0.86^{a}	0.29^{b}	0.22^{b}	0.81^{a}	0.27^{b}	0.17^{b}	0.02	**.002**	.058	.793
LA	g/100 g FAME	10.7^{b}	12.9^{a}	13.9^{a}	11.3	12.8	13.7	0.52	**<.001**	.757	.678
LC n-6 PUFA	g/100 g FAME	3.84^{c}	1.35^{b}	0.69^{a}	3.19^{c*}	1.38^{b}	0.69^{a}	0.07	**<.001**	**.005**	**.003**
Residual nitrite	mg/100 g	-	-	-	4.87^{c}	3.64^{b}	1.98^{a}	0.078	**<.001**		
Total Fe	mg/100 g	0.54	0.55	0.61	0.46	0.49	0.49	0.033	.238	**.004**	.495
Haem-Fe	mg/100 g	0.26	0.25	0.26	0.29	0.31	0.26	0.118	.627	.291	.672
pH	-	5.6	5.6	5.6	5.5	5.5	5.5	0.00		**<.001**	

Data (total n = 12) were analyzed using a linear model with the fixed effects of fat content (F), nitrite-curing (NC) and their interaction term (F×NC); RMSE = root mean square error; a, b, c = means for different fat content (within curing treatment) with different superscripts are significantly different ($P<0.05$); * = significantly different from uncured equivalent ($P<0.05$); SFA = saturated fatty acids; MUFA = monounsaturated fatty acids; PUFA = polyunsaturated fatty acids; ALA = α-linolenic acid (C18:3, n-3); LC n-3 PUFA = long chain omega-3 polyunsaturated fatty acids (C20:5, n-3; C22:5, n-3; C22–6, n-3); LA = linoleic acid (C18:2, n-6); LC n-6 PUFA = Long chain omega-6 polyunsaturated fatty acids (C20:4, n-6; C22:4, n-6; C22:5, n-6); FAME = fatty acid methyl esters.

Table 3. Lipid aldehyde concentrations in uncured and nitrite-cured pork containing different amounts of fat (1, 5, 20%) before and after *in vitro* digestion.

Nitrite-curing		**Uncured**			**Nitrite-cured**				**P-Values**		
Fat content (%)		**1**	**5**	**20**	**1**	**5**	**20**	**RMSE**	**F**	**NC**	**F×NC**
	Phase										
MDA	BD	4.0^{b}	5.4^{a}	5.3^{a}	2.0^{*}	2.0^{*}	1.9^{*}	0.19	**<.001**	**<.001**	**<.001**
(nmol/ml)	D	9.1^{b}	13.3^{a}	12.6^{a}	8.2^{*}	8.4^{*}	8.0^{*}	0.51	**<.001**	**<.001**	**<.001**
	C	15.5^{b}	18.0^{a}	16.4^{b}	14.7	14.3^{*}	13.4^{*}	0.85	**<.001**	**<.001**	**<.001**
4-HNE	BD	58^{b}	221^{a}	290^{a}	*nd*	*nd*	*nd*	38.1	**.019**		
(pmol/ml)	D	3.2^{c}	143^{b}	192^{a}	*nd*	11.5^{b*}	77.2^{a*}	31.6	**<.001**	**<.001**	**<.001**
	C	13.2^{b}	28.2^{a}	35.5^{a}	14.1	19.5	23.3	10.6	**.005**	.079	.335
Pentanal	BD	87^{b}	172^{a}	192^{a}	38	32^{*}	45^{*}	15.1	**.005**	**<.001**	**.007**
(pmol/ml)	D	65^{b}	220^{a}	211^{a}	56^{b}	91^{ab*}	124^{a*}	30.7	**<.001**	**<.001**	**<.001**
	C	73^{b}	115^{ab}	123^{a}	75^{b}	89^{ab}	121^{a}	25.3	**<.001**	.291	.352
Hexanal	BD	286^{b}	1162^{a}	1425^{a}	75	77^{*}	68^{*}	155.5	**.005**	**<.001**	**.005**
(pmol/ml)	D	158^{b}	581^{a}	604^{a}	106	154^{*}	219^{*}	126.3	**<.001**	**<.001**	**.002**
	C	121^{b}	229^{a}	252^{a}	116	156	200	61.4	**<.001**	**.044**	.384
Heptanal	BD	18.4	18.4	24.4	*nd*	*nd*	*nd*	2.91	.202		
(pmol/ml)	D	14.5^{b}	37.7^{a}	27.1^{x}	9.7	13.4^{*}	11.3^{*}	7.86	**<.001**	**<.001**	**.021**
	C	38.2	90.6	90.5	28.5^{b}	74.7^{ab}	105.8^{a}	35.70	**<.001**	.779	.537
Nonanal	BD	20.2	14.9	18.6	6.5^{*}	10.2	5.8^{*}	2.92	.838	**<.001**	.128
(pmol/ml)	D	18.6	18.4	12.9	18.6^{a}	13.1^{ab}	10.4^{b}	3.42	**<.001**	**.029**	.179
	C	11.7^{b}	20.2^{a}	24.3^{a}	12.4	15.4	19.4	4.70	**<.001**	.064	.261

Malondialdehyde (MDA) was measured colorimetrically and expressed as nmol/ml digest. 4-hydroxy-nonenal (4-HNE) and the simple aldehydes were measured through HPLC-fluorescence and expressed as pmol/ml. Aldehydes in meat before digestion (BD) (total n = 12) were analyzed using a linear model with the fixed effects of fat content (F), nitrite-curing (NC) and their interaction term (F×NC). Aldehydes in duodenal (D) digests (total n = 36) and colonic (C) digests (total n = 36) were analyzed using a mixed model with the fixed effects of F, NC and F×NC and the random effect of incubation run. RMSE = root mean square error; a, b, c = means for different fat content (within curing treatment) with different superscripts are significantly different ($P<0.05$); * = significantly different from uncured equivalent ($P<0.05$); *nd* = not detected.

Table 4. Protein oxidation in uncured and nitrite-cured pork containing different amounts of fat (1, 5, 20%) before and after *in vitro* digestion.

Nitrite-curing		Uncured			Nitrite-cured				P-Values		
Fat content (%)		**1**	**5**	**20**	**1**	**5**	**20**	**RMSE**	**F**	**NC**	**F×NC**
	Phase										
PCC	BD	1.49	1.74	1.36	1.00	0.76^{*}	1.28	0.261	.838	**<.001**	**.031**
(nmol DNPH/	D	1.84^{b}	2.45^{ab}	2.92^{a}	2.02	1.91	2.22	0.566	**.007**	**.026**	.054
mg protein)	C	4.42	4.10	4.70	4.40	3.49	4.60	0.770	**.035**	.358	.601
Protein	BD	6.70	6.75	6.40	6.60	6.25	5.80	0.304	.227	.120	.580
(mg/ml)	D	2.10	2.15	1.91	1.87	1.83	1.56	0.327	.137	**.011**	.890
	C	1.23^{b}	1.59^{a}	1.23^{b}	1.30^{a}	1.21^{ab*}	0.94^{b}	0.198	**.002**	**.006**	**.022**

Protein carbonyl compounds (PCC) and protein in meat before digestion (BD) (total n = 12) were analyzed using a linear model with the fixed effects of fat content (F), nitrite-curing (NC) and their interaction term (F×NC). Aldehydes in duodenal (D) digests (total n = 36) and colonic (C) digests (total n = 36) were analyzed using a mixed model with the fixed effects of F, NC and F×NC and the random effect of incubation run. RMSE = root mean square error; a, b = means for different fat content (within curing treatment) with different superscripts are significantly different ($P<0.05$); * = significantly different from uncured equivalent ($P<0.05$).

Table 5. NOC-induced DNA adduct formation by uncured and nitrite-cured pork containing different amounts of fat (1, 5, 20%) before and after *in vitro* digestion.

Nitrite-curing		Uncured			Nitrite-cured				P-Values		
Fat content (%)		**1**	**5**	**20**	**1**	**5**	**20**	**RMSE**	**F**	**NC**	**F×NC**
	Phase										
O^6-C-MeG	BD	*nd*	*nd*	*nd*	*nd*	*nd*	*nd*	-			
(ng/ml)	D	*nd*	*nd*	*nd*	*nd*	*nd*	*nd*	-			
	C1	*nd*	*nd*	*nd*	*nd*	*nd*	*nd*	-			
	C2	46.8^{c}	50.6^{b}	57.8^{a}	48.9^{a}	44.6^{b*}	50.8^{a*}	0.90	**<.001**	**<.001**	**<.001**
	C3	441^{b}	486^{b}	697^{a}	544^{b}	541^{b}	783^{a}	55.2	**<.001**	**.043**	.824

O^6-carboxy-methylguanine (O^6-C-MeG) was not detected (*nd*) in meat before digestion (BD) (total n = 12) and after duodenal (D) digestion (total n = 36). O^6-C-MeG in colonic (C1, C2, C3) digests were analyzed separately (total n = 12 per fecal inoculum), due to the very high variation between fecal inocula, using a linear model with the fixed effects of fat content (F), nitrite-curing (NC) and their interaction term (F×NC). RMSE = root mean square error; a, b, c = means for different fat content (within curing treatment) with different superscripts are significantly different ($P<0.05$); * = significantly different from uncured equivalent ($P<0.05$).

using inoculum 3. The DNA adduct O^6-MeG was not detected in any digestive fluid.

In the blank (no meat) incubations, no O^6-C-MeG was detected when incubated with fecal inoculum 1 but high DNA adduct concentrations were measured when fecal inoculum 2 (101.0±10.6 ng/ml) and 3 (82.8±26.1 ng/ml) were applied. It should be noted that these blank incubations were performed in a separate run and are therefore not fully comparable to the test incubations.

6. Short chain fatty acids and NH_3

Since the blank (no meat) incubations resulted in higher O^6-C-MeG formation compared to the meat digests when the second fecal inoculum was used, we wondered if this might be caused by differences in the fermentation process. Therefore, we repeated 3 blank incubations and 3 digestions of uncured pork containing 5% fat, using fecal inoculum 2. There was no detection of O^6-C-MeG in the blank or meat digests just after addition of the fecal inoculum. After 72 h of fermentation, the blank incubations contained 118.6±26.2 ng O^6-C-MeG/ml whereas the meat digests contained only 56.5±4.9 ng O^6-C-MeG/ml, in line with our previous findings. Significantly higher concentrations of acetate (56.7±9.0 μmol/ml vs. 33.1±0.6 μmol/ml), propionate (24.7±0.7 vs. 14.9±0.3 μmol/ml), butyrate (10.6±1.0 vs. 3.4±0.4 μmol/ml) and NH_3 (34.2±3.1 vs. 18.7±0.8 μmol/ml) were found in the meat digests, compared to the blank digests. Repeated incubations with fecal inoculum 3 confirmed these observations (data not shown).

Discussion

The present *in vitro* digestion study using pork model products allowed to investigate the effects of crucial factors that reflect the variability in composition and properties of meat products, i.e. nitrite-curing and fat content, on oxidation and nitrosation processes during digestion. By adding known pro-oxidants and antioxidants to the applied digestive juices, the *in vivo* situation was mimicked as close as possible. As expected, higher fat contents enhanced the formation of oxidation products and the NOC-specific DNA adduct O^6-C-MeG during digestion. Nitrite-curing on the other hand resulted in clearly lower concentrations of oxidation products before, during and at the end of the *in vitro* digestion, whereas the effect on the formation of O^6-C-MeG proved subjective for inter-individual variation. Previously, Corpet [3] suggested that the formation of oxidation products and NOCs are amongst those that could explain for the association between high red meat consumption and CRC.

In accordance to Hur *et al.* [29] who used a similar *in vitro* digestion model for beef patties, we observed a significant increase in MDA concentrations throughout the duodenal digestive simulation. Previously, it was reported that MDA in the small intestine is absorbed into the blood stream [30] after which it can reach several organs. Free MDA could react with DNA, resulting in the formation of the MDA-specific DNA adduct pyrimido [1,2-α] purine-10(3H)-one-2′-deoxyribose (M1dG) [31]. In contrast to MDA, highest concentrations of 4-HNE were observed in meat before digestion, after which they decreased throughout the digestion. After subtraction of the MDA values present in the applied fecal inocula, also MDA concentrations decreased from the duodenal to the colonic step. This decrease of MDA and 4-HNE during the colonic simulation could be due to reaction with proteins leading to the formation of Schiff bases or with bacterial DNA leading to DNA-adducts [31].

The antioxidative properties of nitrite were already very clear before digestion since MDA, 4-HNE, volatile simple aldehydes and PCC were clearly lower or even undetected in cured meats compared to uncured meats. Nitrite is a known antioxidant trough oxygen sequestration and may act as a precursor of the heat-stable NO-myoglobin by which the release of Fe^{2+} during heating is inhibited [32]. Consequently, less Fe^{2+} is available to catalyze the Fenton reaction, which is responsible for the initiation of oxidation processes. Since all meats were sampled fresh and oxidation in fresh meat is generally negligible, the higher lipid aldehyde and PCC concentrations in uncured meats must originate from processing (mincing, adding fat, heating). The clearly lower residual nitrite, found in the nitrite-cured meat samples when higher amounts of subcutaneous pork fat were added, could be explained by interaction of nitrite with unsaturated FA [33]. Addition of subcutaneous pork fat to meat samples resulted in an expected higher concentration of lipid aldehydes in meat, since more substrate is available for oxidation. Except for 4-HNE, the expected differences in lipid aldehydes between the 5 and 20% fat meat samples throughout digestion were not observed. Fat content of grounded beef varying between 10, 15 and 20% also had little effect on lipid oxidation parameters in the meat [34].

The lower values of oxidation products of nitrite-cured meats compared to uncured equivalents in duodenal and colonic fluids are in agreement with recently published work by Chenni *et al.* [35] who found that intake of nitrite through drinking water (1 g/l) reduced (25%) haem-induced lipid peroxidation in the colon of rats. This effect was not observed to be significant at lower doses (0.17 g/l nitrite and 0.23 g/l nitrate). Nitric oxide (NO) is able to react with ROS generating peroxynitrite, which can induce lipid peroxidation. However, NO can also react with lipophilic peroxyl radicals, generating far more stable alkyl peroxynitrates. Consequently, it was concluded that a 1:1 ratio of NO to ROS enhances lipid peroxidation, while an excess of NO results in inhibition [36]. The reaction between nitrite and unsaturated FA leads to lower residual nitrite levels in the 20% fat meat samples and hence could modify the NO:ROS ratio and induce lipid oxidation. This could explain the higher HNE, pentanal and hexanal concentrations in the cured 20% fat meat sample compared to the cured 1 and 5% fat meat samples.

Also increased protein oxidation was observed throughout the digestion of the meat samples. The higher PCC concentrations after the colonic digestive simulation could be largely attributed to proteins in the fecal inoculum and SHIME medium. No significant differences in PCC concentrations according to fat content were noticed before digestion. It was previously described that lipid radicals may damage proteins by the binding of lipid components such as MDA and 4-HNE to the protein [37]. This could explain the higher PCC concentrations in the uncured 20% fat treatment after duodenum digestion. The lower PCC concentrations in cured meat samples before and after duodenal digestive simulations correspond with the associated lower concentrations of lipid oxidation products.

Next to higher PCC formation, we also observed a significantly higher amount of residual protein in uncured samples, indicating lower protein digestion. These findings agree with Santé-Lhoutellier *et al.* [38] who found a highly significant negative correlation between PCC concentrations and proteolytic susceptibility to pepsin. As mentioned before, MDA and 4-HNE can also react with proteins, leading to the formation of Schiff bases, which are known to play a role in protein aggregation. Previously, it was shown that a higher amount of proteins reaching the colonic fermentation, resulted in a higher formation of potentially toxic protein fermentation products such as ammonium, phenol, pcresol and indol. However, higher formation of these products was not associated with enhanced colon cancer promotion in rats [39].

Previously, it was reported that haem-Fe is responsible for endogenous intestinal *N*-nitrosation [40]. Our results demonstrate that the fat content in meat products enhances the haem-induced intestinal *N*-nitrosation by detecting higher concentrations of the NOC-specific DNA adduct O^6-C-MeG when a higher fat content was present in the digested meat. Salivary nitrite or nitrite-cured meats are sources for NO formation. Both NO and O_2 preferentially diffuse in a lipid environment resulting in accumulation of both reactants in the lipid fraction to form nitrosating species. The rate of this reaction was described to be 300 times faster in a lipid compared to an aqueous environment [41], which could explain the facilitating role of fat in the formation of NOCs.

However, the effect of nitrite-curing of meat on O^6-C-MeG formation was inconsistent in our results, being either promoting or protective depending on the applied fecal inoculum. Possibly, the effect of nitrite-curing depends on the incubation conditions (e.g. O_2 tension), the bacterial composition of the fecal inoculum and interactions with other dietary compounds or metabolites formed during fermentation. This certainly warrants further investigation. However, the effect of nitrite-curing was perceived to be minor compared to the promoting effect of fat content for the meat products examined in the present study.

The formation of the NOC-specific DNA adduct O^6-C-MeG was also highly dependent on the applied fecal inoculum. A difference in total anaerobic bacteria in the colonic fluids, fermentation rate or bacterial composition of the used inocula could explain the differences in the magnitude of detection. More research is required to elucidate the underlying mechanisms causing these differences.

When O^6-C-MeG was measured in the colonic digests, blank incubations without meat displayed high values after 72 h of fermentation. Since no O^6-C-MeG was detected just after addition of the fecal inoculum, its formation must have occurred during the fermentation. The sometimes higher values for the blank incubations than the meat digests is surprising since one expects a higher fermentation rate and more bacterial growth in the meat digests due to the higher supply of nutrients (protein, glycogen, B vitamins,...). Indeed, meat digests contained approximately 2-fold higher concentrations of NH_3, acetate and propionate, and 3-fold higher concentrations of butyrate compared to the blank digests. However, it has been shown in rats on a high protein diet that high butyrate concentrations in the colon decreased DNA damage in the colonocytes [42]. Butyrate was also able to decrease H_2O_2-induced DNA damage in human colonocytes [43]. Therefore, it seems likely that the 3-fold higher butyrate production during fermentation of the meat digests interfered in the genotoxic activity of compounds. The values of O^6-C-MeG in the blank digests can thus not be simply subtracted from the values of the meat digests.

In conclusion, our results indicate that addition of fat favors the formation of oxidation products and the NOC-specific DNA adduct O^6-C-MeG during the digestion of pork. Nitrite-curing of meat inhibited lipid and protein oxidation but this inhibition was less pronounced throughout digestion when meat in the incubation fluids contained 20% fat. The effect of nitrite-curing on O^6-C-MeG formation was contradictory in our results and requires more research. The measurement of O^6-C-MeG was highly variable between fecal inocula originating from different volunteers. In this research, we simulated the passage of meat through the gastrointestinal tract as close as possible to the *in vivo* situation using static *in vitro* incubations. Several *in vivo* experiments have been conducted towards this subject but these studies do not always gain insights in some mechanistic pathways as the presented *in vitro* work does. However, since the *in vivo* situation is always more complex than *in vitro* conditions, the outcomes in this study should be confirmed *in vivo*.

Acknowledgments

We would like to thank S. Lescouhier, D. Baeyens and E. Claeys for the preparation and characterization of meat samples. C. Boterdaele is thanked for her assistance in performing the incubations. L. Hemeryck is thanked for her assistance in the analysis of the NOC-specific DNA adducts.

Author Contributions

Conceived and designed the experiments: TVH KR LV SDS. Performed the experiments: TVH EV. Analyzed the data: TVH. Contributed reagents/materials/analysis tools: JVB LV. Wrote the paper: TVH SDS. Read and commented on the draft manuscript: EV JVB KR LV.

References

1. Chan DS, Lau R, Aune D, Vieira R, Greenwood DC, et al. (2011). Red and processed meat and colorectal cancer incidence: meta-analysis of prospective studies. PLOS ONE 6: e20456.
2. Larsson SC, Wolk A (2006). Meat consumption and risk of colorectal cancer: A meta-analysis of prospective studies. Int J Cancer 119: 2657–2664.
3. Corpet DE (2011). Red meat and colon cancer: Should we become vegetarians, or can we make meat safer? Meat Sci 89: 310–316.
4. Skrzydlewska E, Sulkowski S, Koda M, Zalewski B, Kanczuga-Koda L, et al. (2005). Lipid peroxidation and antioxidant status in colorectal cancer. World J. Gastroenterol 11: 403–406.
5. Yeh CC, Lai CY, Hsieh LL, Tang R, Wu FY, et al. (2010). Protein carbonyl levels, glutathione S-transferase polymorphisms and risk of colorectal cancer. Carcinogenesis 31: 228–233.
6. Lewin MH, Bailey N, Bandaletova T, Bowman R, Cross AJ, et al. (2006). Red meat enhances the colonic formation of the DNA adduct O6-carboxymethyl guanine: implications for colorectal cancer risk. Cancer Res 66: 1859–1865.
7. Sesink AL, Termont DS, Kleibeuker JH, Van der Meer R (2000). Red meat and colon cancer: dietary haem, but not fat, has cytotoxic and hyperproliferative effects on rat colonic epithelium. Carcinogenesis 21: 1909–1915.
8. Lai C, Dunn DM, Miller MF, Pence BC (1997). Non-promoting effects of iron from beef in the rat colon carcinogenesis model. Cancer Let 112: 87–91.
9. Mirvish SS, Haorah J, Zhou L, Clapper ML, Harrison KL, et al. (2002). Total *N*-nitroso compounds and their precursors in hot dogs and in the gastrointestinal tract and feces of rats and mice: possible etiologic agents for colon cancer. J Nutr 132: 3526S–3529S.
10. Pierre FH, Santarelli RL, Allam O, Taché S, Naud N, et al. (2010). Freeze-dried ham promotes azoxymethane-induced mucin-depleted foci and aberrant crypt foci in rat colon. Nutr Cancer 62: 567–573.
11. Santarelli RL, Vendeuvre JL, Naud N, Taché S, Guéraud F, et al. (2010). Meat processing and colon carcinogenesis: cooked, nitrite-treated, and oxidized high-heme cured meat promotes mucin-depleted foci in rats. Cancer Prev Res 3: 852–864.
12. Joosen AM, Kuhnle GG, Aspinall SM, Barrow TM, Lecommandeur E, et al. (2009). Effect of processed and red meat on endogenous nitrosation and DNA damage. Carcinogenesis 30: 1402–1407.
13. Versantfoort CHM, Oomen AG, Van de Kamp E, Rompelberg CJM, Sips AJAM (2005). Applicability of an in vitro digestion model in assessing the bioaccessibility of mycotoxins from food. Food Chem Toxicol 43: 31–40.
14. Van de Wiele T, Vanhaecke L, Boeckaert C, Peru K, Headley J, et al. (2005). Human colon microbiota transform polycyclic aromatic hydrocarbons to estrogenic metabolites. Environ Health Persp 113: 6.
15. Güven Y, Satman I, Dinççag N, Alptekin S (1996). Salivary peroxidase activity in whole saliva of patients with insulin-dependent (type-1) diabetes mellitus. J Clin Periodontol 23: 879–88.
16. Takahama U, Yamamoto A, Hirota S, Oniki T (2003). Quercetin-dependent reduction of salivary nitrite to nitric oxide under acidic conditions and interaction between quercetin and ascorbic acid during the reduction. J Agr Food Chem 51: 6014–6020.
17. Dabrowska-Ufniarz E, Dzieniszewski J, Jarosz M, Wartanowicz M (2002). Vitamin C concentration in gastric juice in patients with precancerous lesions of the stomach and gastric cancer. Med Sci Monitor 8: CR96–CR103.

18. Nalini S, Ramakrishna BS, Mohanty A, Balasubramanian KA (1992). Hydroxyl radical formation in human gastric juice. J Gastroen Hepatol 7: 497–501.
19. Molly K, Woestyne MV, Smet ID, Verstraete W (1994). Validation of the simulator of the human intestinal microbial ecosystem (SHIME) reactor using microorganism-associated activities. Microb Ecol Health D 7: 191–200.
20. Folch J, Lees M, Sloane-Stanley GH (1957). A simple method for the isolation and purification of total lipids from animal tissues. J Biol Chem 226: 497–509.
21. Raes K, De Smet S, Demeyer D (2001). Effect of double-muscling in Belgian Blue young bulls on the intramuscular fatty acid composition with emphasis on conjugated linoleic acid and polyunsaturated fatty acids. Anim Sci 73: 253–260.
22. Hornsey H (1956). The colour of cooked cured pork - Estimation of the Nitric oxide-Haem Pigments. J Sci Food Agric 7: 534–547.
23. Grotto D, Santa Maria LD, Boeira S, Valentini J, Charão MF, et al. (2007). Rapid quantification of malondialdehyde in plasma by high performance liquid chromatography–visible detection. J Pharmaceut Biomed 43: 619–624.
24. Holley AE, Walker MK, Cheeseman KH, Slater TF (1993). Measurement of n-alkanals and hydroxyalkenals in biological samples. Free Radical Bio Med 15: 281–289.
25. Ganhão R, Morcuende D, Estévez M (2010). Protein oxidation in emulsified cooked burger patties with added fruit extracts: Influence on colour and texture deterioration during chill storage. Meat Sci 85: 402–409.
26. Vanden Bussche J, Moore SA, Pasmans F, Kuhnle GGC, Vanhaecke L (2012). An approach based on ultrahigh pressure liquid chromatography-tandem mass spectrometry to quantify O^6-methyl and O^6-carboxymethylguanine DNA adducts in intestinal cell lines. J Chromatogr A 1257: 25–33.
27. Moore SA, Xeniou O, Zeng ZT, Humphreys E, Burr S, et al. (2010). Optimizing immunoslot blot assays and application to low DNA adduct levels using an amplification approach. Anal Biochem 403: 67–73.
28. Chaney AL, Marbach EP (1962). Modified reagents for determination of urea and ammonia. Clin Chem 8: 130.
29. Hur SJ, Lim BO, Park GB, Joo ST (2009). Effects of various fiber additions on lipid digestion during in vitro digestion of beef patties. J Food Sci 74: C653–C657.
30. Gorelik S, Ligumsky M, Kohen R, Kanner J (2008). A novel function of red wine polyphenols in humans: prevention of absorption of cytotoxic lipid peroxidation products. FASEB J 22: 41–46.
31. Nair U, Bartsch H, Nair J (2007). Lipid peroxidation-induced DNA damage in cancer-prone inflammatory diseases: a review of published adduct types and levels in humans. Free Radical Biol Med 43: 1109–1120.
32. Honikel KO (2008). The use and control of nitrate and nitrite for the processing of meat products. Meat Sci 78: 68–76.
33. Trostchansky A, Rubbo H (2008). Nitrated fatty acids: mechanisms of formation, chemical characterization, and biological properties. Free Radical Biol Med 44: 1887–1896.
34. Ismail HA, Lee EJ, Ko KY, Ahn DU (2009). Fat content influences the color, lipid oxidation, and volatiles of irradiated ground beef. J Food Sci 74: C432–C440.
35. Chenni FZ, Taché S, Naud N, Guéraud F, Hobbs DA, et al. (2013). Heme-Induced Biomarkers Associated with Red Meat Promotion of colon Cancer Are Not Modulated by the Intake of Nitrite. Nutr Cancer 65: 227–233.
36. Darley-Usmar V, Wiseman H, Halliwell B (1995). Nitric oxide and oxygen radicals: a question of balance. FEBS Lett 369: 131–135.
37. Dean R, Fu S, Stocker R, Davies M (1997). Biochemistry and pathology of radical-mediated protein oxidation. Biochem J 324: 1–18.
38. Santé-Lhoutellier V, Astruc T, Marinova P, Greve E, Gatellier P (2008). Effect of meat cooking on physicochemical state and *in vitro* digestibility of myofibrillar proteins. J Agr Food Chem 56: 1488–1494.
39. Corpet DE, Yin Y, Zhang XM, Remesy C, Stamp D, et al. (1995). Colonic protein fermentation and promotion of colon carcinogenesis by thermolyzed casein. Nutr Cancer 23: 271–276.
40. Cross AJ, Pollock JR, Bingham SA (2003). Haem, not protein or inorganic iron, is responsible for endogenous intestinal N-nitrosation arising from red meat. Cancer Res 63: 2358–2360.
41. Liu X, Miller MJ, Joshi MS, Thomas DD, Lancaster JR (1998). Accelerated reaction of nitric oxide with O2 within the hydrophobic interior of biological membranes. P Natl Acad Sci USA 95: 2175–2179.
42. Bajka BH, Clarke JM, Cobiac L, Topping DL (2008). Butyrylated starch protects colonocyte DNA against dietary protein-induced damage in rats. Carcinogenesis 29: 2169–2174.
43. Rosignoli P, Fabiani R, De Bartolomeo A, Spinozzi F, Agea E, et al. (2001). Protective activity of butyrate on hydrogen peroxide-induced DNA damage in isolated human colonocytes and HT29 tumour cells. Carcinogenesis 22: 1675–1680.

9

Suitable Habitats for Endangered Frugivorous Mammals: Small-Scale Comparison, Regeneration Forest and Chimpanzee Density in Kibale National Park, Uganda

Sarah Bortolamiol[1,2,6]*, Marianne Cohen[1,3], Kevin Potts[4], Flora Pennec[2], Protase Rwaburindore[5], John Kasenene[5], Andrew Seguya[7], Quentin Vignaud[2,3], Sabrina Krief[2,6]

1 UMR 7533 Laboratoire Dynamiques Sociales et Recomposition des Espaces, Paris Diderot University (Sorbonne Paris Cité), Paris, France, **2** UMR 7206 Eco-Anthropologie et Ethnobiologie (MNHN/CNRS/Paris Diderot), Paris, France, **3** Pole Image, Paris Diderot University (Sorbonne Paris Cité), Paris, France, **4** Department of Biology, Augsburg College, Minneapolis, Minnesota, United States of America, **5** Department of Botany, Makerere University, Kampala, Uganda, **6** Great Ape Conservation Project (PCGS), Sebitoli UWA Station in Kibale National Park, Fort Portal, Uganda, **7** Uganda Wildlife Authority, Kampala, Uganda

Abstract

Landscape patterns and chimpanzee (*Pan troglodytes schweinfurthii*) densities in Kibale National Park show important variation among communities that are geographically close to one another (from 1.5 to 5.1 chimpanzees/km^2). Anthropogenic activities inside the park (past logging activities, current encroachment) and outside its limits (food and cash crops) may impact the amount and distribution of food resources for chimpanzees (frugivorous species) and their spatial distribution within the park. Spatial and temporal patterns of fruit availability were recorded over 18 months at Sebitoli (a site of intermediate chimpanzee density and higher anthropic pressure) with the aim of understanding the factors explaining chimpanzee density there, in comparison to results from two other sites, also in Kibale: Kanyawara (low chimpanzee density) and Ngogo (high density, and furthest from Sebitoli). Because of the post-logging regenerating status of the forest in Sebitoli and Kanyawara, smaller basal area (BA) of fruiting trees most widely consumed by the chimpanzees in Kanyawara and Sebitoli was expected compared to Ngogo (not logged commercially). Due to the distance between sites, spatial and temporal fruit abundance in Sebitoli was expected to be more similar to Kanyawara than to Ngogo. While species functional classes consumed by Sebitoli chimpanzees (foods eaten during periods of high or low fruit abundance) differ from the two other sites, Sebitoli is very similar to Kanyawara in terms of land-cover and consumed species. Among feeding trees, *Ficus* species are particularly important resources for chimpanzees at Sebitoli, where their basal area is higher than at Kanywara or Ngogo. *Ficus* species provided a relatively consistent supply of food for chimpanzees throughout the year, and we suggest that this could help to explain the unusually high density of chimpanzees in such a disturbed site.

Editor: Cédric Sueur, Institut Pluridisciplinaire Hubert Curien, France

Funding: Field trips have been granted by the National Museum of Natural History/ATM 16, ANR JC-JC SAFAPE, Projet pour la Conservation des Grands Singes and Société Francophone de Primatologie. The funders had no role in study design, data collection and analysis, decision to publish, or preparation of the manuscript.

Competing Interests: The authors have declared that no competing interests exist.

* Email: bortolamiol.sarah@gmail.com

Introduction

Factors described as unfavorable to endangered species density, such as habitat fragmentation or anthropogenic activities presence, are not necessarily limiting long-term co-existence of wildlife with human activities [1,2,3]. Our closest relatives, the great apes, are threatened, facing decline of their suitable habitats [4]. Among them, the chimpanzee (*Pan troglodytes*) is classified on the IUCN red list as endangered and has shown a capacity to intermittently cope with human activities [5,6] in the context of increasing proximity between wildlife and human populations [3]. Anti-poaching strategies [7], chimpanzee behavioral flexibility [8], and adaptability to environmental changes could be the main factors influencing their resilience and future capacity for long-term survival. A rough indicator of chimpanzee resilience should be their population density [9].

The availability of food resources influences the geographical distribution and population density limits of a species [10,11]. For example, it has been shown [12] that red colobus *(Procolobus pennantii)* and redtail monkey's group size *(Cercopithecus ascanius)* increased with food resource availability within Kibale National Park. Frugivorous/omnivorous primate (redtail monkeys, blue monkeys – *Cercopithecus mitis*, mangabeys – *Cercopithecus albigena*, l'Hoest monkeys - *Cercopithecus lhoesti*, chimpanzees, baboons - *Papio anubis*) biomass varies among sites within the park (Kanyawara, Ngogo). For example, the biomass of redtail monkeys and mangabeys was 13% greater at Kanyawara than at Ngogo, likely due to different carrying capacity of the two sites, nonequilibrium of the frugivororous community (blue monkeys were out-competed by old-growth specialists at Ngogo) and fruit availability [13,14]. As frugivorous species, chimpanzees are strongly dependent on scarce and patchy food resources [15,16], and thus very vulnerable to habitat disturbance [17]. During periods of fruit scarcity or in response to ecological changes, the flexible fission-fusion social structure exhibited by chimpanzees allows them to reduce party sizes (subgroup) in order to decrease potential feeding competition [18,19,20,21,22,23,24].

Moreover, fruit abundance is variable between seasons [25,26] and years [27,28] in tropical forests. Ripe fruit availability varies within primate habitats, resulting in periods of nutrient deficiency or abundance [15,29]. Food resources can be classified by functional types, since some species provide fruit during times of high fruit abundance (HFA) while others provide fruit during times of low fruit abundance (LFA) [30]. HFA periods tend to offer a higher quantity and diversity of food, and thus frugivorous are able to choose items with preferred nutritional and chemical properties, like digestible carbohydrates and low tannins [31,32]. Further studies have distinguished plant species fruiting during LFA periods as synchronous (sLFA) versus asynchronous (aLFA) fruit producers: the first is sufficiently abundant in the habitat during a particular fruiting season to sustain a frugivorous population [30,33] while the second one is more constantly available but in low abundance.

Among fruit resources, figs are known to be important for chimpanzees wherever they are available [34]. For example, Fig. consumption accounts for 37% up to 90% of monthly feeding time in Kanyawara [35]. *Ficus* species are often cited as fruiting asynchronously and providing continuous and vital supply of fruits across the years for frugivorous species [27], especially during times of fruit scarcity as they serve as important fallback foods at some sites [36].

Studies performed at fine spatial scales are uniquely capable of assessing the adaptability of species to their environment [37], especially the intrinsic capability of mammals to cope with rapid environmental changes. Kibale National Park (KNP), western Uganda, is an interesting study case because it harbors a high density of Eastern chimpanzees (*Pan troglodytes schweinfurthii*, between 500–1000 individuals according to sampling methods [38,39]) varying considerably among communities. Despite the relatively small size of the park, chimpanzee density differs greatly among different study sites [30], as observed for other primates [12,13,14]. The two sites experiencing the most extreme chimpanzee densities among those currently known at Kibale National Park (from 1.5 individuals/km^2 at Kanyawara to 5.1 individuals/km^2 at Ngogo) are separated by only 11 km.

A previous study showed the impact of spatial and temporal heterogeneity of fruit resources on chimpanzee density in the two sites [30]. Ngogo, the site with a high density of chimpanzees, experienced a high density of food plant species during a period of high productivity (HFA); plants fruiting synchronously (sLFA) during periods of low production (LFA) were also a critical component of the resource base. While there was no significant difference for the number of HFA species between sites, the number of sLFA species was higher at Ngogo than Kanyawara. This suggests that sLFA food could be an important factor promoting chimpanzee density.

In this study, we add a third site –Sebitoli-, with the goal of further understanding the link between chimpanzee density, vegetation heterogeneity and spatial and temporal food availability, providing us with a picture of the ability of chimpanzees to adapt to various ecological conditions. Sebitoli site, in the Northern part of the national park, is a very useful third case study, as it is a fragmented habitat, partly in regeneration, and surrounded by an area highly transformed by human population. Inside the forest, a tarmac road cuts through the park, while tea and eucalyptus plantations, as well as gardens, are located at the forest edge [40]. Despite these constraints, the density of chimpanzees is estimated at 4.1 individuals/km^2 (Sebitoli Chimpanzee Project – SCP, unpublished data), which is among the highest in Kibale.

In our study, we test the following hypotheses:

First, according to the small distance between the three sites (< 20 km) we expect low vegetation differences between them, and larger vegetation differences between the two more distant sites (i.e. Sebitoli and Ngogo).

Second, we assume that Sebitoli and Kanyawara are more disturbed than Ngogo because they experienced commercial logging that may have generated gaps and regenerating forests. In addition, both are located on the forest edge and thus constrained by anthropic landscape (gardens, tea and eucalyptus plantations, tea factories). If we assume that the diversity and the food availability influence the chimpanzee party size and density, food resources are expected to be smaller in Kanyawara, medium in Sebitoli and higher in Ngogo.

Third, HFA food as well as sLFA food would be higher in Ngogo (high chimpanzee density) than in Sebitoli (intermediate chimpanzee density site) and lowest in Kanyawara (low chimpanzee density site).

Materials and Methods

Study site

Kibale National Park (795 km^2) is located in Southwestern Uganda (0°13–0°41 N; 30°19–30°32 E; Figure 1). The park, well known for its high diversity of plants and mammals, was described as a mosaic of mature forest (58%), colonizing forest formally used for agriculture (19%), grassland (15%), woodland (6%), lakes and wetlands (2%) [41]. Local landscape is a testimony of the past exploitation of the forest (timber harvest, gardens) by the government and the local communities during the 1970's, creating a heterogeneous landscape that greatly varies between and within sites [42].

Past forest exploitation and current anthropogenic influence reach varying intensities within the three study sites in the park (Table 1). Most of Sebitoli chimpanzee home range edges (0°36–0°40 N; 30°22–30°25 E) are in contact with anthropogenic features (32 kilometers out of 39). The management for forest exploitation defined 51 forestry compartments for the entire Kibale National Park [43]. Sebitoli (N = 11 compartments) has been commercially exploited in four compartments [43]. According to reports, logging led to about 50% of canopy opening in some areas that created forest gaps [44,45], resulting in 35% of current Sebitoli area being harvested [46]. No detail about intensity of logging in Sebitoli has been published. The same proportion of surface area has been harvested in Kanyawara [46] (0°33–0°36 N; 30°20–30°23 E, N = 7 compartments) but contrary to Sebitoli, information of logging activities within the distinct units has been well documented [44,45,47]. From the literature we know that various compartments were lightly logged (K14), heavily logged (K15), and unlogged (K30) compartments [44,45,47,48]. In comparison, Ngogo (0°28–0°30 N; 30°22–30°26 E, N = 3 compartments) seems more homogenous than the two other study sites because it there has been no logging, but historically there have been human settlements, resulting in large grasslands in today's landscape [49]. Therefore, the combination of the features of the three sites gives a precise indication when studying variables influencing chimpanzee densities.

Within Kibale National Park, there is a north-south gradient in elevation causing an increase in temperature and a decrease in rainfall from North to South [45]. The Kanyawara chimpanzee community is located almost in the middle of the two other sites:

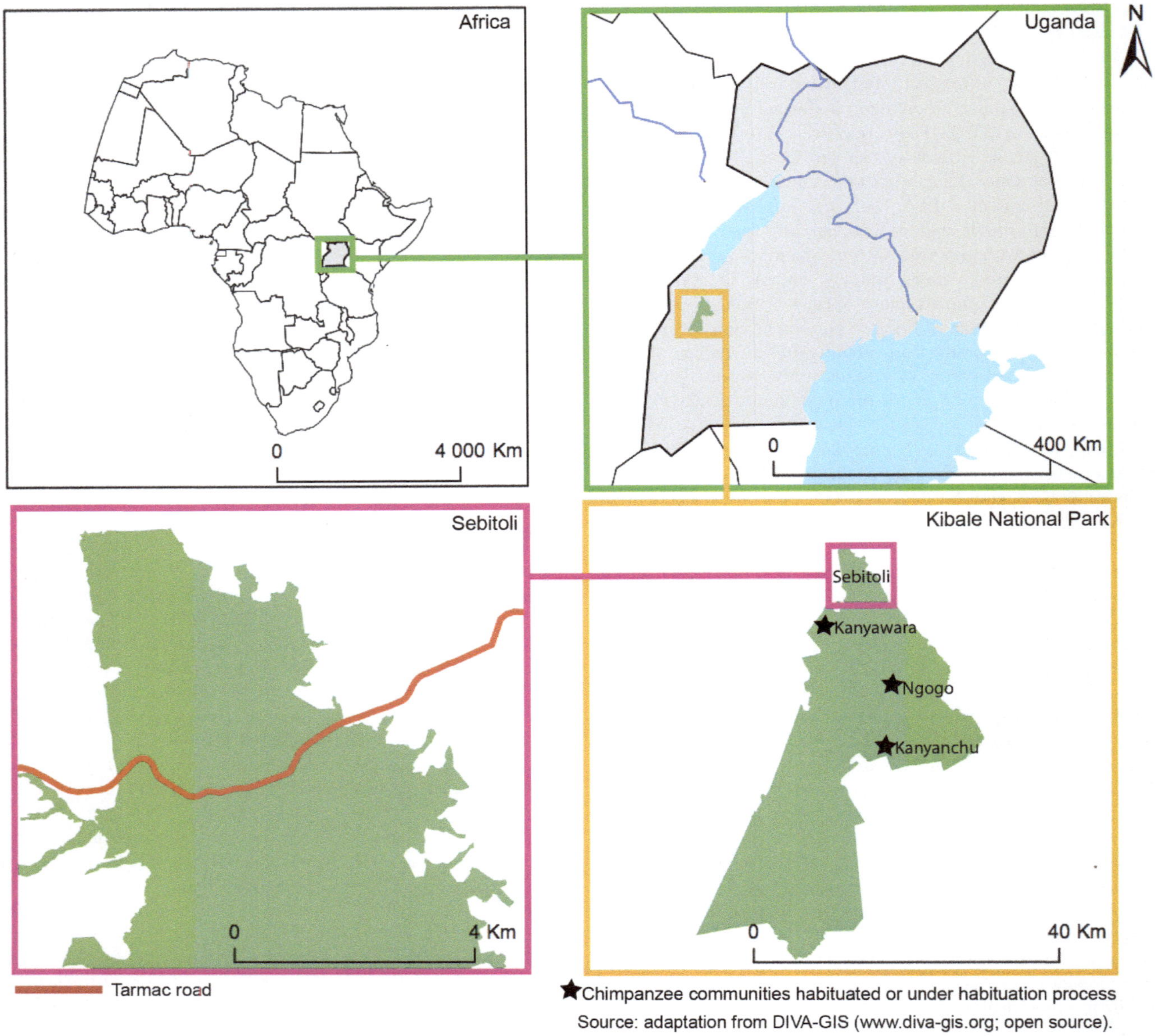

Figure 1. Location of Sebitoli area, Kibale National Park, Western Uganda.

Sebitoli and Ngogo (maximum distance between Sebitoli and Ngogo community centroids: 17 km).

Ethics statement

The studied chimpanzees were observed without any invasive methods or contacts with researchers. Methods used to collect data are in compliance with Uganda Wildlife Authority guidelines and keep to the legal requirements of Uganda. All necessary permits were obtained for this study. The research proposal and the field study is conducted under a "Memorandum of Understanding for research and conservation of chimpanzees in Kibale National Park" between National Museum of Natural History (legal department, SJ445-12), Uganda Wildlife Authority and Makerere University signed July 16th, 2012 for 10 years.

Sebitoli chimpanzee community composition

Chimpanzee habituation in Sebitoli began in 2008 under the Sebitoli Chimpanzee Project.

The field teams of the SCP are composed of two to eight people (Field assistants – FA, researchers and students) and organized in one to four groups. A grid of 80 km of trails is used daily by the research teams. FAs were trained by S Krief to collect data related to chimpanzees and vegetation. Data related to chimpanzees are collected every day, starting at 6 a.m., for 12 hours per day. In this study, four years of Sebitoli data collected by SCP (from February 2nd, 2009 to January 29th, 2013) are analyzed.

Evidence of chimpanzee presence (feces, direct observations, nests, footprints, vocalizations) was used to locate and characterize chimpanzee groups. During the habituation period, chimpanzee location and behaviors were recorded *ad libitum* and contacts, as well as signs of presence, were geo-refereneced (GPS Garmin

Table 1. Past and present anthropogenic influence [30,38,50,51].

	Sebitoli	Kanyawara				Ngogo
		K14 (Lightly logged)	K 15 (Heavily logged)	K 30 (Control)	Total	
	Past					
Timber harvest	x	x	x		x	
Human settlements	x				x	x
Slash-and-burn cultivations	x	x	x	x	x	x
	Present					
Number of tea factories at proximity (>500 m from edge)	3	0	0	0	0	0
Tarmac road	x					
Home range in contact with gardens	81.6%	7.5%	0%	1.2%	47.6%	0%

Oregon™ 300, 400, 450). SCP team recorded the following data systematically: distance between chimpanzee(s) and observers, orientation, tree height, number of individuals, identity (if possible), activities, health status and behaviors, response to observers, level of habituation, food species (item consumed, and its maturity). All GPS points were geo-referenced in the same geodesic system (WGS 84) and cartographic projection (UTM 36 N).

In January 2013, Sebitoli chimpanzee community was estimated to be composed of one hundred individuals, of which 79 were identified, including 28 adult females and 18 adult males (categories according to [52]).

Minimum Convex Polygon method was used to define the Sebitoli chimpanzee home range (MCP-2051 points collected by SCP team during the study period; ET Geowizard software, ArcGIS 9.3). To quantify the Kanyawara chimpanzee home range, MCP method was also used with 2 546 points collected by S Krief and two field assistants during previous research (12 years of data). Finally, MCP generated by SJ Amsler [53] was used to define the Ngogo community (3 901 points, 2003 to 2005 period).

Sebitoli chimpanzee diet

Fresh food-remains and seeds found in fresh feces (less than six hours old) during chimpanzee monitoring, were considered as species consumed by chimpanzees. Due to the habituation process and the *ad libitum* data collection, a feeding bout was considered to begin when at least one chimpanzee of a party was consuming an item of food and to end when all chimpanzees of the party had stopped eating. In addition, party membership was continuously assessed. To estimate the consumption frequency of the different items, the length of feeding bouts related to one item (duration) was multiplied by the number of chimpanzees in the party consuming that food item.

The list of species consumed by chimpanzees was obtained at Sebitoli after 4 years *ad libitum* observations and compared to Kanyawara and Ngogo's data gathered from long-term, published and observed data [30]. We first considered a set of the 18 fruiting species most commonly consumed by the chimpanzee community in each site (some species are common and others are different between sites). We further focused on a set of the top (most consumed) seven species out of the 18, corresponding to 90%, 60–80% and 75% feeding-time at Sebitoli, Kanyawara and Ngogo respectively.

Land-cover composition

Land-cover, not studied in the previous survey [30], was established with identical remote sensing methods for the three sites in a comparative perspective. We used satellite images to evaluate vegetation type diversity, habitat types and their proportions in Sebitoli, Kanyawara and Ngogo. Since land-cover diversity throughout the forest could affect spectral classification inside the forest, as well as its quality, remote sensing analysis was restricted to the forested areas composing each chimpanzee home range. A mask of each site using MCP of respective community home ranges was built. Envi 4.8 was used in remote sensing treatments based on Landsat 7 image (ETM+, orthorectified, 14/03/2001, 30 m) to spectrally determine habitat composition. The following protocol was applied:

1. Principal Component Analysis (PCA) on spectral bands.
2. Unsupervised classification. Five habitat classes were discriminated using K-means method (10 iterations) based on neo-canals obtained from PCA. This allowed us to examine a precise and common classification of habitat types for each study site according to spectral radiometric curves analysis and our knowledge of Sebitoli and Kibale in general. From habitat types defined in literature [41], we can precise the previous classifications by analyzing chlorophyll activity intensity (peak on band 4) and by visual interpretation of woody/non-woody species density gradient to discriminate habitat types that were categorized as follows: Terrestrial Herbaceous Vegetation (THV - herbs and small woody shrubs, abundant and evenly distributed resources belonging to the Zingiberaceae, Marantaceae, Gramineae and Acanthaceae families [16]), degraded forest, regenerating forest, mature forest and grassland areas (mostly represented in Ngogo, very open areas with low chlorophyll activity).

Spatial variation in food availability

Botanical composition was surveyed inside the forest within 63 plots located in Sebitoli chimpanzee home range according to land-cover classes (using an adapted and comparable protocol from [30]). Plots were placed randomly using a stratified sampling method [54] where the number of plots is proportional to surface areas of each land-cover class previously defined with Landsat image.

Nested strip widths of 50 and 20 m were used to enumerate and measure all stems of different size classes and growth forms (even the ones not included in chimpanzee diet).

- All trees and free-standing stems with a diameter at breast height (d.b.h., measure of the diameter of a trunk at 1.30 m) greater than 30 cm (large-size stems) and all strangler figs with a d.b.h. greater than 10 cm were identified and measured in the large size plot (50×50 meters plot).
- All trees and free-standing stems with a d.b.h. between 10 cm and 29 cm (medium-size stems) were identified and measured in the medium-size plot (20×50 meters).

Within the 63 plots, large-size stems (≥30 cm) were recorded in 15.75 ha, and intermediate-size stem (10 to 29 cm) in 6.3 ha. The total proportions of vegetation classes is very similar to previous study [1] but the surface area per d.b.h. class differ mostly for d.b.h. between 30 and 80 cm.

S Bortolamiol and two SCP FA conducted plot censuses. They prepared herbaria in triplicate. One set of herbaria was studied at Makerere University Botany Herbarium Department by P Rwaburindore and J Kasenene.

Temporal variation in food availability

Temporal variations in food availability in the Sebitoli chimpanzee home range were estimated through data obtained from phenological surveys conducted each month by FA between February 2012 and July 2013 (18 months). During the study period, data were collected along 10 trails of 500 meters long each (i.e 5 km in total) dispatched in the Sebitoli chimpanzee home range. 528 individuals of 47 species were monitored at Sebitoli. FA were trained to note the maturity of items (leaves, flowers and fruits) and to give abundance scores (ranging from 0 to 4, 0 representing no fruit and 4 representing a maximum fruit concentration). To analyze resource availability in the forest, food availability of individuals capable of fruiting, bearing unripe and ripe fruits was calculated. Only the feeding species with at least three individuals monitored along the trails that were also represented in vegetation plots were considered. A d.b.h. measurement was taken for all feeding trees on the trail.

Quantifying fruit abundance

In order to compare the density and heterogeneity of fruit-bearing vegetation between sites, the spatial fruit abundance at Sebitoli was determined using a methodology inspired by the one applied to Kanyawara and Ngogo [30]. To sum up the following steps, a schematic representation of basal area and Food Availability Index (FAI) was designed (Figure S1).

(1) Fruit abundance in space. We calculated basal area per hectare of the 18 most consumed species as well as HFA, sLFA or aLFA species in function of their d.b.h. size (G': ≥30 cm d.b.h.; G'': 10 cm ≤ d.b.h. <30 cm on Figure S1).

(2) Fruit abundance in time. Using phenology records, the temporal fluctuation in monthly fruit abundance at Sebitoli was assessed using a 'percent basal area fruiting/ha' method [30,55], and the following formula:

FAI = $\sum$(G(plots) x number of stems bearing fruits per species per month (phenology)).

This method enables a comparison of data across sites by limiting differences in surface area covered by phenology transects and the composition of individual trees monitored.

A monthly score was obtained and classified using a percentile ranking method. Months below the 25th percentile were classified as Low Fruit Abundance (LFA), months higher than the 75th percentile were classified High Fruit Abundance (HFA) and months with an intermediate score were classified Intermediate Fruit Abundance (IFA).

Next, the availability of fruiting species monitored in phenology was classified HFA when more than 30% of individuals were fruiting in HFA months, and less than 20% in LFA months. Species with less than 30% individuals fruiting in HFA months, and more than 20% in LFA months were classified as LFA [1]. For LFA species, a dispersion index - Green Index [56]- was then calculated (PaSsage software) to divide LFA species in 2 categories: synchronous (sLFA) and asynchronous (aLFA).

As our study aims to compare results (see [30]), the same calculation methods were used for species functional classes. However, species fruiting mostly during IFA months did not fit criteria that were just defined in this study. Therefore, IFA species were classfied (N = 6, *Ficus exasperata, Ficus sur, Ficus sansibarica, Prunus africana, Eudenia eminens, Ficus mucuso*) as having LFA or HFA tendencies if any two of the following three criteria applied to the species: percentage of HFA/LFA higher than percentage of LFA/HFA (criteria 1), HFA or LFA percentage deviation closer to the mean (criteria 2) and number HFA/LFA months with no fruit (criteria 3).

Only *Eudenia eminens* could not be classified with this method and was defined as IFA species. Contrary to Ngogo, *Ficus mucuso* are very rare in Sebitoli chimpanzee home range (N = 5 known by SCP in the entire home range) and no individual was recorded in our vegetation plots. However, the fruit of this species is one of the ten most consumed items in the Sebitoli chimpanzee diet, and is likely a very important resource for this community. Therefore, to include this species in the analysis, basal area of *Ficus mucuso* monitored in phenology was used.

Basal area of the 18 species (including top seven fruit-providing species) being most consumed by chimpanzees at each site was compared using Mann-Whitney test followed by Monte-Carlo simulations (10 000 iterations) using XLStats software and Sebitoli, Kanyawara and Ngogo data [30]. Basal areas of HFA, sLFA and aLFA species were also compared. As a unit of the analysis, basal area of stems in each botanical plot was used.

Relation between feeding patch and party size

A feeding patch was defined as an aggregation of food items that allowed uninterrupted feeding for an individual or a party [57]. For most frugivorous species, including chimpanzees, a feeding patch can often be operationally defined as a single tree, where the size of the tree (d.b.h.) represents the size of the feeding patch. The relation between feeding patch size and number of chimpanzees in the party at Sebitoli was tested using a linear regression (XLStats).

Species diversity

Using vegetation plots and Landsat classification, species diversity per hectare of trees was computed by size class (10≤ d.b.h. <30 cm, 30≤ d.b.h. <80 cm, d.b.h. ≥80 cm), for all tree species and for the top 18 species consumed, separately for each of the five land-cover classes. Shannon (H) index was used to measure diversity (Past software, version 2.6). Mean values of H were used as a general indicator to compare sites because there were not enough plots placed in some land-cover classes (especially grasslands at both sites, and THV at Ngogo) to meet the assumptions of standard statistical tests.

Results

Land-cover properties

Sebitoli and Kanyawara land-cover compositions are quite similar (mainly degraded vegetation and regenerating forest), and differ from that of Ngogo (mainly mature and regenerating forest) (Figure 2).

Tree diversity at Sebitoli

We computed and compared vegetation diversity in each land-cover class previously defined at Sebitoli, Kanyawara and Ngogo (Figure 3).

There are clear differences in diversity among tree class sizes. Trees with a d.b.h. greater than or equal to 80 cm were far more diverse at Ngogo in most land-cover class (except for grassland) compared to Sebitoli and Kanyawara. For all trees, and among the 18 most consumed tree species recorded in vegetation plots, species diversity (H) is generally higher at Sebitoli than Kanyawara and Ngogo (Figure 3). Kanyawara is far less diverse for regeneration and mature forest, and is generally less diverse across habitat types compared to Sebitoli.

Sebitoli chimpanzee diet

During the study period, hours spent per year (1490–3344) and number of teams in the forest increased, showing an intensive effort from FA and researchers to locate chimpanzees during the habituation process. The efficiency of chimpanzee habituation is indicated by the increase in visual contact hours per year between observers and chimpanzees (132–1370 hours) and in mean contact time with chimpanzees per year (36–126 minutes), respectively, by multiples of 10 and 4 between February 2009 and January 2013.

Through the study period, observations of feeding bouts (129–561) and time feeding (55–514 hours) increased, which also suggests progress in the habituation process. Mean party size during feeding activities was variable, ranging from 3.56 to 5.35 individuals (range: 1–21).

Using four years of *ad libitum* observations recorded during the habituation process, 89 food items were counted including 17 THV species (23 items; $N_{species} = 9$ for piths, 1 stem, 2 flowers, 6 leaves, 5 fruits) and 52 tree species (66 items; $N_{species} = 4$ for piths, 4 bark, 1 dead wood, 1 wax, 5 flowers, 11 leaves, 40 fruits) (Tables S1, S2) consumed by Sebitoli chimpanzees.

Link between party size and feeding patch size

Only a very small percentage of variation in party size at Sebitoli was explained by feeding patch size (linear regression $R^2 = 0.059$, P-value <0.0001). Also, feeding patch size is smaller at Sebitoli (55.31 cm d.b.h.) than Kanyawara (66.87 cm) and Ngogo (63.38 cm).

Intersites comparison of food resources availability

In order to compare spatial and temporal availability of the 18 fruiting trees most consumed by chimpanzees, we compared the sum of their basal area and functional types (HFA, aLFA, sLFA) in the three communities.

The sum of the basal area of the 18 most consumed fruiting trees is respectively 1.5 and 9.5 times lower at Sebitoli (54 683 cm^2/ha) than at Kanyawara (83 553.9 cm^2/ha) and Ngogo (519 175.9 cm^2/ha) (Figure 4). Among the top 18 species consumed at Sebitoli, 10 species are shared with Kanyawara (six of them shared the same temporal availability with Sebitoli), nine species are shared with Ngogo (two of them shared the same temporal availability with Sebitoli) and there are six species found at all three sites. Seven species at Sebitoli (17 627.3 cm^2/ha) and Kanyawara (8 666.8 cm^2/ha) belong to the *Ficus* genus whereas there are only four *Ficus* species among the top 18 food species at Ngogo (10 708.5 cm^2/ha).

Among the 18 most consumed species, the proportion of HFA species is greater at Sebitoli (N = 11) than at Kanyawara (N = 8) and Ngogo (N = 9). Also, there are no sLFA species at Sebitoli while there are three at Kanyawara and six at Ngogo. One species was classified as IFA at Sebitoli and showed no particular pattern of fruiting. aLFA species were more various at Kanaywara (N = 7) than Sebitoli (N = 6) or Ngogo (N = 3). Finally, at Sebitoli, five *Ficus* species out of seven are classified HFA while there is one out of four at Ngogo and one out of seven at Kanyawara. Other *Ficus* species were aLFA at the three sites.

According to the Mann-Whitney tests (Table 2), Ngogo shows generally higher mean and median basal area per hectare than Sebitoli and Kanyawara for the top 18, the top seven and the HFA species. However, Sebitoli shows significantly higher mean basal areas for overall (11 529.6 cm^2/ha), intermediate (5 378.8 cm^2/ha) and small size stems (3 152.4 cm^2/ha) of aLFA compared to Kanyawara (6 798.0 cm^2/ha, 2 453.6 cm^2/ha, 1 441.8 cm^2/ha

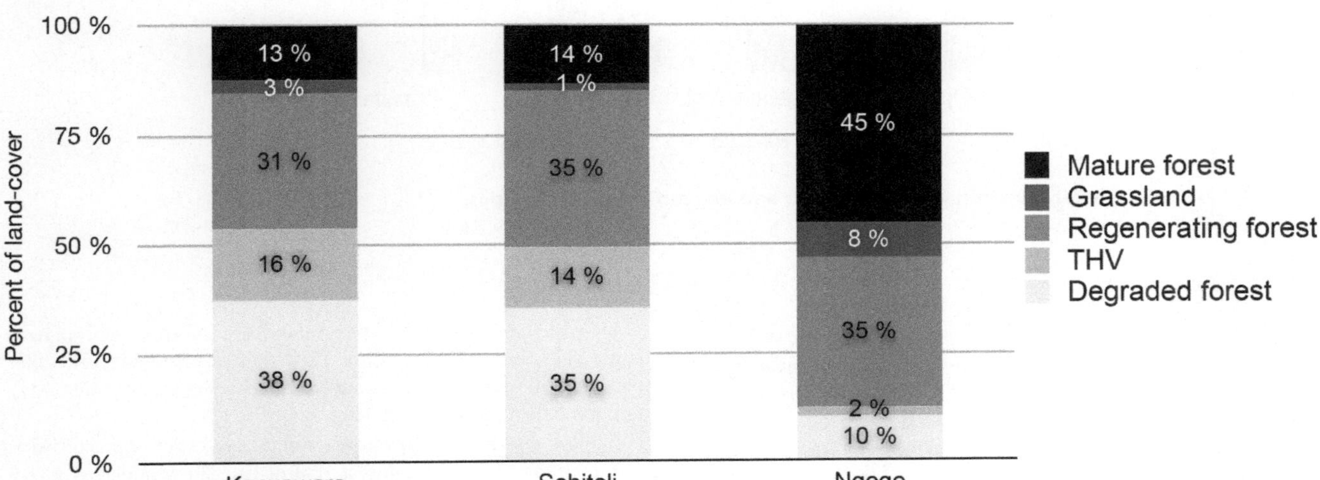

Figure 2. Sebitoli land-cover in comparison with Ngogo and Kanyawara.

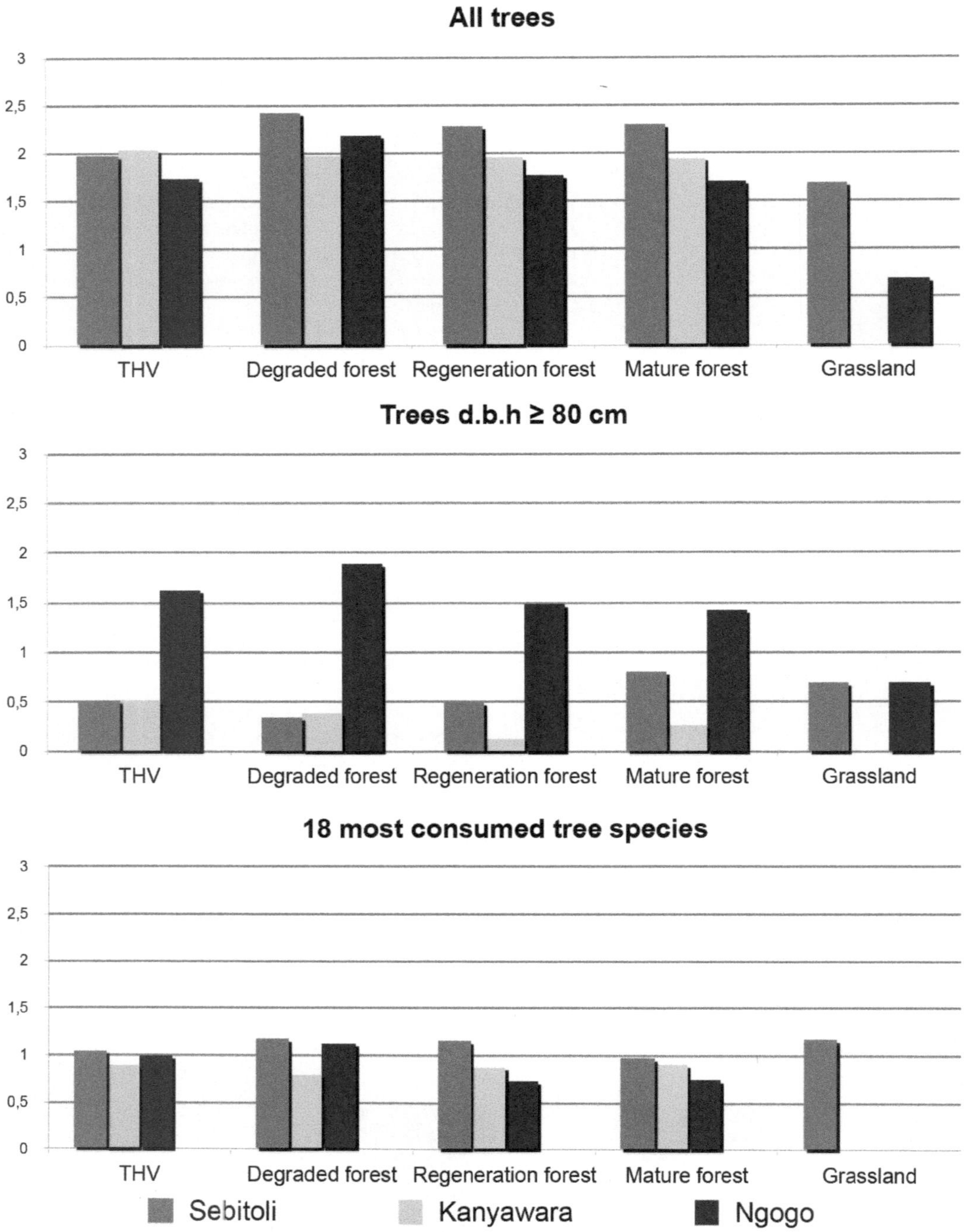

	Mean H trees
Sebitoli	2.13
Kanyawara	1.58
Ngogo	1.61

	Mean H d.b.h
Sebitoli	0.57
Kanyawara	0.26
Ngogo	1.42

	Mean H 18 sp.
Sebitoli	1.11
Kanyawara	0.70
Ngogo	0.72

Figure 3. Diversity index in function of habitat types and vegetation characteristics.

respectively) and Ngogo (4 439.1 cm^2/ha, 0 cm^2/ha, 0 cm^2/ha respectively).

Between Sebitoli and Kanyawara, there was only one aLFA size category showing a significant difference between sites (small stems, P-value <0.0001). The difference was more pronounced between Kanyawara and Ngogo, for which seven size categories showed significant differences (each P-value <0.0001). This trend was even more pronounced between Sebitoli and Ngogo as nine categories were signicantly different (P-value <0.0001). Finally, standard errors (SE) were consistently lower at Sebitoli than Kanyawara and Ngogo.

Discussion

Despite their proximity and similar sizes, the three chimpanzee study sites in Kibale National Park that we studied here differ considerably in terms of food-resource species availability (1), temporal fluctuation (2) and tree maturity (3).

Sebitoli and Kanyawara have similar land-cover characteristics, but Sebitoli is essentially a cul-de-sac surrounded by tea plantations and crossed by a road. Basal area of the 18 most commonly consumed species by chimpanzees were 9.5 times higher at Ngogo than at Sebitoli. Our results confirm that the sites

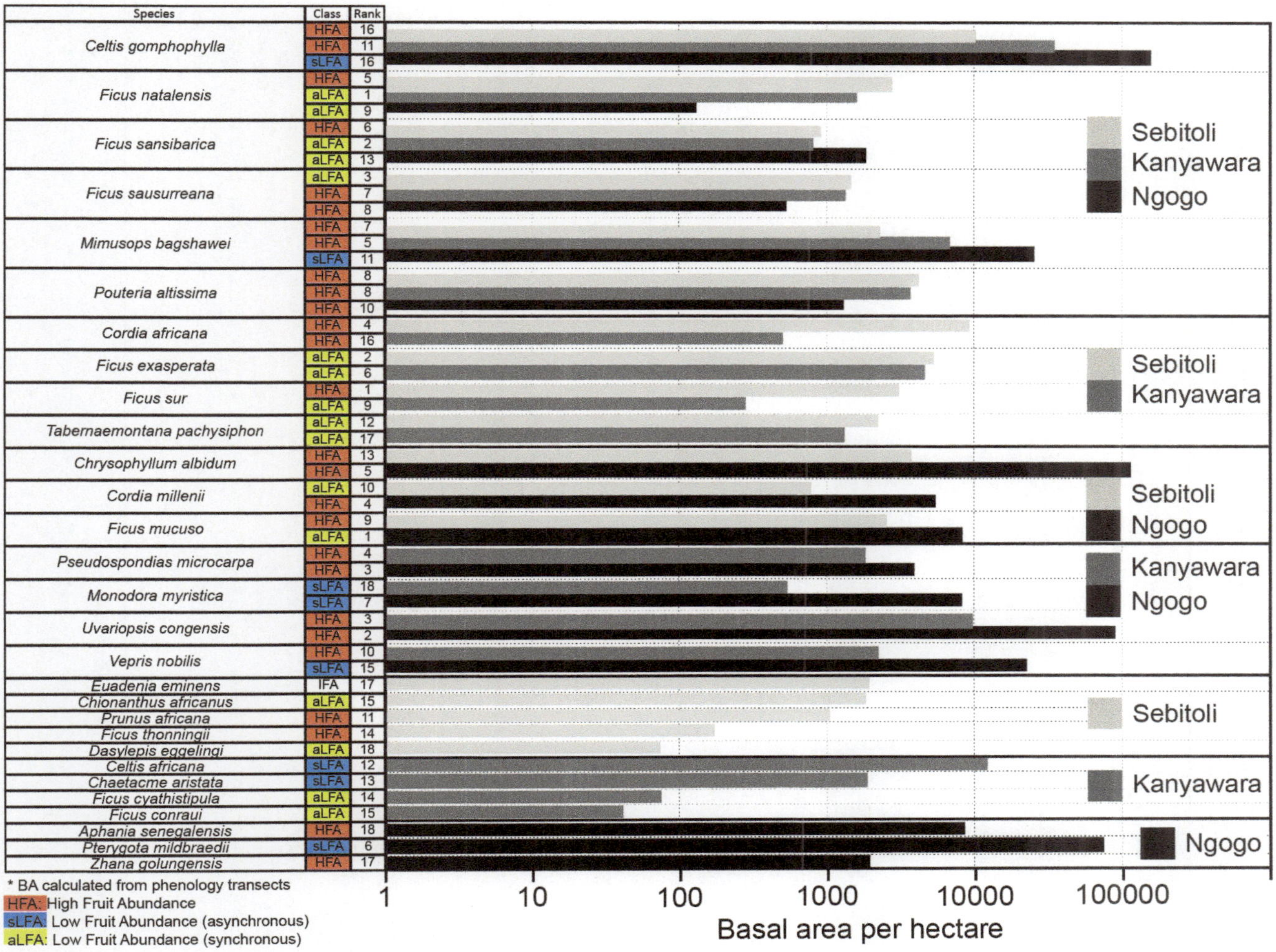

Figure 4. Sum of 18 most consumed species basal area, fruit availability and consumption rank at Sebitoli, Kanyawara and Ngogo (data for Kanyawara and Ngogo from [30]**).** *Morus lactea* (sLFA) and *Treculia africana* (HFA) at Ngogo were absent from plots but present in Ngogo chimpanzee diet.

furthest from one another are also the most distinct in terms of landscape-scale vegetation characteristics (i.e. Sebitoli and Ngogo, hypothesis 1 - confirmed).

Sebitoli harbors a higher density of chimpanzees than Kanyawara. Nevertheless, during our study period, food patch sizes and party sizes were small at Sebitoli compared to Kanyawara and Ngogo [58]. However, our results suggest that it is possible that chimpanzee density is more closely related to diet composition than to food abundance, per se, with *Ficus* and tree species diversity playing key functions. Among the most consumed species at Sebitoli, five of the top seven species and eight of the top 18 species are *Ficus* species. Those *Ficus*, being important to sustain chimpanzee diet year-round [59], may have developed after forest exploitation in Sebitoli, which, as Kanyawara, was affected by such actions. From Sebitoli vegetation plots, 8 species of *Ficus* were censussed (N = 69 individuals) and most individuals were hosted in degraded (N = 24) and regeneration (N = 23) forests. Also, *Ficus* species do not behave the same way: some species such as *Ficus sur* may have multiplied after forest exploitation because their d.b.h. is smaller (min: 35, max: 104, mean 62.3, SD: 22.47) compared to species such as *Ficus saussureana* (min: 95, max: 141, mean: 118, SD: 32.53) that are generally larger and may have prospered after logging. They represent the main food resource for Sebitoli chimpanzees because they are abundant (HFA) and available all year long (IFA, aLFA). Also, tree species diversity is generally higher at Sebitoli than at Kanyawara and Ngogo for all trees in each habitat types as well as for consumed species (Hypothesis 2 – partly confirmed).

Finally, while sLFA species were described as possibly promoting high chimpanzee density at Ngogo compared to Kanyawara, they are totally absent from Sebitoli (Hypothesis 3 – partly confirmed).

Landscape differences and chimpanzee diet

We found larger differences in floristic composition between more distant sites, Sebitoli has more species in common with Kanyawara (closer study site) than Ngogo. While Sebitoli and Kanyawara are similar in terms of land-cover composition, Fig. trees are more dense and diverse at Sebitoli. Also, *Ficus* basal area (among the 18 most heavily consumed items) is higher at Sebitoli than at Kanywara and Ngogo. Sebitoli and Kanyawara border the forest edge (Figure 1) while Ngogo is located in the middle of the forest. Gaps and edges caused by logging activities can favor sunlight, fruit production of the tree crowns and increase average

Table 2. The Mann-Whitney test results on basal area of 18 species being most consumed by chimpanzees (data for Kanyawara and Ngogo from [30]), top seven food species and the different categories of food resources.

		Ngogo			Kanyawara			Sebitoli			Mann-Whitney tests						
	Category	Mean BA/ha (cm^2 ha−1)	Mediane BA/ha (cm^2 ha−1)	SE	Mean BA/ha (cm^2 ha−1)	Mediane BA/ha (cm^2 ha−1)	SE	Mean BA/ha (cm^2 ha−1)	Mediane BA/ha (cm^2 ha−1)	SE	MWU KN	P-value KN	MWU SK	P-value S/K	MWU SN	P-value S/N	Direction S/N/K
Top 18	Overall	157875.2	132622.4	16511.7	83752.5	74038.4	8409.3	54683.0	45238.9	5698.3	834.0	0.0000	1162.0	0.0062	661.5	**<0.0001**	N>K>S
	Large trees	39919.0	22698.0	8461.0	14807.7	0.0	3989.7	21451.2	0.0	1082.8	1063.0	0.0450	1725.5	0.5848	1376.5	0.1172	N>S≈K
	Intermediate trees	57128.6	43568.5	6156.8	43181.9	32114.3	5037.4	24074.6	19267.4	794.1	1085.0	0.1150	1109.0	0.0030	868.0	**<0.0001**	N≈K>S
	Small trees	60827.6	52400.2	6422.4	25763.0	20998.5	4140.0	9157.2	7647.0	113.5	681.5	**<0.0001**	1160.0	0.0064	345.5	**<0.0001**	N>K>S
Top seven	Overall	104763.9	88911.3	13462.7	25567.5	1836.2	6390.6	26360.8	7450.9	4766.8	626.0	**<0.0001**	1838.0	0.2396	815.0	**<0.0001**	N>S≈K
	Large trees	26213.3	0.0	5769.5	9039.6	0.0	2561.0	14190.6	0.0	1017.3	910.0	0.0010	1628.0	0.9490	1301.0	0.0298	N>S≈K
	Intermediate trees	32620.2	20434.2	4655.9	5476.5	0.0	1905.9	11168.2	4071.5	623.0	278.0	**<0.0001**	2117.0	0.0024	1007.0	0.0004	N>S>K
	Small trees	45930.5	27354.3	6733.2	11051.3	0.0	3568.9	1002.0	0.0	35.3	329.5	**<0.0001**	1392.0	0.0614	527.0	**<0.0001**	N>K≈S
HFA	Overall	72055.3	65737.5	9489.5	62455.8	58738.3	7412.0	37485.0	29303.2	5306.4	1285.5	0.6600	1116.5	0.0026	1220.5	0.0220	N≈K>S
	Large trees	5677.9	0.0	2072.4	10214.1	0.0	3913.7	17410.5	0.0	1065.0	1394.0	0.6290	1884.5	0.0726	1968.0	0.0190	S≈K≈N
	Intermediate trees	20447.0	8073.9	3751.2	33014.3	21384.9	4305.7	15530.0	7543.0	632.4	1756.0	0.0070	997.0	0.0002	1589.0	0.7716	K>N≈S
	Small trees	45930.5	27354.3	6733.2	19227.4	5291.2	4031.5	4544.4	1539.4	86.9	916.5	0.0030	1212.0	0.0128	736.0	**<0.0001**	N>K>S
sLFA	Overall	81380.7	73868.2	9644.8	14498.7	7228.3	2433.6	0.0	0.0	0.0	340.0	**<0.0001**	-	-	-	-	Only in N
	Large trees	29802.0	0.0	7894.4	1691.0	0.0	959.4	0.0	0.0	0.0	879.5	**<0.0001**	-	-	-	-	Only in N
	Intermediate trees	36681.6	33560.2	4367.1	7714.0	0.0	1553.4	0.0	0.0	0.0	609.5	**<0.0001**	-	-	-	-	Only in N
	Small trees	14897.1	6372.4	2745.9	5093.8	0.0	1283.5	0.0	0.0	0.0	936.0	0.0034	-	-	-	-	N>K
aLFA	Overall	4439.1	0.0	1924.2	6798.0	0.0	1811.8	11529.6	6605.2	1932.3	1646.0	0.0224	2323.0	0.0006	2591.0	**<0.0001**	S>K>N
	Large trees	4439.1	0.0	1924.2	2902.5	0.0	964.3	2998.5	0.0	325.5	1402.0	0.6632	1423.5	0.0518	1488.0	0.1876	N≈S≈K
	Intermediate trees	0.0	0.0	0.0	2453.6	0.0	1065.6	5378.8	0.0	265.5	1508.0	0.0254	2199.0	0.0004	2444.0	**<0.0001**	S>K
	Small trees	0.0	0.0	0.0	1441.8	0.0	574.1	3152.4	1606.1	52.3	1560.0	0.0060	2300.0	**<0.0001**	2626.0	**<0.0001**	S>K
IFA	Overall	-	-	-	-	-	-	1898.4	0.0	482.9	-	-	-	-	-	-	Only in S
	Large trees	-	-	-	-	-	-	319.1	0.0	81.1	-	-	-	-	-	-	Only in S
	Intermediate trees	-	-	-	-	-	-	344.7	0.0	45.6	-	-	-	-	-	-	Only in S
	Small trees	-	-	-	-	-	-	1234.6	0.0	32.2	-	-	-	-	-	-	Only in S

Direction compares BA sum and indicates p-value difference significativity (p-value ≤0.05; < or >) or non-significativity (≈) (SE: Standard Error).

of leaf quality [60] as well as growth of terrestrial herbaceous vegetation and Fig. trees. Previous studies showed that plant species richness was higher in area previously deforested than in non-exploited areas, and these areas were used by primates [41,61,62].

Trees basal area in Kanyawara increased in all compartments between 1989 and 2006 [61] but previous studies showed that growth rates were variable in function of past logging activities: trees in the most heavily logged area had the slowest growth rate of any of the areas and trees in moderately and lightly logged areas had a slightly faster growth rate than either of the unlogged areas [48]. However, in a study related to red colobus monkeys, analysis on each compartment of Kanyawara indicated that the cumulative d.b.h. of food trees increased in the heavily logged ($P = 0.003$) and lightly logged area ($P = 0.008$) but not in the unlogged forest ($P = 0.191$) [61]. Therefore, logging activities impact forest structure and primate feeding trees to different extents.

Some primate species, such as redtail monkeys and red colobus live on forest edges/patches which is possibly due to dietary preferences for second growth forests and their higher abundance in those areas maybe due to colonizing plants [62]. Mean group densities for frugivorous such as redtail monkeys and gray-cheeked mangabeys were higher in lightly logged than unlogged areas in Kanyawara [63]. Kanyawara chimpanzees use forest compartments that were logged in different intensities (K14, K15, K30) and female individuals mostly range in lightly logged (K14) and unlogged (K30) areas [64]. At Budongo, logged areas and forest edges provided 76% of the chimpanzee food while they represent only 60% of chimpanzee home range [65].

The basal area per hectare of *Ficus* species is higher at Sebitoli (15196.31 cm^2) than at Kanyawara (8187.63 cm^2) and Ngogo (5379.87 cm^2) and *Ficus* species represent a higher percentage among all stems at Sebitoli (7.46%) than at Kanyawara (2.81%) and Ngogo (1.56%). Within Kanyawara, *Ficus* density within all stems increased with logging intensity (K30: 1.43%; K14: 2.43%; K15: 2.69%). Their current basal areas in compartments that were logged in the 1970s is more important in lightly logged areas (K14: 16051.19 cm^2) than in unlogged (K30: 5104.61 cm^2) or heavily logged (K15: 3407.09 cm^2). Low intensity selective logging could be compatible with the conservation of primates [61]. It is possible that commercial timber harvesting did not have a major long term influence on the critical resource base of chimpanzees at Kanyawara and Sebitoli and that the differences of feeding resources between sites result from natural heterogeneity and logging activities [45,66]. It was suggested that light penetration to the forest floor was higher at Kanyawara than Ngogo, favouring the establishment of light demanding species [48]. The fact that *Ficus* basal area and stem proportion are more important at Sebitoli than the two other sites within all trees (and then fruit production) is to be considered as a factor of chimpanzee density. Figs represent relatively high quality food necessary to sustain chimpanzees during times of overall fruit scarcity and this could account for the difference in chimpanzee density between Sebitoli and Kanyawara. There are differences between the pulp and the seed component of Fig. trees (higher caloric density) and Kanyawara figs were described as "energy-rich food with adequate protein" [34]. With regard to the nutritional value of figs, researchers have said that "they should be considered as potatoes for humans, a food that will sustain life at maintenance" [67] meaning that figs are a staple food item to chimpanzees.

Perspectives on chimpanzee adaptability to anthropogenic changes

Sebitoli, the site of intermediate chimpanzee density, had a higher density (at least for the seven species most consumed) and diversity of food resources than Kanyawara (low chimpanzee density). As at Kanyawara, Sebitoli was logged and the lower standard error values in basal areas among stems compared to Kanyawara and Ngogo suggest that most of the forest at Sebitoli is in the same successional stage (smaller d.b.h. compared to Ngogo). Therefore, it is possible that since food patch size (d.b.h.) is smaller at Sebitoli compared to Kanyawara and Ngogo (largely attributable to past forest exploitation), fruiting species can sustain fewer chimpanzees on a tree. Using a linear regression, we found no dependence between the feeding party size (FPS) and food patch size at Sebitoli during the study period. While food patch size explained a large part of the variance in FPS at Ngogo (80%), it explained far less of this variance at Kanyawara (22.7%) [58] and it only explained 5% of the variance in FSP at Sebitoli. Indeed, if fruit resources are consistently available through the year and high-quality patches sparsely distributed, no relationship between FPS and patch size should exist [15].

In the three sites, chimpanzees have long coped with various forms of anthropogenic change (e.g. agriculture, fire, logging). Increasing fragmentation [2] and proximity between natural and anthropogenic landscapes have resulted in close co-existence between wild animals and human populations. Some individuals from different chimpanzee communities are known to cross roads passing through their home range (Bossou, Guinea: [6]; Sebitoli: SCP unpublished data), to raid crops in neighborhood gardens [5; SCP unpublished data], and even deactivate snares set by poachers [68].

The fact that adult chimpanzees continue to observe and learn the use of unfamiliar feeding items from conspecifics with potentially better fitness (males and females between 25 and 40 years old) [69] suggest that chimpanzee adaptation to novel environments is a potentially long-term process based on social transmission. Investigating behavioral and genetic characteristics of migrating females would enable us to monitor the ability of chimpanzees to adapt to environmental changes and their capacity for resiliency, especially under such intense anthropogenic constraints as they currently face (roads, human settlements, threats of snare injuries, etc.).

Inter-sites variations in temporal food availability for chimpanzees

Comparisons between sites within the same forest block are not as common as comparisons between primate populations inhabiting different forests [13,42]. Based on our results, we can conclude that both the density and the temporal availability of food resources for chimpanzees may impact on chimpanzee density in KNP. HFA and sLFA species apparently contribute to chimpanzee density at Ngogo [30]. According to our study, sLFA species do not seem to play a role in Sebitoli chimpanzee density because they are absent from the chimpanzee diet. They may be difficult to identify at Sebitoli because they are scattered and not abundant, and therefore very difficult to census in the entire home range. However, particular skills developed by chimpanzees suggest they are able to categorize food resources based on specific functional classes (synchronous. asynchronous) [70]. Therefore, chimpanzees are able to gather information on diet availability and botanical features.

Five *Ficus* species at Sebitoli mostly fruit during high fruit abundance periods (that were initially classified as intermediate fruit abundance). Like tree diversity and *Ficus* species density, temporal availability of food resources (very short periods of relatively low or high fruit abundance, intermediate fruit availability, asynchronous species fruiting during time of low fruit availability) may also be a major factor explaining chimpanzee density at Sebitoli. Species providing fruits during periods of high fruit abundance (when fruit diversity is frequently high) at Sebitoli (N = 11), as at Ngogo (N = 9), seem to favor chimpanzee density. At some chimpanzee study sites, high quality foods are available across seasons [71,72] and chimpanzees show only limited consumption of relatively low-quality fallback foods such as THV [73]. Chimpanzees can maintain high quality diets year round in cases of low seasonal variations (which is the case of Sebitoli) and high-quality fallback foods. Finally, in disturbed habitat such as regenerating forest that experienced logging activities in the past in Kibale, THV can reach high proportions and consequently offer a large diversity of terrestrial herbaceous vegetation as fallback food.

Conclusion

In the site of Sebitoli, deeply impacted by human past and current activities, chimpanzees are dependent upon Fig. species, and we suggest that the high density of chimpanzees at the site is explained at least partially by temporal fruit availability as well as tree diversity. Owing to their fission-fusion social system, chimpanzees are capable of behaviorally coping with the restrictions on density imposed by the features of this relatively early stage regenerating forest (e.g., forage in small parties when using a small feeding patch in a site where biomass of feeding trees is low). The issue whether chimpanzees communities show a general capacity for resilience to anthropogenic influence and whether they take advantage of disturbed areas (THV, regenerating areas, crops) resulting from human activities inside and outside protected areas deserves further exploration in the future. The high density of chimpanzees at the Sebitoli site is surprising, given its geographical constraints, and past to present exploitation. However, our results suggest that chimpanzees may be able to circumvent the effects of these anthropogenic factors, and therefore their long-term impact may be relatively limited.

Between 1990 and 2000, forest cover decreased by 0.8% in Africa and Cental America, by 0.3% in Asia and Oceania and by 0.4% in South America while it increased in Europe (0.4%) and North America (0.1%) [74]. Primate populations and habitats are therefore highly subject to forest change. Empirical and quantitative information on their capacity for recovery, and the mechanisms through which they recover, is needed in a context of population growth and environment quality management to assess the system equilibrium. Integrating small scale analysis, inter-site comparisons and interdisciplinary methods in nature conservation plans could lead to a better understanding of possible co-existence between wildlife sustainability and human needs.

Supporting Information

Figure S1 Summary of methodology for classifying food ressources.
(TIF)

Table S1 THV species consumed by Sebitoli chimpanzees.
(DOC)

Table S2 Direction compares BA sum and indicates p-value difference significativity (p-value ≤0.05; < or >) or non-significativity (≈) (SE: Standard Error).
(DOC)

Acknowledgments

We are grateful to Uganda Wildlife Authority and Uganda National Council for Science and Technology for giving us the authorization to conduct this survey; Makerere University, Paris-Diderot University, Pôle Image for help with data analysis. We deeply thank J.M Krief co-director of Sebitoli Chimpanzee Project and the field assistants for their work in KNP, particularly Japan Musinguzi, Ronald Musinguzi, Emmanuel Balinda, Christopher Aliganyira, Deogratius Kyomuhangi, John Tweheyo, Joseph Alinaitwe, Denis Sebugwaho and Nicolas Kwezi. Finally we thank colleagues from Paris Diderot, Pole Image, National Museum of Natural History for their worthy comments on this manuscrit. We are indebted to Colin Chapman and an anonymous reviewers for their most valuable comments on the review process.

Author Contributions

Conceived and designed the experiments: SB SK FP MC. Performed the experiments: SB PR JK SK. Analyzed the data: SB KP FP QV MC SK. Contributed reagents/materials/analysis tools: SB MC PR JK AS SK. Wrote the paper: SB MC KP SK.

References

1. Carter NH, Shrestha BK, Karki JB, Pradhan NMB, Liu J (2012) Coexistence between wildlife and humans at fine spatial scales. PNAS 109: 15360–15365.
2. Marsh KL (2003) Primates in fragments – Ecology in conservation. New York: Kluwer Academic/Plenum. 428 p.
3. Hartter J, Ryan SJ, Southworth J, Chapman CA (2011) Landscapes as continuous entities: forest disturbance and recovery in the Albertine Rift landscape. Landsc Ecol 26(6): 877–890.
4. Caldecott JO, Miles J (2005) Atlas Mondial des Grands Singes et de leur Conservation. Paris: UNESCO. 492 p.
5. Naughton-Treves L, Treves A, Chapman CA, Wrangham RW (1998) Temporal patterns of crop-raiding by primates: linking food availability in croplands and adjacent forest. J Appl Ecol 35: 596–606.
6. Hockings KJ, Anderson JR, Matsuzawa T (2006) Road crossing in chimpanzees: a risky business. Curr Biol 16(17): 668–670.
7. Quiatt D, Reynold V, Stokes EJ (2002) Snare injuries to chimpanzees (*Pan troglodytes*) at 10 study sites in east and west Africa. Afr J Ecol 40: 303–305.
8. Hockings KJ (2011) Behavioral flexibility and division of roles in chimpanzee road-crossing. In: Matsuzawa T, Humle T, Sugiyama Y, editors. The Chimpanzees of Bossou and Nimba. Japan: Springer. 221–229.
9. Ives AR (1995) Measuring resilience in stochastic systems. Ecol Monogr 65(2): 217–233.
10. Cant JGH (1980) What limits primates? Primates 21: 538–544.
11. Brown JH (1981) Two decades of Homage to Santa-Rosalia – toward a genera theory of diversity. Am Zool 21: 877–888.
12. Chapman CA, Chapman LJ (2000) Constraints on group size in Red Colobus and red-tailed Guenons: Examining the generality of the Ecological Contraints Model. Int J Primatol 21(4): 565–585.
13. Butynski TM (1990) Comparative ecology of blue monkeys (*Cercopithecus mitis*) in high and low density subpopulations. Ecol Monogr 60: 1–26.
14. Mitani JC, Struhsaker TT, Lwanga JS (2000) Primate community dynamics in old growth forest over 23.5 years at Ngogo, Kibale National Park, Uganda: Implications for conservation and census methods. Int J Primatol 21: 269–286.
15. Chapman CA, Wrangham RW, Chapman LJ (1995) Ecological constraints on group size: an analysis of spider monkey and chimpanzee subgroups. Behav Ecol Sociobiol 36: 59–70.
16. Wrangham RW, Chapman CA, Clark-Arcadi AP, Isabirye-Basuta G (1996) Social ecology of Kanyawara chimpanzees: implications for understanding the costs of great ape groups. In: McGrew WC, Marchant LF, Nishida T, editors. Great Ape Societies. Cambridge: Cambridge University Press. 45–57.
17. Junker J, Blake S, Boesch C, Campbell G, Du Toit L, et al. (2012) Recent decline in suitable environmental conditions for African great apes. Diversity and Distributions 18(11): 1077–1091.
18. Anderson DP, Nordheim EV, Moermond TC, Gone Bi ZB, Boesch C (2005) Factors influencing tree phenology in Taï National Park, Côte d'Ivoire. Biotropica 37(4): 631–640.
19. Goodall J (1986) The chimpanzees of Gombe: patterns of behavior. Cambridge: Harvard University Press. 673 p.

20. Matsumoto-Oda A, Hosaka K, Huffman MA, Kawanaka K (1998) Factors affecting party size in chimpanzees of the Mahale Mountains. Int J Primatol 19: 999–1011.
21. Matsumoto-Oda A, Hayashi Y (1999) Nutritionnal aspects of fruit choice by Chimpanzes. Folia Primatol 70: 154–162.
22. Mitani JC, Watts D, Lwanga J (2002) Ecological and social correlates of chimpanzee party size and composition. In: Boesch C, Hohmann G, Marchant L, editors. Behavioral Diversity in Chimpanzees and Bonobos. Cambridge: Cambridge University Press. 102–111.
23. Mitani JC, Watts DP (2005) Correlates of territorial boundary patrol behaviour in wild chimpanzees. Anim Behav 70: 1079–1086.
24. Wrangham RW (2000) Why are male chimpanzees more gregarious than mothers? A scramble competition hypothesis. In: Kappeler PM, editor. Primate males: causes and consequences of variation in group composition. Cambridge: Cambridge University Press 248–258.
25. Van Schaik CP, Terborgh JW, Wright SJ (1993) The phenology of tropical forests: adaptive significance and consequences for primary consumers. Annu Rev Ecol Evol Syst 24: 353–377.
26. Puig H (2001) La forêt tropicale humide. Paris: Belin. 447 p.
27. Leighton M, Leighton DR (1983) Vertebrate responses to fruiting seasonality within a Bornean rain forest. In: Sutton SL, Whitmore TC, Chadwick AC, editors. Tropical rain forest: ecology and management. Oxford: Blackwell Scientific Publications. 181–196.
28. Tutin CEG, Fernandez M, Rogers ME, Williamson EA, McGrew WC (1991) Foraging profiles of sympatric lowland gorillas and chimpanzees in the Lopé Reserve, Gabon. Philos Trans R Soc London 334: 179–186.
29. Wrangham RW, Conklin NL, Hunt KD (1998) Dietary response of chimpanzees and cercopithecines to seasonal variation in fruit abundance, I. Antifeedants. Int J Primatol 19: 949–970.
30. Potts K, Chapman CA, Lwanga JS (2009) Floristic heterogeneity between forested sites in Kibale National Park, Uganda: insights into the fine-scale determinants of density in a large-bodied frugivorous primate. J Anim Ecol 78: 1269–1277.
31. Reynolds V, Plumptre AJ, Greenham J, Harborne J (1998) Condensed tannins and sugars in the diet of chimpanzees (*Pan troglodytes schweinfurthii*) in the Budongo Forest, Uganda. Oecologia 115: 331–336.
32. Remis MJ (2002) Food preferences among captive western gorillas (*Gorilla gorilla gorilla*) and Chimpanzees (*Pan troglodytes*). Int J Primatol 23: 231–249.
33. Chapman CA, Chapman LJ, Zanne AE, Poulsen JR, Clark CJ (2005) A 12-year phenological record of fruiting: implications for frugivore populations and indicators of climate change. In: Dew JL, Boubli JP, editors. Tropical Fruits and Frugivores: the Search for Strong Interactors. Dordrecht: Springer. 75–92.
34. Wrangham RW, Conklin NL, Etot G, Obua J, Hunt KD, et al. (1993) The Value of Figs to Chimpanzees. Int J Primatol 14(2): 243–256.
35. Thompson ME, Wrangham RW (2008) Diet and reproductive function in wild female chimpanzees (*Pan troglodytes schweinfurthii*) at Kibale National Park, Uganda. Am J Phys Anthropol 135(2): 171–181.
36. Tutin CEG, Fernandez M (1993) Composition of the diet of chimpanzees and comparisons with that of sympatric lowland gorillas in the lopé reserve, Gabon. Am J Primatol 30(3): 195–211.
37. Wiens JA (1989) Spatial scaling in Ecology. Funct Ecol 3(4): 385–397.
38. Uganda Wildlife Authority (2005) Ground census of mammals in Kibale National Park. Report, Kampala, Uganda.
39. Wanyama F, Muhabwe R, Plumptre AJ, Chapman CA, Rothman JM (2010) Censusing large mammals in Kibale National Park: evaluation of the intensity of sampling required to determine change. Afr J Ecol 48(4): 953–961.
40. Narat V, Cibot M, Bokika Ngawolo JC, Dumez R, Krief S (2012) Etude préliminaire de l'influence des disponibilités alimentaires et des activités humaines sur l'utilisation spatial de l'habitat par les chimpanzés et les bonobos. Primatologie (4): 4–10.
41. Chapman CA, Lambert JE (2000) Habitat alteration and the conservation of African primates: case study of Kibale National Park, Uganda. Am J Primatol 50: 169–185.
42. Chapman CA, Chapman LJ, Wrangham RW, Isabirye-Basuta G, Ben-David K (1997) Spatial and temporal variability in the structure of a tropical forest. Afr J Ecol 35: 287–302.
43. Osmaston HA (1959) Working plan for the Kibale and Itwara Forests. Entebbe: Ugandan Forest Department. 142 p.
44. Kasenene JM (1980) Plant regeneration and rodent populations in selectively felled and unfelled areas of the Kibale Forest, Uganda. Ph.D. Thesis. Makerere University, Kampala, Uganda.
45. Struhsaker TT (1997) Ecology of an African rain forest: logging in Kibale and the conflict between conservation and exploitation. Gainesville: University Press of Florida. 432 p.
46. Struhsaker T (1975) The Red Colobus Monkey. Chicago: University of Chicago Press. 311 p.
47. Skorupa JP (1988) The effect of selective timber harvesting on rain forest primates in Kibale Forest, Uganda. PhD Dissertation, University of California, California, USA.
48. Chapman CA, Chapman LJ (1997) Forest regeneration in logged and unlogged forests of Kibale National Park, Uganda. Biotropica 29: 396–412.
49. Lwanga JS (2006) Spatial distribution of primates in a mosaic of colonizing and old growth forest at Ngogo, Kibale National Park, Uganda. Primates 47: 230–238.
50. Mulley BG, Unruh JD (2004) The role of off-farm employment in tropical forest conservation: labor, migration, and smallholder attitudes toward land in western Uganda. J Environ Manage 71: 193–205.
51. Hartter J (2007) Landscape change around Kibale National Park, Uganda: Impacts on land cover, land use, and livelihoods. Gainsesville: University of Florida. 176 p.
52. Pontzer H, Wrangham RW (2006) Ontogeny of ranging in wild Chimpanzees. Int J Primatol 27: 295–309.
53. Amsler SJ (2009) Ranging behavior and territoriality in Chimpanzees at Ngogo, Kibale National Park, Uganda. Ph.D. Thesis. University of Michigan, Ann Arbor, United States of America.
54. Smith PG (1983) Quantitative Plant Ecology. Washington DC: Butterworth Press. 359 p.
55. Cannon CH, Curran LM, Marshall AJ, Leighton M (2007) Long-term reproductive behaviour of woody plants across seven Bornean forest types in the Gunung Palung National Park (Indonesia): suprannual synchrony, temporal productivity, and fruiting diversity. Ecol Lett 10: 956–969.
56. Green RH (1966) Measurment of non-randomness in spatial distributions. Res Popul Ecol 8: 1–7.
57. Chapman CA, White FJ, Wrangham RW (1994) Party size in chimpanzees and bonobos. In: Wrangham RW, McGrew WC, de Waal FMD. Heltne PG, editors. Chimpanzee cultures. Cambridge: Harvard University Press. 41.
58. Potts KB, Watts DP, Wrangham RW (2011) Comparative Feeding Ecology of Two Communities of Chimpanzees (*Pan troglodytes*) in Kibale National Park, Uganda. Int J Primatol 32: 669–690.
59. Tweheyo M, Lye Kåre A (2003) Phenology of figs in Budongo Forest Uganda and its importance for the chimpanzee diet. Afr J Ecol 41: 306–316.
60. Ganzhorn JU (1995) Low-level forest disturbance effects on primary production, leaf chemistry, and lemur populations. Ecology 76: 2084–2096.
61. Chapman CA, Struhsaker TT, Skorupa JP, Snaith TV, Rothman JM (2010) Understanding long-term primate community dynamics: implications of forest change. Ecol Appl 20(1): 179–191.
62. Onderdonk DA, Chapman CA (2000) Coping with forest fragmentation: The primates of Kibale National Park, Uganda. Int J Primatol 21: 587–611.
63. Chapman CA, Balcomb SR, Gillespie TR, Skorupa JP, Struhsaker TT (2000) Long term effects of logging on african primate communities: a 28-year comparison from Kibale national Park. Conserv Biol 14(1): 207–217.
64. Thompson ME, Kahlenberg SM, Gilby IC, Wrangham R (2007) Core area quality is associated with variance in reproductive success among female chimpanzees at Kibale National Park. Anim Behav 73: 501–512.
65. Tweheyo M, Lye Kare A, Weladjic RB (2004) Chimpanzee diet and habitat selection in the Budongo Forest Reserve, Uganda. For Ecol Mgmt 188(1–3): 267–278.
66. Potts KB (2011) The Long-term impact of timber harvesting on the resource base of Chimpanzees in Kibale National Park, Uganda. Biotropica 43: 256–264.
67. Conklin NL, Wrangham RW (1994) The value of Figs to a Hind-gut Fermenting Frugivore: a Nutritional Analysis. Biochem Syst Ecol 22(2): 137–151.
68. Ohashi G, Matsuzawa T (2010) Deactivation of Snares by wild chimpanzees. Primates 52(1): 1–5.
69. Masi S, Gustafsson E, Saint Jalme M, Narat V, Todd A, et al. (2011) Unusual feeding behavior in wild great apes, a window to understand origins of self-medication in humans: Role of sociality and physiology on learning process. Physiol Behav 105: 337–349.
70. Jammaat KRL, Ban SD, Boesch C (2013) Taï chimpanzees use botanical skills to discover fruit: whart we can learn from their mistakes. Anim Cogn 16: 852–860.
71. Stanford CB, Nkurunugi JB (2003) Behavioral ecology of sympatric Chimpanzees and Gorillas in Bwindi Impenetrable National Park, Uganda: Diet. Int J Primatol 24(4): 901–918.
72. Newton-Fisher NE (1999) The diet of chimpanzees in the Budongo Forest Reserve, Uganda. Afr J Ecol 37: 344–354.
73. Yamakoshi G (1998) Dietary responses to fruit scarcity of wild chimpanzees at Bossou, Guinea: possible implications for ecological importance of tool use. Am J Phys Anthropol 106: 283–295.
74. Food and Agriculture Organization (2000) The Global Forest Resources Assessment 2000, Rome: FAO. 377 p.

10

Diet and Diversification in the Evolution of Coral Reef Fishes

Fabio L. Lobato[1], Diego R. Barneche[2], Alexandre C. Siqueira[1], Ana M. R. Liedke[1], Alberto Lindner[1], Marcio R. Pie[3], David R. Bellwood[4], Sergio R. Floeter[1]*

1 Departamento de Ecologia e Zoologia, Universidade Federal de Santa Catarina, Florianópolis, SC, Brazil, **2** Department of Biological Sciences, Macquarie University, Sydney, NSW, Australia, **3** Setor de Ciências Biológicas, Universidade Federal do Paraná, Curitiba, PR, Brazil, **4** Australian Research Council Centre of Excellence for Coral Reef Studies, and School of Marine and Tropical Biology, James Cook University, Townsville, QLD, Australia

Abstract

The disparity in species richness among evolutionary lineages is one of the oldest and most intriguing issues in evolutionary biology. Although geographical factors have been traditionally thought to promote speciation, recent studies have underscored the importance of ecological interactions as one of the main drivers of diversification. Here, we test if differences in species richness of closely related lineages match predictions based on the concept of density-dependent diversification. As radiation progresses, ecological niche-space would become increasingly saturated, resulting in fewer opportunities for speciation. To assess this hypothesis, we tested whether reef fish niche shifts toward usage of low-quality food resources (i.e. relatively low energy/protein per unit mass), such as algae, detritus, sponges and corals are accompanied by rapid net diversification. Using available molecular information, we reconstructed phylogenies of four major reef fish clades (Acanthuroidei, Chaetodontidae, Labridae and Pomacentridae) to estimate the timing of radiations of their subclades. We found that the evolution of species-rich clades was associated with a switch to low quality food in three of the four clades analyzed, which is consistent with a density-dependent model of diversification. We suggest that ecological opportunity may play an important role in understanding the diversification of reef-fish lineages.

Editor: Sebastian C. A. Ferse, Leibniz Center for Tropical Marine Ecology, Germany

Funding: This work benefited from the Computational Biology Service Unit - Cornell University (CBSU Web Computing Interface), funded by Microsoft Corporation. Marcio R. Pie and Sergio R. Floeter were supported by CNPq (http://www.cnpq.br/) (MRP: 304897/2012-4; SRF: 309472/2011-3). David R. Bellwood was supported by the Australian Research Council (http://www.arc.gov.au/). The funders had no role in study design, data collection and analysis, decision to publish, or preparation of the manuscript.

Competing Interests: The authors have declared that no competing interests exist.

* Email: sergio.floeter@ufsc.br

Introduction

Explaining the wide differences in species richness among different evolutionary lineages has been a major goal of evolutionary biology since Darwin and still remains one of the greatest challenges of modern biology [1]. The disparate numbers of extant species among clades results from unequal rates of speciation and extinction through time, and recent methodological advances have helped to elucidate the influence of geographical, environmental and biological factors on diversification (e.g., [2–4]). For instance, some methods have focused on testing how diversification rates are affected by niche availability in biological communities [4,5]. In this sense, the concept of density-dependent diversification, also referred to as 'diversity-dependent' diversification [6,7], suggests that speciation rates are faster when there are abundant resources and few competitors [8]. Thus, as niche space becomes saturated over time, speciation rates decline [8–11]. Evidence for a diversity-dependent diversification scenario involves recurrent explosive radiations following mass extinction events, and the subsequent decline in diversification rates through time [6]. This general pattern in the fossil record has also been identified in recent phylogenies (e.g., [12,13]).

We used molecular phylogenies to test the hypothesis of diversity-dependent diversification in reef fishes, one of the most speciose vertebrate assemblages dating back at least to the early Tertiary (50 Ma) [14]. Reef fishes are remarkable for their use of different micro-habitats and food resources across tropical and temperate seas [15–17]. In the trophic context, food resources such as algae and sessile invertebrates (e.g. sponges and cnidarians) are abundant but usually present 1) relatively low nutritional value per unit mass [18–21], 2) structural and chemical defenses against grazing [22–25], and 3) are less digestible compared to mobile invertebrates (e.g. polychaetes, molluscs, crustaceans, echinoderms) and fishes [26–28]. The use of low-quality diets would impose specific morphological, physiological, and behavioral constraints on fishes during their evolution, as a result of the energetic costs of this novel feeding mode [29,30]. Harmelin-Vivien [16] proposed that the relative stability in the tropics, both between seasons and over geological times, may have shaped the evolutionary processes at molecular, organism and community levels leading to a more efficient use of low-quality food resources among tropical reef fish communities. Harmelin-Vivien hypothesized that increasing species richness in the tropics would have led to high competitive pressures among fishes using high-quality diets [16]. In this case, a shift to a nutrient-poor diet that is underutilized by other species would offer a competitive advantage, leading to the rise of recently derived lineages using relatively low-quality diets. To address this hypothesis, we examined the relationship between the trophic status and rates of diversification of reef fishes.

We focused on four representative clades with good phylogenetic resolution (Chaetodontidae, Labridae, Pomacentridae and Acanthuroidei; see [31]) and examined net speciation rates. Specifically, we tested whether niche shifts to the use of relatively low-quality food resources, such as algae and corals are accompanied by increased net diversification of these lineages. Our results show that both predictions – net speciation rates decrease with time and increase following niche shifts to low-quality diets within lineages – are met in three of the four clades analyzed (in the Labridae the changes were recorded but were not restricted to clades with a low quality diet), suggesting that density-dependent diversification may be a general phenomenon in reef fish evolution.

Materials and Methods

Reef fish groups

We focused on three speciose families in the "consensus" (archetypical) reef fish families (*sensu* [31]): Labridae, Pomacentridae and Chaetodontidae; and a suborder containing three other reef fish families, the Acanthuroidei. These clades were chosen because they represent important elements in the reef environments and have recent phylogenetic data available to be explored. The Labridae (wrasses and parrotfishes) is a diverse group (~575 species) with great disparity in body shape, size, coloration, and habitat preference, being most common in shallow habitats such as coral and rocky reefs [32]. Although most labrid species feed on a variety of hard-shelled invertebrates, some lineages use other types of resources, such as algae, detritus, plankton, coral mucus, ectoparasites, and fish [32,33].

The Pomacentridae (damselfishes and anemonefishes) is one of the four most speciose reef fish families with approximately 380 species [34]. Despite showing great diversity and abundance, damselfishes exhibit a low degree of trophic diversity when compared to the Labridae [15,32]. This relatively restricted ecological diversity seems to be associated with limited morphological variation [35], and similar biomechanical character states have converged many times during their radiation, leading to convergence on food habits such as herbivory, omnivory and planktivory [36].

The Chaetodontidae (butterflyfishes and bannerfishes) includes over 120 species with spectacular coloration and considerable ecological and morphological diversity [37,38]. Found on tropical reefs around the world, they prey on a range of taxa, ranging from obligate or facultative coral feeders to omnivores or sessile invertebrate feeders [38,39].

The Acanthuroidei is a monophyletic suborder that includes the families Acanthuridae (surgeonfishes), Zanclidae (Moorish idol), and Luvaridae (Louvar) [40]. Common in tropical and subtropical seas worldwide, acanthuroids feed mostly by biting attached prey, although zooplanktivory has also evolved within the group [41]. They present a wide variety of morphological and physiological modifications of the jaws and intestines [42–44].

Taxon sampling and sequence alignment

The taxon sampling and molecular data in this study were obtained from previous phylogenetic studies regarding the four abovementioned groups. DNA sequences were downloaded from Genbank following accession numbers in (1) Tang *et al.* [45] for Acanthuroidei, (2) Fessler & Westneat [46] for Chaetodontidae, (3) Westneat & Alfaro [47] for Labridae and (4) Cooper *et al.* [48] for Pomacentridae. Taxon sampling was composed of: (1) 9 acanthuroids; (2) 71 chaetodontids; (3) 84 labrids; (4) 104 pomacentrids.

The sampled Chaetodontidae and Pomacentridae include all currently recognized genera (Table 1). In the suborder Acanthuroidei, all families and genera are represented in the phylogeny. The missing genera in the labrid phylogeny correspond to 12% of labrid species and are mostly monotypic genera (Table 1). Sequences for outgroup species were also downloaded according to the respective references. Sequences downloaded for each species correspond to fragments of (1) two mitochondrial genes (12s, 16s) for acanthuroids, (2) three mitochondrial (12s, 16s, ND3) and two nuclear (Tmo4C4, RAG2) genes for chaetodontids, (3) two mitochondrial (12s and 16s) and two nuclear (Tmo4C4, RAG2) genes for labrids, and (4) three mitochondrial (12s, 16s, ND3) and three nuclear (RAG1, RAG2, bmp4) genes for pomacentrids.

ClustalX 2.0 [49] was used to generate initial alignments for all gene sequences, which were edited using MacClade 4.0 [50]. After sequence edition, the whole datasets consisted of 1,341 bp for Acanthuroidei; 3,106 bp for Chaetodontidae; 2,736 bp for Labridae; and 4,129 bp for Pomacentridae.

Phylogenetic analysis

We inferred the phylogenetic relationships within each family through Bayesian Inference (BI) in MrBayes 3.1.2 using the GTR+ Γ model [51,52]. Data was partitioned by gene in Chaetodontidae and Pomacentridae; for Acanthuroidei, both genes were set as a single partition and for Labridae the mitochondrial genes were set as single partition while the nuclear genes were considered as independent partitions. These partitions were chosen using Bayes factors by comparing the following partitioning schemes: 1. all genes apart; 2. mitochondrial genes apart and nuclear genes as a single partition; 3. nuclear genes apart and mitochondrial genes as a single partition; 4. nuclear and mitochondrial genes as single partitions but apart from each other; 5. all genes as a single partition.

To infer each tree using Bayesian Inference, two independent Markov Chain Monte Carlo (MCMC) runs (each with four chains), were implemented simultaneously for 10 million generations, with trees sampled and saved every 1,000 generations (10,000 trees saved per run) using MrBayes [51]. Default settings were used for all other parameters. All trees prior to stationarity and convergence of the runs were discarded. Stationarity was assigned starting at the leveling off of log likelihood scores and convergence was assumed when the value for the standard deviation of split frequencies remained below 0.01. We computed a majority rule consensus tree (50%) and posterior probabilities of clades with the post-burnin trees. All runs were conducted on the CBSU Web Computing Interface (accessed online at http://cbsuapps.tc.cornell.edu/mrbayes.aspx), and results were analyzed with Tracer 1.5 [53].

Dates estimation and fossil calibration

Divergence times of lineages in all four groups of study were estimated using BEAST 1.5.4 [54]. Rates of lineage splitting were estimated independently from an uncorrelated exponential distribution (UCED) or lognormal distribution (UCLD) given that previous studies tend not to demonstrate autocorrelation of these rates and times of divergence [55–57]. We specified a Yule (pure birth) prior to rates of cladogenesis, given that it assumes only a constant speciation rate across the phylogeny. However, given the high effective sample size values for the estimated parameters, the choice of prior is likely to have no influence on the resulting estimates. The partitions described above were assumed to have

Table 1. Number of sampled and missing species from phylogenetic reconstructions (Fig. 1) according to the total number of species in each subclade.

Tree	Subclades	N° species sampled	N° species missing	Total N° species	% species not represented due to missing genera	% species using LQD
Acanthuroidei	Luvaridae	1	0	1	0	0
	Zanclidae	1	0	1	0	0
	Acanthuridae	7	74	81	0	77
	Total	**9**	**74**	**83**	**0**	**76**
Chaetodontidae	Bannerfishes	17	9	26	0	0
	Prognathodes	2	9	11	0	0
	Chaetodon	52	39	91	0	99
	Total	**71**	**57**	**128**	**0**	**71**
Labridae	Labridae 1b	2	10	12	58	92
	Labridae 2b	6	90	96	10	100
	Labridae 2g	7	19	25	48	36
	Other labrids	69	414	484	9	2
	Total	**84**	**533**	**617**	**12**	**17**
Pomacentridae	*Lepidozygus*	1	0	1	0	0
	Pomacentridae 1	19	48	67	0	100
	Pomacentridae 2	21	88	109	0	0
	Pomacentridae 3	9	11	20	0	0
	Pomacentridae 4	54	130	184	0	60
	Total	**104**	**277**	**381**	**0**	**48**

Percentage of species not represented in the analyses due to missing genera and the percentage of species using Low-quality diet (LQD) in each subclade are also shown.

evolved according to a GTR model with Γ-distributed rate heterogeneity, which was selected based on the Akaike Information Criterion (AIC) values using Modeltest 3.7 [58]. We assigned hard lower bounds and 95% soft upper bounds to the prior distributions of all fossil calibrations points using lognormal distributions. For all calibration points, the hard lower bounds were based on the age of the oldest fossil record of the clade, following the corresponding studies (Table 2).

Since the vast majority of reported chaetodontid fossils are demonstrably erroneous [59], in the case of Chaetodontidae tree we followed Bellwood *et al.* [39] to assign an 95% soft upper bound of 65 Ma at the outgroup node, which is represented by a range of putative outgroup taxa in the reef fish families Zanclidae, Drepaneidae, Ephippidae, Kyphosidae, Scatophagidae and Pomacanthidae [46]. This age represents the transition of fish faunas at the K/T boundary [46,60,61] beyond which there is no fossil record of modern reef fish families. For the same reason, we set the 95% soft upper bound of 65 Ma at the root of Pomacentridae; at the origin of Acanthuridae in the Acanthuroid tree; at the origin of the Labridae 1 clade and at the origin of the Labridae 2 group in the labrid tree (Table 2). The labrid root received the same soft upper bounds but with ln (mean) closer to 65 Ma than 50 Ma. Only in the Labridae 2b node, the 95% soft upper bound was

Table 2. Lognormal distribution, priors and references for the calibration points.

Tree	node	hard-lower bound (Ma)	95% soft-upper bound (Ma)	ln(mean)	ln(SD)	References
Acanthuroidei	Acanthuridae	50	65	1.0	1.04	Bellwood, 1996 [14]
Chaetodontidae	Outgroup	50	65	1.0	1.04	Bellwood *et al.*, 2010 [25]
Labridae	Labridae 2b	15	50	1.5	1.25	Bellwood, 1990 [95]; Smith *et al.*, 2008 [96]
	Labridae 1	50	65	1.0	1.04	Bellwood, 1990 [95]; Cowman *et al.*, 2009 [72]
	Labridae 2	50	65	1.0	1.04	Bannikov & Sorbini, 1995 [48]; Cowman *et al.*, 2009 [72]
	root	50	65	1.0	0.8	Bellwood, 1990 [95]
Pomacentridae	root	50	65	1.0	0.8	Bellwood, 1990 [95]

placed at 50 Ma, marking the oldest fossil record of the Labridae [62].

For each of the four groups we used CBSU Web Computing Interface to run three independent analyses of 10 million generations, sampling trees every 500 generations. Resulting log files were examined using Tracer 1.5 [53] to ensure convergence. After excluding the first 10% burnin, tree files were combined using LogCombiner [54]. With the resulting file, we computed a maximum clade credibility tree using TreeAnnotator [54] to display mean node ages and highest posterior density (HPD) intervals at 95% (upper and lower) for each node.

Character optimization

While it is self-evident that all diets are nutritionally adequate, there are fundamental differences in food composition (i.e. C/N ratio per unit mass) [63,64], and in the way that nutrition is acquired (i.e. feeding behavior) [15]. We provide a simple binary classification for trophic modes termed low quality and high quality diets: 1) The low quality diet was based on food items that are mainly consumed by herbivores, corallivores and coral mucus feeders, which have significantly more carbohydrate in its composition, high ash content, and relatively low nitrogen per unit mass (i.e. sponge tissues, plant material, detritus, etc.). These items generally present physiological challenges for digestion or relatively inaccessible organic components as a result of structural features and secondary metabolites [22–25]. 2) The high quality diet was based on food items that are mainly consumed by piscivores, zooplanktivores and mobile invertebrate feeders, which have relatively high protein/carbohydrate ratio per unit mass [64,65]. These items also present few physiological challenges for digestion (i.e. fish, crustaceans, annelids, echinoderms, mollusks, etc.), assuming that rigid covering shells and crustacean exoskeletons could be overcome [15].

We have classified all species according to their trophic modes and mapped them onto the BI trees using parsimony, as implemented in Mesquite 2.75 [66]. These traits were also optimized with MP (Maximum Parsimony) analysis to identify the independent evolution of trophic modes.

Diversification statistics

All diversification statistics were performed in R [67] using APE 3.0-11 [68], GEIGER 1.99-3.1 [69], and LASER 2.4-1 [70] packages. In order to look for general patterns of declining species-level diversification rate, we applied the constant-rates (CR) test [71] to estimate the γ statistic in each of the four BEAST chronograms. The CR test uses a measure of the relative positions of internal nodes within a phylogeny as basis for calculating the value of γ, which is then used to test the null hypothesis of constant per-lineage speciation and extinction rates through time. Within a completely sampled phylogeny the γ values fit a standard normal distribution with mean = 0, considering a Yule process [71]. Decreases in rates of cladogenesis over time are detected by significantly negative γ values. The incomplete sampling in our analysis will tend to underestimate the number of nodes toward the present, and the CR test may therefore detect a false slowdown in diversification rate. To correct such bias, we performed a Monte Carlo Constant Rates (MCCR) test [71] in which complete phylogenies are simulated under the Yule process by randomly selecting a subsample from the reconstructed topologies and removing them from the analyses. This procedure generates a corrected null distribution allowing the estimation of the significance of negative γ values, which makes the results conservative to extinction. The observed γ values were compared to the 95% confidence interval of a null distribution based on 10,000 topologies simulated for each of the four groups.

We estimated global diversification rate (r**G**) for each of the four groups using the method of Margallon & Sanderson (eqn. 8–11 in [72]). This method calculates the 95% confidence interval of expected species richness for a lineage with origin at time (t) and evolving under a given r**G** and ε, and then compares those estimates with the observed species richness. The estimation considers extinction rates (ε), thus, we estimated r**G** under different values of ε (0.0, 0.5, 0.9 and 0.99). Subclades were defined at the highest monophyletic clades in which species share the same trophic mode. The species richness of such lineages was measured based on valid names listed in the Catalog of Fishes [73] and crown ages were obtained from BEAST chronograms. For lineages with a single species sampled we used stem ages. It is important to use methods with different approaches to correct for possible equivocal interpretation of the results given the limitations of each method. The method of moments' estimator basically considers the relationship between species richness and age. Thus, we used the Relative Cladogenesis (RC) statistic [74] and the method described in [75] to look for significant shifts in net diversification rates. The RC test identifies lineages with significantly faster or slower rates of cladogenesis using a chronogram to calculate the probability that an internal node with n descendent tips get partitioned into two subclades of size *r* and *s*, using a broken-stick distribution as the null expectation [74]. To apply Rabosky's method [75], we first reduced the trees at the level of the subclades of interest by pruning all but one species per subclade from the chronograms. Then, we assigned species richness to each terminal branch as a phenotype vector [70]. This method uses a birth–death estimator based on phylogenetic and taxonomic data to estimate diversification rate and compute the respective likelihood. It contrasts the likelihood of the data under a model with equal diversification rates for all lineages (constant model) to the likelihood under a model where an ancestral diversification rate r1 shifts to a new rate r2 along some branch in the tree (flexible model) [76,77]. For the flexible model, the tree is sequentially split at each branch and r is optimized to the resulting pair of subtrees. The node resulting in the maximum combined likelihood for the bipartite tree is the ML estimate of the shift point. Analyses were conducted under extinction fractions of $\varepsilon = 0.0$, 0.5, 0.9 and 0.99. To contrast the models we used the likelihood ratio test statistic (χ^2 distributed with 2 *d.f.*). Our hypothesis predicts that the flexible model would be more likely than the constant model especially when assigning higher net diversification rates at the origin of clades containing low-quality diet feeders. However, it does not necessarily mean that the net diversification rates have increased at that node. Alternatively, the clade could have retained an ancestral but elevated rate, while another clade or clades exhibited a decline in net diversification. To test these scenarios, we used a constrained version of the two-rate model ('rate-decrease model'), where the highest net diversification rate must occur in the tree bipartition containing the root node, such that no net rate increase is allowed on the path from the root to the clade assigned by the shifting point [78,79].

Results

Phylogenetic Inferences

Bayesian inferences produced highly resolved topologies, very close to those found in the original articles. All phylogenies were well supported and presented good resolution for optimization. For all four clades, stationarity and convergence were reached before 10% of the generations. Valid estimations from Mr. Bayes

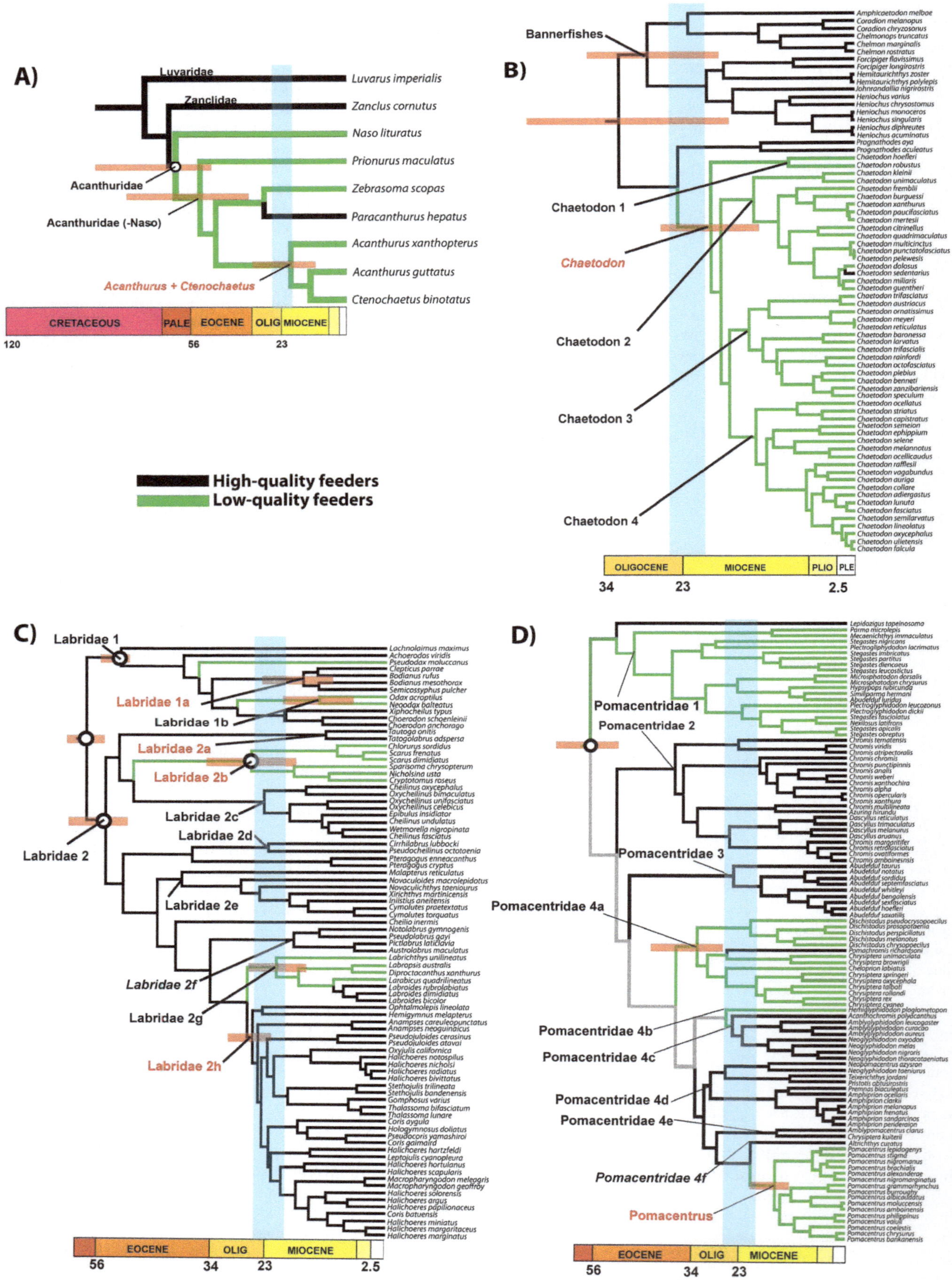
A)
Luvaridae
Zanclidae
Luvarus imperialis
Zanclus cornutus
Naso lituratus
Prionurus maculatus
Zebrasoma scopas
Paracanthurus hepatus
Acanthurus xanthopterus
Acanthurus guttatus
Ctenochaetus binotatus
Acanthuridae
Acanthuridae (-Naso)
Acanthurus + Ctenochaetus
CRETACEOUS
PALE
EOCENE
OLIG
MIOCENE
120
56
23
High-quality feeders
Low-quality feeders
B)
Bannerfishes
Chaetodon 1
Chaetodon
Chaetodon 2
Chaetodon 3
Chaetodon 4
OLIGOCENE
MIOCENE
PLIO
PLE
34
23
2.5
C)
Labridae 1
Labridae 1a
Labridae 1b
Labridae 2a
Labridae 2b
Labridae 2c
Labridae 2d
Labridae 2
Labridae 2e
Labridae 2f
Labridae 2g
Labridae 2h
EOCENE
OLIG
MIOCENE
56
34
23
2.5
D)
Pomacentridae 1
Pomacentridae 2
Pomacentridae 3
Pomacentridae 4a
Pomacentridae 4b
Pomacentridae 4c
Pomacentridae 4d
Pomacentridae 4e
Pomacentridae 4f
Pomacentrus
EOCENE
OLIG
MIOCENE
56
34
23

Figure 1. BEAST chronogram showing optimized character under diet quality of: A) Acanthuroidei; B) Chaetodontidae; C) Labridae; D) Pomacentridae. Black branches represent high-quality feeders, green branches represent low-quality feeders and gray branches mean equivocal character. Red names represent subclades that showed significant higher than expected species richness under rG conditioned to different extinction rates. Bars on nodes represent the 95% HPD of subclades mean age. White dots indicate calibration points. The blue bar represents the expansion of IWP reefs in the Oligo-Miocene period among 25–20 Ma [2,5,80].

runs were indicated by good effective sample sizes (which shows that the MCMC simulation had an adequate length) in the resulting statistics compiled with Tracer. All resulting phylogenies are shown in Figure 1, and the supporting statistics are presented in Table S1 of the appendix.

Dates estimation and character optimization

Mean evolutionary rate, Yule process birth rate, coefficients of variation and mean covariance are presented in Table 3 and the resulting chronograms are shown in Figure 1. The coefficients of variation (CV) are used to assess the overall degree of rate heterogeneity across the trees. The resulting posterior densities from the CV were different from zero, indicating significant rate heterogeneity (unclock-like behavior) in all four groups. The mean covariance (MC) was used to assess the degree of autocorrelation of rates across lineages. In all four phylogenies the resulting posterior densities from MC were close to zero, suggesting that branches with fast rates and slow rates are next to each other.

In the Acanthuroidei, the 95% HPD interval was high for all ages at nodes corresponding to basal relationships. However, the family Acanthuridae had the origin estimated at 61 Ma (95% HPD: 86–50 Ma) (Fig. 1A). Character optimization indicated that the low-quality food habit has evolved once in the suborder at about 52 Ma in the family Acanthuridae (95% HPD: 76–34 Ma) (Fig. 1A). The origin of the most speciose clade, formed by the genera *Acanthurus* + *Ctenochaetus* was 20 Ma (95% HPD: 31–10 Ma).

The origin of chaetodontid outgroup (taxonomically related reef fish families) was estimated at 55 Ma (95% HPD: 65–50 Ma) as we set in our prior. As expected, the family Chaetodontidae seems to be a relatively young family originated at 33 Ma (95% HPD: 45–21 Ma) (Fig. 1B). The relatively low-quality food habit (mainly corallivory) arose at about 20 Ma (95% HPD: 28–13) within the clade *Chaetodon*. The specialization of obligate corallivores appears shortly thereafter at about 15 Ma (95% HPD: 24–12 Ma), in the clade *Chaetodon* 3 (Fig. 1B).

For the labrid tree, three clades used for calibration had age estimates close to the age of the oldest fossil: labrid root = 58 Ma (95% HPD: 62–55 Ma), Labridae 1 = 51 Ma (95% HPD: 53–50), and Labridae 2 = 54 Ma (95% HPD: 59–50) (Fig. 1C). Character optimization indicated that four lineages have arisen that exploit low-quality diets, all independently and at different times, using different food items, although most of the radiation was during the Miocene (Fig. 1C).

The origin of Pomacentridae estimated at 52 Ma (95% HPD: 61–50 Ma) was very close to the age of the oldest fossil of the family used to set a hard lower bound prior (Fig. 1D). The exploitation of low-quality resources appears at the first split in Pomacentridae 1 + *Lepidozygus*. There are three other clades with low-quality diets: Pomacentridae 4a (stem age = 31 Ma, 95% HPD: 39–25), Pomacentridae 4b (25 Ma, 95% HPD: 32–19 Ma) and the genus *Pomacentrus* (15 Ma, 95% HPD: 19–11 Ma), from which only *Pomacentrus* seems to have arisen after the Oligo-Miocene transition (Fig. 1D).

Net diversification rates

Estimated global net diversification rates (r**G**) decreased with increasing extinction rates, as already noted in the method description. Significantly higher than expected species richness under r**G** conditioned to different ε values are found in Figure 2 (Table S1). It corresponds to: (1) *Acanthurus* + *Ctenochaetus* (Acanthuroidei, Fig. 1A); (2) *Chaetodon* (Chaetodontidae, Fig. 1B); (3) Labridae 1a, (4) Labridae 2a, (5) Labridae 2b and (6) Labridae 2 h (Labridae, Fig. 1C); and (7) *Pomacentrus* (Pomacentridae, Fig. 1D). In the Acanthuroidei, we looked for the species richness formed by the clade Acanthuridae to conduct the test since all species, except *Paracanthurus hepatus*, share the same trophic character in this monophyletic group, and we obtained significant values of p only under $\varepsilon = 0.0$. Acanthuridae (-*Naso*) has a mean age of 52 Ma, however, 75% of these species belong to the subclade formed by *Acanthurus* + *Ctenochaetus*, which originated about 20 Ma. Therefore, we believe that all influence that led to higher than expected number of extant species in Acanthuridae

Table 3. Mean evolutionary rate (MER), Yule process birth rate (Yule), coefficient of variance (CV) and mean covariance (MC) for each of the ultrametric trees reconstructed using BEAST.

Tree	MER	Yule	CV	MC
	95% HPD	95% HPD	95% HPD	95% HPD
Acanthuroidei	1.24E-3	1.19E-2	0.54	−0.11
	8.2E-4–1.6E-3	6.1E-3–1.8E-2	0.3–0.7	−0.4–0.1
Chaetodontidae	5.51E-3	8.4E-2	0.37	−1.3E-2
	3.9E-3–7.2E-3	5.6E-2–0.1	0.2–0.4	−0.1–0.1
Labridae	3.89E-3	4.7E-2	0.48	7.3E-2
	3.4E-4–4.3E-3	3.6E-2–5.8E-2	0.4–0.5	−0.07–0.2
Pomacentridae	2,66E-3	5.1E-2	0.47	8.7E-2
	2E-4–3.2E-3	3.9E-3–6.5E-2	0.4–0.5	−0.04–0.2

95% HPD = high-posterior density interval of 95% for each value estimated.

(-*Naso*) came exclusively from the effects of the *Acanthurus* + *Ctenochaetus* diversification. We applied the test considering *Acanthurus* + *Ctenochaetus* species richness and we obtained significant values of p under even higher extinction rates ($\varepsilon = 0.0$ to $\varepsilon = 0.99$). For Labridae 2 h (Labridae) and *Pomacentrus* (Pomacentridae) we obtained significant values of p under $\varepsilon = 0.0$ to $\varepsilon = 0.9$. The remaining clades showed significant p values under $\varepsilon = 0.0$ to $\varepsilon = 0.5$ (Table S1). From these seven speciose clades, RC tests indicated higher than expected rates of cladogenesis in *Chaetodon* (Chaetodontidae), *Pomacentrus* (Pomacentridae), Labridae 1a and Labridae 2b (Labridae).

The comparisons between a constant model and a flexible model showed that the flexible model provided the best explanation for elevated net diversification rate at clades *Acanthurus* + *Ctenochaetus* in Acanthuroidei ($\varepsilon = 0.0$ to $\varepsilon = 0.5$), *Chaetodon* in Chaetodontidae ($\varepsilon = 0.0$), Labridae 2 h in Labridae ($\varepsilon = 0.0$ to $\varepsilon = 0.99$) and *Pomacentrus* in Pomacentridae ($\varepsilon = 0.0$ to $\varepsilon = 0.5$) (Table S2).

Discussion

Low-quality diets and net diversification rates

Patterns of diversification in the Acanthuroidei, Chaetodontidae and Pomacentridae are all concordant with the hypothesis of density-dependent diversification. Clades that shifted towards a new low-quality diet, and originated during the expansion of IWP coral reefs in the Oligo-Miocene period (25–20 Ma) [2,5,80] (Fig. 1, blue line), have a higher than expected number of extant species. These clades are: *Acanthurus* + *Ctenochaetus* in the Acanthuroidei (Fig.1A), *Chaetodon* in the Chaetodontidae (Fig. 1B) and *Pomacentrus* in the Pomacentridae (Fig. 1D). With exception of the Acanthuroidei, these shifts in the rate of diversification have been previously reported [5,38]. However, this is the first study to quantitatively examine the contribution of trophic modes across all three groups.

It is reasonable to attribute the high diversity found in *Chaetodon*, *Pomacentrus* and *Acanthurus* + *Ctenochaetus* to Oligo-Miocene tectonic events and the expansion of reefs in the IWP [2,5,80]. This pattern would be expected considering that most species analyzed in this study are from the IWP and that the origin and diversification of most reef fish lineages took place within regions of the Tethys Sea that later became this biogeographic region during this period [81]. However, many lineages with diets based on high-quality food resources with origins and subsequent radiations close to the Oligo-Miocene boundary did not produce significantly more speciose clades (see Fig. 2 and *Prognathodes* in Chaetodontidae, Fig. 1B; Pomacentridae 3, Pomacentridae 4c, Pomacentridae 4e and Pomacentridae 4f in Pomacentridae, Fig. 1D). Cowman & Bellwood [5] reported that families with a higher proportion of coral-dwelling species had higher rates of diversification following a possible cryptic extinction event. It is now clear that reef systems have been major drivers in reef fish evolution most likely by providing broader range of niches to be exploited [4,56]. Our

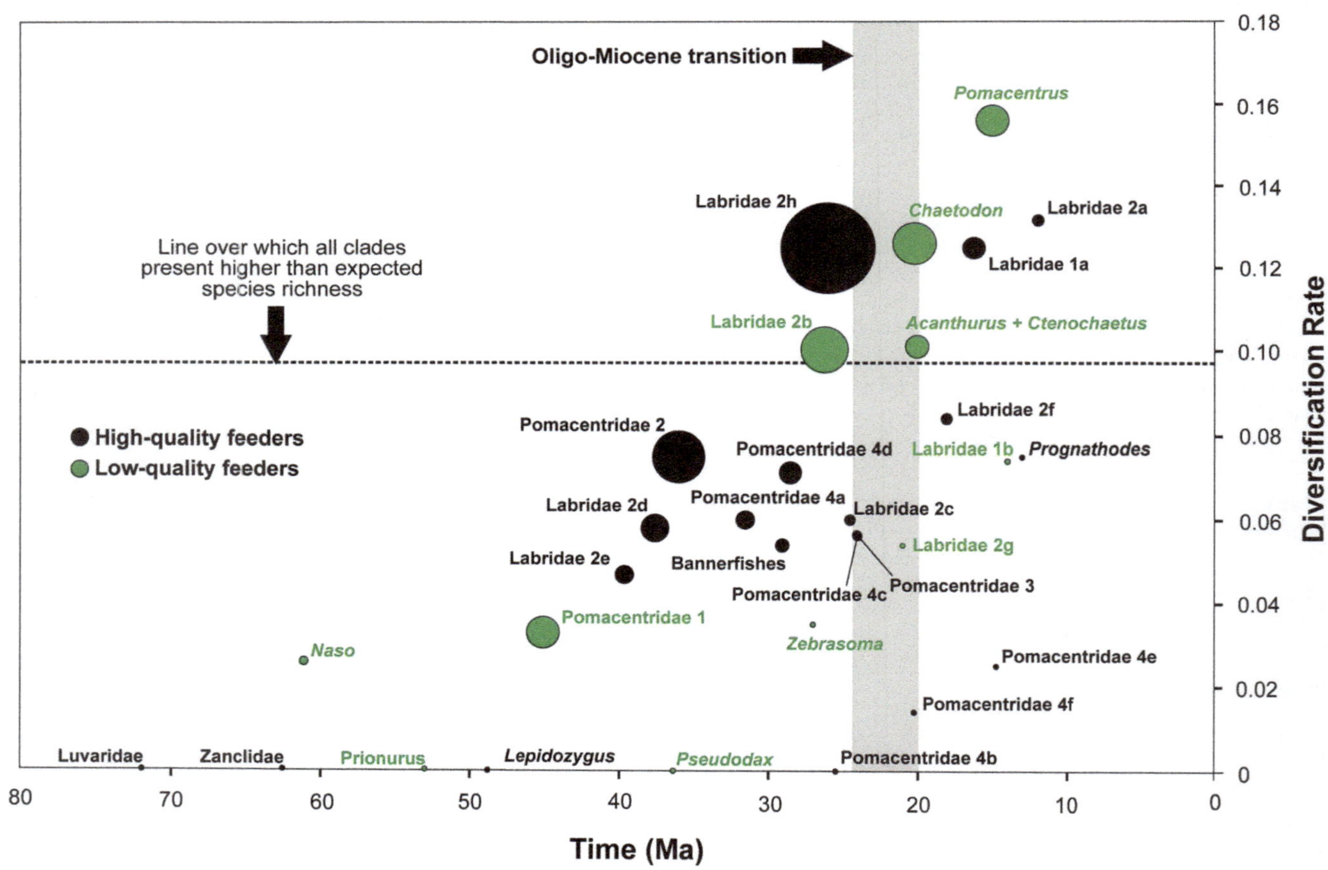

Figure 2. Individual net diversification rate (rG) of subclades *vs.* subclades ages. Black circles represent high-quality feeders, green circles represent low-quality feeders. Dashed line represents the **rG** value over which all clades showed significant higher than expected species richness. Crown ages are according to mean node ages in BEAST analysis. Circle sizes are proportional to the number of species in each clade.

results suggest that exploitation of under-used and abundant 'low-quality' food resources may have played a significant role in this context. Ecological or trophic opportunism may have been a key factor contributing to high diversification rates on specific reef fish groups.

Our results show remarkable parallels to recent studies of fossil surgeonfishes (Acanthuridae) and rabbitfishes (Siganidae) [82] which report a marked change in the trophic status of these fishes in the Oligocene to early Miocene, with the suggestion that the early formation of modern coral reef fish faunas was associated with the exploitation of underutilized EAM (epilithic algal matrix) resources on coral reef flats. The movement onto reef flats was part of a general increase in the exploitation of low-quality trophic resources at that time.

Within the Labridae, the low-quality feeders of the subclade Labridae 2b, which encompasses *Scarus* and *Chlorurus*, showed higher than expected net speciation rates. Several explanations for the relatively high rates of diversification in this subclade have been proposed, including the presence of an intermandibular joint [83], which may be related to the efficient exploitation of a low-quality diet. Relatively high rates of diversification may also reflect vicariance and social factors which may also enhance speciation within the subclade [84]. However, two other subclades of Labridae with low-quality diets that originated during, or after, the Oligo-Miocene transition (Labridae 1b, Labridae 2g), did not presented higher than expected net diversification rates. These results suggest that patterns of diversification within the Labridae may also be influenced by variables such as limited or constrained morphological diversity in Labridae 2g [85], or being a temperate lineage (Labridae 1b) [86]. Moreover, three high-quality diet subclades (Labridae 1a, Labridae 2a and Labridae 2h), presented higher than expected net diversification rates (Fig. 1C, Fig. 2). Clearly, while some labrid groups may have been influenced by a shift to low quality diets, other factors are important and have driven diversification in a range of subclades exploiting a range of trophic modes. These factors may also include biogeographic phenomena such as the expansion of reefs in the Indo-Australian Archipelago or an associated shift in the distribution of reef fishes into the Central Indo-Pacific [2,5,84,87].

It is hard to determine whether low-quality diets are taxonomically more diverse than high-quality diets, given that fishes often exploit complex resources rather than specific food items [88,89]. The key to exploitation of these resources, however, appears to be the possession of the appropriate morphological and physiological modifications to be able to harvest and process low-quality (and often particulate) resources. Indeed, recent fossil evidence has highlighted the Oligocene/Miocene as a key time for the acquisition of morphological features that enable the exploitation of low-quality diets in fishes [90], and the invasion of new areas with extensive availability of low-quality material on coral reefs [82]. These shifts to low-quality diets are associated with the appearance of jaws for scraping in parrotfishes [4,83,91], long-toothed morphologies for selectively harvesting soft tissues or particulates in chaetodontids, acanthurids and blennies [90], and a change on head or body shape to permit exploitation of exposed locations in surgeonfishes [82]. These shifts are likely to be supported by a range of physiological changes in the gut to accommodate the new challenges presented by low-quality diets [26,29,92]. Overall, our results and previous work all point to the Oligocene to early Miocene as a key period in the evolution of reef fishes, marked by a transition to low-quality diets. This trophic shift also appears to have been associated with relatively high rates of diversification.

Competitive interactions and the origin of low-energy diets

There is a central conceptual difference between the present study and that of Harmelin-Vivien [16] in terms of the evolutionary role of decreased competition due to the use of low-quality food resources. For Harmelin-Vivien [16], the rise of low-quality diets is an adaptive response to high levels of competition. In our study, high levels of competition are not necessarily related to the rise of lineages exploiting low-quality diets, but it may be related to the higher net diversification rates in these lineages.

Evolutionary delayed origins of low-energy diets seems to be a widespread pattern within marine communities and has already been described for major metazoan clades such as Crustacea, Mollusca and Echinodermata in different phylogenetic scales [93]. These other clades might have also contributed to high levels of competition on Oligocene/Miocene coral reefs, given that some of these lineages expanded during this period [2] and that they have the ability to compete with fishes for food resources. Within fishes delayed origins of low-quality diets has previously been reported in the Labridae [87] and Chaetodontidae [38]. We now expand this to other major fish groups, showing that the nature and timing of these trophic shifts varies considerably, and that these shifts did not just occur in the Oligocene-Miocene.

The patterns seen in the Acanthuroidei, Chaetodontidae and Labridae are all consistent with the suggestion that the use of low-quality food resources is a derived condition which has evolved independently at least once in each clade [94]. However, the origin of this condition does not appear to be temporally congruent among clades, as suggested by Harmelin-Vivien [16]. In the Acanthuroidei, the origin of low-quality diets in the Acanthuridae coincides with the origin of many other reef fish families (approximately 65–50 Ma), and occurs much earlier than the main period of diversification in reef fishes in the Miocene [5] when most modern reef fish genera arose (Fig. 1A). These results are robust even considering the missing species in the analyses, because all recognized genera are included and the percentage of species using low-quality diets in each subclade are proportional to those used in the reconstructions (Table 1). The Pomacentridae displays the same temporal pattern, with low-quality diet apparently represented at the root of the tree, with the possibility of several independent convergences to a high or low-quality diet (Fig. 1D) [35,36]. It should be noted that in Pomacentridae the different food habits (herbivory, omnivory and zooplanktivory) are likely to be found in all lineages, varying only in the relative contribution of zooplankton and algae to the total ingested biomass.

By contrast, chaetodontid (and to some extent labrid) evolution seems to agree quite well with Harmelin-Vivien's [16] predictions, where the use of relatively low-quality food resources would be a derived condition that arose when reef communities experienced high species richness, suggested by the origin and radiation of *Chaetodon* during the Miocene (Fig. 1B). The reconstruction of ancestral trophic character states suggests that the first butterflyfish may have had the ability to use low-quality food items but could count on a little contribution of high-quality food resources in their diet. Only later did some lineages become more restricted, feeding exclusively on corals, with at least four independent origins of this feeding mode [38]. A similar pattern is seen in the labrids with two independent herbivorous lineages [87].

In the Chaetodontidae, as in Pomacentridae, feeding behaviour appears to be similar among lineages. All *Chaetodon* spp. bite the substratum to ingest food, and are primarily distinguished from each other by the surface they bite. However, the dietary differentiation among chaetodontid lineages seems to transition evolutionarily from high to low-quality diets (possibly due to competitive interactions [16]), while in pomacentrids, low-quality diets are found among early diverging, intermediate and young lineages.

The observations in the present study support recent findings that suggest that reef fishes have experienced two major phases of trophic development in the Cenozoic: an early phase in the Paleogene and a later phase in the Oligocene-Miocene [82,87,90]. Interestingly, the exploitation of low-quality foods was involved in both phases with the Acanthuridae and Pomacentridae exploiting these resources in the Paleogene and the Chaetodontidae and Labridae transitioning primarily in the Neogene. Clearly, the exploitation of low-quality resources is a shift that has been a repeated feature in reef fishes over the last 60 million years.

Conclusions

Our study suggests that the diversification of reef fish lineages may be shaped by ecological opportunity. We present a new perspective in which the emergence of low-quality feeding modes may underpin diversification in a broad range of reef fish families. Our study reinforces the idea of density-dependent diversification influencing the radiation of clades. Moreover, we suggest that trophic shifts have not necessarily induced increasing net rates of diversification in speciose clades, but that they may have reduced declines. Species-rich clades may, therefore, have maintained diversification over time while other clades decreased when niches became saturated. Overall, our study emphasizes the importance of trophic opportunism and low-quality diets in the evolution of reef fishes.

Supporting Information

Table S1 Subclades with higher than expected number of extant species indicated by global diversification rate. Subclades with higher than expected number of extant species indicated by the test of Magallon & Sanderson [63]. **rG** = estimated global diversification rate under different values of extinction rate (**ε**). ***p***<0.05 indicates significant speciose subclades. **NS** = not significant. Subclade labeled in bold = subclades with species using low-quality diets.
(DOCX)

Table S2 Likelihoods and Akaike Information Criterion for constant and flexible models of diversification under different extinction rates. Likelihoods (LH) and Akaike Information Criterion (**AIC**) for constant and flexible models of diversification under different extinction rates (**ε**). **r** is the constant diversification rate estimated across all lineages. p<0.05 indicates significant higher likelihood estimated for the flexible model, in which a diversification rate **r1** shift to **r2** at the subclade indicated. **NS** indicates that the flexible model was not significant assuming shifts in any of the subclades. Rate decreasing scenario was not significant in any case, except in Pomacentridae over ε = 0.5, which was not considered due the equivocal phylogenetic position of *Lepidozygus*.
(DOCX)

Acknowledgments

We thank Tandy Warnow and the whole team of the Cyberinfrastructure for Phylogenetic Research (CIPRES) project (http://www.phylo.org) which allowed us to run much faster analysis. This work also benefited from the Computational Biology Service Unit - Cornell University (CBSU Web Computing Interface). We thank Enrico Rezende, Mariana Bender and Geerat J. Vermeij for discussions and comments on earlier drafts, and two anonymous reviewers for helpful suggestions.

Author Contributions

Conceived and designed the experiments: FLL DRB MRP SRF. Performed the experiments: FLL AL MRP SRF. Analyzed the data: FLL DRB ACS AMRL AL MRP DRB SRF. Contributed reagents/ materials/analysis tools: FLL ACS MRP SRF. Wrote the paper: FLL DRB ACS MRP DRB SRF.

References

1. Ricklefs RE (2007) Estimating diversification rates from phylogenetic information. Ecol Lett 22: 601–610.
2. Renema W, Bellwood DR, Braga JC, Bromfield K, Hall R, et al. (2008) Hopping hotspots: global shifts in marine biodiversity. Science 321: 654–657.
3. Rabosky DL (2009) Ecological limits and diversification rate: alternative paradigms to explain the variation in species richness among clades and regions. Ecol Lett 12: 735–743.
4. Price SA, Holzman R, Near TJ, Wainwright PC (2011) Coral reefs promote the evolution of morphological diversity and ecological novelty in labrid fishes. Ecol Lett 14: 462–469.
5. Cowman PF, Bellwood DR (2011) Coral reefs as drivers of cladogenesis: expanding coral reefs, cryptic extinction events, and the development of biodiversity hotspots. J Evol Biol 24(12): 2543–2562.
6. Sepkoski JJ (1998) Rates of speciation in the fossil record. Philos Trans R Soc Lond B, Biol Sci 353: 315–326.
7. Espeland M, Murienne J (2011) Diversity dynamics in New Caledonia: towards the end of the Museum model? BMC Evol Biol 11: 254.
8. Rabosky DL, Lovette IJ (2008) Density-dependent diversification in North American wood warblers. Philos Trans R Soc Lond B, Biol Sci 275: 2363–2371.
9. Walker TD, Valentine JW (1984) Equilibrium models of evolutionary diversity and the number of empty niches. Am Nat 124: 887–899.
10. Phillimore AB, Price TD (2008) Density-dependent cladogenesis in birds. PLoS Biol 6: 483–489.
11. White JW, Samhouri JF, Stier AC, Wormald CL, Hamilton SL, et al. (2010) Synthesizing mechanisms of density dependence in reef fishes: behavior, habitat configuration, and observational scale. Ecology 91: 1949–1961.
12. Ricklefs RE (2003) Global diversification rates of passerine birds. Philos Trans R Soc Lond B, Biol Sci 270: 2285–2291.
13. Rüber L, Zardoya R (2005) Rapid cladogenesis in marine fishes revisited. Evolution 59: 1119–1127.
14. Bellwood DR (1996) The Eocene fishes of Monte Bolca: the earliest coral reef fish assemblage. Coral Reefs 15: 11–19.
15. Wainwright PC, Bellwood DR (2002) Ecomorphology of feeding in coral reef fishes. In: Sale PF, editor. Coral reef fishes: dynamics and diversity on a complex ecosystem. San Diego: Academic Press. pp. 33–55.
16. Harmelin-Vivien ML (2002) Energetics and fish diversity on coral reefs. In: Sale PF, editor. Coral reef fishes: dynamics and diversity on a complex ecosystem. San Diego: Academic Press. pp. 265–274.
17. Floeter SR, Ferreira CEL, Dominici-Arosemena A, Zalmon IR (2004) Latitudinal gradients in Atlantic reef fish communities: trophic structure and spatial use patterns. J Fish Biol 64: 1680–1699.
18. Bruggemann JH, Begeman J, Bosna EM, Verbug P, Breeman AM (1994) Foraging by the stoplight parrotfish *Sparisoma viride*. II. Intake and assimilation of food, protein, and energy. Mar Ecol Prog Ser 112: 57–71.
19. Bowen SH, Lutz EV, Ahlgren MO (1995) Dietary protein as determinants of food quality: trophic strategies compared. Ecology 76: 899–907.
20. Ferreira CEL, Peret AC, Coutinho R (1998) Seasonal grazing rates and food processing by tropical herbivorous fishes. J Fish Biol 53: 222–235.
21. Horn MH (1998) Feeding and digestion. In: Evans DH, editor. The Physiology of Fishes. New York: CRC Press. pp. 41–60.
22. Hay ME (1991) Fish–seaweed interactions on coral reefs: effects of herbivorous fishes and adaptations of their prey. In: Sale PF, editor. The Ecology of Fishes on Coral Reefs. San Diego: Academic Press. pp. 96–119.
23. Paul VJ (1992) Chemical defenses of benthic marine invertebrates. In: Sale PF, editor. Ecological Roles of Marine Natural Products. Ithaca: Comstock. pp. 164–188.
24. Burns E, Ilan M (2003) Comparison of anti-predatory defenses of Red Sea and Caribbean sponges. II. Physical defence. Mar Ecol Prog Ser 252: 115–123.
25. Burns E, Ifrach I, Carmeli S, Pawlik JR, Ilan M (2003) Comparison of antipredatory defenses of Red Sea and Caribbean sponges. II. Chemical defence. Mar Ecol Prog Ser 252: 105–114.
26. Horn MH (1989) Biology of marine herbivorous fishes. Oceanogr Mar Biol Annu Rev 27: 167–272.

27. Choat JH, Bellwood DR (1991) Reef fishes: their history and evolution. In: Sale PF, editor. The Ecology of fishes on Coral Reefs. San Diego: Academic Press. pp. 39–60.
28. Meylan A (1991) Nutritional characteristics of sponges in the diet of the hawksbill turtle, *Eretmochelys imbricata*. In: Rützler K, editor. New Perspectives in Sponge Biology. Washington: Smithsonian Institution Press. pp. 472–477.
29. Choat JH, Clements KD (1998) Vertebrate herbivores in marine and terrestrial environments: a nutritional ecology perspective. Annu Rev Ecol Syst 29: 375–403.
30. Choat JH, Clements KD (2002) The trophic status of herbivorous fishes on coral reefs 1: dietary analyses. Mar Biol 140: 613–623.
31. Bellwood DR (1998) What are coral reef fishes?—Comment on the report by D.R. Robertson: Do coral reef fish faunas have a distinctive taxonomic structure? (Coral Reefs 17: 179–196). Coral Reefs 17: 187–189.
32. Wainwright PC, Bellwood DR, Westneat MW, Grubich JR, Hoey AS (2004) A functional morphospace for the skull of labrid fishes: patterns of diversity in complex biomechanical systems. Biol J Linn Soc lond 82: 1–25.
33. Kuiter RH (2010) Labridae fishes: Wrasses. Seaford: Aquatic Photographics. 390 p.
34. Froese R, Pauly D (2014) FishBase: World Wide Web electronic publication. Available: www.fishbase.org. Accessed 2014 Jan 17.
35. Cooper WJ, Westneat MW (2009) Form and function of damselfish skulls: rapid and repeated evolution into a limited number of trophic niches. BMC Evol Biol 9: 24.
36. Frédérich B, Sorenson L, Santini F, Slater GJ, Alfaro ME (2013) Iterative Ecological Radiation and Convergence during the Evolutionary History of Damselfishes (Pomacentridae). Am Nat 81: 94–113.
37. Ferry-Graham LA, Wainwright PC, Hulsey CD, Bellwood DR (2001) Evolution and mechanics of long jaws in butterflyfishes (Family Chaetodontidae). J Morphol 248: 120–143.
38. Bellwood DR, Klanten S, Cowman PF, Pratchett MS, Konow N, et al. (2010) Evolutionary history of the butterflyfishes (f: Chaetodontidae) and the rise of coral feeding fishes. J Evol Biol 23: 335–349.
39. Kuiter RH (2002) Butterflyfishes, bannerfishes and their relatives: a comprehensive guide to Chaetodontidae and Microcanthidae. Chorleywood: TMC Publishing. 180 p.
40. Near TJ, Dornburg RI, Eytan BP, Keck WL, Smith KL, et al. (2013) Phylogeny and tempo of diversification in the superradiation of spiny-rayed fishes. Proc Natl Acad Sci U S A 101: 12738–21743.
41. Klanten SO, van Herwerden L, Choat JH, Blair D (2004) Patterns of lineage diversification in the genus *Naso* (Acanthuridae). Mol Phylogenet Evol 32: 221–235.
42. Jones RS (1968) Ecological relationships in Hawaiian and Johnston Island acanthurids (surgeonfishes). Micronesica 4: 310–361.
43. Purcell SW, Bellwood DR (1993) A functional analysis of food procurement in two surgeonfish species, *Acanthurus nigrofuscus* and *Ctenochaetus striatus* (Acanthuridae). Environ Biol Fishes 37: 139–159.
44. Konow N, Bellwood DR, Wainwright PC, Kerr AM (2008) Evolution of novel jaw joints promote trophic diversity in coral reef fishes. Biol J Linn Soc Lond 93: 545–555.
45. Tang KL, Berendzen PB, Wiley EO, Morrissey JF, Winterbottom R, et al. (1999) The phylogenetic relationships of the suborder Acanthuroidei (Teleostei: Perciformes) based on molecular and morphological evidence. Mol Phylogenet Evol 11: 415–425.
46. Fessler JL, Westneat MW (2007) Molecular phylogenetics of the butterflyfishes (Chaetodontidae): taxonomy and biogeography of a global coral reef fish family. Mol Phylogenet Evol 45: 50–68.
47. Westneat MW, Alfaro ME (2005) Phylogenetic relationships and evolutionary history of the reef fish family Labridae. Mol Phylogenet Evol 36: 370–390.
48. Cooper WJ, Smith LL, Westneat MW (2009) Exploring the radiation of a diverse reef fish family: phylogenetics of the damselfishes (Pomacentridae), with new classifications based on molecular analyses of all genera. Mol Phylogenet Evol 52: 1–16.
49. Thompson JD, Gibson TJ, Plewniak F, Jeanmougin F, Higgins DG (1997) The ClustalX windows interface: flexible strategies for multiple sequence alignment aided by quality analysis tools. Nucleic Acids Res 24: 4876–4882.
50. Maddison DR, Maddison WP (2000) MacClade 4: analysis of phylogeny and character evolution, Version 4.0. Sunderland: Sinauer Associates, Massachusetts, MA. 492 p.
51. Huelsenbeck JP, Ronquist FR (2001) Mrbayes: Bayesian inference of phylogeny. Bioinformatics 17: 754–755.
52. Huelsenbeck JP, Ronquist F, Nielsen R, Bollback JP (2001) Bayesian inference of phylogeny and its impact on evolutionary biology. Science 294: 2310–2314.
53. Rambaut A, Drummond AJ (2007) Tracer. Available: http://tree.bio.ed.ac.uk/software/tracer/. Accessed 2012 Feb 7.
54. Drummond AJ, Rambaut A (2007) Bayesian evolution analysis by sampling trees. BMC Evol Biol 7: 214.
55. Drummond AJ, Ho SYW, Phillips MJ, Rambaut A (2006) Relaxed phylogenetics and dating with confidence. PLoS Biol 4: 699–710.
56. Alfaro ME, Santini F, Brock CD (2007) Do reefs drive diversification in marine teleosts? Evidence from the pufferfish and their allies (Order Tetraodontiforms). Evolution 61: 2104–2126.
57. Brown JW, Rest JS, García-Moreno J, Sorenson MD, Mindell DP (2008) Strong mitochondrial DNA support for a Cretaceous origin of modern avian lineages. BMC Evol Biol 6: 6.
58. Posada D, Crandall KA (1998) Modeltest: Testing the model of DNA substitution. Bioinformatics 14:817–818.
59. Bannikov AF (2004) Fishes from the Eocene of Bolca, northern Italy, previously classified with the Chaetodontidae (Perciformes). Studi e Ricerche sui Giacimenti Terziari di Bolca 13: 55–74.
60. Bellwood DR, Wainwright PC (2002) The history and biogeography of fishes on coral reefs. In: Sale PF, editor. Coral reef fishes: dynamics and diversity on a complex ecosystem. San Diego: Academic Press. pp. 5–32.
61. Bellwood DR, van Herwerden L, Konow N (2004) Evolution and biogeography of marine angelfishes (Pisces: Pomacanthidae). Mol Phylogenet Evol 33: 140–155.
62. Bannikov AF, Sorbini L (1990) *Eocoris bloti*, a new genus and species of labrid fish (Perciformes, Labroidei) from the Eocene of Monte Bolca, Italy. Studi e Recereche sui Giacimenti Terziari di Bolca 6: 133–148.
63. Brey T, Rumohr H, Ankar S (1988) Energy content of macrobenthic invertebrates: general conversion factors from weight to energy. J Exp Mar Biol Ecol 117: 271–278.
64. Brey T, Müller-Wiegmann C, Zittier ZMC, Hagen W (2010) Body composition in aquatic organisms - A global data bank of relationships between mass, elemental composition and energy content. J Sea Res 64: 334–340.
65. Bowen SH, Lutz EV, Ahlgren MO (1995) Dietary protein as determinants of food quality: trophic strategies compared. Ecology 76: 899–907.
66. Maddison WP, Maddison DR (2011) Mesquite: a modular system for evolutionary analysis. Available: http://mesquiteproject.org/. Accessed 2012 Jun 10.
67. R Development Core Team (2013) R: A language and environment for statistical computing. R Foundation for Statistical Computing, Vienna, Austria. Available: http://www.R-project.org/. Accessed 2013 Jan 20.
68. Paradis E, Claude J, Strimmer K (2004) APE: analyses of phylogenetics and evolution in R language. Bioinformatics 20: 289–290.
69. Harmon LJ, Weir JT, Brock CD, Glor RE, Challenger W (2008) GEIGER: investigating evolutionary radiations. Bioinformatics 24: 129–131.
70. Rabosky DL (2006) LASER: a maximum likelihood toolkit for detecting temporal shifts in diversification rates from molecular phylogenies. Evol Bioinform Online 2: 273–276.
71. Pybus OG, Harvey PH (2000) Testing macro-evolutionary models using incomplete molecular phylogenies. Philos Trans R Soc Lond B, Biol Sci 267: 2267–2272.
72. Magallon S, Sanderson MJ (2001) Absolute diversification rates in angiosperm clades. Evolution 55: 1762–1780.
73. Eschmeyer WN (2012) Catalog of Fishes. Available: http://researcharchive.calacademy.org/research/ichthyology/catalog/fishcatmain.asp. Accessed 2012 Jan 10.
74. Nee S, Mooers O, Harvey PH (1992) Tempo and mode of evolution revealed from molecular phylogenies. Proc Natl Acad Sci USA 89: 8322–8326.
75. Rabosky DL (2007) Likelihood methods for detecting temporal shifts in diversification rates. Evolution 60: 1152–1164.
76. Sanderson MJ (1994) Reconstructing the evolution of genes and organisms using maximum likelihood. In: Fambrough D, editor. Molecular evolution of physiological processes. New York: Rockefeller. pp. 13–26.
77. Sanderson MJ, Wojciechowski MF (1996) Diversification rates in a temperate legume clade: are there "so many species" of *Astragalus* (Fabaceae)? Am J Bot 83: 1488–1502.
78. Rabosky DL, Donnellan SC, Talaba AL, Lovette IJ (2007) Exceptional among-lineage variation in diversification rates during the radiation of Australia's largest vertebrate clade. Philos Trans R Soc Lond B, Biol Sci 274: 2915–2923.
79. Kazancioglu E, Near TJ, Hanel R, Wainwright PC (2009) Influence of sexual selection and feeding functional morphology on diversification rate of parrotfishes (Scaridae). Philos Trans R Soc Lond B, Biol Sci 276: 3439–3446.
80. Williams ST, Duda TF (2008) Did tectonic activity stimulate speciation in the Oligo-Miocene Indo-West Pacific? Evolution 62: 1618–1634.
81. Cowman PF, Bellwood DR (2013) The historical biogeography of coral reef fishes: global patterns of origination and dispersal. J Biogeogr 40: 209–224.
82. Bellwood DR, Goatley CHR, Brandl SJ, Bellwood O (2014) Fifty million years of herbivory on coral reefs: fossils, fish and functional innovations. Philos Trans R Soc Lond B, Biol Sci 281: 20133046.
83. Price SA, Tavera JJ, Near TJ, Wainwright PC (2010) Functional innovations and morphological diversification in parrotfish. Evolution 64: 3057–3068.
84. Choat JH, Klanten OS, van Herwerden L, Robertson DR, Clements KD (2012) Patterns and processes in the evolutionary history of parrotfishes (family Labridae). Biol J Linn Soc 107: 529–557.
85. Hoey AS, Bellwood DR, Barnett A (2012) To feed or to breed: morphological constraints of mouthbrooding in coral reef cardinalfishes. Philos Trans R Soc Lond B, Biol Sci 279: 2426–2432.
86. Clements KD, Alfaro ME, Fessler J, Westneat MW (2004) Relationships of the Temperate Australasian Labrid Fish Tribe Odacini (Perciformes: Teleostei). Mol Phylogenet Evol 32: 575–587.
87. Cowman PF, Bellwood DR, van Herwerden L (2009) Dating the evolutionary origins of wrasse lineages (Labridae) and the rise of trophic novelty on coral reefs. Mol Phylogenet Evol 52: 621–631.

88. Wilson S, Bellwood DR, Choat JH, Furnas M (2003) Detritus in coral reef ecosystems and its use by coral reef fishes. Oceanogr Mar Biol 41: 279–309.
89. Kramer MJ, Bellwood O, Bellwood DR (2013) The trophic importance of algal turfs for coral reef fishes: the crustacean link. Coral Reefs 32: 575–583.
90. Bellwood DR, Hoey AS, Bellwood O, Goatley CHR (2014) Evolution of long-toothed fishes and the changing nature of fish–benthos interactions on coral reefs. Nat Commun 5: 3144.
91. Streelman JT, Alfaro ME, Westneat MW, Bellwood DR, Karl SA (2002) Evolutionary history of the parrotfishes: biogeography, ecomorphology, and comparative diversity. Evolution 56: 961–971.
92. Elliott J, Bellwood DR (2003) Alimentary tract morphology and diet in three coral reef fish families. J Fish Biol 63: 1598–1609.
93. Vermeij GJ, Lindberg DR (2000) Delayed herbivory and the assembly of marine ecosystems. Paleobiology 26: 419–430.
94. Kotrschal K (1988) Evolutionary patterns in tropical marine reef fish feeding. J Zoolog Syst Evol Res 26: 51–64.
95. Bellwood DR (1990) A new fossil fish *Phyllopharyngodon longipinnis* gen. et sp. nov. (family Labridae) from the Eocene, Monte Bolca, Italy. Studi e Ricerche sui Giacimenti Terziari di Bolca 6: 149–160.
96. Smith LL, Fessler JL, Alfaro ME, Streelman JT, Westneat MW (2008) Phylogenetic relationships and the evolution of regulatory gene sequences in the parrotfishes. Mol Phylogenet Evol 49: 136–152.

11

A Predictive Model of the Dynamics of Body Weight and Food Intake in Rats Submitted to Caloric Restrictions

Marine Jacquier[1,2]*, **Fabien Crauste**[1,2], **Christophe O. Soulage**[3], **Hédi A. Soula**[3,4]

1 Université de Lyon, Université Lyon 1, CNRS UMR 5208, Institut Camille Jordan, Villeurbanne-Cedex, France, **2** Inria Team Dracula, Inria Center Grenoble Rhône-Alpes, Grenoble Rhône-Alpes, France, **3** CarMeN, INSERM U1060, Université de Lyon, INSA-Lyon, Univ. Lyon-1, Villeurbanne, France, **4** Project-Team Beagle, Inria Center Grenoble Rhône-Alpes, Grenoble Rhône-Alpes, France

Abstract

Dynamics of body weight and food intake can be studied by temporally perturbing food availability. This perturbation can be obtained by modifying the amount of available food over time while keeping the overall food quantity constant. To describe food intake dynamics, we developed a mathematical model that describes body weight, fat mass, fat-free mass, energy expenditure and food intake dynamics in rats. In addition, the model considers regulation of food intake by leptin, ghrelin and glucose. We tested our model on rats experiencing temporally variable food availability. Our model is able to predict body weight and food intake variations by taking into account energy expenditure dynamics based on a memory of the previous food intake. This model allowed us to estimate this memory lag to approximately 8 days. It also explains how important variations in food availability during periods longer than these 8 days can induce body weight gains.

Editor: Mihai Covasa, INRA, France

Funding: This work was funded by the authors' institutions: INSA Lyon, University Lyon 1, Inria and Inserm. The funders had no role in study design, data collection and analysis, decision to publish, or preparation of the manuscript.

Competing Interests: The authors have declared that no competing interests exist.

* Email: marine.jacquier@inria.fr

Introduction

Body weight regulation has become a major concern in our societies. A classical case of body weight dysregulation – obesity – is characterized by an excessive accumulation of white adipose tissue due to an energy imbalance between the energy derived from consumed food and the energy expended to maintain life [1–3]. Because obesity is recognized as an important health hazard [4], the causes of this imbalance have been extensively investigated in the past several years [5,6] with findings pointing out to peripheral as well as central mechanisms controlling food intake [7–9]. While feeding behavior – especially in human – can be difficult to assess, food intake behavior can be modulated by numerous factors, including but not restricted to nutrient signals – meal size and composition – and also orexigenic and anorexigenic hormones [10]. Among these hormones, ghrelin [11–13], cholecystokinin (CCK) [14], peptide YY [14], glucagon-like peptide-1 (GLP-1) [14] and leptin [15], have been identified as the main endocrine regulators of food intake. Anorexigenic gut peptides (CCK, GLP-1 and peptide YY) are produced in response to the presence of nutrients in the gastro-intestinal tract; their production is sensitive to changes in food composition such as an increase in fat content [16,17]. An increased level of ghrelin triggers feeding behavior and ghrelin production is decreased during the course of a meal [18]. On the other hand, leptin, a hormone secreted by adipose cells in proportion to white adipose tissue accretion, is known to trigger satiety [19].

All these hormones control the energy input. Yet, adaptation of the basal energy expenditure is another mechanism regulating food intake. It aims at reducing the difference between energy intake and the energy needed by the organism [20]. The latter can be modified by changes in activity and/or by adaptive thermogenesis (particularly in brown adipose tissue) [8,21,22]. In cases of overfeeding, thermogenesis is increased and ATP is wasted by completing futile cycles [23], while when underfeeding, energy expenditure is reduced to vital mechanisms [24]. This adaptation can prevent weight loss despite a reduced energy intake [22]. However it is not instantaneous and can be sustained, leading to important weight gains in individuals previously submitted to a strict diet. This is observed in humans and explains why body weight does not decrease linearly in time despite a constant reduction in caloric intake [25].

In normal conditions, these mechanisms should control weight variations. However some perturbations can destabilize this control. Our objective is to investigate mathematically whether variations in food availability could be the origin of such a destabilization.

Numerous mathematical or computational models describing metabolism regulation and body characteristics evolution exist in the literature. These models focus on different modelling scales, from cell to organism and from seconds to years [26]. Some models have been applied to animal subjects. Tam et al. [27] focused on physiological effects of leptin on energy homeostasis and food intake in mice. Guo and Hall [28,29] predicted dynamics of body weight and composition with respect to energy use in mice. Van Leeuwen et al. [30] studied the effect of food restriction on survival and body growth in mice. Other models have been applied to humans and were focused on energy use [31,32] or relationships between fat mass and fat-free mass [33,34]. These models were used to describe either normal conditions, overfeeding or starvation [35,36].

From the modelling point of view, feeding behavior and hunger have been relatively ignored. Although some results on the feeding dynamics correlate with body mass index [37], no other modelling work has ever studied the impact of food availability dynamics on the feeding behavior and body weight regulation.

In this paper, we propose a mathematical model of body weight dynamics (divided in fat mass and fat-free mass), taking into account hunger, defined throughout this manuscript as the amount of food needed by the organism, leptin, ghrelin and glucose variations. Food intake is assumed to be regulated by the available amount of food and by hunger. As we focus on the influence of available and consumed food, we have chosen to consider only leptin (as an indicator of fat storage), ghrelin (representative of the volume of food intake) and glucose (proportional to the energy content of the diet) amongst all the factors influencing food intake. Unlike other published models, this system includes a memory of past food intake to model the adaptation of energy expenditure to caloric restrictions.

To challenge the model and find relevant parameter values, we conducted a simple feeding experiment on rats. One group received *Ad libitum* food. The time course of the available food for the three other groups was modified with three different frequencies, while maintaining an isocaloric diet during the entire experiment. We show that low frequency perturbations are very likely to induce weight gains and that our model is able to predict this feature.

Materials and Methods

Experimental Procedures

Animal care. Animal experiments were performed under the authorization n°69-266-0501 (INSA-Lyon, DDPP-DSV, Direction Départementale de la Protection des Populations - Services Vétérinaires du Rhône), according to the guidelines laid down by the French Ministère de l'Agriculture (n° 87–848) and the E.U. Council Directive for the Care and Use of Laboratory Animals of November 24th, 1986 (86/609/EEC). COS (n° 69266257) holds a special license to experiment on living vertebrates issued by the French Ministry of Agriculture and Veterinary Service Department.

Thirty twelve-week-old Wistar rats were purchased from Janvier SA (Le Genest-Saint-Isle, France) and housed in an air-conditioned room at 24 ± 1°C with a LD (light/dark) 12:12 cycle (light on at 6:30 am) with free access to food (2016C, 12.6 kJ/g, 66% carbohydrates, 12% fat, 22% proteins, Harlan, Gannat, France) and water.

Rats were randomly separated into 5 groups (D0, AL, H0, H1 and H4) of 6 individuals (no significant difference of initial body weight was found between these groups: *p-value* = 0.26). Each rat was identified and housed individually throughout the protocol.

The group D0 was sacrificed on the first day of the experiment (as described below), so the initial biometric data of the rats are available, including body weight, body length, white adipose tissue mass, brown adipose tissue mass, muscles and organs weights (see Table 1). At the end of the experiment (i.e. 8 weeks) the other rats were sacrificed to obtain the same data. Blood samples were collected at the same time for further analyses. The total body lipid content can easily and accurately be predicted from the gravimetric determination of the retroperitoneal fat deposits [38]. Thus the retroperitoneal fat pads weights (rWAT) were used to estimate the total body lipid content (L in grams), using the formula $L = 7.96\text{rWAT} + 3.13$ [38].

Rats from groups AL, H0, H1 and H4 were individually housed and received chow diet for 8 weeks in different quantities each day (see Fig. 1). The control group AL received *Ad libitum* food (approximately 25 g per rat per day). *Ad libitum* food also corresponds to the diet before the beginning of the experiment in each group. The other groups (H0, H1, H4) were submitted to a restriction in caloric availability corresponding to 80% of *Ad libitum* diet. This reduction should theoretically avoid leftovers, as this amount is below normal consumption, in order to have a better control on food intake.

The pattern of food distribution was not the same for these three groups. Group H0 received the same amount of food every day for 8 weeks. For the H1 group the food was randomly allocated for each week of the experiment. Group H4 was submitted to an important restriction for 4 weeks followed by an excess of food for the remaining 4 weeks. The amount of food given each day is reported in Fig. 1. The remaining food was measured and removed each day to determine the food really consumed (see Fig. 2 B). Great care was taken to ensure that most of the food was either eaten or removed and not wasted. In a preliminary experiment, we determined that food spillage only accounts for $6.9 \pm 1{,}0$% of the total food intake. Therefore it was considered to be negligible.

During the experiment, the beginning of the week (the day the food availability was changed) was set on Tuesday and rats were weighted every Friday morning. This protocol tends to minimize and to separate the effects of stress due to changes in food availability and stress due to weighting.

Sacrifice, blood and tissue collection. Animals were deeply anesthetized with sodium pentobarbital (60 mg/kg ip), blood ($\sim$5 mL) was collected through puncture of vena cava on heparinized syringe and centrifuged 2 min at 8000 g. Plasma samples were snap frozen in liquid nitrogen and stored at -80°C until analysis. Liver, heart, kidneys, gastrocnemius muscles, epididymal, retroperitoneal and subcutaneous inguinal white adipose tissue (WAT) were dissected out according to anatomical landmarks, weighed to the nearest milligram, snap frozen in liquid nitrogen and stored at -80°C. Total WAT mass was calculated as the sum of the mass of epididymal, retroperitoneal and subcutaneous inguinal WAT deposits.

Individual data is freely available upon request.

Biochemical analysis. Plasma ghrelin and leptin assays were performed using immunoassays (acylated rat/mouse ghrelin #A05117 and rat/mouse leptin EIA #A05176, Cayman, SpiBio, Montigny le Bretonneux, France) according to the manufacturer's recommendations. The detection limit and intra-assay coefficient of variation for ghrelin were 0.2 pg.mL^{-1} and 11%, respectively. The detection limit and intra-assay coefficient of variation for leptin were 50 pg.mL^{-1} and 4%, respectively. Blood glucose was measured using an automatic glucose monitor (Optium Xceed, Abbott, Rungis, France). All assays were performed at least in duplicate (see Table 2).

Individual data is freely available upon request.

Mathematical Model

In this section, the mathematical model is described (See Table 3 for a description of all variables and Fig. 3 for a schematic representation of the system). This model focuses on fat mass and fat-free mass evolutions regulated by hunger and available food. Hunger is defined as the amount of food the system would consume were there no constraint on food availability. There exist multiple factors influencing food intake [7–10,14,39], yet we focus on 3 of them: leptin, ghrelin and glucose (which is highly correlated with insulin) as they regulate hunger at different time scales [8].

Table 1. Biometric data.

	D0	AL	H0	H1	H4
Body weight (g)	333.8±15.9	493±46.7	410.5±24.1	404.8±40.5	444.5±16.4
Body length (cm)	22.9±0.53	26.4±0.51	25.4±0.66	25.1±0.75	26±0.67
rWAT (g)	4.24±1.49	9.77±2.30	8.82±3.80	7.63±1.56	9.58±2.61
Total WAT (g)	17±4.6	33.3±9.4	29.2±9.7	28.2±4.7	32.9±5.4
iBAT (mg)	287±39	425±199	365±71	367±64	390±153
Kidneys (g)	2.37±0.59	3.11±0.22	2.56±0.04	2.69±0.35	2.70±0.34
Heart (g)	0.96±0.09	1.40±0.13	1.16±0.05	1.24±0.12	1.19±1.13
Soleus (g)	235±48	248±37	172±33	203±24	183±45
EDL (g)	110±37	165±44	193±18	188±12	192±51

Each column gives biometric data for the 5 groups: for all groups except D0 (group sacrificed on the first day of the experiment), data have been obtained at the end of the experiments.
WAT = White Adipose Tissue, rWAT = retroperitoneal White Adipose Tissue, iBAT = interscapular Brown Adipose Tissue, EDL = Extensor digitorum longus.

Fat mass (S, in grams) and fat-free mass (W, in grams) are assumed to be produced depending on the instantaneous difference (Δ_E) between energy intake and energy expenditure. To model this phenomenon we adapted the equations in [28,29] previously developed for a mouse model and we used the same notations: ρ_S and ρ_W denote the energy densities for fat mass and fat-free mass respectively (kJ.g^{-1}) and Δ_E the instantaneous difference of energy (kJ.min^{-1}). Evolutions of S and W are given by:

$$\frac{dS}{dt} = \frac{\Delta_E}{\rho_W x + \rho_S}, \qquad (1)$$

$$\frac{dW}{dt} = \frac{\Delta_E x}{\rho_W x + \rho_S}, \qquad (2)$$

where $x \equiv dW/dS = \zeta + \psi.\exp(\kappa.S)$ [28,29].

Energy intake (EI) is supposed to be a function of the caloric content of the diet. This food consumption per minute, denoted by $c(a,h)$ (kJ.min^{-1}), is assumed to be a function of hunger h (kJ) and available food a (kJ). We assume $c(a,h)$ is equal to the minimum of a and h per unit of time. Hunger was defined as the amount of food needed by the system (see above). Hence, food consumption is either equal to hunger, when enough food is available or to the available food a.

Several formulae describe energy expenditure [34,40], using linear dependencies on body weight, fat mass and fat-free mass. In the current model, the energy expenditure (EE) is assumed to be a function of the caloric content of the body (expressed as a function of fat mass and fat-free mass) with a rate of energy expenditure R. The result is the amount of Joules lost per minute. We then define the energy balance Δ_E as:

$$\Delta_E = EI - EE = c(a,h) - R(\rho_W W + \rho_S S + \xi),$$

where $EI = c(a,h)$ and $EE = R(\rho_W W + \rho_S S + \xi)$.

One can note that fat-free mass has a negative feedback on itself and that fat-mass may have either a positive or negative feedback on itself, depending on the value of Δ_E. Fat mass can have a positive feedback on fat-free mass, via x (see equation (2)), since creation of fat mass leads to the creation of lean mass [33].

The evolution of the amount of available food a (in kJ) depends on the input of food in the system f (usually a given amount each day) and the consumption c. The available food a satisfies

$$\frac{da}{dt} = f(t) - c(a,h). \qquad (3)$$

In order to describe variations in appetite, the model should take into account the evolution of factors influencing hunger. As previously mentioned, we focus on leptin, glucose and ghrelin concentration. The total plasma leptin l (in ng) is assumed to be produced proportionally to the fat mass [27],

$$\frac{dl}{dt} = \gamma_2 S - \gamma_1 l. \qquad (4)$$

Group	Week 1	Week 2	Week 3	Week 4	Week 5	Week 6	Week 7	Week 8
AL	*Ad libitum*							
H0	20 g	20 g	20 g	20 g	20 g	20 g	20 g	20 g
H1	15 g	25 g	10 g	10 g	30 g	35 g	5 g	30 g
H4	10 g	10 g	10 g	10 g	30 g	30 g	30 g	30 g

Figure 1. Daily available food per rat in each group. Changes of quantities occur each week, except for group AL which was not submitted to caloric restriction. At the end of the 8-weeks experiment, each rat in groups H0, H1 and H4 will have received 1120 g of food. Consumed food is not always equal to this amount but is recorded every day.

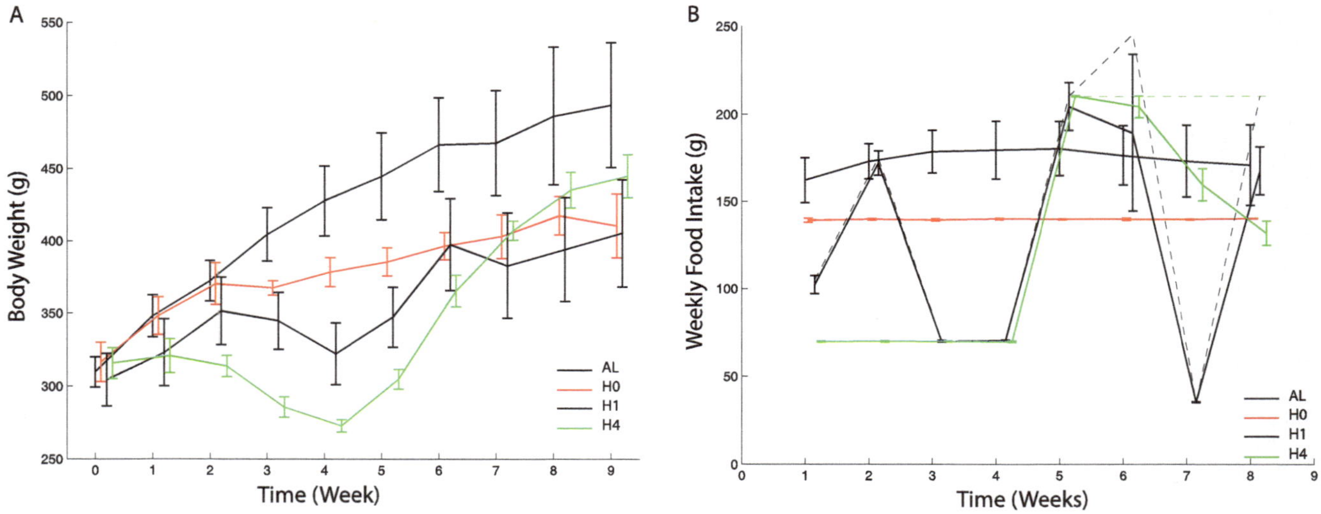

Figure 2. Body weight and food intake evolution. A) Temporal evolution of body weights (in grams) for each group (mean $\pm$ sd): AL (black), H0 (red), H1(blue) and H4 (green). A small offset has been added to the time points to ease the reading. **B)** Evolution of consumed food (straight lines, mean $\pm$ sd) weekly by each rat (in each group: AL (black), H0 (red), H1(blue) and H4 (green)) compared to the available food (dashed lines). Group H0 consumed all its available food for the duration of the experiment while groups H1 and H4 had leftovers.

Total glucose u (g) and ghrelin concentration e (pg.mL^{-1}) in plasma depend on the diet composition [18]. The glucose level increases with food intake as follows:

$$\frac{du}{dt} = \mu_1 c(a,h) - \mu_2 u. \tag{5}$$

Ghrelin production is inhibited in the presence of food in the stomach [41],

$$\frac{de}{dt} = \frac{v_2}{1 + v_1 c(a,h)} - v_3 e. \tag{6}$$

The hunger h is regulated in the central nervous system, integrating signals from the rest of the body via circulating hormones [7,8]. Regulation of hunger is a complex system. The amount of circulating leptin as an indicator of body adiposity leads to a decrease in hunger [8], so we assume hunger decreases when leptin increases. The ghrelin concentration decreases when the stomach is full and the hunger follows the same variations [12] so we assume hunger increases when ghrelin increases. The effect of leptin and ghrelin is opposite, though they both have an action in the arcuate nucleus [18]. The hunger h is also supposed to be a decreasing function of glucose level u [42]. The hunger h was defined as the amount of Joules required by the system at any time, so the evolution of h is given by:

$$\frac{dh}{dt} = \frac{\alpha_1 e}{1 + \alpha_2 l} - \beta(\alpha_3 + u)h. \tag{7}$$

System (1)–(7) takes regulations at short and long time scales into account. Variables directly linked to daily food intake such as ghrelin concentration and glucose level have an influence on a daily basis whereas leptin has an influence on a longer time scale.

Adaptation of Energy Expenditure

The previously described model is well adapted when food is available *Ad libitum*. As the food consumed is always equal to hunger, the organism does not need to change relatively to environmental conditions and its rate of energy expenditure R is therefore constant. In the case of caloric restrictions, energy expenditure is lowered to maintain the energy balance [43]. To take this phenomenon into account, we assume that the rate of energy expenditure R depends on the food consumed, with a memory effect.

The rate of energy expenditure R is known to adapt to the past food intake $c(a,h)$ [24]. As the food is supposed to be available on

Table 2. Plasma hormones and glucose assays.

	D0	AL	H0	H1	H4
Ghrelin (pg.mL^{-1})	nd	43.30 $\pm$ 17.75	25.66 $\pm$ 14.65	78.48 $\pm$ 97.96	18.01 $\pm$ 9.88
Leptin (ng.mL^{-1})	4.34$\pm$1.78	7.53$\pm$2.72	3.60$\pm$1.66	5.19$\pm$1.66	7.07$\pm$3.66
Glucose (mg.dL^{-1})	140.7$\pm$11.6	148.7$\pm$24.1	132.2$\pm$8.9	121.4$\pm$14.8	144.3$\pm$21.2

Ghrelin, leptin and glucose concentrations in plasma in the control group and at the end of the experiment for groups AL, H0, H1 and H4 (mean $\pm$ sd, nd: not determined).

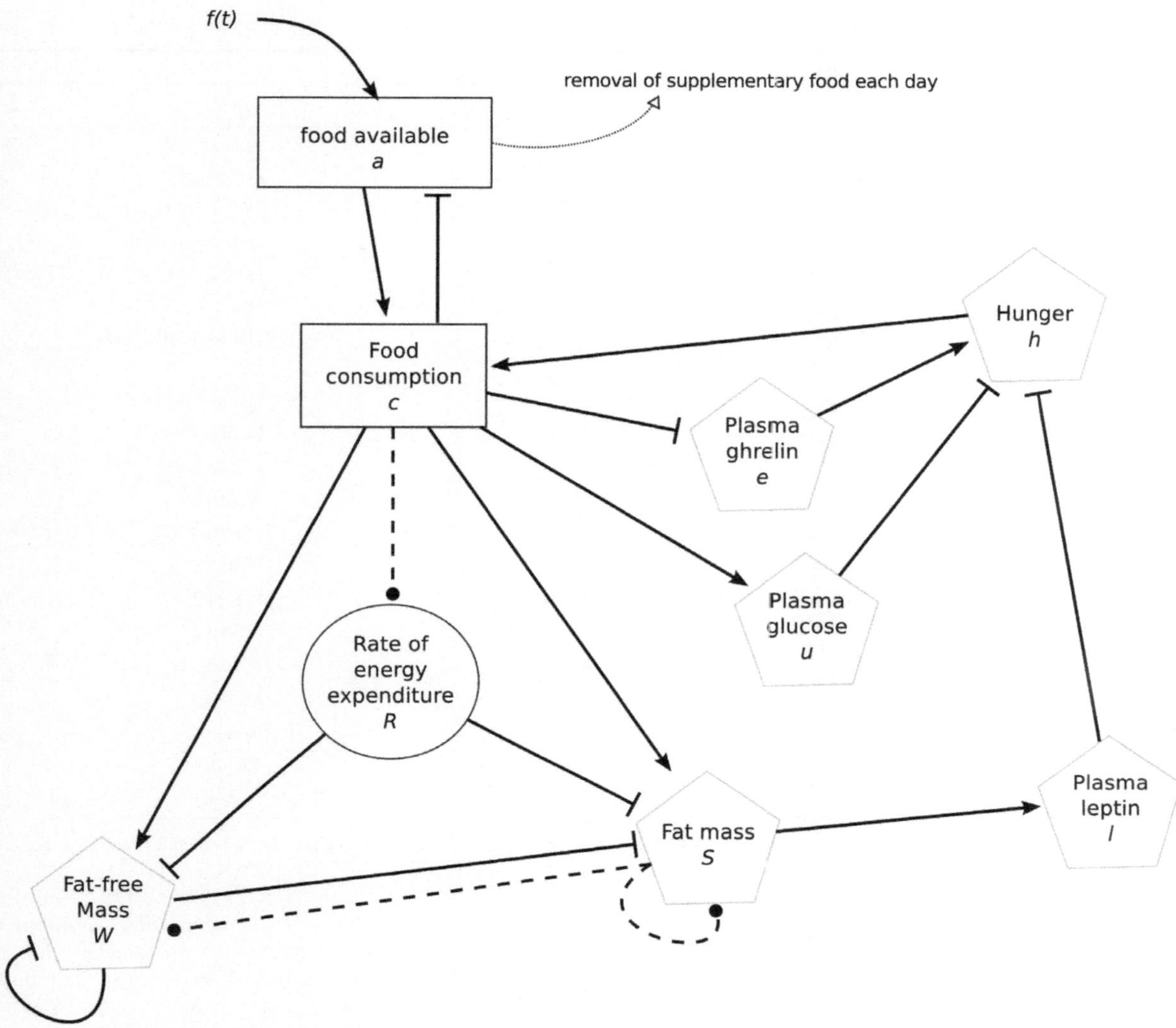

Figure 3. Schematic representation of the model. Positive influences are represented by straight lines with arrows and negative influences by bar-headed lines. Relations whose effect can vary in time are represented by dashed lines with a dot at the end.

a daily basis, the mean food intake in the last τ days is compared to the mean food intake in the last τ' days (with $\tau' > \tau$) to define the value of R. The "reference" food (food consumed between times $t-\tau'$ and t) is slowly modified accordingly, so R is constant if the food intake doesn't change for at least τ' days. When food intake varies on short periods of time, the rate of energy expenditure R is progressively modified to reduce the difference between these mean food intakes, with a rate of adaptation equal to ϵ, as follows:

$$\frac{dR}{dt} = \epsilon\left(\frac{1}{\tau}\int_{t-\tau}^{t} c(a(v),h(v))dv - \frac{1}{\tau'}\int_{t-\tau'}^{t} c(a(v),h(v))dv\right). \quad (8)$$

This equation needs an initial condition R_0 which corresponds to the value of the rate of energy expenditure with a constant food intake equal to hunger (*Ad libitum* case).

Other factors influence energy expenditure [20,39] such as plasma leptin, environment and aging [43,44]. Nevertheless this model focuses only on the effect of caloric variations as it is the easiest parameter to measure and manipulate experimentally.

Parameter Estimation

System (1)–(3) use 21 parameters whose values are essential to the relevance of the simulation results. Amongst these, the 4

Table 3. Model variables.

Name	Symbol	Unit
food available	a	kJ
hunger	h	kJ
plasma ghrelin	e	pg.mL^{-1}
plasma glucose	u	g
plasma leptin	l	ng
fat mass	S	g
fat-free mass	W	g
rate of energy expenditure	R	min^{-1}

Variables of the model with associated units and symbols.

Table 4. Model parameters.

Parameter	Value	Unit	
ν_1	1.52	min.kJ^{-1}	experiments
ν_2	0.4025	pg.mL^{-1}.min^{-1}	experiments
ν_3	0.007	min^{-1}	[46]
μ_1	0.039	g.kJ^{-1}	diet composition
μ_2	0.007	min^{-1}	[47]
γ_1	0.074	min^{-1}	[48]
γ_2	0.126	ng.g^{-1}.min^{-1}	[48] and experiments
ρ_W	7.5	kJ.g^{-1}	[29]
ρ_S	39.3	kJ.g^{-1}	[29]
ξ	1964.4	kJ	fit step 1
ζ	2.2	–	fit step 1
ψ	1.6×10^{-9}	–	fit step 1
κ	0.269	g^{-1}	fit step 1
R_0	2.525×10^{-5}	min^{-1}	fit step 1
α_1	4.02×10^{-8}	mL.kJ.min^{-1}.pg^{-1}	fit step 2
α_2	1.66×10^{-4}	ng^{-1}	fit step 2
α_3	5.03×10^{-4}	g	fit step 2
β	5.99×10^{-6}	min^{-1}.g^{-1}	fit step 2
ϵ	9.05×10^{-9}	kJ^{-1}	fit step 3
τ	1	day	fit step 3
τ'	8	day	fit step 3

Values of the parameters used in the model and associated units. When the parameter is taken from the literature, the corresponding reference is indicated.

parameters of hormone production and degradation are taken from the literature (see Table 4 for a summary of units and origins of parameters of the model). Food-relative parameters depend on the composition of the chow diet.

To estimate the 12 remaining parameters, we used the final fat mass and the evolution of body weight of each individual rat from groups AL and H1. Parameter values were obtained by minimizing the residual sum of squares (RSS) of observed data compared to simulation results using the Nelder-Mead algorithm [45]. We then used these parameter values to test the predictive capacity of our model against data from groups H0 and H4.

In the AL case, *Ad libitum* food implies that food intake c is always equal to h and the rate of energy expenditure R is constant. Consequently, energy expenditure only depends on fat mass S and fat-free mass W. We have access to the experimentally consumed food, so we use this value to explicitly determine the evolution of h. Hence equations (1) and (2) are decoupled from the other equations and we consider them as an independent subsystem.

In a first step, applying the minimization algorithm to this subsystem leads to an estimation of the 4 parameter values relative to equations (1) and (2). Then, in a second step, we estimate the remaining parameter values using equations (1), (2), (4), (5), (6) and (7) and the previously determined parameters. To estimate the parameters relative to h in equation (7) we once again use data from group AL. However, this time, c was determined by the values of a corresponding to *Ad libitum* food and h is given by (7). As R is supposed to be constant over group AL, the system used here was composed by all equations except (8). Finally, those parameters relative to the rate of energy expenditure R, were estimated in a third step, using experimental data from hypocaloric group H1. We then used the whole system of equations and parameter values previously estimated for AL.

Parameter estimation is detailed as follows:

Step 1. Only equations (1) and (2) are used. The input of the system is the experimentally determined consumed food c for group AL. We assume R is equal to R_0 when Ad libitum food is

Table 5. Approximate bayesian computation of parameters.

	ϵ (kJ^{-1})	τ (day)	τ' (day)
mean	1.01×10^{-8}	1.3	8.4
standard deviation	0.74×10^{-8}	0.9	6.1

Mean and standard deviation of selected runs of the ABC ($RSS < 1.3\ RSS_{opti}$) for parameters relative to the memory of the system (ϵ, τ and τ'). Mean values are close to parameter values estimated with the optimisation process but with an important standard deviation around these values.

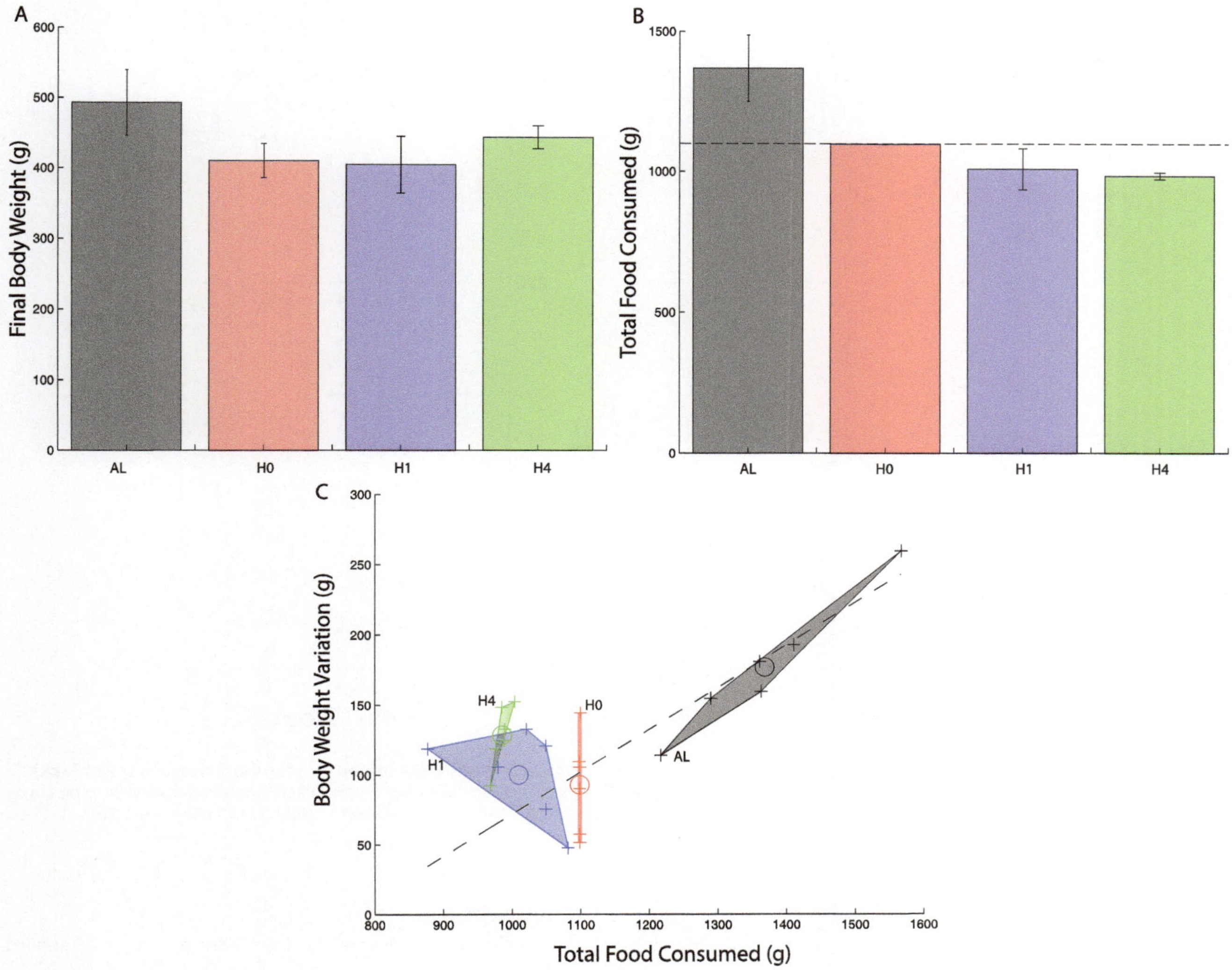

Figure 4. Final experimental body weight and food intake. A) Final body weights at the end of the experiment for all groups. All hypocaloric groups (H0, H1, H4) are significantly different from group AL. Within hypocaloric groups, H4 is significantly different from H0. **B)** Total amount of food consumed in grams at the end of experiment (8 Weeks) for all groups (mean $\pm$ standard deviation). All hypocaloric groups (H0, H1, H4) consumed significantly less food than group AL. Within hypocaloric groups, H4 is significantly different from H0 and H1. Dashed line is the amount of the total food that was available for the hypocaloric group. **C)** Variation of body weight from the start to the end of the experiment versus the total amount of food consumed. Crosses indicate individual points, open circles are the averages and the whole group is described by its convex hull. The dashed line is the linear regression for the group AL ($p=0.005$ and $R^2=0.88$). The slope is 0.3, indicating that the weight gain is equal to 30% of the weight of the consumed food.

available. As we have a value for c, it is not necessary to describe the variations of hunger and hormones so the only dynamical variables of the subsystem are S and W. The RSS between outputs of the model (predicted body weight and fat mass) and experimental data (body weight and fat mass) is minimized for each individual rat from group AL. This leads to an estimation of the parameters ξ, κ, ψ, ζ and the basal rate of energy expenditure $R=R_0$.

Step 2. Equations (1), (2), (4), (5), (6) and (7) are used with experimental data from group AL. Parameter values determined at step 1 are used at this step. The rate of energy expenditure R is still supposed to be constant as the food is Ad libitum, with $R=R_0$ determined in the previous step. In this step, $c(a,h)$ is supposed to be equal to h as a is always higher than h (to take unlimited food into account). This leads to an estimation of the parameter values relative to the hunger h: α_1, α_2, α_3 and β.

Step 3. For the last step, the whole system is used. Both the pattern of food availability and experimental data from group H1 are used, with five initial days of Ad libitum food to be consistent with the experiment. Parameters determined at steps 1 and 2 are used. As the H1 rats are supposed to adapt to the reduced and varying amount of food available, this allows to estimate the parameters associated with energy expenditure variations: ϵ, τ and τ' in equation (8). Initial condition for R is chosen to be equal to R_0 determined at step 1 as initial food is Ad libitum.

Akaike Information Criteria (AIC) was computed to compare the ability of the current model and of a model without memory (using equations (1)-(7) and R constant as for the AL case) to

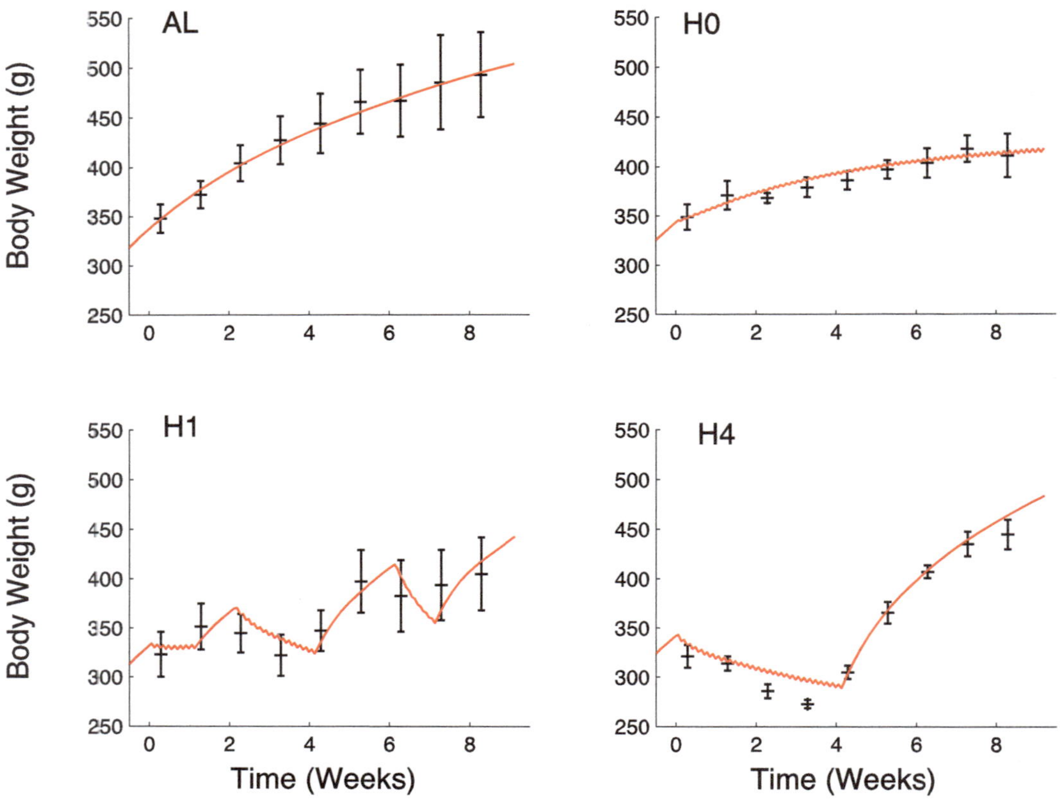

Figure 5. Simulated evolution of body weight (red line) compared to experimental data (mean ± standard deviation in black). In each group, the food input matches the experimental patterns and the first 5 days of the simulation were conducted with *Ad libitum* diet to be closer to the experiment. Parameter values were estimated with data from groups AL and H1 and predictions were made with these parameter values on groups H0 and H4. Top left: AL; top right: H0; bottom left: H1; bottom right: H4.

reproduce the data. $AIC = n \ln(RSS/n) + 2k$ with n the number of points used to evaluate the results, RSS the residual sum of squares and k the number of estimated parameters.

Approximate bayesian computation (ABC) was used to calculate a distribution of the computed parameter values, starting with uniform sampling around optimized parameters. Runs with a residual sum of squares smaller than a certain level RSS_{opti} (defined using the result of the optimization process) were selected; here the threshold was equal to 1.3 RSS_{opti} (see Table 5 for means and standard deviations of these distributions).

Predictions

Following the estimation procedure (see previous paragraphs), the model was tested with the patterns of food input corresponding to the two other groups of rats (H0 and H4) to evaluate its predictive capacity. Parameter values determined for groups AL and H1 were used. As all the rats were supposed to be similar (same origin and age), we used the same parameter values for each group.

If another group (H0 or H4) was chosen at step 3 of the estimation procedure instead of H1, the set of parameters associated with R was different. However the RSS for each set of parameters were close from one another. Hence, the simulated data will be better for the chosen group than it will for the other groups. The data from each group could be fitted individually to have better results but this would suppress the predictive capacity of the model.

Statistical Analysis

All results are presented in the form: mean ± standard deviation.

Normality of the samples was tested using Shapiro-Wilks test. Statistical comparison was performed using Mann-Whitney test for two groups, and an analysis of variance (ANOVA) for more than two groups. All analyses were performed using the R software (www.R-project.org).

Results

Food Availability Modifies Body Weight Dynamics

We present in this section the results of the experiments performed on rats – see the "Materials and Methods" section for details. In addition to a control group (called AL for *Ad libitum*, $n = 6$), three groups of 6 rats had their food availability modified during the 8 week long experiment. All rats experienced *Ad Libitum* feeding conditions prior to the experiment. Fig. 1 describes the available food time course for groups H0, H1 and H4 characterised by periods of variations of 0, 1 and 4 weeks respectively. In order to ensure a controlled total food intake, these groups were hypocaloric (around 80% of AL's average intake). Group H0 was daily fed with a constant amount of food with no variations. Group H1 was daily fed with random and uncorrelated amounts of food around the average. The feeding pattern of group H4 basically corresponds to a fasting experiment for 4 weeks (less than 60% of the AL's average intake) followed by a refeeding in the following month. In the three hypocaloric groups, the total

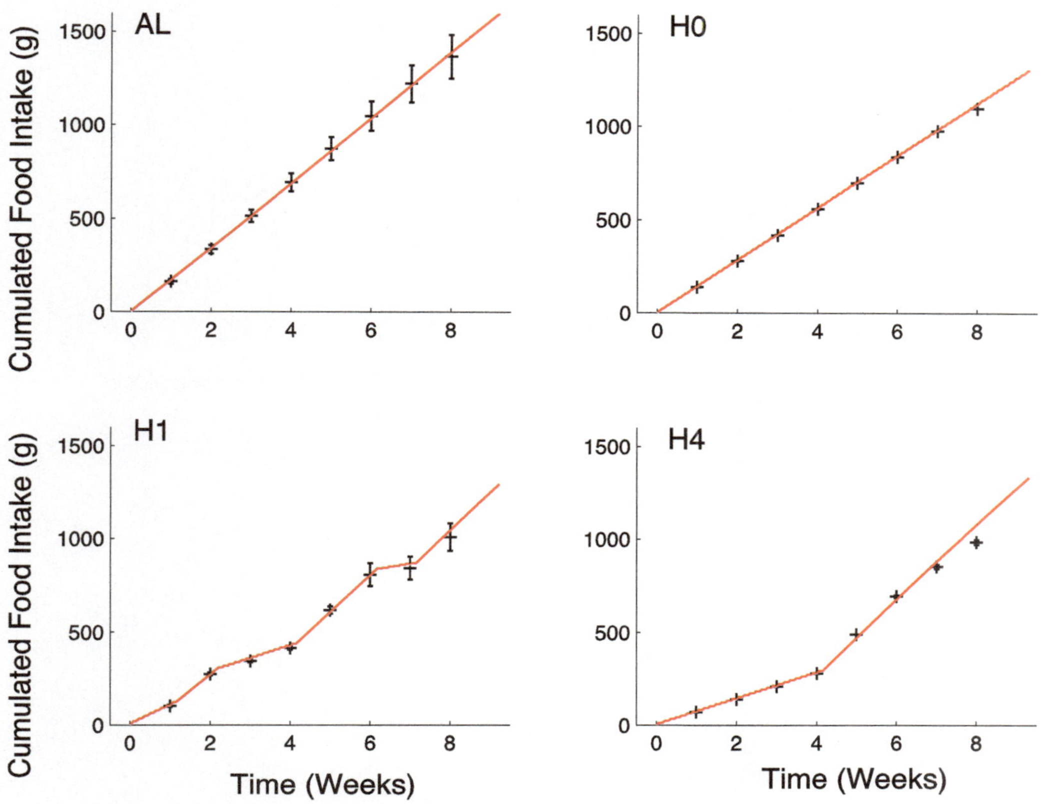

Figure 6. Evolution of cumulated food intake predicted by the model (red curve) compared to experimental data (black crosses: mean ± sd). Available food in the simulation corresponds to experimental patterns in each group, with *Ad libitum* diet in each group at the beginning. Results from groups AL and H1 correspond to the parameter estimation process while results for groups H0 and H4 correspond to predictions. Top left: AL; top right: H0; bottom left: H1; bottom right: H4.

amount of food provided to each rat during the whole experiment was the same (1120 g in 8 weeks corresponding to 14.07 MJ – see Fig. 1).

At the end of the experiment, individuals were sacrificed and fat mass, muscles masses and some organ masses were collected and weighted. Table 1 displays the values along with an initial control group sacrificed on the first day of the experiment (called D0 for "day 0"). As expected, body weight is smaller for the groups with reduced food (H0, H1 and H4) compared to group AL ($p=0.00086$) and different between the 4 groups ($p=0.0008$ for the ANOVA). There is no significant evidence that distributions of body weights in each group are not normal ($p-values$ between 0.21 and 0.97).

As shown on Fig. 4 A, a difference in final body weight exists within hypocaloric groups H0, H1 and H4, the corresponding $p-value$ is slightly above the 5% threshold ($p-value=0.0636$). Pairwise comparison yields significant differences between H0 and H4 ($p-value=0.02056$) whereas total food consumption (see Fig. 4 B) is significantly different between the two groups ($p-value=0.005$), in the *opposite direction*. Rats in group H4 have a higher body weight although they ate less food than rats from group H0. No such differences are observed for group H1.

These results suggest that an energy expenditure adaptation occurs according to the amount of food consumed. This is summarized on Fig. 4 C which shows the variations of body weight during the experiment as a function of the total amount of food consumed. All data points are plotted and the convex hull has been coloured according to each group. Data for group AL closely follows a linear pattern with slope 0.3 which indicates that each gram of food consumed turns into 0.3 grams of body weight. The other groups do not follow the same pattern. Strikingly group H4 is well above the line indicating that its individuals ate less food but

Table 6. Akaike Information Criteria.

	H0	H4	H1
AIC with memory	375	368	445
AIC without memory	382	413	448

AIC (Akaike Information Criteria) for groups H0, H4 and H1 to compare results of the model with and without memory. $AIC=n\ln(RSS/n)+2k$ with n the number of points used to evaluate the results, RSS the residual sum of square and k the number of parameters estimated. AIC is smaller in the model with memory, even if there are more parameters: this model is more adapted to explain these data.

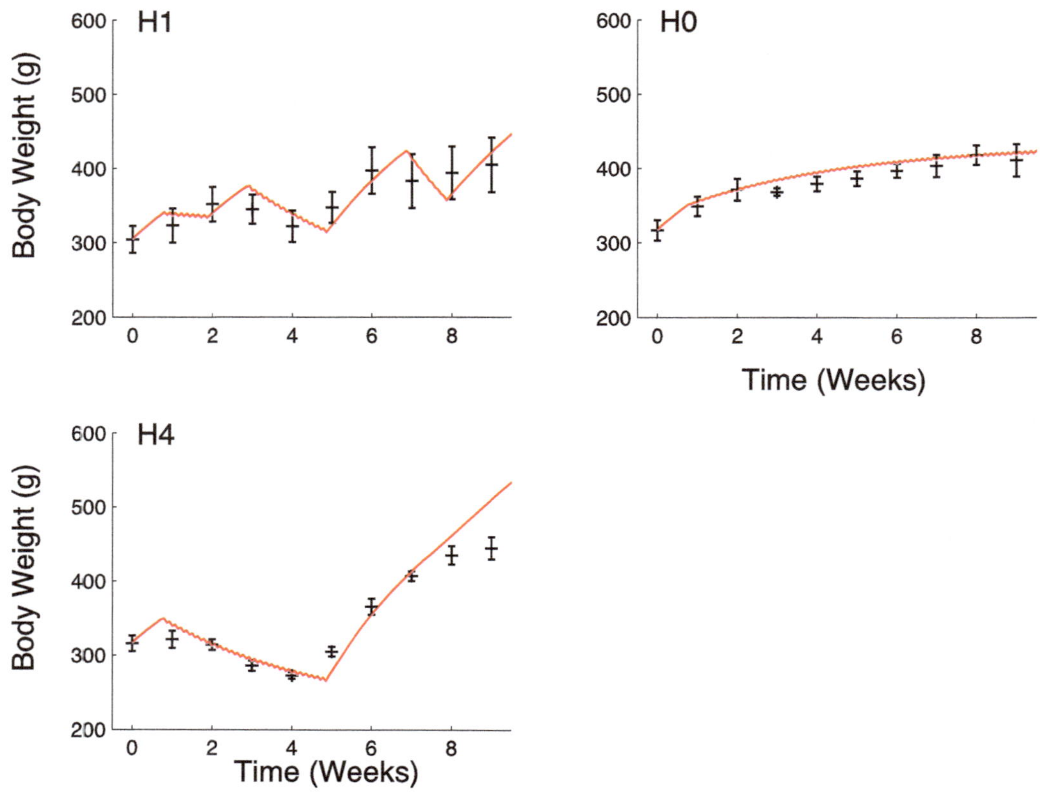

Figure 7. Predicted body weight with a constant rate of energy expenditure *R* compared to experimental results. Simulation for group H1 corresponds to the parameter estimation without memory (estimation of R_0 and other parameter values obtained for group AL). Predicted body weight in this case does not match experimental results. In particular, body weight is slightly overestimated for group H0 while in cases H1 and H4, the amplitude of variations is too important due to the absence of adaptation to food intake.

that a bigger fraction of it turned into body weight. The H1 pattern is somewhat similar but less significantly.

Body weight evolution is displayed on Fig. 2 A and is consistent with the food intake in Fig. 2 B albeit with a delay, as the increase or decrease is associated with the food intake in the previous week. As observed in previous studies, when presented with various amounts of food, rats adapt their eating pattern depending on past eating behavior. Our main experimental result is that rats adapt their energy expenditure by taking efficiently advantage of the available food when in fasting conditions and using more energy when overfed. This behavior results in different body weights for the same caloric intakes.

Mathematical Model of Food Intake and Body Weight Evolution

We show in this section the predictive power of our model of feeding behavior and food intake dynamics. The model and the equations are presented in details in the "Materials and Methods" section.

Our model describes the evolution of hunger, leptin, ghrelin, plasma glucose which is correlated with insulin, energy expenditure and body weight, composed of fat and lean mass (see Table 3 for a list of the variables and their units). This model allows to describe hunger, defined as the amount of food needed by the organism, by computing the dynamics of food intake in the short term. Energy expenditure is described as a function of the rate of energy expenditure, fat-mass and fat-free mass. It includes a delay equation describing the variations of the rate of energy expenditure *R*. The evolution of *R* depends on the comparison of short-term food intake with long-term food intake (see equation (8)). Fig. 3 describes the components of the model and Table 4 describes the parameters as well as their units. The fitting procedure used to determine some parameter values is fully described in the "Materials and Methods" section. It uses only AL and H1 as training data sets.

Fig. 5.AL and 5.H1 show the results of the parameter estimation on groups AL and H1, illustrated on body weight evolution. Simulations are accurate for both groups, as expected from the parameter estimation process. In addition, the model correctly predicts the results on the validating data sets: good matches are obtained for both H0 (Fig. 5.H0) and H4 (Fig. 5.H4). Variations of predicted body weight for group H4 correlate with modifications of food availability and are close to experimental values. Small daily oscillations are observed in groups H0, H1 and H4, especially when available food is below hunger. These oscillations correspond to a daily pattern of food intake: while food is available, it is consumed, resulting in an increase in body weight, then the consumption is equal to 0 and the body weight decreases. In the case of group H4, the predicted body weight at the end of the period of restriction (week 4) is slightly higher than the actual data. As the amplitude of the restriction is important, the adaptation could be less efficient in reality than it is in the model. There are also other phenomena such as environmental conditions, excluded here for simplicity, that could influence this adaptation.

Food availability is the only input of the model (see "Materials and Methods" section). It is defined according to the experimental

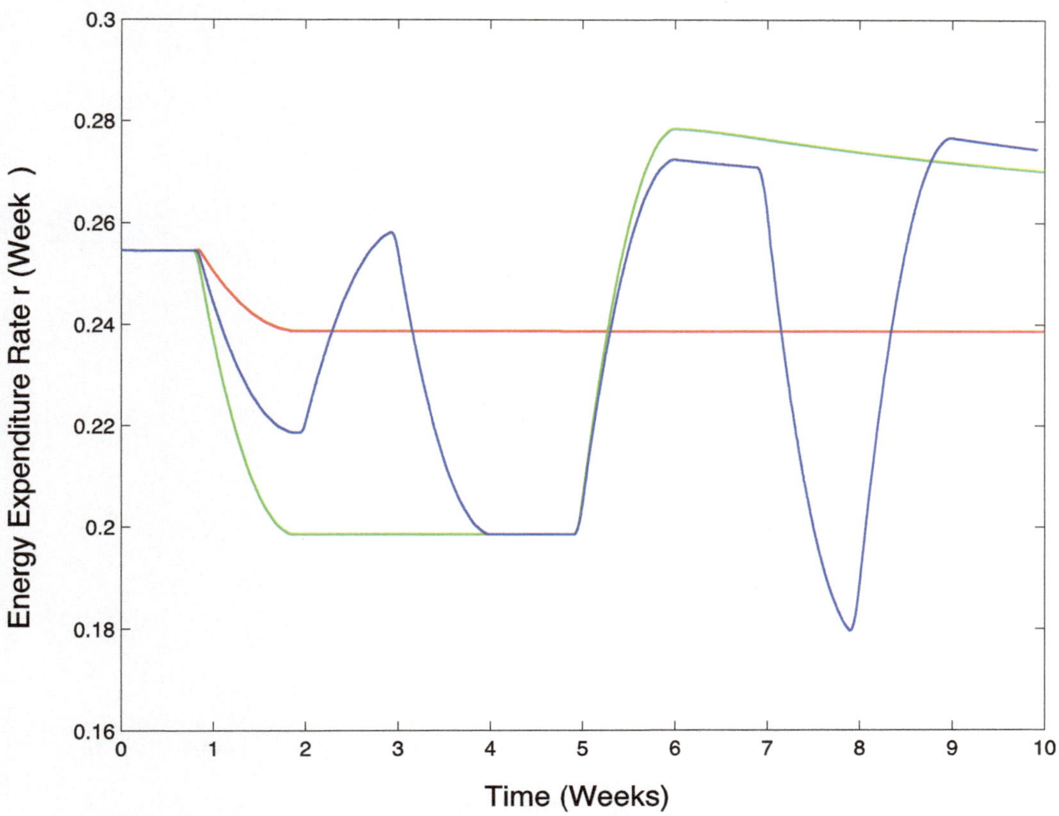

Figure 8. Predicted rate of energy expenditure variations in the cases H0 (red), H1(blue) and H4 (green), starting from the same initial condition. *R* value is stabilizing to a different value after a few days if the food pattern is followed for a long enough time (>8 days). Changes occur when the food availability is modified.

pattern, including the five days of *Ad libitum* diet at the beginning. Our model correctly predicts food intake pattern, as shown on Fig. 6. In particular, for groups H1 and H4, the model predicts leftover food as observed in reality. In all cases, predicted food intake is a close match to the experimental data.

A Metabolic Memory is Necessary to Explain the Observed Data

The hypothesis that adaptation of the rate of energy expenditure is performed with a memory is included in equation (8) – namely the variable R is modified with a memory of the food intake in the past. As explained in the previous section, this model leads to an accurate reproduction of the experimental data. To test the relevance of this memory in the system, simulations were run with a constant value of R equal to the initial value R_0 of the rate of energy expenditure. The value of R_0 was obtained using the estimation procedure described in the section "Materials and Methods" without any memory of the past food intake and data from group H1. The model without memory was then applied to groups H0 and H4.

The values of the residual sum of squares are higher without memory than in the simulations with a non-constant R for groups H0, H1 and H4. Moreover the data are no longer well explained and predicted without memory (see Fig. 7). Akaike Information Criteria allows us to objectively compare these two different models (see Table 6). For each group, AIC is lower with memory than without, indicating that this model better explains our data despite the extra parameters to estimate. One may notice that better results could be obtained for the model without memory, by evaluating R_0 in each group separately, but the model would not be predictive anymore. For group AL, the memory did not impact the score, as expected: the rats are not submitted to caloric restrictions so they don't need to adapt their rate of energy expenditure to avoid weight variations.

Hypothesis to Explain Body Weight Differences

The main result here is derived from the evolution of the rate of energy expenditure. The variations of R are subjected to a delay equation that takes memory of past food intake into account. The model predicts the memory to be around 8 days (see Table 4).

The important weight gain in group H4 during the last 4 weeks is then explained by the lag in the refeeding period when energy expenditure is still low (see Fig. 8) while food intake is at its highest (see Fig. 2 B). Due to the delay in the adaptation of the rate of energy expenditure, the difference between energy intake and energy expenditure is maximal during this period. In the H1 case, also submitted to important caloric variations, the period of 1 week is too short to modify the rate of energy expenditure in the same way as for group H4. The adaptation is then mitigated and the observed weight gain is less important than it is for group H4.

The model was applied for 16 weeks (see Fig. 9), with H0 food pattern following H0, H1 or H4 experiment. With the same amount of food during the last 8 weeks for the three groups, the final predicted body weight tends to the same value regardless of the food pattern in the first 8 weeks. The lower food consumption for groups starting with H1 or H4 patterns does not impact this

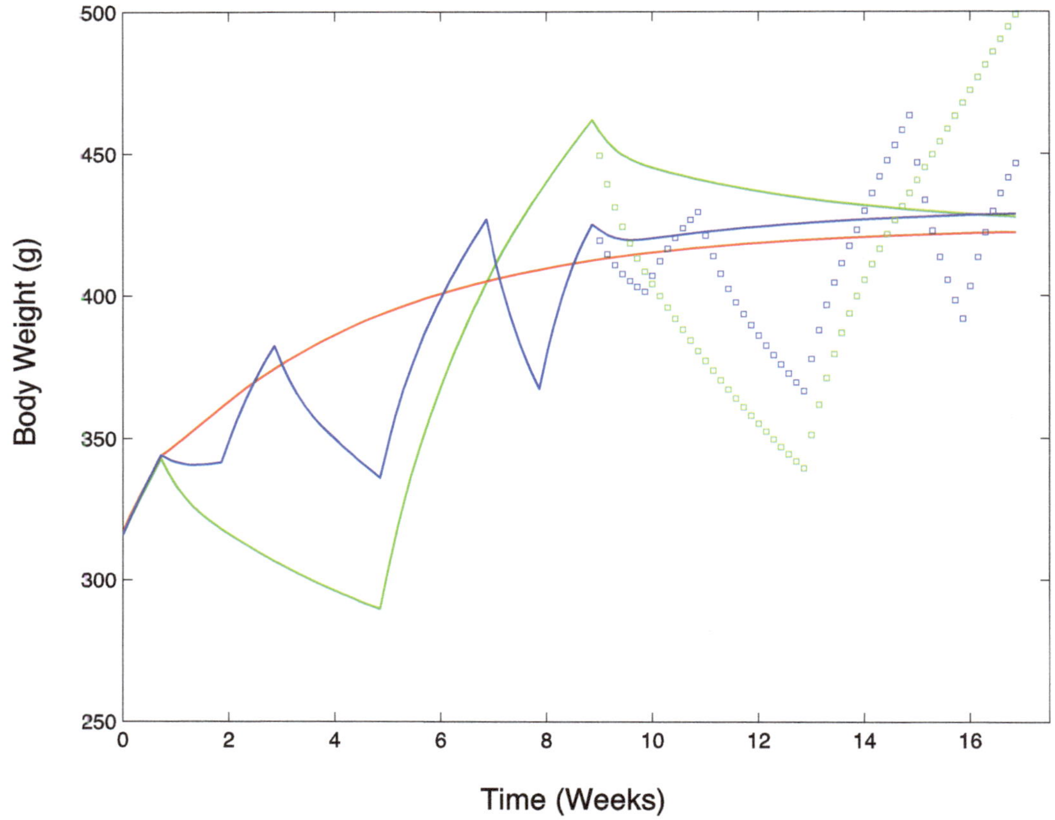

Figure 9. Predicted body weight for a 16 week experiment with different combinations of food availability patterns. In blue H1 followed by H0 (line) or H1 (squares), in green H4 followed by H0 (line) or H4 (squares) and in red twice H0. In cases with H0 in the last 8 weeks (lines), the body weight tends to the same value, whatever the past variations.

evolution. The adaptation to a constant amount of food intake leads to a fixed body weight after some time. Applying twice the same pattern (meaning the H1 diet for 16 weeks or the H4 diet for 16 weeks) leads to increases in body weights and fat mass, which reach elevated values(see Fig. 9). These variations with large amplitudes could have deleterious effects on the biological system, such as development of leptin or insulin resistances.

Discussion

In this work, we showed that food availability fluctuations can trigger body weight variations that cannot be explained by differences in the overall energy intake. In our experiment, rats submitted to the same quantity of food but distributed differently over time exhibited significant weight differences. These differences were strongest when the period of variation was high – one month of low food availability followed by one month of important food availability.

In order to explain these results, we presented a new model of body weight dynamics, describing hunger (defined as the amount of food needed by the organism), hormones and food availability dynamics. This model includes a delay equation describing variations of the rate of energy expenditure, which is adapting according to the memory of food intake. This delay equation was shown to be crucial.

After estimating the parameter values that best fit our experimental data, we showed that our model was able to both explain and predict food intake and body weight dynamics from our experimental results. We also showed that without the memory of food intake, the model cannot correctly reproduce the experimental data, which stresses that this adaptation is essential, in particular when food availability is low. Indeed, our model predicts that a period of caloric restriction leads to an increase in hunger and a decrease in the rate of energy expenditure. Ending these restrictions triggers a higher food consumption and a larger energy storage, with an increased rate of energy expenditure matching the food intake pattern. However this increase takes time to occur and during this delay period, a high amount of food is consumed while the energy expenditure remains low. We estimated a lag of 8 days which explains why quicker variations did not lead to any increase in weight. This provides a simple explanation for weight variations. A similar phenomenon is observed in humans and could explain why people submitted to very strict diets tend to gain more fat when they stop dieting, as their bodies have adapted to the reduced food consumption [25].

Although individual variability may play an important role when describing body weight variations and food intake dynamics, we did not focus on this aspect and rather considered an average behavior. The model proved its efficiency to describe the data. From the experimental results (Fig. 2), one may note that individual variability is globally initially low and increases with the duration of the experiment. Consequently, validation of the model's predictions on the evolution of body weight during a period of time greater than 8 weeks should be supported by additional experiments and could benefit from considering variability.

The model has largely ignored some phenomena such as aging processes which affect the rate of energy expenditure, appetite or sensitivity of the system to stimuli. Indeed feeding behavior can be extremely complex especially regarding food content and palatability. Also, leptin and insulin resistances are not included in this model but are known to have an influence on the regulation of appetite and storage of fat mass following an important weight gain. Including some of these phenomena could result in a better description of the system and help enhancing our understanding of the mechanisms behind these adaptations. Nevertheless, the approach developed in this work, based on innovative mathematics and the use of a simple model, proved to be relevant to describe this physiological system.

Acknowledgments

The authors thank the reviewers for their helpful comments and Dr. David Parsons for his help in writing the manuscript.

Author Contributions

Conceived and designed the experiments: COS HAS. Performed the experiments: COS MJ. Analyzed the data: MJ. Wrote the paper: MJ FC COS HAS.

References

1. Flier JS (2004) Obesity wars: molecular progress confronts an expanding epidemic. Cell 116: 337–350.
2. Kahn SE, Hull RL, Utzschneider KM (2006) Mechanisms linking obesity to insulin resistance and type 2 diabetes. Nature 444: 840–846.
3. Abrams P, Katz LEL (2011) Metabolic effects of obesity causing disease in childhood. Curr Opin Endocrinol Diabetes Obes 18: 23–27.
4. (2000) Obesity: preventing and managing the global epidemic. report of a who consultation. World Health Organ Tech Rep Ser 894: i–xii, 1–253.
5. Barsh GS, Farooqi IS, O'Rahilly S (2000) Genetics of body-weight regulation. Nature 404: 644–651.
6. Friedman JM (2000) Obesity in the new millennium. Nature 404: 632–634.
7. Morton GJ, Cummings DE, Baskin DG, Barsh GS, Schwartz MW (2006) Central nervous system control of food intake and body weight. Nature 443: 289–295.
8. Schwartz MW, Woods SC, Porte D, Seeley RJ, Baskin DG (2000) Central nervous system control of food intake. Nature 404: 661–671.
9. Woods SC, Schwartz MW, Baskin DG, Seeley RJ (2000) Food intake and the regulation of body weight. Annu Rev Psychol 51: 255–277.
10. Crespo CS, Cachero AP, Jimnez LP, Barrios V, Ferreiro EA (2014) Peptides and food intake. Front Endocrinol (Lausanne) 5: 58.
11. Wren AM, Seal LJ, Cohen MA, Brynes AE, Frost GS, et al. (2001) Ghrelin enhances appetite and increases food intake in humans. J Clin Endocrinol Metab 86: 5992.
12. Cummings DE, Shannon MH (2003) Roles for ghrelin in the regulation of appetite and body weight. Arch Surg 138: 389–396.
13. Higgins SC, Gueorguiev M, Korbonits M (2007) Ghrelin, the peripheral hunger hormone. Ann Med 39: 116–136.
14. Duca FA, Covasa M (2012) Current and emerging concepts on the role of peripheral signals in the control of food intake and development of obesity. Br J Nutr 108: 778–793.
15. Stephens TW, Basinski M, Bristow PK, Bue-Valleskey JM, Burgett SG, et al. (1995) The role of neuropeptide y in the antiobesity action of the obese gene product. Nature 377: 530–532.
16. Covasa M (2010) Deficits in gastrointestinal responses controlling food intake and body weight. Am J Physiol Regul Integr Comp Physiol 299: R1423–R1439.
17. Duca FA, Zhong L, Covasa M (2013) Reduced cck signaling in obese-prone rats fed a high fat diet. Horm Behav 64: 812–817.
18. Beck B, Musse N, Stricker-Krongrad A (2002) Ghrelin, macronutrient intake and dietary preferences in long-evans rats. Biochem Biophys Res Commun 292: 1031–1035.
19. Friedman JM, Halaas JL (1998) Leptin and the regulation of body weight in mammals. Nature 395: 763–770.
20. Garrow JS (1987) Energy balance in man–an overview. Am J Clin Nutr 45: 1114–1119.
21. Lowell BB, Spiegelman BM (2000) Towards a molecular understanding of adaptive thermogenesis. Nature 404: 652–660.
22. Tremblay A, Royer MM, Chaput JP, Doucet E (2013) Adaptive thermogenesis can make a difference in the ability of obese individuals to lose body weight. Int J Obes (Lond) 37: 759–764.
23. Wijers SLJ, Saris WHM, van Marken Lichtenbelt WD (2009) Recent advances in adaptive thermogenesis: potential implications for the treatment of obesity. Obes Rev 10: 218–226.
24. Evans SA, Parsons AD, Overton JM (2005) Homeostatic responses to caloric restriction: influence of background metabolic rate. J Appl Physiol (1985) 99: 1336–1342.
25. Hall KD, Sacks G, Chandramohan D, Chow CC, Wang YC, et al. (2011) Quantification of the effect of energy imbalance on bodyweight. Lancet 378: 826–837.
26. de Graaf AA, Freidig AP, Roos BD, Jamshidi N, Heinemann M, et al. (2009) Nutritional systems biology modeling: from molecular mechanisms to physiology. PLoS Comput Biol 5: e1000554.
27. Tam J, Fukumura D, Jain RK (2009) A mathematical model of murine metabolic regulation by leptin: energy balance and defense of a stable body weight. Cell Metab 9: 52–63.
28. Guo J, Hall KD (2009) Estimating the continuous-time dynamics of energy and fat metabolism in mice. PLoS Comput Biol 5: e1000511.
29. Guo J, Hall KD (2011) Predicting changes of body weight, body fat, energy expenditure and metabolic fuel selection in c57bl/6 mice. PLoS One 6: e15961.
30. van Leeuwen IMM, Kelpin FDL, Kooijman SALM (2002) A mathematical model that accounts for the effects of caloric restriction on body weight and longevity. Biogerontology 3: 373–381.
31. Chow CC, Hall KD (2008) The dynamics of human body weight change. PLoS Comput Biol 4: e1000045.
32. Hall KD (2010) Predicting metabolic adaptation, body weight change, and energy intake in humans. Am J Physiol Endocrinol Metab 298: E449–E466.
33. Hall KD (2007) Body fat and fat-free mass inter-relationships: Forbes's theory revisited. Br J Nutr 97: 1059–1063.
34. Horgan GW (2011) The behaviour of a neutral model of weight regulated only by body mass. J Theor Biol 270: 1–6.
35. Hall KD (2006) Computational model of in vivo human energy metabolism during semistarvation and refeeding. Am J Physiol Endocrinol Metab 291: E23–E37.
36. Hall KD (2010) Mathematical modelling of energy expenditure during tissue deposition. Br J Nutr 104: 4–7.
37. Periwal V, Chow CC (2006) Patterns in food intake correlate with body mass index. Am J Physiol Endocrinol Metab 291: E929–E936.
38. Newby FD, DiGirolamo M, Cotsonis GA, Kutner MH (1990) Model of spontaneous obesity in aging male wistar rats. Am J Physiol 259: R1117–R1125.
39. Woods SC, Seeley RJ, Porte D, Schwartz MW (1998) Signals that regulate food intake and energy homeostasis. Science 280: 1378–1383.
40. Nelson KM, Weinsier RL, Long CL, Schutz Y (1992) Prediction of resting energy expenditure from fat-free mass and fat mass. Am J Clin Nutr 56: 848–856.
41. Cummings DE (2006) Ghrelin and the short- and long-term regulation of appetite and body weight. Physiol Behav 89: 71–84.
42. Campfield LA, Smith FJ (1990) Transient declines in blood glucose signal meal initiation. Int J Obes 14 Suppl 3: 15–31; discussion 31–4.
43. McCarter RJ, Palmer J (1992) Energy metabolism and aging: a lifelong study of fischer 344 rats. Am J Physiol 263: E448–E452.
44. Greenberg JA, Boozer CN (2000) Metabolic mass, metabolic rate, caloric restriction, and aging in male fischer 344 rats. Mech Ageing Dev 113: 37–48.
45. Nelder JA, Mead R (1965) A simplex method for function minimization. The Computer Journal 7: 308–313.
46. Vestergaard ET, Hansen TK, Gormsen LC, Jakobsen P, Moller N, et al. (2007) Constant intra- venous ghrelin infusion in healthy young men: clinical pharmacokinetics and metabolic effects. Am J Physiol Endocrinol Metab 292: E1829–E1836.
47. Cobelli C, Toffolo G, Ferrannini E (1984) A model of glucose kinetics and their control by insulin, compartmental and noncompartmental approaches. Mathematical Biosciences 72: 291–315.
48. Zeng J, Patterson BW, Klein S, Martin DR, Dagogo-Jack S, et al. (1997) Whole body leptin kinetics and renal metabolism in vivo. Am J Physiol 273: E1102–E1106.

Behavioral and Neural Correlates of Acute and Scheduled Hunger in C57BL/6 Mice

Christian M. Gallardo[1]⁹, Cynthia T. Hsu[1]⁹, Keith M. Gunapala[1], Maksim Parfyonov[2], Chris H. Chang[3], Ralph E. Mistlberger[2], Andrew D. Steele[1,4]*

1 Division of Biology, California Institute of Technology, Pasadena, California, United States of America, **2** Department of Psychology, Simon Fraser University, Burnaby, British Columbia, Canada, **3** W.M. Keck Science Department, Claremont McKenna College, Pitzer College, Scripps College, Claremont, California, United States of America, **4** Biological Sciences Department, California State Polytechnic University Pomona, Pomona, California, United States of America

Abstract

In rodents, daily feeding schedules induce food anticipatory activity (FAA) rhythms with formal properties suggesting mediation by food-entrained circadian oscillators (FEOs). The search for the neuronal substrate of FEOs responsible for FAA is an active area of research, but studies spanning several decades have yet to identify unequivocally a brain region required for FAA. Variability of results across studies leads to questions about underlying biology versus methodology. Here we describe in C57BL/6 male mice the effects of varying the 'dose' of caloric restriction (0%, 60%, 80%, 110%) on the expression of FAA as measured by a video-based analysis system, and on the induction of c-Fos in brain regions that have been implicated in FAA. We determined that more severe caloric restriction (60%) leads to a faster onset of FAA with increased magnitude. Using the 60% caloric restriction, we found little evidence for unique signatures of neuronal activation in the brains of mice anticipating a daily mealtime compared to mice that were fasted acutely or fed ad-libitum–even in regions such as the dorsomedial and ventrolateral hypothalamus, nucleus accumbens, and cerebellum that have previously been implicated in FAA. These results underscore the importance of feeding schedule parameters in determining quantitative features of FAA in mice, and demonstrate dissociations between behavioral FAA and neural activity in brain areas thought to harbor FEOs or participate in their entrainment or output.

Editor: Paul A. Bartell, Pennsylvania State University, United States of America

Funding: Funding for these studies was provided by the Broad Fellows Program in Brain Circuitry at Caltech, an Ellison Medical Foundation New Scholar Award to ADS, a Grants Program in Eating Disorders Research award from the Klarman Family Foundation to ADS. The funders had no role in study design, data collection and analysis, decision to publish, or preparation of the manuscript.

Competing Interests: The authors have declared that no competing interests exist.

* E-mail: adsteele@csupomona.edu

⁹ These authors contributed equally to this work.

Introduction

Circadian regulation of organismal physiology and health is a rapidly expanding area of research [1,2,3,4]. Numerous studies have examined the entraining properties of light on the "master" clock, the suprachiasmatic nucleus (SCN), which is a cluster of ~10,000 neurons in the most ventral and medial portion of the rostral hypothalamus with connections to many nearby nuclei involved in coordinating metabolism, wakefulness, and body temperature [5,6,7,8]. Clearly, light inputs via the SCN can coordinate feeding behavior but the question of whether feeding behavior itself can be an important zeitgeber (entraining stimulus) has received increasing attention in recent years [1,9].

If nocturnal rodents are fed during the day, the rest phase of their circadian rest-activity cycle, they show activity preceding the scheduled feeding time, termed "food anticipatory activity" (FAA), in addition to their normal nighttime activity [10]. In SCN-lesioned animals, which are arrhythmic when food is available *ad libitum* (AL), activity converges to a single peak preceding scheduled feeding, suggesting the presence of a timing mechanism that coordinates activity with feeding independent of the SCN [11,12]. Formal properties of FAA in SCN-ablated and intact rodents are consistent with mediation by one or more food-entrainable circadian oscillators (FEO). Despite many years of investigation, the location of the FEO(s) necessary for FAA remains uncertain and food anticipatory rhythms are surprisingly robust to knockouts of known circadian clock genes [13,14,15,16,17]. The role of hunger related inputs assessed using gene knockout studies is no less murky [18,19,20,21,22,23,24].

A number of *ex vivo* neuronal activation studies have been undertaken to delineate the neuronal circuitry of FAA. Measures have included mRNA or protein expression of immediate early genes, such as *c-Fos*, or clock components like *Period 1 or 2*, or metabolic markers such as 2-deoxyglucose uptake in brain sections of rats or mice on daily feeding schedules [25,26,27,28,29,30,31,32,33]. These studies have broadly implicated several hypothalamic and a few extrahypothalamic regions as involved in FAA, with some variability in results across studies.

One potential cause of variable results is variation in the method and extent of food restriction. Previous studies mapping neural correlates of FAA have used limited-duration feeding schedules, in which rats or mice are permitted to eat as much as they can during a fixed mealtime, usually in the 2–6 h range. Here we present the results from experiments that utilized limited-amount feeding schedules, in which mice were provided once daily with an amount of food corresponding to some percentage of daily AL caloric intake. Mice on limited amount caloric restriction (CR) feeding schedules can eat for a more extended period of time, but still exhibit robust FAA. The first objective of this study was to determine the extent to which daytime FAA and nocturnal activity (which together determine the magnitude of commonly used metrics of FAA) depend on the degree of CR. We found that the rapidity and magnitude of FAA induction increases with the degree of CR, and established a 60% CR feeding schedule as optimal for inducing high amplitude FAA that is stable over many weeks. We then used a 60% CR schedule and immunohistochemical staining of the immediate early gene product c-Fos to map the neural correlates of CR at 5 time points before and after scheduled food access or an acute fast. We examined c-Fos expression in a number of brain regions implicated in FAA, including the nucleus accumbens, dorsomedial, ventromedial and lateral hypothalamus, and the cerebellum. Surprisingly, these areas did not exhibit significantly elevated c-Fos expression 1 and 2.5 h prior to scheduled daily food access, by comparison with acute fasting and AL food access conditions, although expression was marked 2 h after meal onset. These results indicate that limited-amount CR schedules can dissociate behavioral FAA from a commonly used correlate of neural activity in brain regions observed to be activated prior to limited-time feeding schedules.

Materials and Methods

Ethics Statement

These experiments were approved by the California Institute of Technology Institutional Animal Care and Use Committee under protocol #1567.

Behavioral Analysis

Video-based activity data was analyzed using HomeCageScan 3.0; behavioral definitions were as described previously [34,35]. High intensity activity was defined as walking, jumping, rearing, and hanging behaviors. Activity data were accumulated in 60-minute time bins and evaluated for statistically significant changes using non-parametric tests such as the Mann-Whitney Test using GraphPad Instat. All graphs were made with GraphPad Prism 4; medians are reported +/− interquartile ranges. Sample sizes are indicated in the Figure legends.

Acute Fasting Experiment

For acute fasting experiments male C57BL/6J at least 10 weeks of age were purchased from Jackson Labs (Bar Harbor, ME). These mice were maintained on a 13:11 LD cycle and single-housed for 4–6 days with AL access to food (Laboratory Rodent Chow Type 5001) and water prior to being placed on special feeding protocols. Daily food intake was measured over a 48 h period beginning at least three days after single housing and used to compute the amount of food delivered during CR (see below). For the experiment n = 13 mice were fasted and n = 15 mice were AL control. These mice were video recorded for 24 hours and the videos were analyzed using HomeCageScan 3.0.

Dose-response Experiment

Male C57BL/6J mice from Jackson Labs were singly housed four days after arrival. Body weight measurements were taken at days −10, −3, 3, 7, 14, 21, 28, 35, and 42, with Day 0 marking the start of special feeding conditions (approximately twelve days after single-housing).

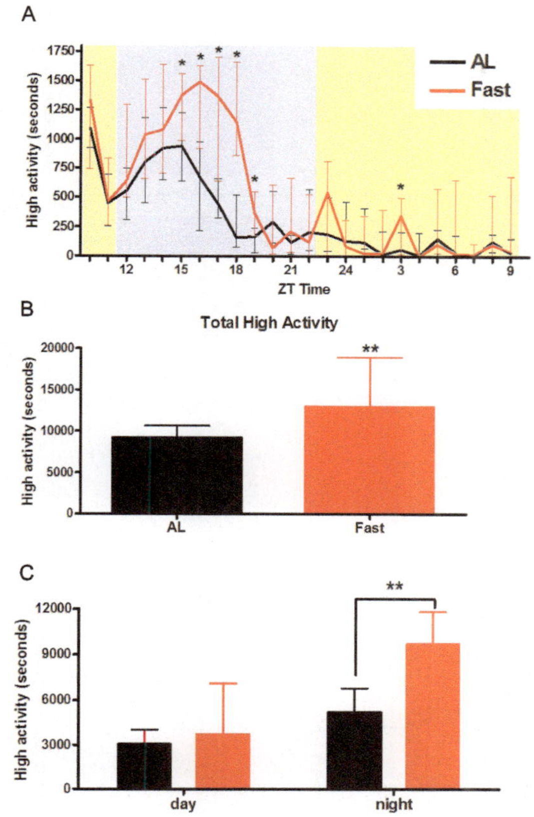

Figure 1. High activity profiles, and total diurnal and nocturnal activity of ad libitum and acutely fasted mice. (A) The seconds of high activity per hour in a 24 hour video recording of AL mice (black) or acutely fasted mice (red). The light phase is shown in yellow (ZT 10–12) followed by 11 hours of darkness indicated in gray (ZT 12–23) followed by light (ZT 24–9) (B) The total high activity summed across the 24 hour recording for AL and fasted mice. (C) The total high activity during the light and dark periods. n = 13 fasted and n = 15 AL. Values represent medians +/− IQ range. The statistical significance was tested using Mann-Whitney test; **denotes $p<0.01$.

Mice were given AL food and water until day 0 of the study. Approximately one week prior to day 0, food intake was measured for forty-two mice over the course of two days. Starting from day 0, 2 hours prior to lights-off (Zeitgeber Time 10, where ZT12 is lights-off by convention) eight mice were given AL access to food, eight were given 110% of the mean food intake for all mice, eight were given 80% of the mean food intake for all mice, and ten were given 60% of the mean food intake for all mice. All mice were recorded for 23.5–24 hours once a week starting with day 0 and ending at day 42. Mice were fed and recorded at ZT 10. Water remained freely available throughout the study though we noted that mice did most of their drinking behavior during the 2 hours after meal presentation.

Neural Correlates of Acute and Scheduled Hunger

Mice were divided into three groups: AL, CR, and Fast (no food for the indicated time before perfusions). Mice in AL and Fast groups had free access to chow and water. Mice in the CR group were provided with 60% of their AL levels. On the last day of the scheduled feeding (day 28), mice were euthanized with carbon dioxide and perfused transcardially with 10 mL of 0.1 M PBS at 5 time points relative to scheduled feeding: time point

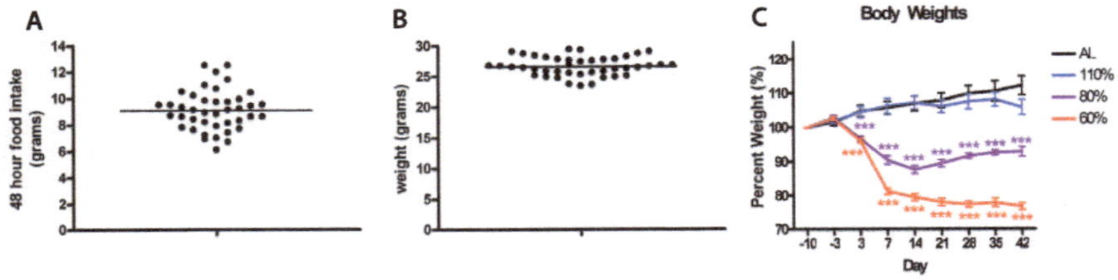

Figure 2. Food intake and body weight distribution and normalized body weights of mice on different food restriction amounts. (A) Individual measurements of food intake over a 48 hour period for individual mice divided by 2 to give a 24 hour food intake (n=42). (B) Individual measurements of body weight prior to any dietary change (day−10) (n=42). (C) Mean body weight measurements +/− SEM of each treatment group over the duration of the experiment. Mice fed AL (black; n=8), 110% (blue, n=8), 80% (purple; n=8) and 60% (red; n=10) show dose-dependent changes in body weight depending on food availability. Significance was tested with Tukey-Kramer multiple comparisons test with one-way ANOVA post-test for all treatment groups vs. AL controls for each respective day. ***denotes $p<0.001$.

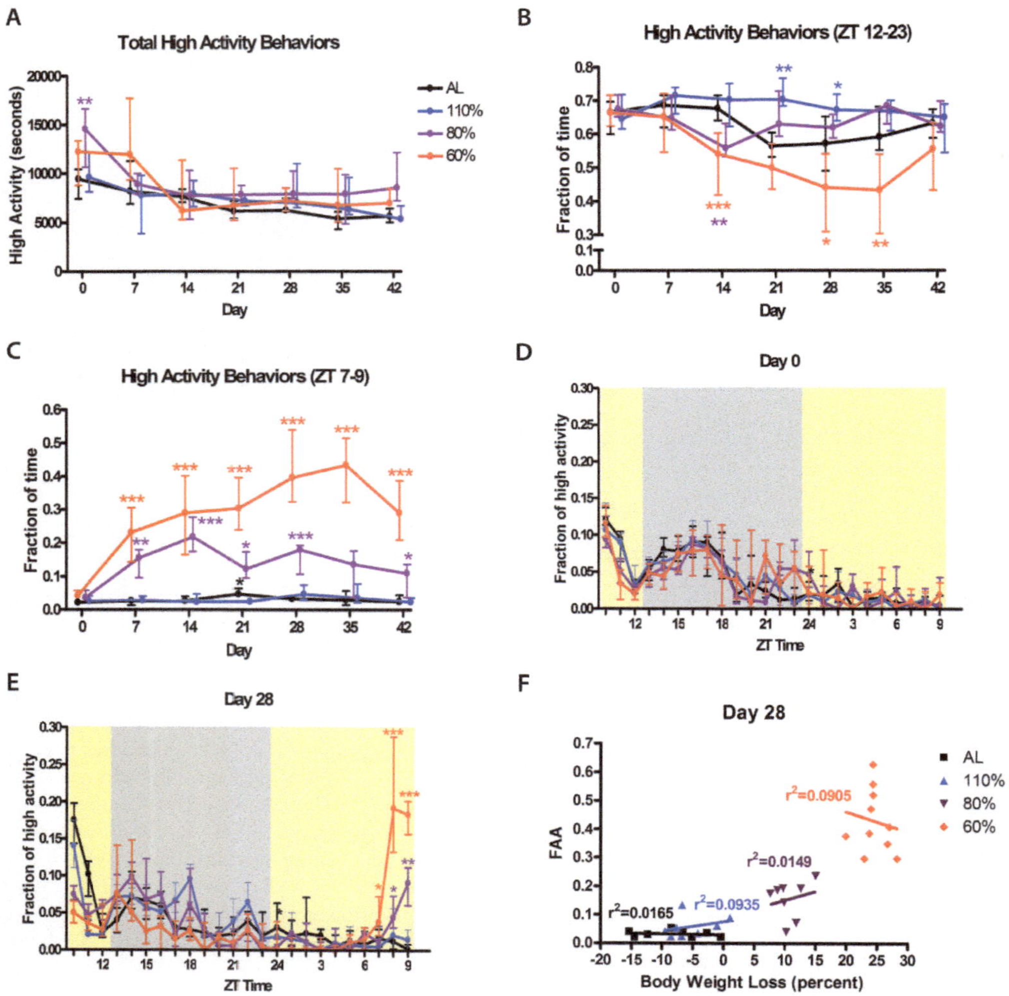

Figure 3. High activity behaviors of mice in on different food restriction amounts. (A) The total amount of high activity behaviors (in seconds) during weekly 24 hour video recordings for mice on AL, 110%, 80%, and 60% CR. (B) Normalized nocturnal high activity behaviors during weekly 24 hour video recordings for mice on AL, 110%, 80%, and 60% CR. (C) Fraction of time spent on high activity behaviors in the 3 hours preceding meal presentation (ZT 7–9). (D) Normalized fraction of time per hour spent on high activity behavior during the 24-recording of day 0 (D) and (E) day 28 of dose-response experiment. Values represent medians +/− IQ range, with high activity values normalized to total daily activity (significance tested with Mann-Whitney test with Dunn's post test for all treatment groups vs. AL controls for each respective day). *denotes $p<0.05$, **denotes $p<0.01$, and ***denotes $p<0.001$. n=8 for all groups except for 60% CR where n=10. (F) Correlation and linear regression of normalized food anticipatory activity in the 3 hours preceding scheduled feeding with % body weight loss.

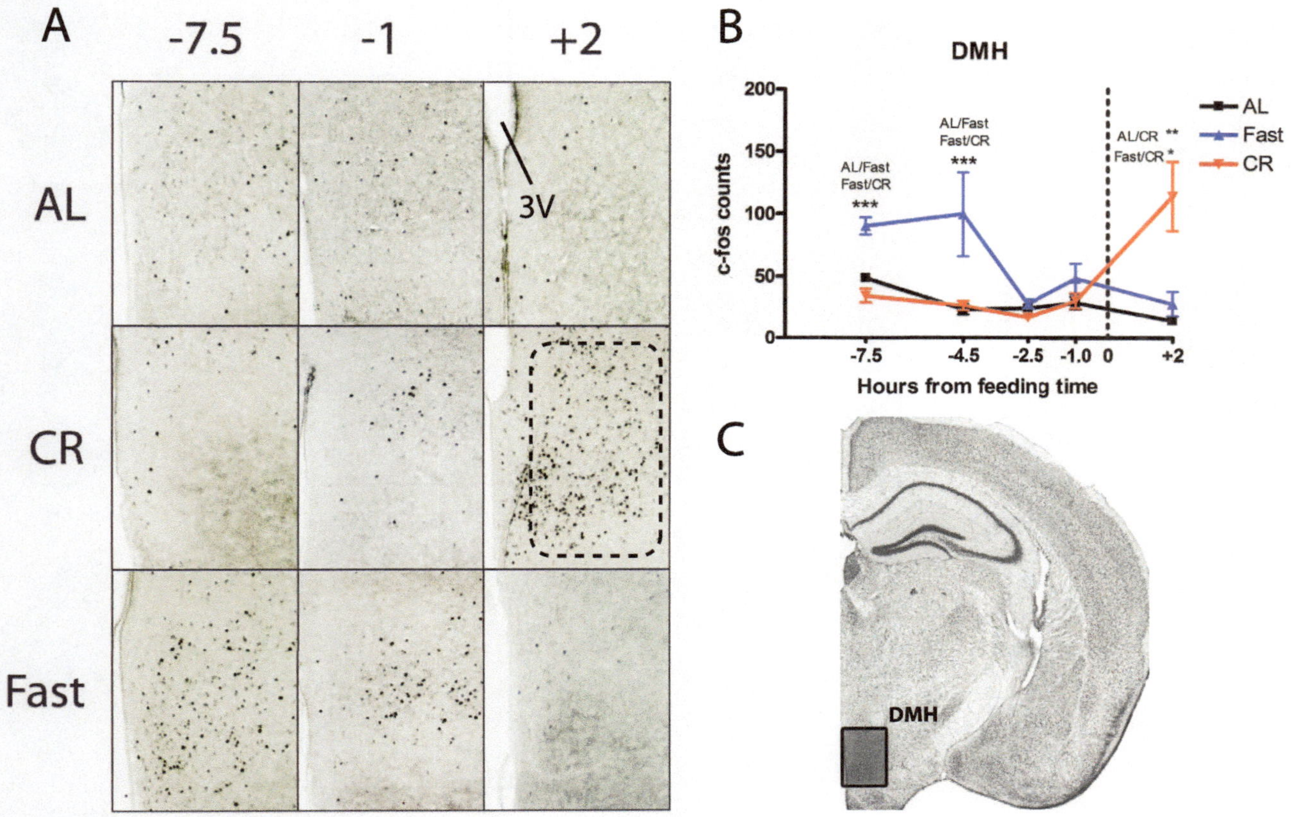

Figure 4. c-Fos protein expression in the dorsomedial hypothalamus of calorie-restricted, acutely fasted, and AL control mice. (A) Representative images of c-Fos staining the DMH of mice at −7.5, −1 hours before feeding and +2 hours after feeding. (B) Mean (±SEM) number of c-Fos-immunoreactive nuclei in the DMH of AL controls (blue), fasted (blue), and CR (red) at 5 time points relative to feeding. TP 0 represents time of expected meal presentation as highlighted by the vertical dotted line on the x-axis. (C) Representative coronal brain map with Nissl stain showing location of region under study. (Adapted from Paxinos and Franklin 2007) [57]. Sample sizes for TP−7.5 thru +2 are n = 6, 11, 11, 9, 5 for AL groups, n = 6, 11, 8, 9, 5 for CR groups, and n = 4, 4, 4, 4, 4 for Fasted groups.

(TP) −7.5, −4.5, −2.5, −1, +2. Biological samples sizes for were n = 2 per group at TP −7.5; n = 4 for AL and CR and n = 2 for fasted at TP −4.5; n = 4 for AL and CR and n = 2 for fasted at TP −2.5; n = 3 for AL and CR and n = 2 for fasted at TP −1; and n = 2 for all groups at TP +2. The brains were removed from mice and immersion fixed in 10% buffered formalin (Sigma) for at least 24 h. They were then bisected in a saggital plane and half-brains were sent to NeuroScience Associates (Knoxville, TN). Samples were then treated with 20% glycerol and 2% dimethylsulfoxide to prevent freeze-artifacts and embedded with up to 32 hemi-brains in a block of gelatin matrix using MultiBrain Technology™. The block of embedded tissue was allowed to cure and then was rapidly frozen by immersion in isopentane chilled to −70°C with crushed dry ice. Blocks were mounted on a freezing stage of an AO 860 sliding microtome and sectioned coronally at 35 μm thickness. All sections cut were collected sequentially into a 4×6 array of containers filled with 'antigen preserve' (buffered ethylene glycol). At the completion of sectioning, each container holds a serial set of one-of-every-24th section (e.g. one section every 840 μm). For Immunostaining every 6th section was used.

For immunochemistry, the sections were stained free-floating. All incubation solutions from the blocking serum use Tris buffered saline (TBS) with Triton X100 (TX) as the vehicle; all rinses are with TBS. After a hydrogen peroxide treatment and blocking serum, the sections were immunostained with a primary anti-c-Fos (Novus, rabbit anti c-Fos) 1:10,000 antibody overnight at room temperature. Vehicle solution contains 0.3% TritonX-100 for permeabilization. To visualize the location of binding site of the primary antibody an avidin-biotin-HRP complex (details in Vectastain elite ABC kit, Vector, Burlingame, CA) is applied. After rinses, the sections were treated with diaminobenzidine tetrahydrochloride (DAB) using nickel enchancemnet and hydrogen peroxide to create a visible reaction product and mounted on gelatinized (subbed) glass slides, air dried, dehydrated in alcohols, cleared in xylene and cover slipped.

c-Fos stained sections were examined under a Nikon Eclipse TE2000-U light microscope coupled to a computer with NIS-Elements BR 3.0 software. Image saturation was avoided by adjusting exposure time with the brain slice with the highest c-Fos signal. Expression analysis of c-Fos protein was done for the following regions: SCN (0.48 to 0.655 caudal to bregma), nucleus accumbens core (NAc) (0.745 to 0.445 rostral to bregma),

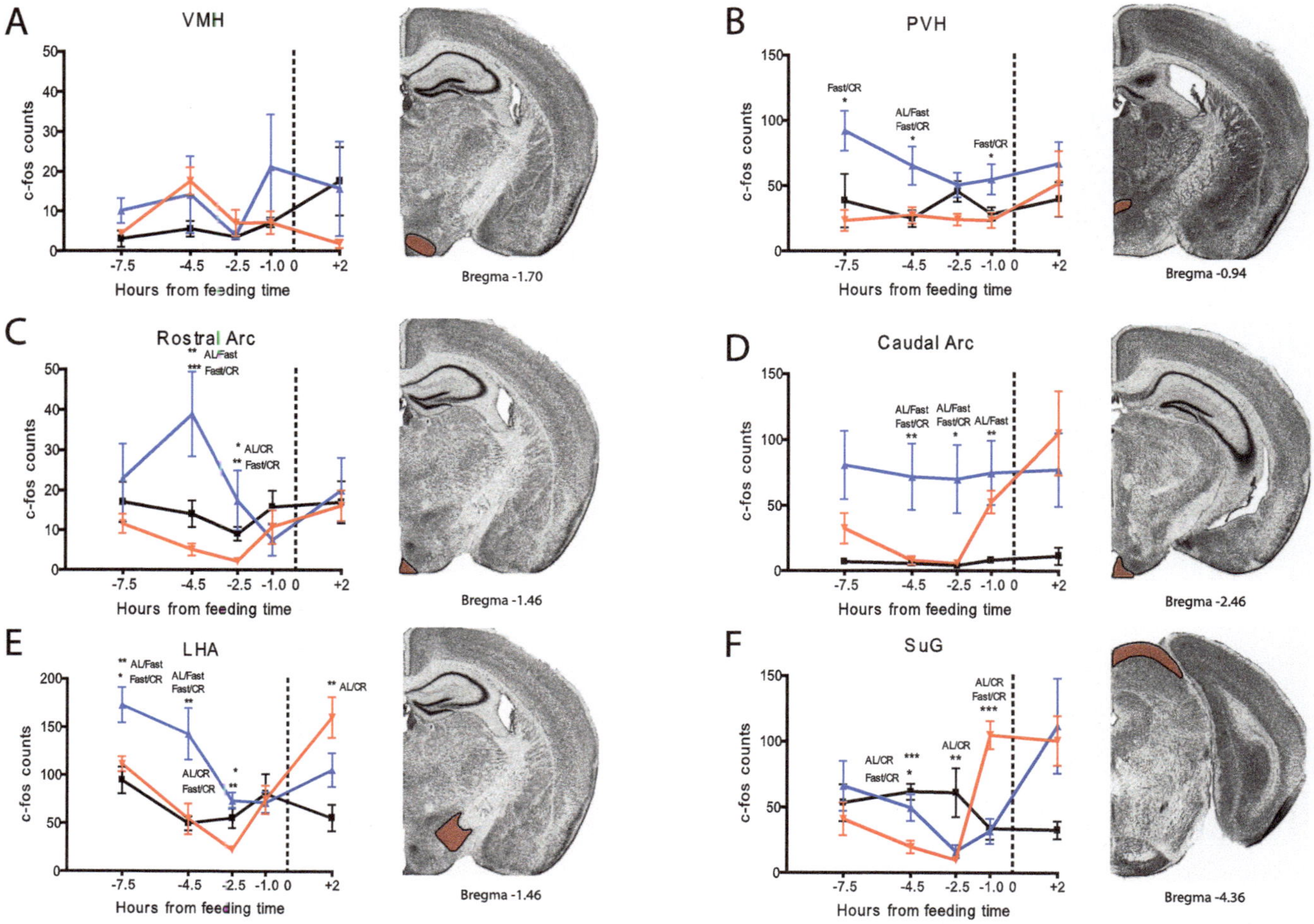

Figure 5. c-Fos induction in VMH, PVH, LHA, Rostral and Caudal Arc, and SuG of calorie-restricted, acutely fasted, and AL control mice. Mean (±SEM) number of c-Fos-immunoreactive nuclei in the several brain nuclei of AL controls (blue), fasted (blue), and CR (red) at 5 time points relative to feeding. TP 0 represents time of expected meal presentation as highlighted by the vertical dotted line on the x-axis. (A) Mean (+/− SEM) c-fos counts for the ventral medial hypothalamus (VMH). (B) c-Fos counts for the paraventricular nucleus (PVH). (C) c-fos counts for the rostral arcuate nucleus. (D) c-fos counts for the caudal arcuate nucleus. (E) c-fos counts for the lateral hypothalamus (LHA). (F) c-fos counts for the superior colliculus gray layer (SuG). Sample sizes for TP−7.5 thru +2 are n = 2–6, 7–12, 7–12, 6–9, 4–6 for AL groups, n = 3–6, 4–12, 5–12, 4–9 for CR groups, and n = 5–6, 5–6, 2–6, 6, 5–6 for Fast groups. Representative images of each neuroanatomical location are shown (from Paxinos and Franklin).

paraventricular hypothalamus (PVH) (0.48 to 0.655 caudal to bregma), Rostral arcuate (Arc) (1.055 to 1.855 caudal to bregma), caudal arcuate (Arc) (2.055 to 2.255 caudal to bregma), ventromedial hypothalamus (VMH) (1.255 to 1.755 caudal to bregma), dorsomedial hypothalamus (DMH) (1.255 to 1.755 caudal to bregma), lateral hypothalamus (LHA) (1.255 to 1.755 caudal to bregma), cerebellum (6.355 to 7.055 caudal to bregma), and superior colliculus (SuG) (3.68 to 4.45 caudal to bregma). Cells immunopositive for c-Fos protein were counted using 10x and 4x lenses. The mean number of c-Fos-positive cells per time point was calculated from individual unilateral counts at three contiguous bregma depths (with at least 3 replicates per time point). Counts were done automatically by software after setting an ROI and threshold levels for each brain region, with threshold levels kept constant in between counts of a specific brain region. ROIs were defined in slices based on visible landmarks and comparison with mouse brain atlas of Paxinos and Franklin (2007). Representative images were captured using the CCD camera while doing automated counts. Tukey-Kramer parametric regressions were used to establish statistical differences between groups (AL, CR, Fast).

Results

Acute Food Deprivation Increases Nocturnal Activity

We tested the home cage behavioral response to acute food deprivation in C57BL/6 male mice. At ZT10 (2 hours before lights-off) we removed all food from the cage of n = 13 mice and left in ample food for n = 15 mice and monitored these mice for 24 hours. The fasted mice showed a strong increase in 'high' activity behaviors (defined as jumping, hanging, rearing, and walking), particularly in the middle-to late night hours of ZT 15–18 (Figure 1A). The total high activity over 24 hours was significantly increased in the fasted group compared to the AL control group during the 24-hour video recording (Figure 1B; p = 0.0044, Mann-Whitney). Activity during the 13 hour lights on period was not increased in fasted mice; however, nighttime activity almost doubled in fasted mice compared to AL controls, showing a statistically significant increase (Figure 1C; $p<0.01$, Mann-Whitney).

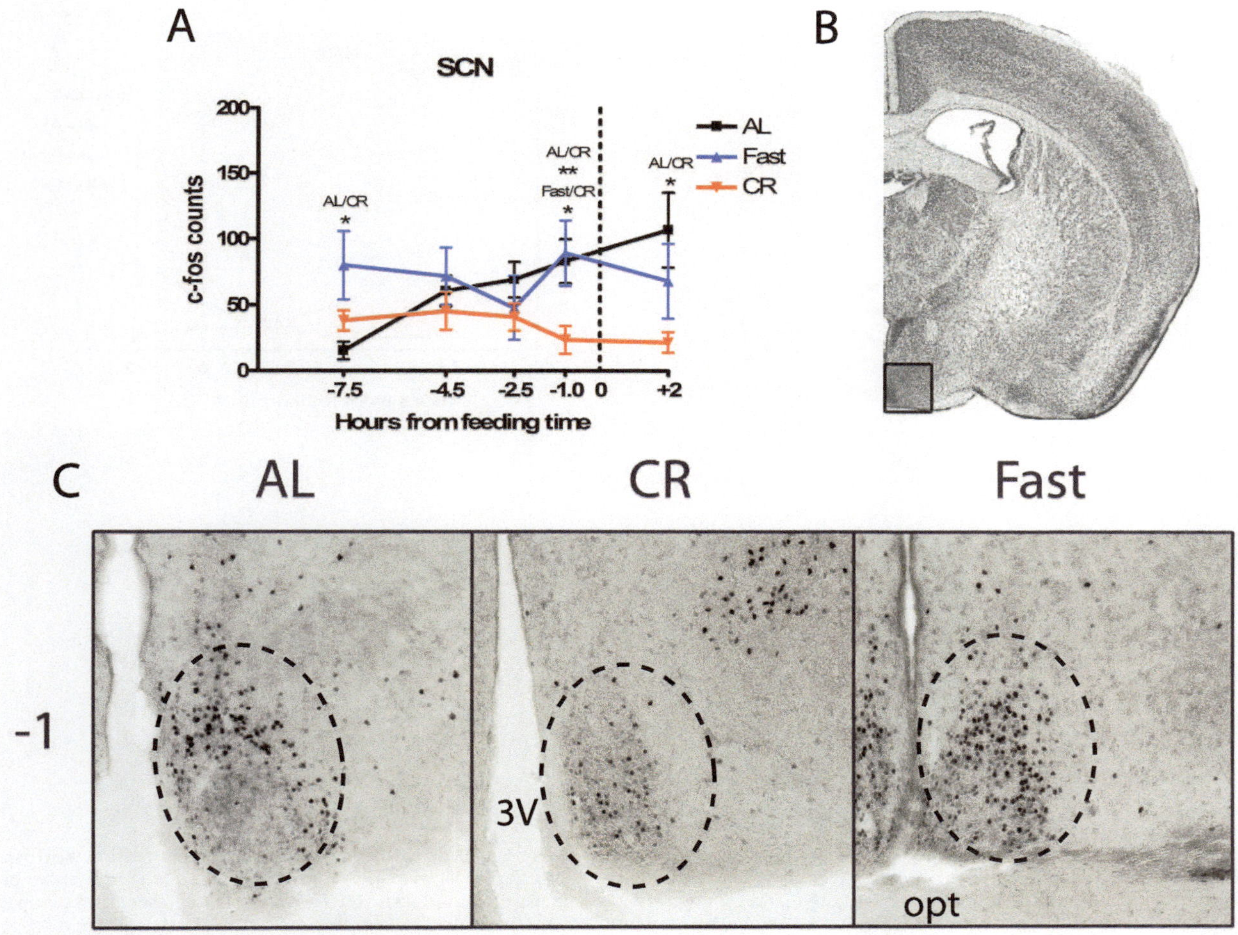

Figure 6. c-Fos protein expression in the in the suprachiasmatic nucleus (SCN) of calorie-restricted, acutely fasted, and AL control mice. (A) Mean (±SEM) number of c-Fos-immunoreactive nuclei in the SCN of AL controls, fasted, and CR at 5 time points measured relative to feeding. (B) Representative coronal brain map with Nissl stain showing location of region under study adapted from Paxinos and Franklin. (C) Representative micrographs at TP−1 of FOS expression in the SCN. Sample sizes for TP−7.5 thru +2 are n = 6, 11, 12, 8, 6 for AL groups, n = 5, 12, 11, 11, 6 for CR groups, and n = 6, 6, 6, 6, 6 for Fast groups.

Nocturnal Activity Decreases While FAA Increases with Increased Magnitude of CR

There is evidence that CR increases activity overall but it has not been examined in detail using C57BL/6J male mice under the same time scales typically employed by our laboratory [36,37,38]. To that end, we tested the effect of varying the percentage of food delivered on a timed CR schedule in C57BL/6J male mice and assayed their overall, nocturnal, and preprandial high activity behaviors.

We measured food intake over 48 hours for all mice used in this study, finding a broad range of values from 3 to 6 grams per day (mean 4.6+/−0.1 SEM; Figure 2A). Body weight showed some variability as well but not as much as food intake. The smallest mouse weighed 23.4 grams while the largest mouse weighed 29.3 grams (mean weight 26.6+/−0.2 grams; Figure 2B). Rather than scale the percent CR on an individual mouse basis, which would be cumbersome, we restricted based on the population average. For mice fed an AL diet we delivered an additional pellet to their cage daily at ZT 10 to control for the disturbance of feeding while for another group we delivered 110% of AL food intake (in pilot studies we observed FAA in some mice for 100% diets). Mice that were fed 60% of the mean food intake exhibited a precipitous decrease in weight until day 7, when the decrease tapered to ~80% of day −3 baseline values (Figure 2C). Mice fed 60% CR also had significantly lower percent weight than those fed 80% CR starting on day 7 and lasting the duration of scheduled feeding experiments ($p<0.001$). Mice that were fed 80% CR had a significant decrease in weight from day −3 to day 14 ($p<0.001$); however, they also had a significant weight gain from day 14 to day 28 ($p<0.001$). Mice fed 110% of the mean food intake showed a modest increase in body weight that was similar to that of AL controls, until day 14, when body weight stabilized to around 105% of baseline value. Mice fed 110% did not show any statistically significant difference from mice fed AL in the percent change in weight relative to day −3. Mice fed AL had a significant change in weight between day −3 and day 14 ($p<0.05$), day 3 and 35 ($p<0.05$), day 3 and 42 ($p<0.01$), and day 7 and day 42 ($p<0.01$) (Repeated Measures ANOVA with Tukey-Kramer Multiple Comparison's Test).

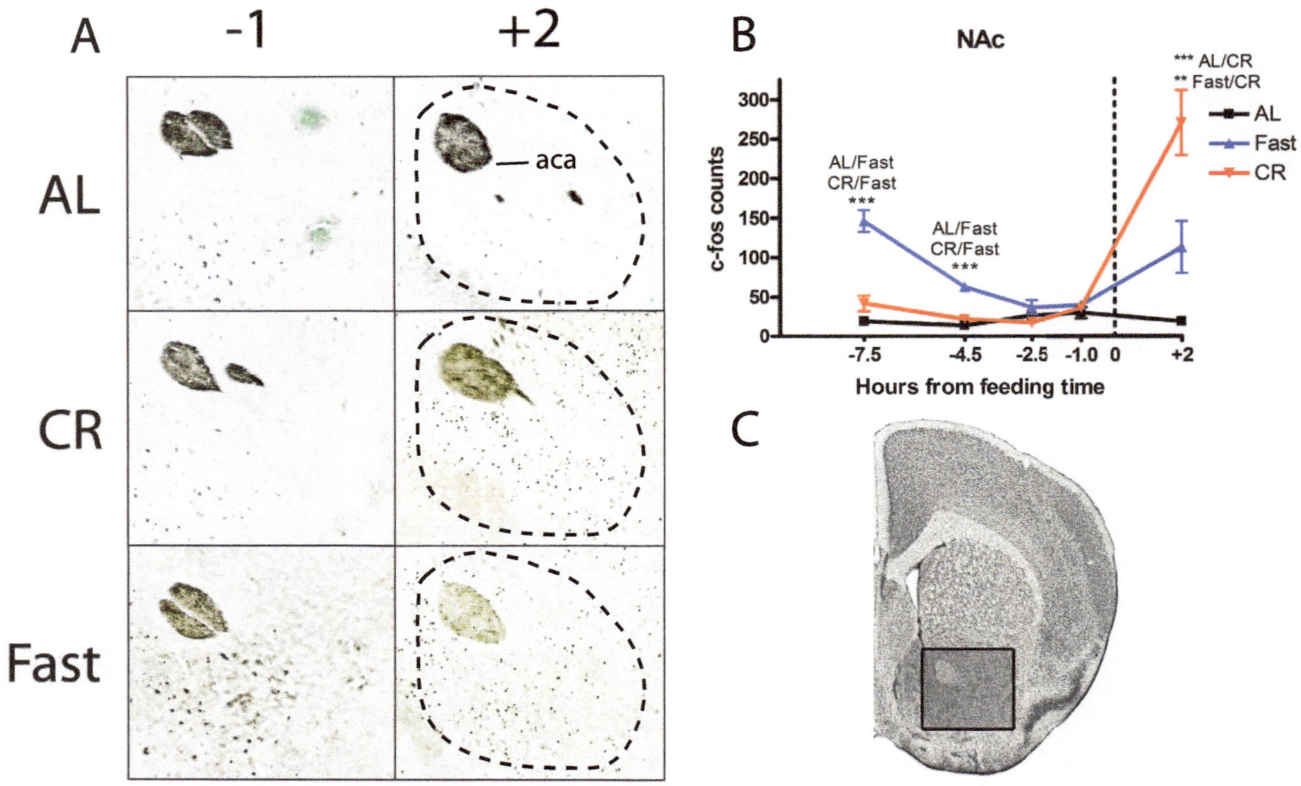

Figure 7. c-Fos protein expression in the in the nucleus accumbens core (NAc Core) of calorie-restricted, acutely fasted, and AL control mice. (A) Representative micrographs of c-Fos staining in the core of the nucleus accumenbs at TP−1 and +2. (B) Mean (±SEM) number of c-Fos-immunoreactive nuclei in the NAc Core of AL, fasted, and CR mice at 5 time points measured relative to feeding. (C) Representative coronal brain map with Nissl stain showing location of region under study. (Adapted from Paxinos and Franklin). Sample sizes for TP−7.5 thru +2 are n = 4, 8, 8, 6, 4 for AL groups, n = 4, 8, 8, 6, 4 for CR groups, and n = 4, 4, 4, 4, 4 for Fast groups.

Overall, the total amount of high activity behaviors (in seconds) of mice on CR was not higher than that of AL controls (Figure 3A). In fact, we were surprised to observe that activity was significantly elevated only at one time point for 80% CR–the first day of the modified diet ("day 0")–and that at no other points were mice on CR more active than those on AL or 110% AL control diets (Figure 3A). Despite this lack of a major difference in overall activity, we followed our standard practice of normalizing high activity by dividing the seconds of high activity in each hourly bin by the total high activity for that day, resulting in a fraction of high activity per hour. When binning for high activity behaviors during the 11 hours of darkness (ZT 12–23), mice in the 60% CR group showed a clear decrease in normalized nocturnal high activity, reaching its lowest points on days 28 and 35 (Figure 3B). Even when taking into account the slight decrease in dark cycle activity in AL controls over time, the decrease in nighttime activity in the 60% CR groups was statistically significant on days 14, 28, and 35 ($p<0.001$, $p<0.05$, and $p<0.01$ respectively). Conversely mice fed 110% of the baseline food intake showed a distinctly more constant fraction of nighttime activity compared to AL controls with statistically significant differences on days 21 and 28 ($p<0.01$ and $p<0.5$ respectively). Mice in the 80% CR group displayed a transient decrease in nighttime activity relative to the AL controls at day 14 but then showed a similar amount of nocturnal activity at all later time points (Figure 3B).

Preprandial high activity behaviors for CR groups during the 3 hours preceding scheduled meal time (ZT 7–9) showed a dose-dependent increase in the fraction of high activity compared to AL controls, with mice on 60% CR exhibiting an overall greater magnitude of FAA compared to those on 80% CR (Figure 3C). Mice on 60% CR showed FAA that was statistically significant ($p<0.001$) on all days following the start of restricted feeding schedules (Figure 3C). Mice on 80% CR displayed FAA fairly consistently but at a lesser magnitude than the mice on 60% CR. In this group, FAA was statistically significant on CR days 14 and 28 at $p<0.001$, on days 7, 21 and 42 at $p<0.05$, but not on day 35, although some individual mice did exhibit preprandial high activity behaviors on that day. The mean fraction of high activity that was observed during the FAA window in both AL mice and the mice fed 110% of baseline was consistently below 5% for all days. There was no statistically significant difference between the AL controls and the mice fed 110% at any time point except day 21 when AL mice showed an increase in activity ($p<0.05$). Waveforms of normalized activity are shown for the first day (Day 0) and the 28th day of modified diet (Figure 3D–E). We also tested for a correlation between percentage of weight loss and FAA within treatement groups but found no evidence for linear relationships as r^2 values were very low; for example, the r^2 value from a linear regression between % weight loss and FAA among mice on 60% CR was only 0.09 (Figure 3F). Similar analyses was performed for each day of the experiment with a similar result (Supplemental Figure 1).

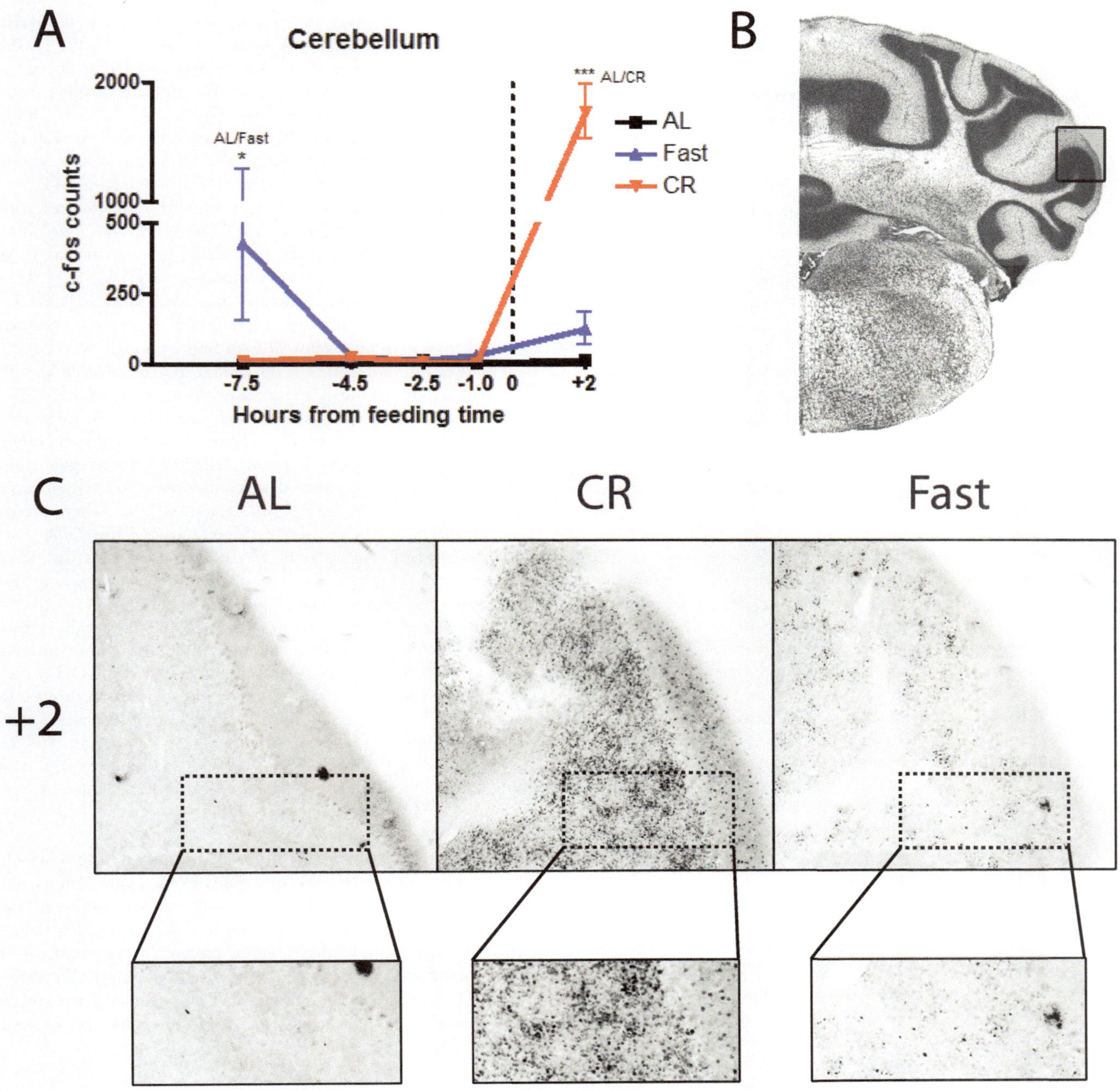

Figure 8. c-Fos protein expression in the in the ansiform lobule crus 2 of the cerebellum of calorie-restricted mice, acutely fasted, and AL control mice. (A) Mean (±SEM) number of c-Fos-immunoreactive nuclei in the NAc Core of AL controls, fasted and CR mice at 5 time points measured relative to feeding. CR mice show a prodigious increase ($p<0.001$) in FOS protein expression at TP+2 (note the split y-axis). Fasted show significant induction of FOS protein at TP−7.5 ($p<0.05$). AL control mice do not show any appreciable induction in the expression of FOS protein at any time point. (B) Representative coronal brain map with Nissl stain showing location of the ansiform lobule crus 2 of the Cerebellum adapted from Paxinos and Franklin. (C) Representative micrographs at TP+2 of FOS expression. Insets show high magnifications of c-Fos labeling in the lobule. Sample sizes for TP−7.5 thru +2 are n=6, 15, 10, 8, 3 for AL groups, n=6, 12, 12, 9, 6 for CR groups, and n=3, 5, 5, 5, 3 for Fast groups.

Neural Correlates of Acute and Scheduled Hunger

To determine the patterns of neural activity in mice on CR feeding schedules, additional C57BL/6J male mice were obtained and assigned to one of three groups: 1) 60% CR feeding at ZT 10 for 28 days 2) AL controls given an extra food pellet at ZT 10 daily to control for disturbances and 3) fasted controls treated identically to group 2 until the last day of the experiment, day 29, when food was removed 24 h prior to euthanasia. The acutely fasted mice control for c-Fos activation in response to hunger and any nonspecific wakefulness or activity. Based on our observations in the present study (Figure 3) and those of our prior studies [18,28,39] with C57BL/6J male mice, FAA begins ~3 hours prior to scheduled meal time. On the final day of the experiment, day 29, brain samples were taken from n = 2–4 mice from each group at ZT 2.5 (7.5 hours prior to meal time, indicated as TP −7.5 in the Figures), ZT 5.5 (TP −4.5), ZT 7.5 (TP −2.5), ZT 9 (TP −1), and ZT 11 (2 hours after meal time, labeled as TP +2). The mice at +2 were fed their meal so signals at this time point are either due to entrainment or feeding itself. Brains were fixed, cut into 35 micron sections, and every 6th section was immunostained for c-Fos (see Materials and Methods).

Subsequently, these sections were examined microscopically, focusing on patterns of c-Fos induction in regions of the hypothalamus that have been implicated in metabolism, circadian rhythm, and/or food entrainment. We began by examining the dorsomedial hypothalamus (DMH), which has been reported to express c-Fos and the circadian clock proteins Per1 and Per2 in association with restricted feeding schedules in which food access is limited to 4–6 h in the mid-light period [26,31] [40,41]. Counting both the pars compacta and the ventral DMH revealed essentially no c-Fos induction prior to scheduled meal time in mice on CR diets (Figure 4). Most of the c-Fos induction in the fasting group was seen at time point (TP) −7.5 (7.5 hours prior to scheduled meal time) and −4.5 hours where c-Fos was significantly higher in the DMH of fasted mice versus those on Al or on CR ($p<0.001$). The most striking group difference in c-Fos activation occurred 2 hours after meal time when there were at least twice as many c-Fos positive nuclei in the CR samples compared to the AL or fasted groups (Figure 4; $p<0.05$ for CR versus fasted; $p<0.01$ for CR versus AL).

We continued by examining other hypothalamic structures that have been implicated in FAA, hunger sensing, or both. The ventromedial hypothalamus (VMH) was implicated as a mediator of FAA by Ribeiro and colleagues using mice [32] but our cell counts in this region showed no significant group differences at any time point (Figure 5A). We next examined the paraventricular nucleus of the hypothalamus (PVH), a structure that showed c-Fos activation prior to a scheduled daytime meal in rats [41]. Our results clearly indicate an increase in c-Fos expression in this region in fasted mice but no change in the mice on CR feeding (Figure 5B). We examined the arcuate nucleus (Arc) separately in terms of rostral and caudal axes [42]. AL and CR samples showed similar c-Fos expression before mealtime in the rostral Arc, but fasted mice showed a significant increase at −4.5 and −2.5 hours before feeding (Figure 5C; $p<0.05$ AL vs. CR and $p<0.01$ Fast vs. CR). In the caudal Arc we observed increased c-Fos expression in the CR group one hour prior to mealtime relative to earlier time points, but not relative to the AL controls (Figure 5D). Interestingly, the caudal Arc showed strong and continued activation in fasted mice at all time points, including after feeding at +2 hours. The lateral hypothalamus (LHA) showed an activation pattern similar to that of the PVH with fasted samples significantly elevated over AL and CR at −7.5 and −4.5 hours prior to feeding (Figure 5E). A notable difference occurred after feeding, when CR samples showed a large increase in c-Fos expression compared to AL samples in the LHA, similar to what was observed in the DMH (Figure 5E). During our initial survey we noted that the gray layer of the superior colliculus (SuG) showed strong c-Fos induction one hour prior to feeding (Figure 5F). The CR group showed a strong and statistically significant c-Fos induction in the SuG one hour prior to meal time when values surged from about 10 cells per section to more than 100 ($p<0.001$ at TP −1 comparing CR to AL or to fast; Figure 5F). In contrast, the fasted mice showed an increase in staining in the SuG only after feeding. Given its role in visual processing, this region may be a correlate of arousal rather than a mediator of FAA.

The last hypothalamic structure that we examined was the SCN, which despite being ruled out as a circadian clock necessary for FAA, may be a modulator of FAA and is thought to compete with the FEO for control over the arousal state of the animal. CR treatment groups show a significantly lower preprandial c-Fos induction at TP −1 compared to both fasted and AL mice ($p<0.05$ and $p<0.01$ respectively) (Figure 6). Suppressed c-Fos induction in the CR mice continued into the post-prandial time point, with AL mice showing significantly higher c-Fos induction compared to the CR group ($p<0.05$), and the fasted group showing a trend for more c-Fos cells compared to the CR group.

We continued our search for neural correlates of food entrainment outside of the hypothalamus by examining the nucleus accumbens core (NAc), an area involved in reward and the motivational drive for caloric intake. One prior study in rats implicates the NAc in food entrainment [43]. Our c-Fos counting results in the NAc were similar to those obtained in the DHM and LHA. There was no preprandial c-Fos induction in mice on CR (Figure 7). In contrast, fasted mice showed a significant increase in c-Fos expression at −7.5 and −4.5 hours before feeding ($p<0.001$ fast versus AL or CR). The NAc showed a massive increase in c-Fos staining after feeding in CR mice and in fasted mice as well but not as large of an increase ($p<0.001$ CR versus AL, $p<0.01$ CR versus fasted; Figure 7).

The final structure that we examined was the cerebellum, which may contain FEOs [44]. We quantified c-Fos expression in the ansiform lobule crus 2 of the cerebellum. We observed no preprandial increase in c-Fos staining in CR samples (Figure 8). However, after feeding there was a massive increase in c-Fos immunostaining in the cerebellum (Figure 8) ($p<0.001$ CR versus AL, at TP +2). Although we quantified only the ansiform lobule crus 2, visual inspection of other areas of the cerebellum showed similar changes.

Discussion

In this study we observed that acute fasting specifically increases nocturnal activity. We have determined that timed 60 and 80% CR feeding induces robust FAA in the hours before feeding and that this increased activity before meal time comes at the expense of nocturnal activity. The results of our dose response study emphasize the important role of caloric intake in eliciting FAA. Although mice on a relatively modest CR such as 80% CR will exhibit FAA, this difference becomes small after 14 days of scheduled feeding. In addition, suppression of nocturnal activity of mice on 80% CR ceases after only 14 days of CR. This shows that mice on a modest CR not only exhibit reduced FAA relative to mice on a more severely restricted diet but also exhibit daily activity patterns that may gradually become more like those of mice on an AL diet over the course of an experiment. Our results suggest that a 60% CR is ideal for maintaining consistency in behavior across individual mice as well as over the course of experiments lasting several weeks. Whether the increased FAA in 60% CR mice relative to 80% CR is due to effects downstream from FEOs driving FAA or also involves an increase in the strength of food as a Zeitgeber is an open question that would require range of entrainment or meal-shift re-entrainment experiments to assess.

Using the 60% CR protocol we then examined neural correlates of daily feeding or acute fasting using c-Fos immunostaining. Surprisingly, we observed very little evidence for preprandial activation of brain regions in mice on CR schedules, but did observe dramatic activations of many brains regions in CR groups when samples were taken two hours after meal onset. These results are striking in the magnitude of the differences before and after mealtime, and in the discrepancies with previous studies that have reported c-Fos activation of a number of these structures in rats or mice on limited-time as opposed to limited-amount feeding schedules. One factor that could be explored in future studies is the number of days of restricted feeding prior to c-Fos assessment. Mice in our study were adapted to restricted feeding schedules for 1 month, while previous studies have typically used 10, 14 or 21 days. c-Fos in some brain regions may be activated by metabolic factors that eventually adapt to long-term caloric restriction. This may also explain the increased c-Fos expression noted in the acute 24 h fasting groups in most brain regions sampled in our study.

The DMH has been the focus of numerous studies of FAA employing lesion and clock gene or immediate early gene mapping methods [40,45,46,47,48]. At least three studies using limited-duration daytime feeding schedules reported significant increases of c-Fos prior to mealtime in rats or mice [41]. Our data, by contrast, reveal no preprandial induction in the DMH of mice maintained on a 60% CR schedule but strong postprandial c-Fos induction (consistent with postprandial data from Poulin and Timofeeva, 2008) and strong induction in fasted groups at the very early preprandial time points, suggesting a predominantly satiety-sensing or meal processing role for the DMH in our model. While the DMH has been ruled out as necessary for FAA, it has been proposed as a source of inhibitory inputs to the SCN pacemaker, which promote the expression of FAA by suppressing sleep-promoting SCN output during the day (the sleep phase in nocturnal rodents) [40,47,49]. Our immunohistochemical data do not provide strong support for a DMH-SCN intrahypothalamic gate model given the visibly low c-Fos induction in the DMH in both CR and AL groups at all preprandial time points.

On the other hand, we did observe significantly lower c-Fos induction in the SCN prior to mealtime in the CR groups compared to Fast/AL groups. This result is consistent with the model that FAA may be facilitated by inhibition of the SCN to permit locomotor activity in the usual sleep phase of the circadian cycle. This model is further supported by evidence that FAA is enhanced by SCN-ablation in rats [50]. We previously observed that AL fed mice can anticipate a daily palatable meal of cheese or high fat diet and that this was associated with a modest increase in c-Fos expression in the SCN [28] This suggests that mice can anticipate a daily meal without SCN inhibition (or, more precisely, without a reduction of c-Fos protein in the SCN). A difference in pre-meal SCN activity between CR and palatable feeding schedules may explain in whole or in part why FAA is much greater in mice on the CR schedules.

The nucleus accumbens, part of the reward system, has been another target of interest regarding a role in promoting FAA. Mendoza and colleagues [43] observed c-Fos induction in the NAc prior to mealtime, and found that lesions restricted to the NAc suppressed FAA in rats. An earlier study in which the entire NAc was removed did not observe reduced FAA in food restricted rats, indicating that while components of the NAc may participate in expression of FAA, the structure cannot be the source of signals critical for timing FAA [51]. A modulatory role for the NAc is also suggested by the results of recent studies of ghrelin-deficient mice, which expressed less FAA in some studies, and have reduced c-Fos expression in the mesolimbic dopamine pathway under restricted feeding conditions [29]. Our c-Fos data are not consistent with a critical role for the NAc given the extremely low preprandial c-Fos induction in mice on CR. On the contrary, the strong induction of c-Fos 2 hours after meal onset is more consistent with a role for the NAc in processing stimuli related to food intake, including its reward properties. The NAc may be more important for anticipating palatable food [30,52], although this remains to be tested directly.

In conclusion, the results of our study underscore the importance of feeding schedule parameters for the expression of behavioral and neural correlates of FAA in mice. Mice provided food at the same time every day may show weak FAA if CR is modest. This raises the possibility that neural, genetic or endocrine manipulations could reduce FAA without impinging on the food-entrainable clock mechanism, by reducing metabolic activity and thereby effectively reducing the degree of CR expressed relative to caloric needs. The results of our study also raise questions about the role of several hypothalamic structures thought to be important for induction of FAA. We established that a 60% CR schedule induces robust FAA in mice, but using this schedule failed to observe food anticipatory increases in c-Fos in the DMH, VMH, PVN, Arc, or LHA of mice after ~30 days of restricted feeding. By contrast, most of these structures showed robust elevation of c-Fos 2-h after meal onset. These results demonstrate that neural activity in the hypothalamus and other regions can be dissociated from FAA in CR mice, as has previously been reported in rats and mice anticipating a palatable daily snack without CR [28,30,53]. In the absence of convincing evidence that FAA is eliminated by lesions confined to any one brain structure, many researchers in the field now favor the idea that FAA is regulated by a distributed population of FEOs [2,9,30,33,54,55,56]. This model would seem to predict activation of multiple regions in the brain preceding scheduled meal time, but this was not evident in our study. It is certainly possible that FAA output may involve reductions in activity in some structures (e.g., the SCN) and activation in other structures that is not reflected in marked c-Fos expression, or there may have been c-Fos entrainment in structures not thoroughly examined in this study (e.g., brain stem nuclei). This issue may require alternative measures of neural activity for clarification.

Supporting Information

Figure S1 Correlation of normalized food anticipatory activity in the 3 hours preceding scheduled feeding with % body weight loss at Day 7 (A), Day 14 (B), Day 21 (C), Day 35 (D), and Day 42 (E).
(EPS)

Author Contributions

Conceived and designed the experiments: CMG CTH KMG ADS. Performed the experiments: CMG CTH KMG MP CHC REM ADS. Analyzed the data: CMG CTH REM ADS. Wrote the paper: CMG CTH REM ADS.

References

1. Tahara Y, Shibata S (2013) Chronobiology and nutrition. Neuroscience 253: 78–88.
2. Blum ID, Lamont EW, Abizaid A (2012) Competing clocks: metabolic status moderates signals from the master circadian pacemaker. Neurosci Biobehav Rev 36: 254–270.
3. Challet E, Mendoza J (2010) Metabolic and reward feeding synchronises the rhythmic brain. Cell Tissue Res 341: 1–11.
4. Schroeder AM, Colwell CS (2013) How to fix a broken clock. Trends Pharmacol Sci 34: 605–619.
5. Morin LP, Allen CN (2006) The circadian visual system, 2005. Brain Res Rev 51: 1–60.
6. Morin LP (2013) Neuroanatomy of the extended circadian rhythm system. Exp Neurol 243: 4–20.
7. Deurveilher S, Semba K (2005) Indirect projections from the suprachiasmatic nucleus to major arousal-promoting cell groups in rat: implications for the circadian control of behavioural state. Neuroscience 130: 165–183.
8. Canteras NS, Ribeiro-Barbosa ER, Goto M, Cipolla-Neto J, Swanson LW (2011) The retinohypothalamic tract: comparison of axonal projection patterns from four major targets. Brain Res Rev 65: 150–183.
9. Mistlberger RE (2011) Neurobiology of food anticipatory circadian rhythms. Physiol Behav 104: 535–545.
10. Mistlberger RE (1994) Circadian food-anticipatory activity: formal models and physiological mechanisms. Neurosci Biobehav Rev 18: 171–195.
11. Stephan FK, Swann JM, Sisk CL (1979) Entrainment of circadian rhythms by feeding schedules in rats with suprachiasmatic lesions. Behav Neural Biol 25: 545–554.
12. Stephan FK (1983) Circadian rhythm dissociation induced by periodic feeding in rats with suprachiasmatic lesions. Behav Brain Res 7: 81–98.
13. Takasu NN, Kurosawa G, Tokuda IT, Mochizuki A, Todo T, et al. (2012) Circadian regulation of food-anticipatory activity in molecular clock-deficient mice. PLoS One 7: e48892.
14. Mendoza J, Albrecht U, Challet E (2010) Behavioural food anticipation in clock genes deficient mice: confirming old phenotypes, describing new phenotypes. Genes Brain Behav 9: 467–477.
15. Storch KF, Weitz CJ (2009) Daily rhythms of food-anticipatory behavioral activity do not require the known circadian clock. Proc Natl Acad Sci U S A 106: 6808–6813.
16. Pendergast JS, Nakamura W, Friday RC, Hatanaka F, Takumi T, et al. (2009) Robust food anticipatory activity in BMAL1-deficient mice. PLoS One 4: e4860.
17. Pitts S, Perone E, Silver R (2003) Food-entrained circadian rhythms are sustained in arrhythmic Clk/Clk mutant mice. Am J Physiol Regul Integr Comp Physiol 285: R57–67.
18. Gunapala KM, Gallardo CM, Hsu CT, Steele AD (2011) Single gene deletions of orexin, leptin, neuropeptide Y, and ghrelin do not appreciably alter food anticipatory activity in mice. PLoS One 6: e18377.
19. Akiyama M, Yuasa T, Hayasaka N, Horikawa K, Sakurai T, et al. (2004) Reduced food anticipatory activity in genetically orexin (hypocretin) neuron-ablated mice. Eur J Neurosci 20: 3054–3062.
20. Blum ID, Patterson Z, Khazall R, Lamont EW, Sleeman MW, et al. (2009) Reduced anticipatory locomotor responses to scheduled meals in ghrelin receptor deficient mice. Neuroscience 164: 351–359.
21. Kaur S, Thankachan S, Begum S, Blanco-Centurion C, Sakurai T, et al. (2008) Entrainment of temperature and activity rhythms to restricted feeding in orexin knock out mice. Brain Res 1205: 47–54.
22. LeSauter J, Hoque N, Weintraub M, Pfaff DW, Silver R (2009) Stomach ghrelin-secreting cells as food-entrainable circadian clocks. Proc Natl Acad Sci U S A 106: 13582–13587.
23. Sutton GM, Perez-Tilve D, Nogueiras R, Fang J, Kim JK, et al. (2008) The melanocortin-3 receptor is required for entrainment to meal intake. J Neurosci 28: 12946–12955.
24. Szentirmai E, Kapas L, Sun Y, Smith RG, Krueger JM (2010) Restricted feeding-induced sleep, activity, and body temperature changes in normal and preproghrelin-deficient mice. Am J Physiol Regul Integr Comp Physiol 298: R467–477.
25. de Vasconcelos AP, Bartol-Munier I, Feillet CA, Gourmelen S, Pevet P, et al. (2006) Modifications of local cerebral glucose utilization during circadian food-anticipatory activity. Neuroscience 139: 741–748.
26. Verwey M, Amir S (2011) Nucleus-specific effects of meal duration on daily profiles of Period1 and Period2 protein expression in rats housed under restricted feeding. Neuroscience 192: 304–311.
27. Gravotta L, Gavrila AM, Hood S, Amir S (2011) Global Depletion of Dopamine Using Intracerebroventricular 6-Hydroxydopamine Injection Disrupts Normal Circadian Wheel-Running Patterns and PERIOD2 Expression in the Rat Forebrain. J Mol Neurosci.
28. Gallardo CM, Gunapala KM, King OD, Steele AD (2012) Daily scheduled high fat meals moderately entrain behavioral anticipatory activity, body temperature, and hypothalamic c-Fos activation. PLoS One 7: e41161.
29. Lamont EW, Patterson Z, Rodrigues T, Vallejos O, Blum ID, et al. (2012) Ghrelin-deficient mice have fewer orexin cells and reduced cFOS expression in the mesolimbic dopamine pathway under a restricted feeding paradigm. Neuroscience 218: 12–19.
30. Mendoza J, Angeles-Castellanos M, Escobar C (2005) Entrainment by a palatable meal induces food-anticipatory activity and c-Fos expression in reward-related areas of the brain. Neuroscience 133: 293–303.
31. Mieda M, Williams SC, Richardson JA, Tanaka K, Yanagisawa M (2006) The dorsomedial hypothalamic nucleus as a putative food-entrainable circadian pacemaker. Proc Natl Acad Sci U S A 103: 12150–12155.
32. Ribeiro AC, Sawa E, Carren-LeSauter I, LeSauter J, Silver R, et al. (2007) Two forces for arousal: Pitting hunger versus circadian influences and identifying neurons responsible for changes in behavioral arousal. Proc Natl Acad Sci U S A 104: 20078–20083.
33. Blum ID, Lamont EW, Rodrigues T, Abizaid A (2012) Isolating neural correlates of the pacemaker for food anticipation. PLoS One 7: e36117.
34. Steele AD, Jackson WS, King OD, Lindquist S (2007) The power of automated high-resolution behavior analysis revealed by its application to mouse models of Huntington's and prion diseases. Proc Natl Acad Sci U S A 104: 1983–1988.
35. Gunapala KM, Chang D, Hsu CT, Manaye K, Drenan RM, et al. (2010) Striatal pathology underlies prion infection-mediated hyperactivity in mice. Prion 4: 302–315.
36. Mistlberger RE, Buijs RM, Challet E, Escobar C, Landry GJ, et al. (2009) Food anticipation in Bmal1−/− and AAV-Bmal1 rescued mice: a reply to Fuller, et al. J Circadian Rhythms 7: 11.
37. Chen D, Steele AD, Lindquist S, Guarente L (2005) Increase in activity during calorie restriction requires Sirt1. Science 310: 1641.
38. Boily G, Seifert EL, Bevilacqua L, He XH, Sabourin G, et al. (2008) SirT1 regulates energy metabolism and response to caloric restriction in mice. PLoS One 3: e1759.
39. Luby MD, Hsu CT, Shuster SA, Gallardo CM, Mistlberger RE, et al. (2012) Food anticipatory activity behavior of mice across a wide range of circadian and non-circadian intervals. PLoS One 7: e37992.
40. Acosta-Galvan G, Yi CX, van der Vliet J, Jhamandas JH, Panula P, et al. (2011) Interaction between hypothalamic dorsomedial nucleus and the suprachiasmatic nucleus determines intensity of food anticipatory behavior. Proc Natl Acad Sci U S A 108: 5813–5818.
41. Poulin A-M, Timofeeva E (2008) The dynamics of neuronal activation during food anticipation and feeding in the brain of food-entrained rats. Brain research 1227: 128–141.
42. Balthasar N, Coppari R, McMinn J, Liu SM, Lee CE, et al. (2004) Leptin receptor signaling in POMC neurons is required for normal body weight homeostasis. Neuron 42: 983–991.
43. Mendoza J, Angeles-Castellanos M, Escobar C (2005) Differential role of the accumbens Shell and Core subterritories in food-entrained rhythms of rats. Behav Brain Res 158: 133–142.
44. Mendoza J, Pevet P, Felder-Schmittbuhl MP, Bailly Y, Challet E (2010) The cerebellum harbors a circadian oscillator involved in food anticipation. J Neurosci 30: 1894–1904.
45. Gooley JJ, Schomer A, Saper CB (2006) The dorsomedial hypothalamic nucleus is critical for the expression of food-entrainable circadian rhythms. Nat Neurosci 9: 398–407.
46. Landry GJ, Simon MM, Webb IC, Mistlberger RE (2006) Persistence of a behavioral food-anticipatory circadian rhythm following dorsomedial hypothalamic ablation in rats. Am J Physiol Regul Integr Comp Physiol 290: R1527–1534.
47. Moriya T, Aida R, Kudo T, Akiyama M, Doi M, et al. (2009) The dorsomedial hypothalamic nucleus is not necessary for food-anticipatory circadian rhythms of behavior, temperature or clock gene expression in mice. Eur J Neurosci 29: 1447–1460.
48. Mistlberger RE (2006) Circadian rhythms: perturbing a food-entrained clock. Curr Biol 16: R968–969.
49. Landry GJ, Kent BA, Patton DF, Jaholkowski M, Marchant EG, et al. (2011) Evidence for time-of-day dependent effect of neurotoxic dorsomedial hypothalamic lesions on food anticipatory circadian rhythms in rats. PLoS One 6: e24187.
50. Angeles-Castellanos M, Salgado-Delgado R, Rodriguez K, Buijs R, Escobar C (2010) The suprachiasmatic nucleus participates in food entrainment: a lesion study. Neuroscience 165: 1115–1126.
51. Mistlberger RE, Mumby DG (1992) The limbic system and food-anticipatory circadian rhythms in the rat: ablation and dopamine blocking studies. Behav Brain Res 47: 159–168.
52. Angeles-Castellanos M, Salgado-Delgado R, Rodriguez K, Buijs RM, Escobar C (2008) Expectancy for food or expectancy for chocolate reveals timing systems for metabolism and reward. Neuroscience 155: 297–307.
53. Mendoza J, Angeles-Castellanos M, Escobar C (2005) A daily palatable meal without food deprivation entrains the suprachiasmatic nucleus of rats. Eur J Neurosci 22: 2855–2862.
54. Mistlberger RE, Kent BA, Chan S, Patton DF, Weinberg A, et al. (2012) Circadian clocks for all meal-times: anticipation of 2 daily meals in rats. PLoS One 7: e31772.
55. Escobar C, Cailotto C, Angeles-Castellanos M, Delgado RS, Buijs RM (2009) Peripheral oscillators: the driving force for food-anticipatory activity. Eur J Neurosci 30: 1665–1675.

56. Feillet CA, Mendoza J, Albrecht U, Pevet P, Challet E (2008) Forebrain oscillators ticking with different clock hands. Mol Cell Neurosci 37: 209–221.

57. Paxinos G, Franklin K (2007) The mouse brain in stereotaxic coordinates. El Sevier Academic Press.

13

Rats Eat a Cafeteria-Style Diet to Excess but Eat Smaller Amounts and Less Frequently when Tested with Chow

Timothy South[1]◔, Nathan M. Holmes[2]◔, Sarah I. Martire[2], R. Frederick Westbrook[2], Margaret J. Morris[1]*

1 Department of Pharmacology, School of Medical Sciences, University of New South Wales, Sydney, Australia, **2** Department of Psychology, University of New South Wales, Sydney, Australia

Abstract

Background: Obesity is associated with excessive consumption of palatable, energy dense foods. The present study used an animal model to examine feeding patterns during exposure to and withdrawal from these foods.

Methods: Male Sprague Dawley rats were exposed to standard lab chow only (Chow rats) or a range of cafeteria-style foods eaten by people (Caf rats). After 1, 4, 7 and 10 weeks of diet in their home cage, rats were subjected to 24-hour test sessions in a Comprehensive Lab Animal Monitoring System (CLAMS). In the first two test sessions, Chow rats were exposed to standard lab chow only while Caf rats were exposed to a biscuit and high-fat chow diet. In the final two test sessions, half the rats in each group were switched to the opposing diet. In each session we recorded numbers of bouts, energy consumed per bout, and intervals between bouts across the entire 24 hours.

Results: Relative to Chow rats, Caf rats initiated fewer bouts but consumed more energy per bout; however, their motivation to feed in the CLAMS declined over time, which was attributed to reduced variety of foods relative to their home cage diet. This decline in motivation was especially pronounced among Caf rats switched from the palatable CLAMS diet to standard lab chow only: the reduced energy intake in this group was due to a modest decline in bout frequency and a dramatic decline in bout size.

Conclusions: Exposure to a cafeteria-diet, rich in variety, altered feeding patterns, reduced rats' motivation to consume palatable foods in the absence of variety, and further diminished motivation to feed when palatable foods were withdrawn and replaced with chow. Hence, variety is a key factor in driving excessive consumption of energy dense foods, and therefore, excessive weight gain.

Editor: Silvana Gaetani, Sapienza University of Rome, Italy

Funding: This research was supported by a project grant (568728) from the National Health and Medical Research Council of Australia. The funders had no role in study design, data collection and analysis, decision to publish, or preparation of the manuscript.

Competing Interests: Fred Westbrook has served as an academic editor for PLOS ONE. Note that this does not alter the authors' adherence to all the PLOS ONE policies on sharing data and materials, as detailed online in the guide for authors.

* E-mail: m.morris@unsw.edu.au

◔ These authors contributed equally to this work.

Introduction

The consumption of palatable energy dense foods has increased dramatically over the past forty years. This increased consumption has pushed rates of obesity to epidemic proportions among children, adolescents and adults across the world [1]. Excessive consumption of palatable energy dense foods leads to weight gain, but it is unclear how exposures to these foods influence eating patterns, particularly during the development of obesity. The fact that palatable energy dense foods are hedonically attractive, widely available and relatively cheap means that, compared to forty years ago, people today may eat more frequently (e.g., snacking), consume more each time they eat (e.g., increased portion size), or some combination of these factors. Alternatively, eating patterns may have changed very little in the last forty years: instead, people may have become overweight and obese in record numbers simply because the available foods are more energy dense.

Studies of eating patterns and how they change over time are difficult to conduct in people. It is difficult to ensure compliance, and therefore, to track eating across a prolonged period (like that which leads to obesity). Even when compliance is achieved, the nature of self-report data means it is difficult to verify the type and amount of foods that people eat. For these reasons, animal studies have been used to examine behavioural and biological factors that regulate feeding, and how exposure to palatable energy dense foods changes feeding patterns. In the latter respect, several investigators have reported that rodents, like people, prefer foods that are rich in fat and sugar, eat them to excess and become overweight [2–4]. We have shown that rats exposed to a range of the energy dense foods eaten by people also prefer these foods to chow, eat them to excess, become overweight, and display hallmarks of obesity [5–6]. Martire, Holmes, Westbrook and Morris (2013) recently examined how this cafeteria style diet affected feeding patterns [7]. Across several weeks of diet, rats exposed to the cafeteria diet initiated fewer meals (feeding immediately followed by grooming and sleeping, a sequence indicative of behavioural satiety) than rats exposed to standard lab chow. However during the early stages of diet exposure, rats exposed to the cafeteria diet snacked more than their chow-fed counterparts; and the early levels of snacking were directly related to terminal body weights.

Other evidence suggests that motivation to consume diets of varying palatability changes with extended exposure to a cafeteria-style diet. Naïve rats exposed to palatable foods for the first time consumed twice-as-much energy as rats with a history of exposure to these foods [8]. Conversely, when rats exposed to a cafeteria diet were subsequently switched to standard lab chow, they ate less than rats only fed chow, lost weight, and exhibited signs of hypothalamic-pituitary-adrenal (HPA) axis activation, evident as increased corticotrophin releasing factor (CRF) mRNA expression [8–9]. Whilst previous studies have examined the microstructure of feeding on palatable diets during the development of obesity, few have examined how feeding patterns change when a palatable diet is withdrawn. A notable exception is a study by Rogers (1985) who exposed rats to a diet composed of chow supplemented with white bread, milk chocolate and biscuits and then switched them to chow only [10]. He reported that the rats became hypophagic due to eating fewer meals and eating less on average at each meal. Rogers attributed this change in eating pattern, at least in part, to a negative contrast effect whereby the hedonic value of the chow was reduced because of the prior exposure to the highly palatable bread, chocolate and biscuits.

The present study had two aims. The first was to provide a further examination of feeding patterns among rats exposed to either a cafeteria diet or standard lab chow. Martire et al (2013) showed that exposure to a cafeteria-style diet influences the regularity of meals and snacks; however, the fact that feeding behaviour was examined in the home cage prohibited measurement of the energy density of each meal or snack. Here, we assessed feeding behaviour directed towards standard lab chow or palatable foods (biscuit and high-fat chow) using the Comprehensive Lab Animal Monitoring System (CLAMS), which permitted a more detailed examination of feeding frequency, amounts eaten, and the relationship between these measures. The second aim was to examine changes in feeding patterns among: (1) rats exposed to palatable foods for the first time; and (2) rats maintained on the cafeteria diet and then withdrawn from this diet for the first time (i.e., switched to standard lab chow only). Based on the results reported by South et al (2012), we expected that, relative to controls, rats exposed to palatable foods for the first time in the CLAMS would consume more, while rats withdrawn from the cafeteria diet for the first time in the CLAMS would consume less. Based on the results reported by Rogers (1985), we expected that rats withdrawn from the cafeteria diet would not only eat less but that this would be due to them eating fewer and smaller meals. Conversely, we expected that rats exposed to chow and given palatable foods would eat more and larger meals.

Materials and Methods

1. Animal procedures

Male Sprague–Dawley rats (n = 48) were obtained from a commercial supplier (Animal Resource Centre, Perth, Australia) and maintained in a colony room kept at 23°C and on a 12 h light:12 h dark cycle (lights on at 07:00). Rats were housed in polypropylene cages (20 cm length ×32 cm width ×19 cm height) whose floors were covered with wood shavings. There were three rats per cage. Standard rat chow (CH, 11 kJ/g, energy 12% fat, 21% protein, 65% carbohydrate, Gordon's Specialty Stock feeds, NSW, Australia) and tap water were provided *ad libitum* throughout the experiment. Rats were handled daily and familiarized with the CLAMS in a single four hour session on one of these days. Following this acclimatization to the laboratory, half the rats (n = 24) were assigned to standard chow and half (n = 24) to the cafeteria diet which contained lab chow, modified chow [60% powdered chow mixed with 33% sweetened condensed milk and 7% saturated animal fat (pork lard)], as well as various foods (15.3 kJ/g, energy 32% fat, 14% protein, and 60% carbohydrate) selected from cakes, cookies, dim sims, pasta and meat pies. The foods selected were changed daily but always included one food (meat pies or dim sims) high in protein and two (cakes, biscuits, or pasta) high in carbohydrates and/or sugar. Food was provided daily at 17:00. Food intake was recorded once a week by measuring the amount of food provided at 17.00 hr and that remaining 24 hr later (with spillage taken into account).

Ethics Statement. All procedures were approved by the Animal Care and Ethics Committee of the University of New South Wales and were consistent with guidelines for animal research by the Australian National Health and Medical Research Council.

2. Feeding in the Comprehensive Lab Animal Monitoring System (CLAMS)

All rats were removed from their home cages and placed in individual plexiglass cages (60 cm length ×20 cm width ×20 cm height) of the Comprehensive Lab Animal Monitoring System (CLAMS; Columbus Instruments, Columbus, OH). During CLAMS monitoring, feeding was assessed using ground food placed in 24 metal floor feeders, each attached to the CLAMS plexiglass cages (two feeders/cage). Feeders rested on balances directly linked to a computer for measuring continuous food intake (every thirty seconds). During each of the CLAMS sessions, cumulative food intake was automatically recorded for 24 h. A bout was defined as a period of continuous eating: the minimum bout duration was the resolution at which data were collected in the CLAMS, 30 s; two consecutive 30 s periods in which feeding occurred was defined as a single 60 s bout; three consecutive 30 s periods in which feeding occurred was defined as a single 90 s bout; and so forth.

All rats were tested in the CLAMS apparatus across four sessions. These sessions occurred one, four, seven and 10 weeks after diet exposure, each lasted 24 hours, and commenced at 15:00. In the first two sessions, rats were exposed to foods consistent with their home-cage history. Rats maintained on the cafeteria diet in their home cage, termed 'Caf' rats, were exposed to two palatable (PAL) foods: powdered, sweetened high fat chow (14% Fat, 40% Carbohydrate, 8% Protein) and powdered shortbread cookies (20% Fat, 71% Carbohydrate, 6.5% Protein). Rats maintained on standard lab chow in their home cage, termed 'Chow' rats, were exposed to the same standard lab chow in the CLAMS but in powdered form (4% Fat, 50% Carbohydrate, 14% Protein). In the final two sessions, half of the Caf rats were again exposed to biscuit and high-fat chow (Group Caf-PAL); and half of the Chow rats were again exposed to standard lab chow (Group Chow-CHOW). Remaining Caf rats were exposed to standard lab chow in the CLAMS for the first time (Group Caf-CHOW) and remaining Chow rats were exposed to palatable biscuit and high-fat chow for the first time (Group Chow-PAL; see Table 1). Water was continuously available in the clams.

3. Statistical Analysis

3a. Home cage 24-hour energy intake (kJ) and body weight. During each of the weeks in which rats were subjected

Table 1. Description of groups used in the current experiment.

	Palatable diet in CLAMS	Chow only in CLAMS
Cafeteria diet in home cage	Caf-PAL	Caf-CHOW
Chow only in home cage	Chow-PAL	Chow-CHOW

to CLAMS test sessions, one 24-hour period was selected for measurement of home cage energy intake. This consisted in weighing the food prior to placement in the home cage, and after a period of 24 hours, any food leftover was weighed. The difference in weight of each food was used to calculate total 24-hour energy intake for the three rats in each home cage. The average intake per cage was analyzed by ANOVA with a between-subjects factor of group (Caf versus Chow) and a within-subjects factor of time (across four time points of the study). The body weights of individual rats were also recorded during these same periods and analyzed by ANOVA with a between-subjects factor of group (Caf versus Chow) and a within-subjects factor of time (across four time points of the study).

3b. Feeding in Caf and Chow rats. We conducted three analyses. Analysis 1 examined feeding patterns in Caf and Chow rats, focusing on feeding in Groups Caf-PAL and Chow-CHOW across the four CLAMS test sessions, and within each CLAMS test session. Analysis 2 examined the effect of a diet switch on feeding by Caf and Chow rats. Here, we focused on changes in feeding patterns in Group Chow-PAL relative to Group Caf-PAL, and Group Caf-CHOW relative to Group Chow-CHOW. Analysis 3 examined the more acute effects of a diet switch. We directly compared feeding in Group Chow-PAL during its first exposure to the palatable biscuit and high-fat chow in week 7 with feeding in Group Caf-PAL during its first exposure to the palatable biscuit and high-fat chow in week 1. We also compared feeding in Group Caf-CHOW during its first exposure to standard lab chow in the CLAMS in week 7 with feeding in Group Chow-CHOW during its first exposure to chow in the CLAMS in week 1.

Analyses 1 and 2 progressed in four stages. First, levels of energy intake (kJ) were submitted to ANOVA with a between-subjects factor of group (Caf-PAL vs. Chow-CHOW) and within-subjects factors of test session (Sessions 1–4) and time (blocks of four hours within a session). Second, numbers of bouts and energy intake per bout were submitted to ANOVA with group as a between-subjects factor (Caf-PAL vs. Chow-CHOW) and test session as a within-subjects factor (Sessions 1–4). Third, distributions of inter-bout intervals and bout sizes were generated by pooling these data across rats within groups, and the Kolmogorov-Smirnov (abbreviated to K-S) test was used to assess differences in the distributions between the groups. Finally, average bout size was plotted against average inter-bout interval for individual rats in each group, and Pearson product-moment correlations were used to assess the degree of linearity in the relationship between these variables.

In Analysis 3, single factor ANOVAs were used to separately compare Groups Caf-PAL and Chow-PAL, and Groups Caf-CHOW and Chow-CHOW on each of the following measures: total energy intake, numbers of bouts, and energy intake per bout (bout size). Thereafter, average bout size was plotted against average inter-bout interval for individual rats in each group. The degree of linearity in the relationship between these variables was assessed using Pearson product-moment correlations.

At each stage of each analysis, the criterion for rejection of the null hypothesis was set at alpha = .05.

Results

1. Home cage 24-hour energy intake (kJ) and body weight

Figure 1 shows average energy intake (kJ, 1A) and body weight (1B) for all Caf and all Chow rats across the duration of the experiment. Analysis of the energy intake data confirmed that, overall, Caf rats consumed more energy than Chow rats, $F(1,6) = 228.59$, $p<.01$. Critically, the size of the difference in energy intake between the two groups was most pronounced during the early weeks of diet exposure, evidenced by a statistically significant group x (linear) interaction, $F(1,6) = 6.86$, $p<.05$. However, even in the final week of diet exposure, it is clear that, Caf rats consumed almost double the amount of energy as Chow rats. Analysis of body weight data also showed that, averaged over groups, there was a linear increase in body weight across weeks of the study, $F(1,46) = 2059.77$, $p<.01$, and that the rate of increase was greater for Caf than Chow rats, group x (linear) interaction, $F(1,46) = 93.12$, $p<.01$. Consequently, Caf rats became significantly heavier than Chow rats, $F(1,46) = 49.84$, $p<.01$. In sum, Caf rats consumed more energy and gained weight more rapidly than Chow rats.

2. Feeding in Caf and Chow rats

2a. Changes in energy intake (kJ) between and within 24-hour CLAMS test sessions. Figure 2 shows energy intake (kJ) across blocks of four hours for Caf-PAL and Chow-CHOW rats in each of the CLAMS test sessions. It is clear that Caf rats consumed more kJ than Chow rats when they were first introduced to the CLAMS in week 1 (2A), but that energy intake in the two groups was equivalent thereafter as energy intake declined across and within test sessions (2B–D). The statistical analysis confirmed a significant decline in energy intake between-, $F(1,22) = 37.26$, $p<.01$, and within-sessions, $F(1,22) = 81.27$, $p<.01$. Critically, both of these effects interacted with Group, smaller $F(1,22) = 8.22$, $p<.01$; and the three-way interaction between Group, test and time was also significant, $F(1,22) = 26.94$, $p<.01$.

To determine the source of the three-way interaction, the data from each test session were submitted to ANOVA with factors of Group and time. In Week 1, Caf rats consumed more energy than Chow rats, $F(1,22) = 126.05$, $p<.01$. A significant group x time interaction confirmed that this difference between the two groups was most pronounced during the early stages of the test session, $F(1,22) = 33.01$, $p<.01$. Analyses of the data from each of the remaining test sessions (in weeks 4, 7 and 10) showed that energy intake declined over time, smallest $F(1,22) = 12.54$, $p<.01$. The rate of this decline was equivalent for Caf and Chow rats: the Group x time interaction was not significant, $Fs<1$; and overall, there was no significant difference in energy intake between the two groups, $Fs<2.36$.

2b. Changes in bout number and bout size between sessions. *Number of bouts* Figure 3A shows the total numbers of bouts in each of the CLAMS test sessions for Caf-PAL and Chow-CHOW rats. It is clear that the numbers of bouts declined across

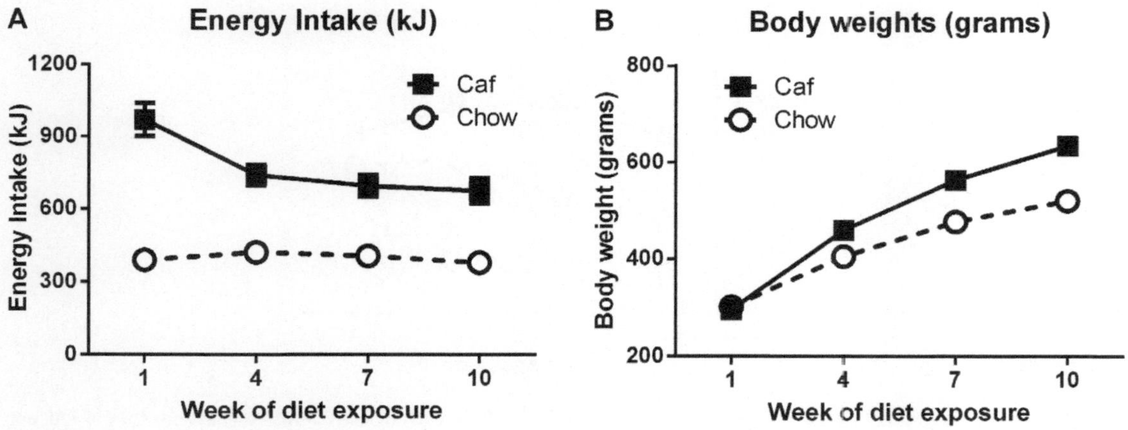

Figure 1. Home cage energy intake. Average home cage 24-hour energy intake (kJ, **A**) and individual body weights of Caf and Chow rats (**B**) across the duration of the experiment. Each data point represents the mean (+SEM) for the particular unit of analysis.

test sessions, and that this decline was more pronounced for Caf-PAL than Chow-CHOW rats. The analysis of these data revealed significant linear and quadratic components to the decline in bout numbers across test sessions, smaller $F(1,22) = 20.02$, $p<.01$, the latter of which interacted with Group, $F(1,22) = 7.06$, $p<.05$. This reflects the finding that Caf-PAL rats had fewer bouts than Chow-CHOW rats in the middle test sessions; indeed, Caf-PAL rats had fewer bouts than Chow-CHOW rats overall, $F(1,22) = 7.32$, $p<.05$.

Bout size Figure 3B shows the average bout size in each of the CLAMS test sessions for Caf-PAL and Chow-CHOW rats. Bout size increased across test sessions, $F(1,22) = 11.73$, $p<.01$, and the rate of this increase was greater for Chow-CHOW than Caf-PAL

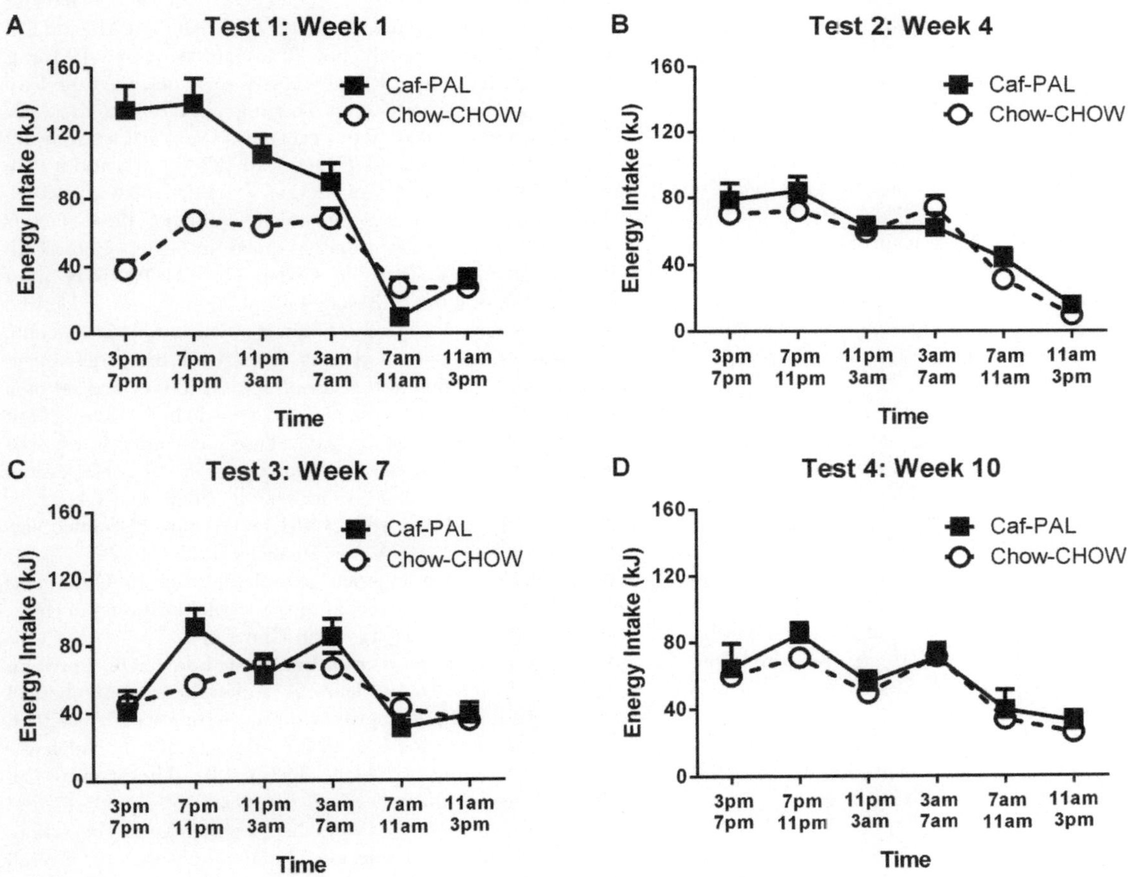

Figure 2. CLAMS energy intake. (**A–D**) Energy intake (kJ) for Caf-PAL and Chow-CHOW rats in each of the 24-hour CLAMS test sessions. Each data point is the mean (+SEM) energy intake in a block of four hours.

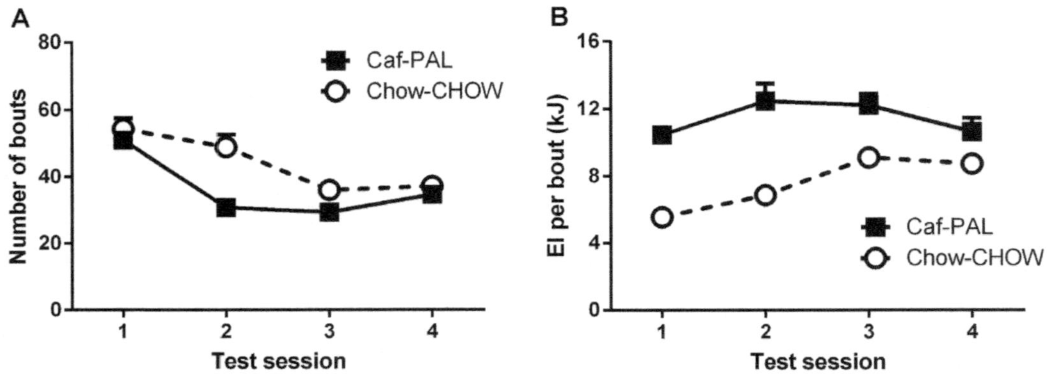

Figure 3. Bout frequency and size. Total numbers of bouts (**A**) and average bout size (**B**) in each of the CLAMS test sessions for Caf-PAL and Chow-CHOW rats. Each data point represents the mean (+SEM) for the entire session.

rats, $F\,(1,22) = 10.76$, $p<.01$. However, overall, Caf-PAL rats had larger bouts than Chow-CHOW rats, $F\,(1,22) = 52.55$, $p<.01$.

In summary, Caf-PAL rats consumed more energy than Chow-CHOW rats in the CLAMS during the early but not late stages of diet exposure. Despite equivalent energy intake during the late stages of diet exposure, the two groups differed in the way energy was obtained: Caf-PAL rats initiated fewer bouts than Chow-CHOW rats, but on average, each bout was higher in energy.

2c. Distributions of waiting times (between bouts) and bout sizes. Figures 4A–D show the distributions of inter-bout intervals and bout sizes for Caf-PAL and Chow-CHOW rats during the first and last test sessions. In the first test session, Caf-PAL rats showed a leftward shift in the distribution of inter-bout intervals (Figure 4A), K-S test $<.001$, and a rightward shift in the distribution of bout sizes (Figure 4B), K-S test $<.001$. These shifts reflect the fact that Caf-PAL rats had proportionally more short inter-bout intervals (<2 min), and proportionally more bouts of larger size.

In the final test session, Caf-PAL rats again showed a leftward shift in the distribution of inter-bout intervals (Figure 4C), K-S test $<.001$, but there was no difference in the distribution of bout sizes between the two groups (Figure 4D), K-S test $>.05$. Inspection of the figure shows that the latter result was due to a rightward shift in the distribution for Chow-CHOW rats from week 1 to week 10: that is, an increase in bout size among Chow-CHOW rats as opposed to a decrease in bout size among Caf-PAL rats.

In summary, exposure to a cafeteria diet in the home cage led to a persistent increase in the number of short inter-bout intervals (< 2 min) relative to chow-fed controls, and a transient increase in the numbers of larger bouts (>10 kJ).

2d. Relationship between energy intake and wait times. Figures 4E and F show average bout size plotted against average inter-bout interval for individual Caf-PAL and Chow-CHOW rats in the first (4E) and final (4F) test sessions. Both groups showed a positive relationship between these variables in each test session: this relationship approached significance in the first test session, $r = .52$ for Caf-PAL rats and $r = .56$ for Chow-CHOW rats, larger $t(10) = 2.12$, $p = .06$, and was highly significant in the final test session, $r = .74$ for Caf-PAL rats and $r = .71$ for Chow-CHOW rats, smaller $t(10) = 3.21$, $p<.01$. Thus, rats that consumed more energy per bout waited longer before initiating the next bout or, alternatively, rats that waited longer between bouts consumed more energy per bout.

3. The effect of a diet switch on feeding in Caf and Chow rats

3a. Changes in energy intake (kJ) between and within 24-hour CLAMS test sessions. Figures 5A and B show energy intake (kJ) across blocks of four hours for each of the four groups during the post-switch test sessions. As noted above, at each of these two time points, Caf-PAL and Chow-CHOW rats were equivalent with respect to both total energy intake, and the pattern of energy intake across 24 hours of testing. Relative to each of these groups, there were clear differences in feeding behaviour among Chow rats tested with palatable foods (Chow-PAL) and Caf rats tested with standard lab chow (Caf-CHOW): Chow-PAL rats consumed the most energy, Caf-CHOW rats consumed the least energy, and these effects were most apparent during the early stages of each test session. Statistical analysis revealed a significant main effect of Caf-vs-Chow, $F(1,44) = 109.22$, $p<.01$, and a two-way Caf-vs-Chow x switch interaction, $F(1,44) = 158.83$, $p<.01$.

Higher-order interactions involving both of these factors confirmed that the elevated energy intake in Group Chow-PAL and reduced energy intake in Group Caf-CHOW were most pronounced during the early stages of each test session, evidenced by significant three-way Caf-vs-Chow x switch x time interaction, $F(1,44) = 79.92$, $p<.01$); and that the size of these differences increased from the first to the second test session, evidenced by a significant four-way Caf vs. Chow x switch x time x test interaction, $F(1,44) = 4.60$, $p = .05$. Post-hoc comparisons confirmed that in the first block of four hours in each test session, Chow-PAL rats consumed more energy than Caf-PAL rats, smaller $F(1,22) = 14.29$, while Caf-CHOW rats consumed less energy than Chow-CHOW rats, smaller $F(1,22) = 16.24$.

In summary, when exposed to palatable foods, Chow rats consumed more energy than Caf rats; and when exposed to chow, Caf rats consumed less energy than Chow rats.

3b. Changes in bout number and bout size between sessions. *Number of bouts* Figure 5C shows the total numbers of bouts for each of the four groups during testing. It is clear that, independently of the foods available at test, Caf rats had fewer bouts than Chow rats, $F(1,44) = 16.98$, $p<.01$. The two-way Caf vs. Chow x switch interaction was significant, $F(1,44) = 5.47$, $p<.05$, as was the three-way Caf vs. Chow x switch x test interaction, $F(1,44) = 6.35$, $p<.05$. These interactions imply that the overall difference in bout numbers between Caf and Chow rats was largely due to low numbers of bouts in Caf rats switched from palatable foods to standard lab chow (Caf-CHOW), especially in the final test session. Post-hoc tests of bout numbers in the final

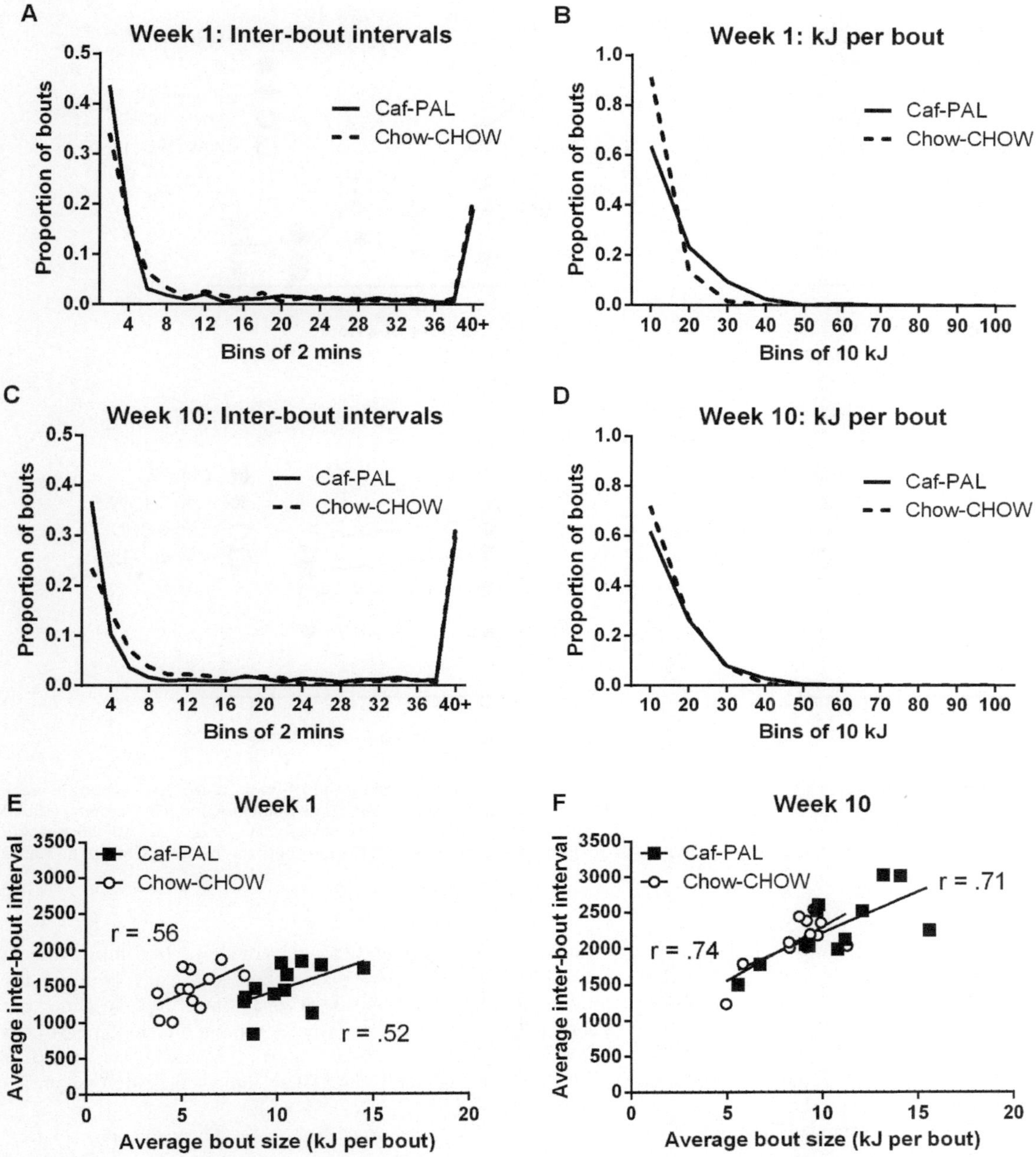

Figure 4. Distributions of inter-bout intervals and bout sizes. (**A & B**) Distributions of inter-bout intervals (A) and bout sizes (B) for Caf-PAL and Chow-CHOW rats during the first CLAMS test session (week 1). (**C & D**) Distributions of inter-bout intervals (C) and bout sizes (D) for Caf-PAL and Chow-CHOW rats during the last CLAMS test session (week 10). (**E & F**) Average bout size (kJ) versus average inter-bout interval for individual Caf-PAL and Chow-CHOW rats in the first (week 1, E) and final (week 10, F) CLAMS test sessions.

session revealed that Caf-CHOW rats had fewer bouts than Chow-CHOW rats, $F(1,22) = 20.36$, but Caf-PAL and Chow-PAL rats did not significantly differ, $F(1,22) = 4.43$.

Bout size Figure 5D shows the average bout size for each of the four groups during testing. It is clear that in both test sessions, Chow-PAL rats had the largest (most energy dense) bouts, Caf-PAL and Chow-CHOW rats had moderately sized bouts, and that Caf-CHOW rats had the smallest bouts. ANOVA revealed a main effect of Caf vs. Lean, $F(1,44) = 22.71$, $p<.01$, which was moderated by a two-way Caf vs. Chow x switch interaction, $F(1,44) = 72.68$, $p<.01$. Post-hoc tests confirmed that average bout size was smaller for Caf-CHOW rats compared to Chow-CHOW rats, $F(1,22) = 39.15$, but Caf-PAL and Chow-PAL rats did not significantly differ, $F(1,22) = 5.46$.

In summary: Caf rats initiated fewer bouts, consumed less energy per bout, and therefore, less energy overall than Chow rats. These differences were largely due to a persistent reduction in consumption of lab chow among Caf rats used to eating a range of palatable foods; and partly due to enhanced consumption of the palatable foods among Chow rats used to eating lab chow.

3c. Distributions of waiting times (between bouts) and bout sizes. Figure 6 shows the distributions of inter-bout

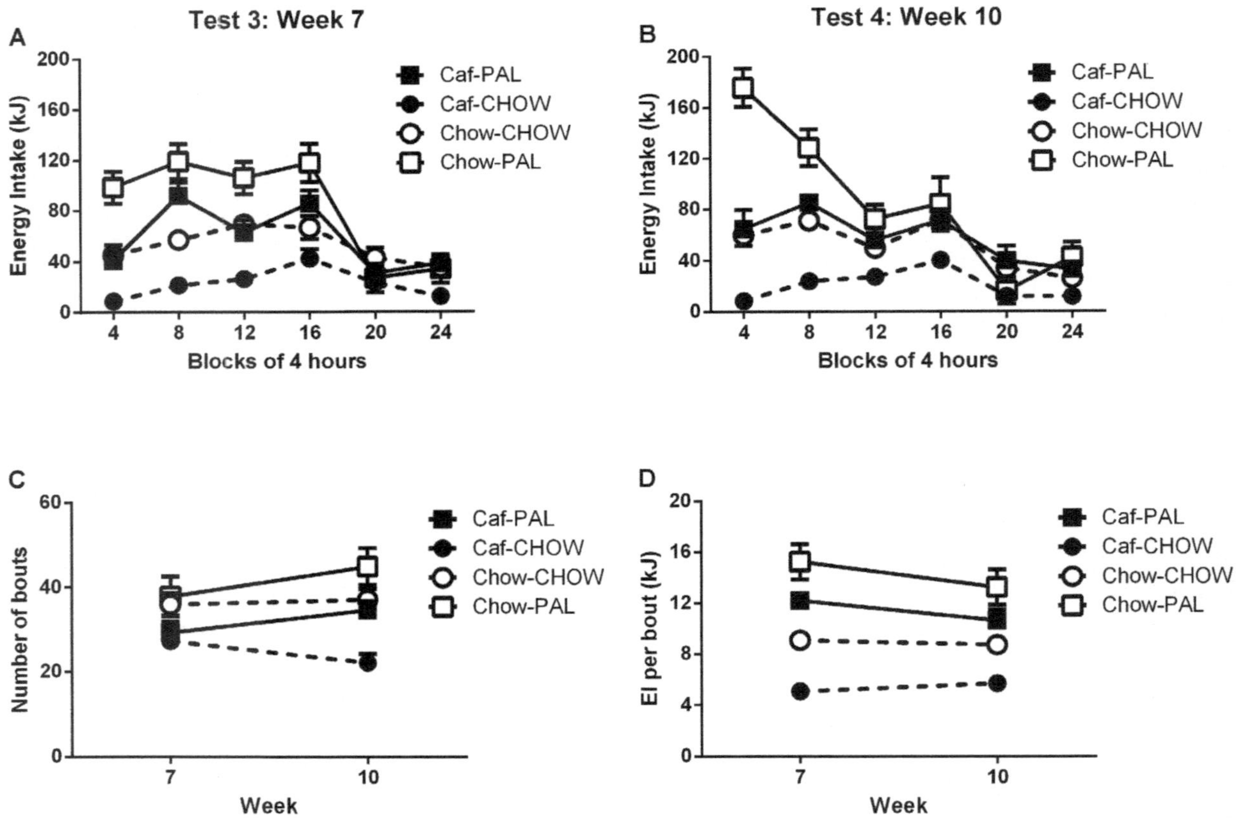

Figure 5. Post-switch CLAMS energy intake. (**A**) Energy intake (kJ) for each of the four groups during the 24-hour CLAMS test sessions in week 7. (**B**) Energy intake (kJ) for each of the four groups during the 24-hour CLAMS test sessions in week 10. Each data point in A and B is the mean (+SEM) energy intake in a block of four hours. (**C**) Total numbers of bouts for each of the four groups during test sessions in weeks 7 and 10. (**D**) Average bout size for each of the four groups during test sessions in weeks 7 and 10. Each data point in C and D represents the mean (+SEM) for an entire session.

intervals (left) and bout sizes (right) for groups tested with either palatable foods (top) or standard lab chow (bottom). The data shown are from the final test session only. Among rats tested with palatable foods, there was a leftward shift in the distribution of inter-bout intervals for Chow-PAL rats relative to Caf-PAL rats (Figure 6A), K-S test $<.001$; and a small but statistically significant rightward shift in the distribution of bout sizes (Figure 6B), K-S test $<.01$. In contrast, among rats tested with standard lab chow, there was a leftward shift in the distribution of bout sizes for Caf-CHOW rats relative to Chow-CHOW rats (Figure 6C), K-S test $<.001$; but there was no difference between these two groups in the distribution of inter-bout intervals (Figure 6D), K-S test $>.05$.

Thus, compared to Caf rats with a history of exposure to palatable foods, Chow rats tested with palatable foods consumed similar sized bouts, but had proportionally more wait times of shorter duration (from one bout to the next); and compared to Chow rats with a history of exposure to chow only, Caf rats tested with chow showed a similar distribution of waiting times to the next bout, but had proportionally more bouts of smaller size.

3d. Consumption of biscuit and high fat chow by rats offered palatable foods. Figure 7 shows the average size (kJ, 7A) and average wait time (7B) to the next bout for Caf-PAL and Chow-PAL rats, separated for bouts consisting of either biscuit only or high-fat chow only. Caf-PAL rats tended to have larger biscuit bouts relative to high-fat chow, especially in the final test session; whereas biscuit and high-fat chow bouts for Chow-PAL rats were similar in terms of their average size. In contrast, among Caf-PAL rats, the average waiting time to the next bout was the same following a bout of biscuit or a bout of high-fat chow; but among Chow-PAL rats, the average waiting time to the next bout was longer following a bout consisting of biscuit versus a bout consisting of high-fat chow. These impressions were supported statistically.

Percent of total energy intake from biscuit The percentage of total energy intake obtained through consumption of biscuit differed between Caf-PAL and Chow-PAL rats: Averaged across the final two test sessions, these percentages were 72% and 49% for Caf-PAL and Chow-PAL rats, respectively. A two-way ANOVA of these data revealed a main effect of group, $F(1,22) = 6.44$, $p<.05$, but no effect of test session and no group x test interaction, $Fs<1$.

Average bout size Averaged across all rats in the two groups, the average size of biscuit bouts was greater than that of high-fat chow, $F(1,22) = 5.91$, $p<.05$. The size of biscuit bouts relative to high-fat chow bouts differed between the two groups, evidenced by a significant two-way food x group interaction, $F(1,22) = 12.29$, $p<.01$; and this difference was most evident in the final test session, evidenced by a significant three-way food x group x test interaction, $F(1,22) = 6.24$, $p<.05$. To identify the source of these interactions, the data from each test session were submitted to ANOVA with factors of group and food. In the first post-switch test session (week 7), there was no overall difference in bout size for biscuit versus high-fat chow, $F(1,22) = 2.4$, no overall difference in

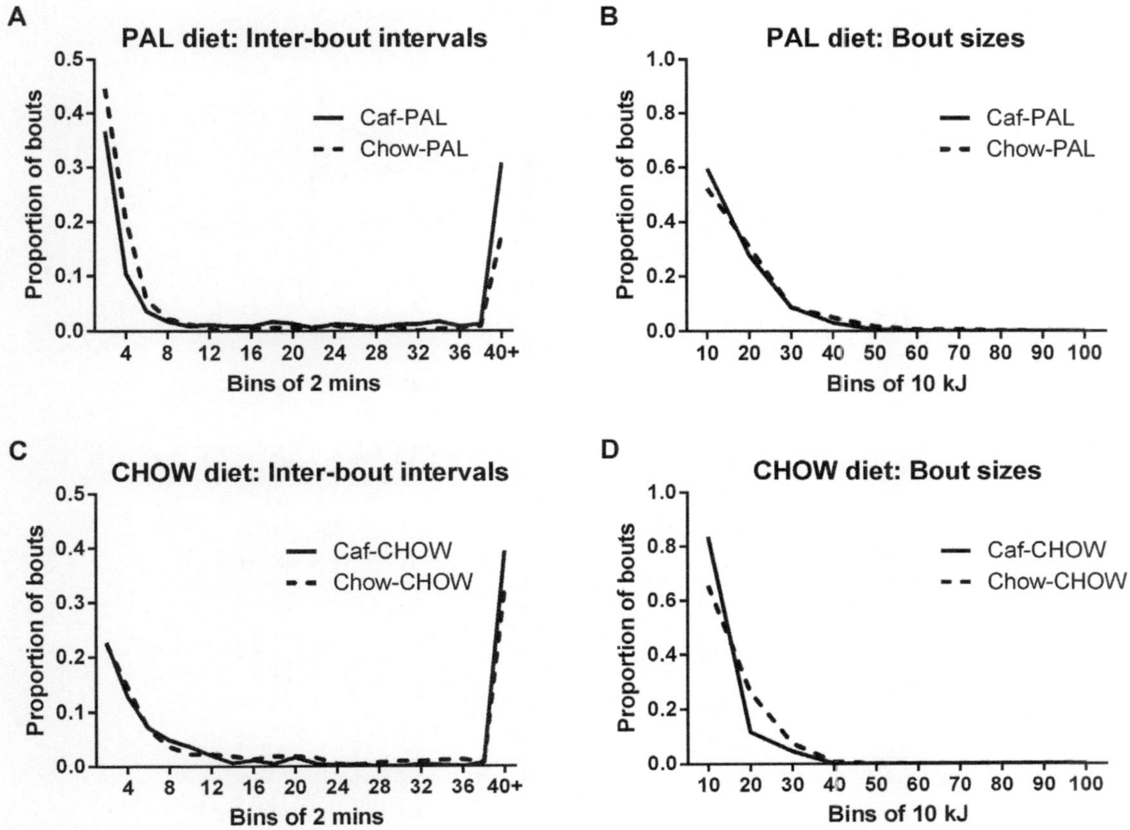

Figure 6. Post-switch distributions of inter-bout intervals and bout sizes. Distributions of inter-bout intervals (left, A & C) and bout sizes (right, B & D) for groups tested with either palatable foods (top, A & B) or standard lab chow (bottom, C & D). The data shown are from the final test session only (in week 10).

bout size between the two groups, $F<1$, and no group x food interaction, $F(1,22) = 4.38$, Fc = 5.76. In the final test session, the main effects of biscuit versus high-fat chow bout, $F(1,22) = 5.34$, and group, $F<1$, were again not significant; but there was a significant interaction between these factors, $F(1,22) = 11.59$, $p < .05$, consistent with larger biscuit bouts than high-fat chow bouts among Caf-PAL rats but not Chow-PAL rats.

Inter-bout intervals Overall, there was no difference in average wait time to the next bout following a bout consisting of biscuit or a bout consisting of high-fat chow, $F(1,22) = 1.44$. However, there was a significant test x food interaction, $F(1,22) = 10.75$, $p<.01$, suggesting that differences in waiting times following a biscuit bout or a high-fat chow bouts changed across testing. Inspection of Figure 7B suggests that this change was due to a decrease in post-high-fat-chow wait times among Caf-PAL rats and an increase in post-biscuit wait times among Chow-PAL rats. However, the two-way food x group interaction only approached significance, $F(1,22) = 3.86$, and the three-way food x group x test interaction was not significant, $F(1,22) = 1.27$.

Figures 7C and D show average bout size plotted against average inter-bout interval for individual Caf-PAL (7C) and Chow-PAL rats (7D) in the final test session, again separated according to bout identity (biscuit or high-fat chow). Among Caf-PAL rats (7C), there was a positive relationship between the amount of biscuit consumed and post-biscuit wait times, $t(10) = 2.62$, $p<.025$; the relationship between amount of high-fat-chow consumed and post-high-fat-chow wait times approached significance, $t(10) = 2.13$, $p = .06$. Chow-PAL rats (7D) also showed a clear positive relationship between amount of high-fat-chow consumed and post-high-fat-chow wait times, $t(10) = 2.30$, $p<.025$; but these rats showed no relationship between the amount of biscuit consumed and post-biscuit wait times, $t<1$.

Figures 7E and F show the corresponding plots for individual Caf-CHOW and Chow-CHOW rats, respectively. Here-Chow-CHOW rats showed a positive relationship between amount of chow consumed and wait times between chow bouts, $t(10) = 3.58$, $p<.01$, whereas Caf-CHOW rats showed no such relationship, $t<1$.

In summary: Caf-PAL rats consumed more biscuit than high-fat chow, both overall and in terms of average bout size, at least by the final session of testing; however, the average waiting times following consumption of either food were equivalent. Chow-PAL rats showed the opposite pattern: they ate equal amounts of biscuit and chow, both overall and in terms of average bout size, but waited longer to the next bout after having eaten biscuit. With the exception of Chow-PAL and Caf-CHOW rats, all groups showed a positive relationship between bout size and wait times: rats that had larger average bout sizes had longer average wait times to the next bout. This relationship was not evident with respect to consumption of biscuit by Chow-PAL rats, or consumption of chow by Caf-CHOW rats.

4. Feeding in switch groups in week 7 relative to Caf and Chow rats in week 1

The top panel of Figure 8 shows total energy intake (8A), numbers of bouts (8B) and bout size (energy intake per bout, 8C)

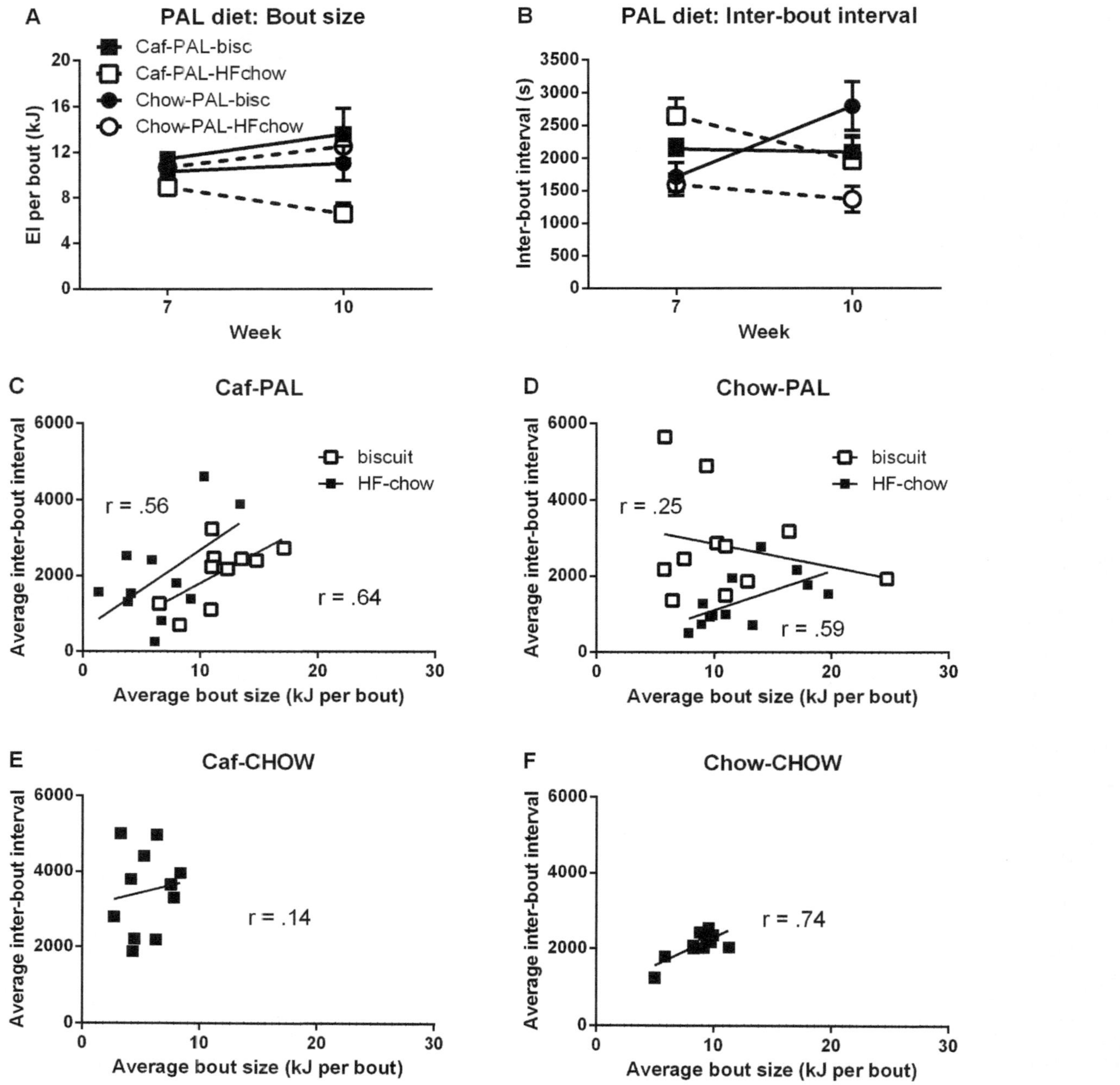

Figure 7. Palatable food consumption in the CLAMS. (**A**) Average bout size (kJ) for Caf-PAL and Chow-PAL rats, separated for bouts consisting of either biscuit only or high-fat chow only. (**B**) Average wait time to the next bout for Caf-PAL and Chow-PAL rats, separated for bouts consisting of either biscuit only or high-fat chow only. Each data point in A and B represents the mean (+SEM) for an entire session. (**C & D**) Average bout size versus average inter-bout interval for individual Caf-PAL (C) and Chow-PAL rats (D) in the final test session, again separated according to bout identity. (**E & F**) Average bout size versus average inter-bout interval for individual Caf-CHOW (E) and Chow-CHOW rats (F) in the final test session.

for Caf-PAL rats in week 1 versus Chow-PAL rats in week 7 (left half of each figure), and Chow-CHOW rats in week 1 versus Caf-CHOW rats in week 7 (right half of each figure). Caf-PAL and Chow-PAL rats consumed the same amount of energy, $F<1$, but differed in the way this energy was obtained: Chow-PAL rats initiated fewer bouts, $F(1,22) = 5.88$, $p<.05$, but consumed more energy in each bout, $F(1,22) = 10.63$, $p<.01$, than Caf-PAL rats. Caf-CHOW rats consumed less energy than Chow-CHOW rats, $F(1,22) = 75.89$, $p<.01$, which was due to the fact that they initiated fewer bouts, $F(1,22) = 52.46$ $p<.01$, rather than consuming smaller bouts, $F<1$.

The bottom panel of Figure 8 shows the total numbers of bouts plotted against average bout size for individual rats in Groups Caf-PAL and Chow-PAL (8D) and Groups Caf-CHOW and Chow-CHOW (8E). With the exception of those in Group Caf-CHOW, rats in each of the other three groups showed a clear negative relationship between the number of total bouts and the average size of a bout, smallest $t(10) = 2.71$, $p<.025$; rats that consumed more energy per bout initiated fewer bouts overall. This

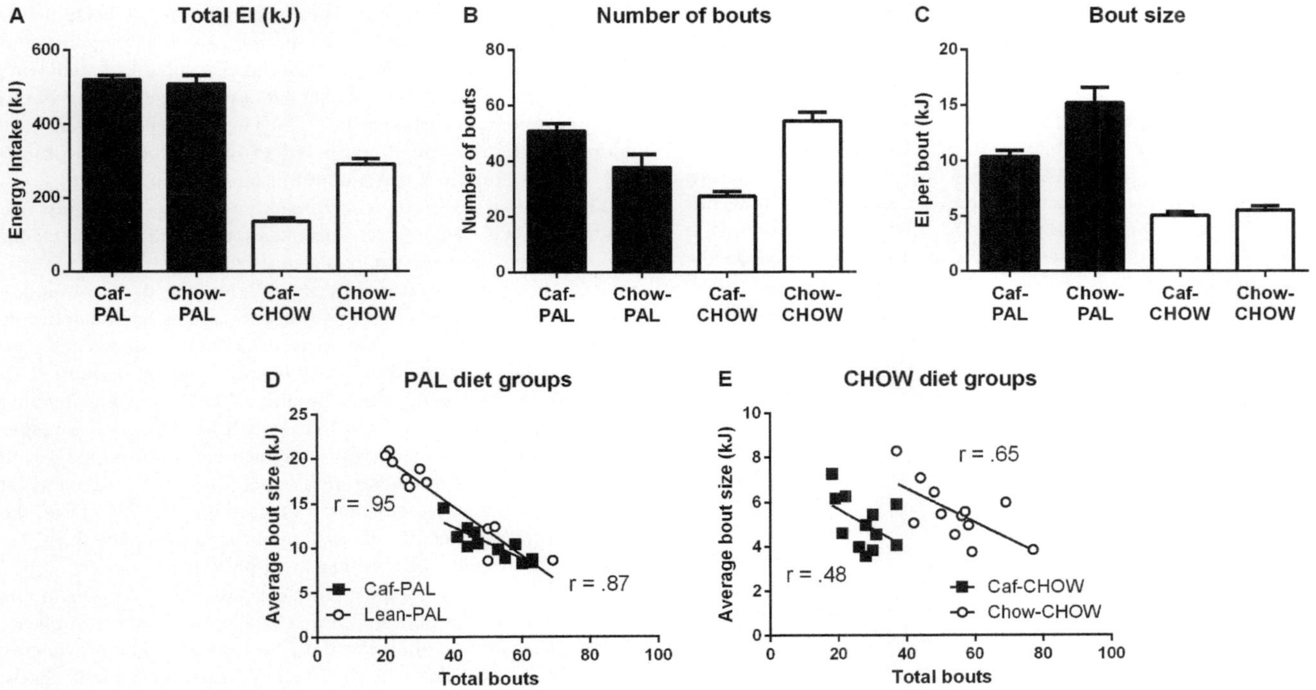

Figure 8. Cross-week comparison of switch effects. (A–C) Total energy intake (kJ, A), numbers of bouts (B) and bout size (kJ per bout, C) for Caf-PAL rats in week 1 versus Chow-PAL rats in week 7 (left half of each figure), and Chow-CHOW rats in week 1 versus Caf-CHOW rats in week 7 (right half of each figure). Each column represents the mean (+SEM) for an entire 24-hour session. **(D & E)** Total number of bouts versus average bout size (kJ) for individual rats in Groups Caf-PAL (week 1) and Chow-PAL (week 7; 8D), and for individual rats in Groups Caf-CHOW (week 7) and Chow-CHOW(week 1, 8E).

relationship was absent among Caf-CHOW rats, $t = 1.73$: the initiation of a bout among these rats was largely independent of how much they in fact consumed during each bout.

Discussion

This study examined changes in feeding patterns among rats with a history of exposure to a cafeteria-style diet, Caf rats, or standard lab chow, Chow rats. We assessed feeding patterns among these rats using the CLAMS, where rats were presented with foods consistent with their home cage history: specifically, Caf rats were presented with palatable biscuit and high-fat chow while Chow rats were presented with standard lab chow. The unit of analysis was individual eating bouts that occurred during 24-hour test sessions at different stages of diet exposure. This unit of analysis avoided arbitrary classification schemes that, in the absence of independent verification criteria (e.g., such as the behavioural satiety sequence [7]), has the potential to obscure rather than clarify how feeding patterns change with exposure to a cafeteria diet.

Among Chow rats consuming chow, the number of feeding bouts declined over time, the average bout size increased, and there was a clear positive relationship between these measures: those rats that had the largest bout sizes waited the longest until the next bout, suggesting that feeding in these rats was regulated by time since the last bout. Compared to Chow rats, Caf rats consuming palatable biscuit and high fat chow initiated fewer bouts [7], but this difference was transient: by the final test session, Caf and Chow rats initiated feeding bouts with the same regularity. In contrast, Caf rats consumed more energy per bout, and this difference persisted across all sessions of testing. These differences in Caf rats relative to Chow rats were reflected in differences in the distributions of inter-bout intervals and bout sizes: in the first and last test sessions, Caf rats showed a leftward shift in the distribution of inter-bout intervals (they were more likely than Chow rats to initiate feeding in the minutes following a prior bout), and a rightward shift in the distribution of bout sizes (they were less likely than Chow rats to have bouts of size 10 kJ or less). In spite of these shifts, the relationship between average bout sizes and average wait times between bouts among Caf rats was the same as that observed among Chow rats: feeding in both groups of Caf rats was regulated by time since the last bout.

Critically, a history of exposure to the cafeteria-style diet dramatically affected motivation to consume diets of varying palatability or variety. First, Caf rats maintained on the cafeteria diet and provided with standard lab chow in the CLAMS dramatically reduced their consumption. Relative to Chow rats fed standard lab chow throughout the study and subjected to an equivalent test history, this reduced consumption was due to fewer bouts, reflecting a rightward shift in the distribution of waiting times between bouts; as well as a decrease in energy consumed per bout, reflecting a leftward shift in the distribution of bout sizes. Relative to Chow rats fed standard lab chow in the first week of CLAMS testing, the reduced consumption in Caf rats provided with chow was specifically due to fewer bouts: Chow rats tested with chow for the first time and Caf rats tested with chow for the first time consumed bouts of the same size. The change in feeding when Caf rats were withdrawn from the cafeteria diet for the first time was perhaps most evident in the absence of any relationship between average bout size and average wait time between bouts. Hence, feeding in this group was not regulated by the time since the previous bout. One obvious possibility is that the history of exposure to the cafeteria diet rendered standard lab chow relatively unpalatable [3,11], and so, in spite of long intervals between bouts that likely engendered hunger, these rats refrained from feeding.

Second, as Caf rats accumulated experience with cafeteria-style foods in their home cage, their motivation to consume biscuit and high-fat chow in the CLAMS test sessions declined: these rats ultimately consumed less of these foods compared to Chow rats exposed to them for the first time (in fact, Caf rats presented with biscuit and high fat chow ultimately consumed these foods to the same modest level as Chow rats fed standard lab chow). Comparisons of Caf and Chow rats exposed to the palatable foods revealed that Caf rats fed less regularly, but when they did feed, they consumed the same amount in energy. Consistent with this, the distribution of waiting times between bouts was shifted to the right for Caf rats, but distributions of bout sizes were not different. When consumption of biscuit and high-fat chow was analyzed separately, Chow rats exposed to biscuit and high-fat chow showed no preference for one over the other, consuming both just as avidly; whereas Caf rats preferred biscuit over high-fat chow. It should also be noted that Chow rats showed a clear positive relationship between the average size of high-fat chow bouts and wait times following these bouts; but there was no relationship between the average size of biscuit bouts and wait times following these bouts. In contrast, Caf rats showed a clear positive relationship between the size of high-fat chow bouts and post-high-fat chow wait times, as well as the size of biscuit bouts and post-biscuit wait times. Taken together, these findings have three important implications. First, the fact that feeding in Caf but not Chow rats following a biscuit bout was regulated by time since the last biscuit bout suggests at least some degree of adaptation to the cafeteria diet. Second, possibly as a consequence of this adaptation, the motivation to consume palatable foods declined among rats exposed to the cafeteria diet. Third, exposure to the cafeteria diet shifted food preferences.

Why did motivation to consume biscuit and high-fat chow decline among Caf rats? There are a number of possible explanations. First, studies have shown that variety in the diet enhances meal size and energy intake among rats exposed to palatable foods [4]. Having been exposed to a range of foods that differed in flavor and texture in their home cages, Caf rats were accustomed to variety, and hence, the relative lack of variety when rats were tested in the CLAMS may have been enough to reduce motivation to feed. Second, rats given chronic access to a cafeteria-style diet become relatively insensitive to reward, indexed by an increase in the threshold at which direct electrical self-stimulation of neural reward circuits was maintained relative to control rats exposed to standard lab chow [2]. The implication of these blunted neural responses is that palatable foods that are normally highly valued and rewarding lose their ability to initiate and maintain behaviors directed towards their procurement.

Diet-induced changes in the rewarding value of palatable foods may occur either because of, or in addition to, increases in circulating levels of anorectic hormones, and therefore, the satiating capacity of energy dense foods. In this respect, previous work in our lab has shown that following two weeks of exposure to the same cafeteria diet as that used in the current experiment, levels of blood glucose and inhibitory feeding signals, insulin and leptin, are significantly elevated [5]. The effects of blood glucose changes on insulin release and its subsequent anorectic effects are well established [12]. In humans, obesity is associated with reduced levels of the stimulatory feeding signal ghrelin [13], while dieting is associated with increases in ghrelin [14]. Ghrelin levels are differentially affected by consumption of different macronutrient components: release of ghrelin is enhanced following consumption of meals containing fat and protein, but reduced by consumption of carbohydrate [15]. Hence, high fat meals have poorer satiation potential compared to high carbohydrate meals [16–18], resulting in less frequent but larger meals [19–20].

The fact that rats in the current study were exposed to just two foods during CLAMS test sessions makes it difficult to make claims about seeking of particular macronutrients (e.g., protein). Nonetheless, the fact that Caf, but not Chow rats demonstrated a preference for biscuit over high-fat chow suggests that chronic exposure to the cafeteria diet biases selection of foods that are higher in fat, carbohydrate, and overall energy (biscuit). This suggestion is consistent with a wealth of evidence showing that obese people prefer palatable foods, such as those rich in sugar [21]. It is also consistent with evidence for meal-skipping and increased snacking on energy-rich foods (those with high and fat content) among adolescents and young adults [22–23]. Thus, the increased prevalence of obesity may be accompanied by an increased prevalence of irregular meal patterns.

While diet-induced changes in food palatability explain many aspects of the present findings, other factors may have also played a role. According to the "Protein Leverage Hypothesis", energy intake is tightly regulated by the levels of protein in available foods, rather than levels of carbohydrate or fat [24–26]. Consistent with this hypothesis, Chow rats accustomed to eating standard lab chow in the home cage and exposed to foods relatively low in protein in the CLAMS (e.g., biscuit and high-fat chow) may have consumed more of the test foods to obtain their usual intake of protein. However, it does not explain why Caf rats accustomed to eating palatable foods in the home cage and exposed to a relatively rich source of protein in the CLAMS (i.e., standard lab chow) consumed less than their Chow counterparts: if the Caf-CHOW rats were simply protein seeking, one may have expected that their energy intake in the CLAMS test sessions should have been equivalent to that of the Chow-CHOW rats.

In summary, the present study has extended previous studies showing that exposure to a cafeteria diet alters feeding patterns such that bout numbers decrease [7], while the energy density of each bout increases. It has also shown that exposure to the diet increases preferences for food that is relatively rich in fat and carbohydrate (biscuit over high-fat chow); and dramatically reduces motivation to consume palatable foods, at least under circumstances where variety is limited. Finally, it has shown that complete withdrawal from cafeteria-style foods diminishes the motivation to feed, and that what feeding does occur is not regulated by factors like time since the last bout [10]. Extrapolation of these findings to people suggests that the affordability, attractiveness and availability of palatable energy dense foods may initially encourage consumption of larger snacks and meals, in terms of both volume, and critically, total energy content. However, over time, it may be the extraordinary variety of energy dense foods that drives over-consumption, and therefore, excessive weight gain.

Author Contributions

Conceived and designed the experiments: RFW MJM. Performed the experiments: TS SIM. Analyzed the data: NMH TS. Wrote the manuscript: TS NMH RFW MJM. Read and approved the final manuscript: TS NMH SIM RFW MJM. Other: TS and NMH.

References

1. Lindberg MA, Dementieva Y, Cavender JMA (2011) Why Has the BMI Gone Up So Drastically in the Last 35 Years? J Addict Med 5: 272–278.
2. Johnson PM, Kenny PJ (2010) Dopamine D2 receptors in addiction-like reward dysfunction and compulsive eating in obese rats. Nat Neurosci 13: 635–641.
3. Rogers PJ, Blundell JE (1984) Meal patterns and food selection during the development of obesity in rats fed a cafeteria diet. Neurosci Biobehav Rev 8: 441–453.
4. Rolls BJ, van Duijvenvoorde PM, Rowe EA (1983) Variety in the diet enhances intake in a meal and contributes to the development of obesity in the rat. Physiol Behav 31: 21–27.
5. Hansen MJ, Jovanovska V, Morris MJ (2004) Adaptive responses in hypothalamic neuropeptide Y in the face of prolonged high-fat feeding in the rat. J Neurochem 88: 909–916.
6. Maniam J, Morris MJ (2010) Palatable cafeteria diet ameliorates anxiety and depression-like symptoms following an adverse early environment. Psychoneuroendocrinology 35: 717–728.
7. Martire SI, Holmes NM, Westbrook RF, Morris MJ (2013) Altered feeding patterns in rats exposed to a palatable cafeteria diet: increased snacking and its implications for development of obesity. PLoS One 8: e60407. doi: 10.1371/journal.pone.0060407
8. South T, Westbrook RF, Morris MJ (2012) Neurological and stress related effects of shifting obese rats from a palatable diet to chow and lean rats from chow to a palatable diet. Physiolo Behav 105: 1052–1057.
9. Goularte JF, Ferreira MBC, Sanvitto GL (2012) Effects of food pattern change and physical exercise on cafeteria diet-induced obesity in female rats. B J Nutr 108: 1511–1518.
10. Rogers PJ (1985) Returning "cafeteria-fed" rats to a chow diet: Negative contrast and effects of obesity on feeding behaviour. Physiol Behav 35: 493–499.
11. Davis JD (1989) The Microstructure of Ingestive Behavior. Ann N Y Acad Sci 575: 106–121. doi: 10.1111/j.1749-6632.1989.tb53236.x
12. Campfield LA (1997) Metabolic and Hormonal Controls of Food Intake: Highlights of the Last 25 Years: 1972–1997. Appetite 29: 135–152.
13. Zhang S, Zhang Q, Zhang L, Li C, Jiang H (2013) Expression of ghrelin and leptin during the development of type 2 diabetes mellitus in a rat model. Mol Med Rep 7: 223–228.
14. Sumithran P, Prendergast LA, Delbridge E, Purcell K, Shulkes A, et al (2011) Long-term persistence of hormonal adaptations to weight loss. N Engl J Med 365: 1597–604.
15. Erdmann J, Topsch R, Lippl F, Gussmann P, Schusdziarra V (2004) Postprandial response of plasma ghrelin levels to various test meals in relation to food intake, plasma insulin, and glucose. J Clin Endocrinol Metab 89: 3048–3054. doi: 10.1210/jc.2003-031610
16. Green SM, Wales JK, Lawton CL, Blundell JE (2000) Comparison of high-fat and high-carbohydrate foods in a meal or snack on short-term fat and energy intakes in obese women. B J Nutr 84: 521–530.
17. Lucas F, Sclafani A (1999) Differential Reinforcing and Satiating Effects of Intragastric Fat and Carbohydrate Infusions in Rats. Physiol Behav 66: 381–388.
18. Warwick ZS, Synowski SJ, Rice KD, Smart AB (2003) Independent effects of diet palatability and fat content on bout size and daily intake in rats. Physiol Behav 80: 253–258.
19. Melhorn SJ, Krause EG, Scott KA, Mooney MR, Johnson JD, et al (2010) Acute exposure to a high-fat diet alters meal patterns and body composition. Physiol Behav 99: 33–39.
20. Synowski SJ, Smart AB, Warwick ZS (2005) Meal size of high-fat food is reliably greater than high-carbohydrate food across externally-evoked single-meal tests and long-term spontaneous feeding in rat. Appetite 45: 191–194.
21. Epstein LH, Carr KA, Lin H, Fletcher KD (2011) Food reinforcement, energy intake, and macronutrient choice. Am J Clin Nutr 94: 12–18.
22. Koletzko B, Toschke AM (2010) Meal patterns and frequencies: do they affect body weight in children and adolescents? Crit Rev Food Sci Nutr 50: 100–105.
23. Zizza C, Siega-Riz AM, Popkin BM (2001) Significant Increase in Young Adults' Snacking between 1977–1978 and 1994–1996 Represents a Cause for Concern! Preventive Med 32: 303–310.
24. Simpson SJ, Raubenheimer D (2005) Obesity: the protein leverage hypothesis. Obes Rev 6: 133–142. doi: 10.1111/j.1467-789X.2005.00178.x
25. Larue-Achagiotis C, Martin C, Verger P, Louis-Sylvestre J (1992) Dietary self-selection vs. complete diet: Body weight gain and meal pattern in rats. Physiol Behav 51: 995–999.
26. Martinez-Cordero C, Kuzawa CW, Sloboda DM, Stewart J, Simpson SJ, et al (2012) "Testing the Protein Leverage Hypothesis in a free-living human population." Appetite 59: 312–315.

14

Effect of Cafeteria Diet History on Cue-, Pellet-Priming-, and Stress-Induced Reinstatement of Food Seeking in Female Rats

Yu-Wei Chen, Kimberly A. Fiscella, Samuel Z. Bacharach, Donna J. Calu*

Intramural Research Program, NIDA/NIH, Baltimore, Maryland, United States of America

Abstract

Background: Relapse to unhealthy eating habits is a major problem in human dietary treatment. The individuals most commonly seeking dietary treatment are overweight or obese women, yet the commonly used rat reinstatement model to study relapse to palatable food seeking during dieting primarily uses normal-weight male rats. To increase the clinical relevance of the relapse to palatable food seeking model, here we pre-expose female rats to a calorically-dense cafeteria diet in the home-cage to make them overweight prior to examining the effect of this diet history on cue-, pellet-priming- and footshock-induced reinstatement of food seeking.

Methods: Post-natal day 32 female Long-Evans rats had seven weeks of home-cage access to either chow only or daily or intermittent cafeteria diet alongside chow. Next, they were trained to self-administer normally preferred 45 mg food pellets accompanied by a tone-light cue. After extinction, all rats were tested for reinstatement induced by discrete cue, pellet-priming, and intermittent footshock under extinction conditions.

Results: Access to daily cafeteria diet and to a lesser degree access to intermittent cafeteria diet decreased food pellet self-administration compared to chow-only. Prior history of these cafeteria diets also reduced extinction responding, cue- and pellet-priming-induced reinstatement. In contrast, modest stress-induced reinstatement was only observed in rats with a history of daily cafeteria diet.

Conclusion: A history of cafeteria diet does not increase the propensity for cue- and pellet-priming-induced relapse in the rat reinstatement model but does appear to make rats more susceptible to footshock stress-induced reinstatement.

Editor: Judith Homberg, Radboud University, Netherlands

Funding: The work was supported by the Intramural Research Program of the National Institute on Drug Abuse. The funders had no role in study design, data collection and analysis, decision to publish, or preparation of the manuscript.

Competing Interests: The authors have declared that no competing interests exist.

* Email: donna.calu@nih.gov

Introduction

Excessive consumption of unhealthy palatable foods is a major public health problem contributing to obesity and obesity-related diseases [1,2]. While many people attempt to control their food intake through dieting, most relapse to maladaptive eating habits within a short time [3–6]. This relapse is often triggered by acute exposure to palatable food, food-associated cues, or stress [6–10]. In order to model this clinical situation, we and the others have adopted the rat reinstatement model [11], which has been used extensively to study relapse to drug seeking [12–14]. In this model, rats are trained to lever-press for palatable food. After extinction of the food-reinforced responding, the rats are tested for reinstatement induced by non-contingent exposure to palatable food, food-associated cues, or stressors [15,16].

The reinstatement procedure, which is relatively simple to implement, has proven to be very suitable for studying relapse to palatable food seeking during dieting because it reliably induces robust reinstatement effects across a variety of reinstating stimuli [16]. Nevertheless, this reinstatement model fails to capture certain aspects of the clinical problem. First, the target population seeking treatment for relapse to unhealthy eating after dieting is primarily comprised of overweight and obese individuals, and the proportion of women taking dietary supplements or seeking dietary treatment is more than twice that of men [17,18]. Yet most preclinical relapse studies to date use normal-weight male rats to study relapse to palatable food seeking [15,19]. Second, in the reinstatement procedure rats are typically given limited access to nutritionally balanced chow during the training and extinction/testing phases in order to promote enhanced motivation in the operant chamber. While humans with unhealthy eating habits generally consume limited amounts of nutritionally balanced foods and greater amounts of calorically-dense palatable foods, during dieting, subjects not only restrict the amount of calorically-dense food they eat but also tend to consume nutritionally balanced foods. These aspects of the human situation are not accurately modeled using standard chow food deprivation throughout the reinstatement procedure.

To increase the clinical relevance of the relapse to palatable food seeking model, we gave young female rats daily or intermittent (Monday, Wednesday, Friday) access to a calorically-dense cafeteria diet in the home-cage prior to and throughout the training period in order to make the rats overweight. Exposure to highly palatable and energy-dense food not only leads to obesity in rodents, but also causes dysregulation of reward processing and stress responses [20–22], both of which implicated in relapse behavior [16,23]. Therefore, to more accurately model human dieting, we terminated access to cafeteria diets at the end of the training phase and examined the effect of diet history on discrete cue-, pellet priming-, and footshock-induced reinstatement of food seeking after extinction.

Materials and Methods

Subjects and apparatus

Female Long-Evans (total N = 24) rats (Charles River Laboratories, Wilmington, MA; 26 days old at time of arrival) were maintained on a reverse 12 h light/dark cycle (lights off at 8 AM) and were given free access to standard laboratory chow and water during the experiment. Rats were individually housed on postnatal day (PND) 30 and were weight matched across groups before being assigned to each diet condition (n = 8 per group). Diet manipulations began on PND 32. Following 50 days of diet exposure, rats began behavioral training. We performed the experiments in accordance to the "Guide for the care and use of laboratory animals" (8th edition, 2011, US National Research Council) and experimental protocols were approved by the Intramural Research Program (NIDA) Animal Care and Use Committee.

Behavioral experiments were conducted in standard self-administration chambers (Med Associates). Each chamber had two levers 9 cm above the floor, but only one lever (the "active," retractable lever) activated the pellet dispenser, which delivered 45 mg food pellets containing 12.7% fat, 66.7% carbohydrate, and 20.6% protein (catalog #1811155; Test Diet). This pellet type was chosen based on pellet preference tests in food-restricted female rats, using six pellet types (obtained from Test Diet and Bioserv) with different compositions of fat (0–35%) and carbohydrate (45–91% sugar pellets) and different flavors (no flavor, banana, chocolate, grape) [15]. Rats were housed in the animal facility and transferred to the self-administration chambers prior to the training sessions, and returned to the facility at the end of the 2-h sessions.

Diet manipulations

The chow only rats received free access to standard laboratory chow (Teklad global 18% protein rodent diet, Harlan Laboratories) (58% carbohydrate, 24% protein, 18% fat).

The daily cafeteria diet rats also had free access to standard laboratory chow in addition to a rotating schedule of highly palatable "cafeteria items." This diet consisted of two items per day—one savory item and one sweet item. Two weeks on this diet allowed for a full rotation of cafeteria diet items including potato chips, corn snacks, chocolate cake, peanut butter cookies, pepperoni, pretzels, chocolate sandwich cookies, chocolate-chip cookies, and breakfast pastries. Both the chow and the cafeteria items were pre-weighed and the savory and sweet items were placed in two separate ceramic ramekins in the rats' home-cages, while the chow was available in the home-cage food hopper. Twenty-four hours later any chow or cafeteria items remaining in the cage were independently weighed to determine daily intake for each item. Daily intake of cafeteria items and chow was monitored Monday through Thursday. The amount of each item consumed per rat was converted to calories (kcal) using data provided by the manufacturers. The intermittent cafeteria diet rats received the same rotation of highly palatable cafeteria items that the daily cafeteria rats received in addition to free access to standard laboratory chow. However, these rats had 24 h of forced abstinence from the cafeteria items every Tuesday, Thursday, Saturday, and Sunday, during which the chow was available. Using the identical procedure described above, daily intake of cafeteria items (Monday, Wednesday, Friday) and chow (every day) was monitored and the caloric intake (kcal) from each item was calculated, except that the consumption was monitored Monday through Saturday. This was due to the intermittent schedule of this diet, in which cafeteria items had to be removed on Saturday morning following the 24 h access that began Friday morning. All rats were weighed daily during home-cage diet exposure and before each training, extinction, and reinstatement testing session.

Training, extinction and reinstatement of food-reinforced responding

The experimental conditions used during training, extinction and reinstatement phases were similar to those used in previous studies in male and female rats [19,24,25], with the exception of food restriction and duration of sessions.

Training and extinction

Behavioral training began with 2 days of magazine training which involved 2-h sessions during which pellets (Test Diet Purified Rodent Tablet (5TUL)) were delivered non-contingently, every 5 min into a food cup located to the right of the active lever. Pellet delivery was accompanied by a compound 5-s tone (2900 Hz)-light (7.5W white light) cue, both located above the active lever. Subsequently, rats were trained to self-administer the pellets on a fixed-ratio-1 (FR-1), 20-s timeout reinforcement schedule. At the start of each 2-h session, the red house light was turned on and the active lever was extended. Reinforced active lever presses resulted in delivery of one pellet, accompanied by the compound 5-s tone-light cue. Active lever presses during the 20-s timeout or presses on the inactive lever had no programmed consequences. Rats underwent 10 training sessions under these conditions. During training, rats were maintained on their respective diets.

Following ten 2-h food self-administration training sessions, all rats underwent no-cue extinction sessions in which active lever presses were no longer reinforced with a food pellet or the tone-light cue. During the extinction phase, in order to mimic human dieting, daily cafeteria and intermittent cafeteria rats were switched to free access chow diet, no longer receiving access to the cafeteria items in the home-cage. Chow rats experienced no change in the free access chow home-cage diet condition.

All rats were given 11 extinction sessions (no cue), and reached an extinction criterion (mean active lever pressing across the last three extinction sessions <20% of extinction day 1 responding) before the cue-induced reinstatement test began. Before the pellet-priming- and footshock-induced reinstatement tests started, all rats underwent another 7 and 2 sessions, respectively, of 2-h extinction, in which responses on the previously active lever led to tone-light cue presentations but no pellets (extinction with cue). On the day of the pellet-priming or footshock-induced reinstatement test, all rats underwent additional within-session extinction, and the reinstatement manipulation started after an extinction criterion was reached (<20 active lever responses within 1 h).

Cue-induced reinstatement

After all rats reached extinction criterion, they underwent one day of cue-induced reinstatement testing. Cue reinstatement testing consisted of a single 2-h session beginning with 1 non-contingent tone-light cue presentation immediately after the session started [26–28]. During the session, active lever presses resulted in tone-light cue but no pellet (20 s timeout). Active lever presses during the 20-s timeout or presses on the inactive lever had no programmed consequences.

Pellet-priming-induced reinstatement

After 7 sessions of 2-h daily extinction (with cue) session, the rats underwent one day of within-session extinction/pellet priming-induced reinstatement testing. The pellet priming test consisted of six 60 min mini-sessions separated by 5 min time out, in which the active lever was retracted and the house light was extinguished. The first 3 mini-sessions were conducted under extinction conditions (with cue) with the third hour serving as the 0 pellet baseline mini-session. At the start of the remaining 3 mini-sessions 1, 2, or 4 pellets were delivered non-contingently (each was separated by 20 s) into the food hopper, in ascending order. The within-session priming procedure is based on previous studies with cocaine priming [29,30].

Footshock-induced reinstatement

The rats underwent 2 additional 2-h daily sessions of extinction with cue between pellet priming- and footshock-induced reinstatement tests. For the test, the rats underwent one day of within-session extinction/footshock-induced reinstatement testing, which consisted of five to six mini-sessions. The testing started with three to four 60 min extinction mini-sessions separated by 5 min time out, in which the active lever was retracted and the house light was extinguished. These mini-sessions were conducted under extinction conditions (with cue), with the third or fourth hour serving as the 0 min duration shock baseline. A 10 min time out in which the active lever was retracted and the house light was extinguished followed this baseline session. After this timeout, rats received 5 min of intermittent footshock (0.18–0.30 mA based on individual shock reactivity; 0.5 s ON and an average of 40 s OFF period, 10–70 s intershock interval) with house light extinguished and lever retracted. Subsequently, the effect of 5-min footshock on reinstatement was assessed in a 60-min session under extinction conditions. After another 10 min time out, they received 10 min of intermittent footshock (0.18–0.30 mA based on individual shock reactivity). Reinstatement effect was again assessed in a 60-min session post-footshock. The within-session footshock-induced reinstatement procedure is based on a previous study with heroin [31] and the shock ON and OFF duration is based on previous studies on footshock-induced reinstatement of drug seeking [32,33].

Statistical analyses

Data were analyzed using the SPSS statistical software (IBM). The factors used in the statistical analyses are described in the Results section below. Results are presented as group means (±SEM). Significant main effects and interaction effects ($p<0.05$) from ANOVAs were followed by post-hoc Fisher PLSD tests when appropriate.

Results

Effect of home-cage diet history on body weight gain

Rats that had daily access to cafeteria items gained significantly more body weight and consumed more calories during the diet exposure, but this difference in body weight disappeared once the diet was no longer available. From PND 32 all rats had home-cage access to their designated diet (daily cafeteria, intermittent cafeteria, chow only) for 64 days before cafeteria diets were removed and extinction began. The cumulative body weight gain and caloric intake during these phases are shown in **Fig. 1**. For the body weight gain during the first phase, when the cafeteria items were available in home-cages (weeks 1 to 9), we analyzed the data using the mixed ANOVA, with the between-subjects factor of Diet Condition and within-subjects factor of Time (weeks 1 to 9). Statistical analysis on cumulative body weight gain showed significant main effects of Diet Condition and Time ($F_{2,21}=6.8$ and $F_{8,168}=839.0$, respectively, $p<0.01$), and a significant interaction of Diet Condition x Time ($F_{16,168}=8.5$, $p<0.01$). Post-hoc analysis, as depicted in **Fig. 1A**, showed that the daily cafeteria group gained significantly more weight than the chow-only group from week 3 to the end of the diet exposure period. Similarly, analysis of caloric intake showed significant main effects of Diet Condition and Time ($F_{2,21}=39.5$ and $F_{8,168}=24.5$, respectively, $p<0.01$), and a significant interaction of Diet Condition x Time ($F_{16,168}=4.8$, $p<0.01$). Post-hoc analysis (**Fig. 1B**) showed that the daily cafeteria group had significantly more caloric intake than chow-only groups from week 1.

Once the cafeteria items were removed (weeks 10–14), a similar analysis on cumulative body weight gain as stated above showed a significant main effect of Time ($F_{4,84}=7.9$, $p<0.01$) and interaction of Diet Condition x Time ($F_{8,64}=17.6$, $p<0.01$), but not Diet Condition ($p=0.29$), suggesting that there was no longer a body weight difference between groups. Post-hoc analysis (**Fig. 1A grey shaded region**) showed that the daily cafeteria group weighed significantly more only during the first week following cessation of cafeteria diet, and there were no group differences during reinstatement testing. A similar analysis on caloric intake after the cessation of cafeteria diet as stated above showed significant main effects of Diet Condition and Time ($F_{2,21}=9.0$ and $F_{4,84}=6.3$, respectively, $p<0.01$) and interaction of Diet Condition x Time ($F_{8,84}=4.7$, $p<0.01$). Post-hoc analysis (**Fig. 1B grey shaded region**) showed that the daily cafeteria group had significantly less caloric intake than the chow-only group for the first three weeks following cessation of cafeteria diet.

Effect of cafeteria diet history on pellet self-administration and extinction

Training. All rats demonstrated reliable food-reinforced responding, but the magnitude and time course of responding over days differed between diet conditions with significantly lower food self-administration in rats in the daily cafeteria diet condition (**Fig. 2**). We analyzed the data using the mixed ANOVA, with the between-subjects factor of Diet Condition and within-subjects factor of Session. Analyses of pellets earned showed a significant main effect of Diet Condition and Session ($F_{2,21}=16.6$ and $F_{9,189}=2.3$, respectively, $p<0.05$), but no significant interaction of Diet Condition x Session ($p=0.96$). Post-hoc differences are depicted in **Fig. 2A**. Analyses on time-out responses on the active lever showed a significant main effect of Diet Condition and Session ($F_{2,21}=9.1$ and $F_{9,189}=5.0$, respectively, $p<0.01$), and a significant interaction of Diet Condition x Session ($F_{18,189}=2.1$, $p<0.01$). A post-hoc analysis comparing the time-out responses between sessions 1 and 10 for each diet condition showed that the

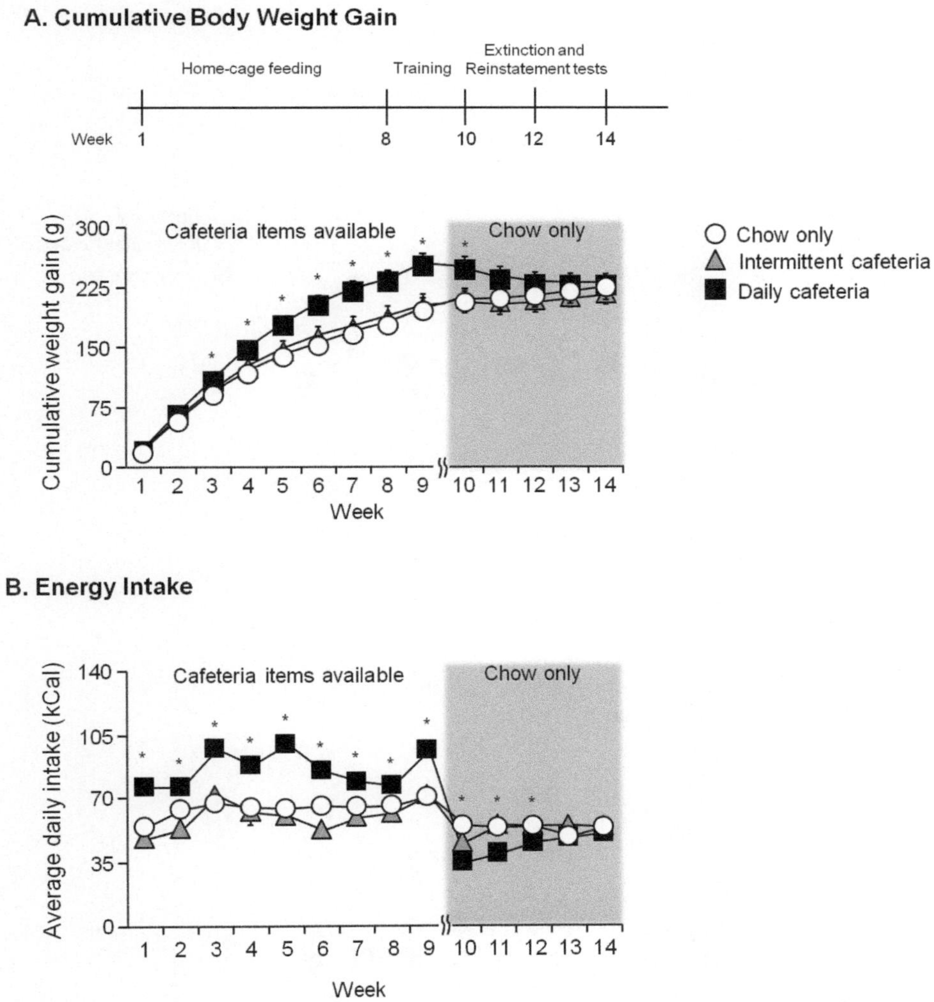

Figure 1. Cumulative body weight gain and average daily caloric intake in rats with different diet conditions. A. Weekly average cumulative body weight gain (mean±SEM) in rats with daily access to a cafeteria diet, intermittent access to a cafeteria diet or daily access to chow-only. Weeks 1–7 correspond to the home-cage access phase and Weeks 8–9 correspond to training phase in which access to home-cage diets remained unchanged. Extinction started on Week 10, from which time the cafeteria items were no longer available. All rats had *ad libitum* chow from Week 10 to the end of testing. Discrete-cue induced reinstatement test occurred in Week 12; pellet-priming- and intermittent footshock-induced reinstatement tests occurred in Week 14. **B.** Daily average caloric intake from diet (mean±SEM). *Different between chow-only and daily cafeteria group, $p<0.05$, $n=8$ per group.

chow-only group, but not the daily or intermittent cafeteria groups, demonstrated escalated time-out responding after 10 days of training ($t_7=2.4$, $p<0.05$) (**Fig. 2B, inset**). Additional analysis showed that while the intermittent group had access to cafeteria items before some training sessions, this did not affect their time-out responding (cafeteria diet available: 168.5±21.0 vs. cafeteria diet not available: 188.0±22.9). Inactive lever pressing data for the training phase are presented in table 1.

Extinction. All rats reduced active lever responding during the extinction phase, both in the absence and presence of the tone-light cue (prior to or after cue-induced reinstatement, respectively), but similar to food self-administration lever responding was significantly lower in the daily cafeteria group (**Fig. 2C**). The analysis using the mixed ANOVA, with the between-subjects factor of Diet Condition, and within-subjects factors of Lever (active, inactive) and Session, showed significant main effects of Diet Condition and Session ($F_{2,21}=8.7$ and $F_{10,210}=72.3$, $p<0.01$) and interactions of Diet Condition x Lever, Diet Condition x Session, and Lever x Session ($F_{2,21}=8.5$, $F_{20,210}=9.0$, and $F_{10,210}=62.2$, respectively, $p<0.01$), and Diet Condition x Lever x Session ($F_{20,210}=6.8$, $p<0.01$). Post-hoc differences between groups were depicted in **Fig. 2C**, and consistent with the level of lever pressing observed during training, chow-only had greater lever responding compared to the daily cafeteria during the early extinction sessions. Inactive lever pressing data for the extinction phase are presented in table 1.

Effects of cafeteria diet history on cue-induced reinstatement

Discrete tone-light cues successfully reinstated active lever responding in all rats, but the magnitude of responding was lower in rats with a history of cafeteria diet (**Fig. 3A**). Data were analyzed using mixed-factor ANOVA, with the between-subjects

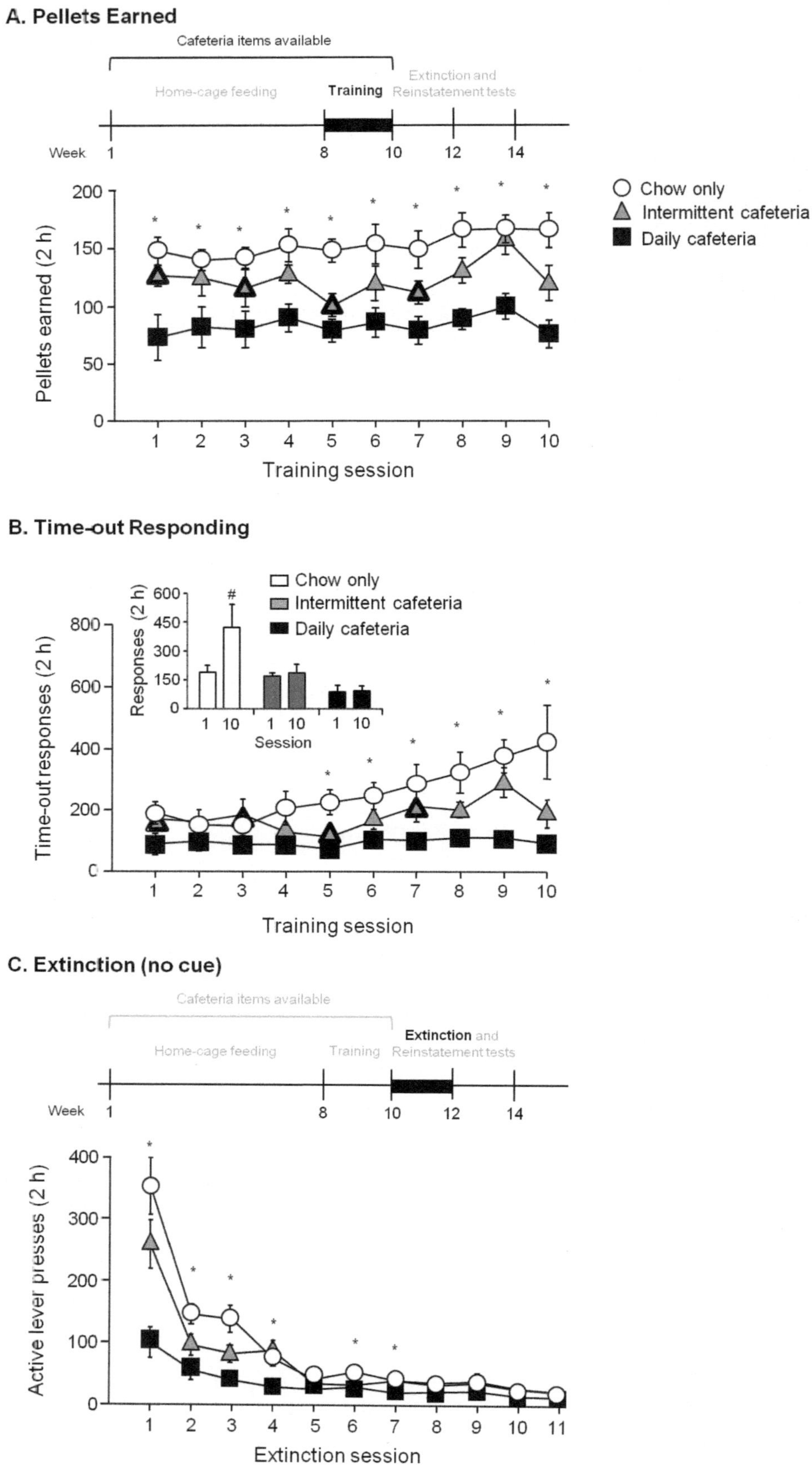
A. Pellets Earned
Cafeteria items available
Home-cage feeding
Training
Extinction and Reinstatement tests
Week 1 8 10 12 14
Pellets earned (2 h)
Training session
Chow only
Intermittent cafeteria
Daily cafeteria
B. Time-out Responding
Time-out responses (2 h)
Responses (2 h)
Session
Chow only
Intermittent cafeteria
Daily cafeteria
Training session
C. Extinction (no cue)
Cafeteria items available
Home-cage feeding
Training
Extinction and Reinstatement tests
Week 1 8 10 12 14
Active lever presses (2 h)
Extinction session

Figure 2. Effect of home-cage diet condition on food self-administration training. A. Reinforcers (pellets) earned (mean±SEM). **B.** Time-out responding during food self-administration training for different diet conditions. Inset: difference in time-out between training sessions 1 and 10 for each diet condition. # Different between sessions 1 and 10 within diet condition, $p<0.05$. **C.** Active lever responding (mean±SEM) under extinction conditions without cue (lever responding had no consequence).*Different between chow-only and daily cafeteria group, $p<0.05$, $n=8$ per group. Data points with heavier outlines indicate days that intermittent group had access to cafeteria items prior to the session.

factor of Diet Condition, within-subjects factor of Lever (active, inactive) and Reinstatement Condition (last day extinction [no cue], cue). We found significant main effects of Lever and Reinstatement Condition ($F_{1,21}=62.6$ and $F_{1,21}=45.0$, respectively, $p<0.01$), but not Diet Condition ($p=0.15$), and significant interactions of Diet Condition x Lever, Diet Condition x Reinstatement Condition, and Lever x Reinstatement Condition ($F_{2,21}=4.9$, $F_{2,21}=5.5$, $F_{1,21}=35.4$, $p<0.05$). A post-hoc comparison showed an approaching significant difference between lever responding in the chow-only compared to the daily cafeteria group ($p=0.06$). Overall, our results showed that while the cue-induced reinstatement effect is observed in all groups, this effect is most pronounced in the chow-only group and least pronounced in the daily cafeteria group.

Effects of cafeteria diet history on pellet priming-induced reinstatement

Similar to the cue-induced reinstatement test, pellet-priming-induced reinstatement was more pronounced in the chow-only group than in the rats with a history of cafeteria diet (**Fig. 3B**). Data were analyzed using mixed-factor ANOVA, with the between-subjects factor of Diet Condition, within-subjects factors of Lever (active, inactive) and Pellet Number (0, 1, 2, 4). The results showed significant main effects of Diet Condition, Lever, and Pellet Number ($F_{2,21}=4.1$, $F_{1,21}=79.1$, and $F_{3,63}=16.5$, respectively, $p<0.05$), as well as significant interactions of Diet Condition x Lever, Lever x Pellet Number, and Diet Condition x Lever x Pellet Number ($F_{2,21}=7.2$, $F_{3,63}=18.6$, $F_{6,63}=2.9$, $p<0.05$). Lever responding across all pellet priming conditions in the chow-only group was significantly higher than either intermittent cafeteria or daily cafeteria groups ($p<0.05$). In order to further understand the effect of Pellet Number on groups with cafeteria diet histories, we performed three separate repeated measures ANOVAs for chow-only, daily cafeteria and intermittent cafeteria groups, using the within-subjects factors of Lever (active, inactive) and Pellet Number (0, 1, 2, 4). Results from the analyses of daily and intermittent cafeteria diet groups showed significant main effects of Lever and Pellet Number (daily cafeteria: $F_{1,7}=16.1$, $F_{3,21}=3.3$, respectively, $p<0.05$; intermittent cafeteria: $F_{1,7}=67.5$, $F_{3,21}=5.9$, respectively, $p<0.01$), and interaction of Lever x Pellet Number ($F_{3,21}=9.9$, $p<0.01$) in the intermittent cafeteria group only. Thus, similar to the effect of discrete cue, the reinstatement induced by pellet priming was most robust in chow-only and least robust in the daily cafeteria rats.

Effects of cafeteria diet history on intermittent footshock-induced reinstatement

Intermittent footshock induced modest reinstatement of lever pressing; this effect was significant in the daily cafeteria group, but not the intermittent cafeteria or chow-only groups (**Fig. 3C**). Data were analyzed using mixed-factor ANOVA, with the between-subjects factor of Diet Condition, within-subjects factor of Lever (active, inactive) and Shock Duration (0, 5, and 10 min). The results showed significant main effects of Lever and Shock Duration ($F_{1,21}=39.0$, $F_{2,42}=4.0$, $p<0.05$), but not Diet Condition ($p=0.93$). In order to further understand the main effect of shock across groups, we performed two separate repeated measures ANOVAs, with Lever (active, inactive) and Shock Duration (0, 5, and 10 min) as within-subjects factors, focusing on rats that previously had access to cafeteria diets. The analysis of the daily cafeteria group only showed a Lever x Shock Duration interaction ($F_{2,14}=3.7$, $p=0.05$), and post-hoc tests on active lever

Table 1. Summary of inactive-lever presses during the training, extinction, and reinstatement testing.

		Chow only	Intermittent cafeteria	Daily cafeteria
Training	day 1	20.3±7.9	22.8±7.1	11.6±7.4
	day 10	10.5±4.8	3.4±1.1	2.5±1.1
Extinction (no cue)	day 1	19.6±8.7	6.3±2.9	4.1±2.3
	day 10	4.4±1.5	7.9±3.5	2.9±1.8
Cue-induced reinstatement	No cue	4.4±1.7	8.5±4.0	16.0±14.9
	Cue	9.1±3.5	6.6±3.4	2.4±2.0
Pellet priming-induced reinstatement	0 pellet	2.8±1.2	1.8±0.9	0.8±0.5
	1 pellet	2.9±1.7	2.5±1.7	1.6±1.2
	2 pellets	1.4±0.7	2.4±1.3	5.6±4.6
	4 pellets	4.6±2.3	1.3±0.6	9.8±7.0
Footshock-induced reinstatement	0 min	3.0±1.1	3.6±1.9	5.3±3.0
	5 min	7.5±2.7	4.3±1.6	8.8±6.0
	10 min	4.6±2.3	13.4±10.8	6.6±2.9

Data are mean±SEM.

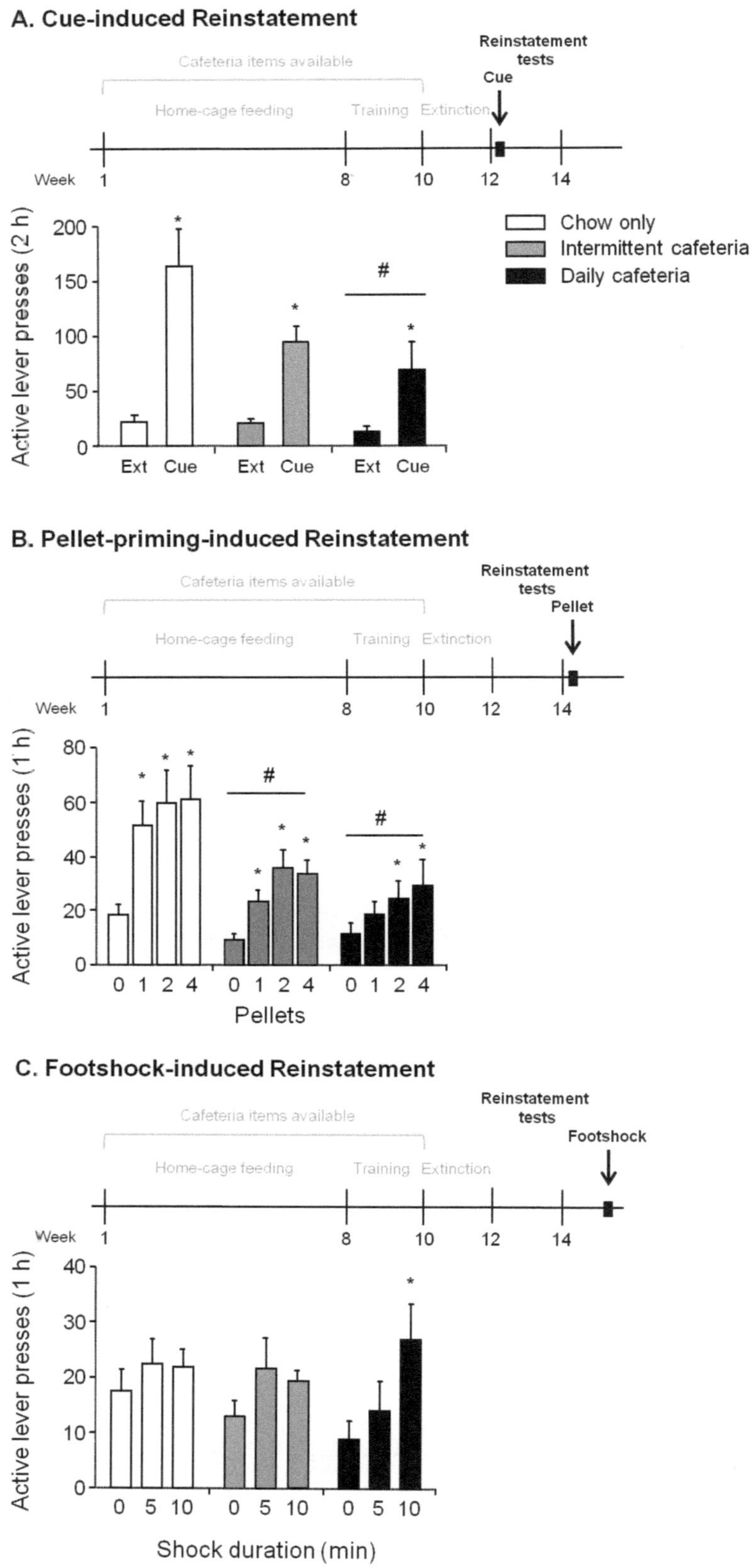

Figure 3. Effect of home-cage diet histories on reinstatement of food seeking. A. Effect of discrete cue presentation on reinstatement. Active lever responding (mean±SEM) under extinction (with cue) conditions following a single non-contingent cue presentation at the start of the session. *Different between the last day of extinction (without cue) and cue-test within subject, $p<0.05$. # Different in overall lever pressing from chow-only group, $p=0.06$. **B.** Effect of pellet priming on reinstatement. Active lever responding (mean±SEM) under extinction conditions (with cue) following 1, 2, and 4 non-contingent pellet deliveries at the beginning of an extinction session. *Different between 0 pellet baseline (last one hour

extinction session) and respective pellet test within subject, $p<0.05$. # Different in overall lever pressing from chow-only group, $p<0.05$. **C.** Effect of intermittent footshock on reinstatement. Active lever responding (mean±SEM) under extinction conditions (with cue) following 5 min and 10 min of intermittent footshock.

responding showed a significant difference between 0 min and 10 min shock ($p<0.05$). A similar analysis of the intermittent cafeteria group failed to show a significant interaction. Thus, in contrast to discrete cue or pellet-priming, the daily cafeteria diet group appears to be more sensitive to intermittent footshock-induced reinstatement than the intermittent cafeteria or chow-only groups.

Discussion

In the present study, we examined reinstatement of food seeking in a more clinically relevant rat model, which used unrestricted female rats that became overweight by prolonged exposure to a cafeteria diet. In agreement with previous reports [34,35], we found that daily exposure to cafeteria diet leads to increased caloric intake and significant weight gain. This diet manipulation, however, led to decreased concurrent self-administration of normally preferred food pellets. After cessation of diet exposure in the home-cage and removal of the preferred food pellets from the operant chambers during the extinction and reinstatement phases, rats with prior history of daily cafeteria diet, and to a lesser degree prior history of intermittent cafeteria diet, showed decreased extinction responding, and cue- and pellet-priming-induced reinstatement. In contrast, modest stress-induced reinstatement was only observed in rats with a history of daily cafeteria diet. Another finding in our study is that, independent of the history of home-cage diet, female rats with free access to standard chow not only demonstrated escalation in time-out responding during pellet self-administration, but also demonstrated robust cue- and pellet-priming-induced reinstatement. The increase in time-out responding is interesting in light of studies using drug or food reinforcers, which have suggested that lever pressing during the non-reinforced period reflects a compulsive reward seeking behavior that may predict the "addiction-prone" phenotype [36,37]. These data extend previous reinstatement studies in food-restricted male or female rats during the extinction and reinstatement phases [15,16] by examining these behaviors in unrestricted female rats.

Female rats with *ad libitum* access to cafeteria diet alongside standard chow show clinically relevant food intake patterns

The present home-cage food access procedures may provide a more clinically relevant picture of food intake prior to and during dieting than is typical of food reinstatement studies [15]. Initially, humans with unhealthy eating habits consume limited amounts of nutritionally balanced foods and greater amounts of calorically-dense palatable foods. Then during dieting human subjects not only restrict the amount of calorically-dense food they eat but also tend to consume nutritionally balanced foods. Traditional home-cage food restriction in reinstatement studies is an experimenter-administered manipulation that forces the rat to consume less nutritionally balanced food in order to accommodate for palatable food consumption. The current procedures (chow and cafeteria diet freely available) allowed the rats to choose how much nutritionally balanced and calorically-dense food to consume. Under these conditions, rats consumed less nutritionally balanced food and more palatable food (in the home-cage), a pattern similar to the unhealthy eating habits observed in humans prior to dieting. Then during extinction and reinstatement, rats fed cafeteria diets were switched to a chow-only diet, a qualitative manipulation that more closely models human dieting than the maintenance of chow restriction commonly used in reinstatement studies.

The current procedures may prove valuable in revealing the involvement of neural mechanisms in reinstatement that are qualitatively different in overweight rats as compared to normal weight rats. Studies show that chronic access to a cafeteria diet leads to metabolic and immune dysfunctions commonly associated with human obesity [34,38]. Furthermore, unhealthy diet histories cause dysregulations in reward processing and stress systems [20,21], both of which are critical in controlling relapse behavior [16,23].

Female rats with cafeteria diet history show modest cue- and pellet-priming-induced reinstatement

We found that rats with prior daily and intermittent cafeteria diet history showed relatively modest discrete cue- and pellet-priming-induced reinstatement effects as compared to rats fed with chow only. This is perhaps not surprising, since both cafeteria groups demonstrated low levels of operant pellet self-administration during the training and extinction phases. These effects may be explained by the successive negative contrast effect, which describes a change in animals' behavior following a downshift in the qualitative or quantitative value of an expected reward [39] and is often observed in the context of instrumental settings when food pellets are used as reward [40,41]. Indeed, since rats compare the present reward with their previous experiences and respond according to its relative value [42], rats that previously had access to highly palatable cafeteria items may not perceive the operant pellet to be as rewarding as the rats fed chow-only.

If the value of outcome is lower for rats with cafeteria diet histories, this might explain the reduced motivation during self-administration and pellet-priming reinstatement testing. Previous work has shown that rats with access to sucrose during adolescence show a lower motivation to self-administer saccharin during adulthood [43]. Further, this less effective reinforcer would presumably support less incentive salience attribution to the pellet-associated cues [44], which may reduce the cue's effectiveness at reinstating behavior. The possible influence of such negative contrast effects in blunting motivation in the operant setting should be carefully considered in studies that seek to make rats overweight using palatable diets prior to assessing motivation for other natural and drug rewards.

Exposure to the daily cafeteria diet may also lead to a depressive-like, anhedonic state, which could contribute to the lack of responding during reinstatement tests observed in cafeteria rats. Exposure to energy dense diets elevates brain stimulation reward threshold in rats [35], and also increases depression-related behaviors in forced swim and sucrose preference tests in mice [45,46]. Withdrawal from palatable food, as experienced by the daily cafeteria rats during the extinction and testing phases of the present study, also leads to depressive-like behaviors in rats using similar diet manipulations [47]. Other studies have found that naltrexone and social defeat, both of which cause anhedonia [48,49], either suppress responding in reinstatement testing [50] or reduce lever responding during extinction [51]. Thus, an anhedonic state associated with withdrawal from cafeteria diets may contribute to the blunted reinstatement effects observed in the present study, another important consideration for future studies.

Female rats with prior cafeteria diet history show modest stress-induced reinstatement

Although rats that previously had daily access to cafeteria diet consistently showed less lever responding during training, extinction and cue- and pellet-priming-induced reinstatement, they were particularly sensitive to stress-induced reinstatement. Indeed, while chow-only rats did not respond to footshock-induced reinstatement of food seeking, a pattern similar to previous findings [52,53], the daily cafeteria group significantly increased lever pressing after 10 min of intermittent footshock. This heightened sensitivity to stress is consistent with studies in rodents showing that extended access to and withdrawal from palatable food causes adaptations in stress circuitry [22,54–57]. In the present study, rats previously fed cafeteria diet, which restrict intake of chow once palatable food is no longer available, show greater sensitivity to stress-induced reinstatement, a finding that parallels the clinical observation that restraint eaters have a greater tendency to overeat when encountering a stressful situation [58,59]. Future studies are needed to determine the underlying mechanisms and related physiological changes of this diet-induced hypersensitivity to stress. For example, while studies have shown that access to or removal of cafeteria diet did not affect baseline corticosterone levels [56], diet history can affect how stress circuitry responds to acute stressors [60].

The stress-effect in the cafeteria group should, however, be interpreted with caution. First, the amount of lever pressing observed in the cafeteria group after footshock, while significantly different than baseline responding, is not as robust as the cue and pellet priming reinstatement effects reported here and footshock stress effect reported previously with heroin and cocaine [31,32,61]. Second, all rats were repeatedly tested across multiple reinstating stimuli, and footshock-induced reinstatement testing was conducted last. However, repeated testing is unlikely to confound our interpretations, since all rats underwent additional extinction sessions before footshock testing, and the baseline lever-pressing for the cafeteria group remained consistent across all reinstatement testing. Similar repeated testing procedures have also been used in various reinstatement studies and reliable results are obtained [25,62–68].

Finally, footshock-induced reinstatement testing occurred 4–5 weeks after the cessation of cafeteria diets. At the time of footshock testing both body weight and caloric intake differences between cafeteria and chow-only groups had disappeared. When examining the impact of historical manipulations such as exposure to or withdrawal from cafeteria diets, it can be argued that it would be ideal to do so at an earlier time point than that used in the present study. However, similar withdrawal periods have been used in drug studies where footshock-induced reinstatement effects were found [31,32,61]. Further, the stress sensitivity observed here could be time-dependent, as is the incubation of drug or sucrose craving [69]. Future studies are needed to determine the time-course of this potentially enhanced sensitivity to stress in cafeteria rats.

Conclusions

Here, we demonstrate that it is possible to study reinstatement of food seeking in a clinically relevant model that makes rats overweight by giving them access to unhealthy foods commonly consumed by humans. Female rats serve as suitable subjects for reinstatement studies, as under the current procedures they demonstrated robust self-administration responding and reinstatement effects without the need for food restriction. Studies have shown that chronic caloric restriction can cause long-lasting changes in the stress- and feeding-related pathways [54], and the level of food restriction may contribute to the differential effect of pharmacological agents on reinstatement of food seeking [15]. A potential concern when using intact female rats is that fluctuations in ovarian hormones across the estrous cycle can influence reinstatement behavior [64,70,71]. In the present study we did not directly track estrous cycle phase, and thus we cannot rule out the possibility that cafeteria diet histories influence the estrous cycle, which might contribute to observed differences in reinstatement behavior between groups. Nevertheless, a previous study has shown that ovarian hormones and estrous cycle phase play relatively insignificant roles in reinstatement of palatable food seeking [72]. Together with a recent study showing that the behavior of female rodents is no more intrinsically variable than that of male rodents, as commonly assumed [73], our results provide a useful procedural validation for future studies that intend to study reinstatement under conditions that more accurately model clinical observations in individuals seeking treatment for relapse to unhealthy eating during dieting.

Acknowledgments

The work was supported by the Intramural Research Program of the National Institute on Drug Abuse. We thank Dr. Yavin Shaham for his insightful comments on the manuscript.

Author Contributions

Conceived and designed the experiments: YWC DJC. Performed the experiments: YWC KAF SZB. Analyzed the data: YWC KAF. Contributed to the writing of the manuscript: YWC KAF DJC.

References

1. Swinburn B, Sacks G, Ravussin E (2009) Increased food energy supply is more than sufficient to explain the US epidemic of obesity. Am J Clin Nutr 90: 1453–1456.
2. Swinburn BA, Sacks G, Lo SK, Westerterp KR, Rush EC, et al. (2009) Estimating the changes in energy flux that characterize the rise in obesity prevalence. Am J Clin Nutr 89: 1723–1728.
3. Kramer FM, Jeffery RW, Forster JL, Snell MK (1989) Long-term follow-up of behavioral treatment for obesity: patterns of weight regain among men and women. Int J Obes 13: 123–136.
4. Peterson CB, Mitchell JE (1999) Psychosocial and pharmacological treatment of eating disorders: a review of research findings. J Clin Psychol 55: 685–697.
5. Skender ML, Goodrick GK, Del Junco DJ, Reeves RS, Darnell L, et al. (1996) Comparison of 2-year weight loss trends in behavioral treatments of obesity: diet, exercise, and combination interventions. J Am Diet Assoc 96: 342–346.
6. McGuire MT, Wing RR, Klem ML, Lang W, Hill JO (1999) What predicts weight regain in a group of successful weight losers? J Consult Clin Psychol 67: 177–185.
7. Grilo CM, Shiffman S, Wing RR (1989) Relapse crises and coping among dieters. J Consult Clin Psychol 57: 488–495.
8. Kayman S, Bruvold W, Stern JS (1990) Maintenance and relapse after weight loss in women: behavioral aspects. Am J Clin Nutr 52: 800–807.
9. Polivy J, Herman CP (1999) Distress and eating: why do dieters overeat? Int J Eat Disord 26: 153–164.
10. Torres SJ, Nowson CA (2007) Relationship between stress, eating behavior, and obesity. Nutrition 23: 887–894.
11. Ghitza UE, Gray SM, Epstein DH, Rice KC, Shaham Y (2006) The anxiogenic drug yohimbine reinstates palatable food seeking in a rat relapse model: a role of CRF(1) receptors. Neuropsychopharmacology 31: 2188–2196.
12. See RE (2002) Neural substrates of conditioned-cued relapse to drug-seeking behavior. Pharmacol Biochem Behav 71: 517–529.

13. Self DW, Nestler EJ (1998) Relapse to drug-seeking: neural and molecular mechanisms. Drug Alcohol Depend 51: 49–60.
14. Shaham Y, Shalev U, Lu L, De Wit H, Stewart J (2003) The reinstatement model of drug relapse: history, methodology and major findings. Psychopharmacology 168: 3–20.
15. Calu DJ, Chen YW, Kawa AB, Nair SG, Shaham Y (2014) The use of the reinstatement model to study relapse to palatable food seeking during dieting. Neuropharmacology 76 Pt B: 395–406.
16. Nair SG, Adams-Deutsch T, Epstein DH, Shaham Y (2009) The neuropharmacology of relapse to food seeking: methodology, main findings, and comparison with relapse to drug seeking. Progress in neurobiology 89: 18–45.
17. Pillitteri JL, Shiffman S, Rohay JM, Harkins AM, Burton SL, et al. (2008) Use of dietary supplements for weight loss in the United States: results of a national survey. Obesity (Silver Spring) 16: 790–796.
18. Davy SR, Benes BA, Driskell JA (2006) Sex differences in dieting trends, eating habits, and nutrition beliefs of a group of midwestern college students. J Am Diet Assoc 106: 1673–1677.
19. Nair SG, Navarre BM, Cifani C, Pickens CL, Bossert JM, et al. (2011) Role of dorsal medial prefrontal cortex dopamine D1-family receptors in relapse to high-fat food seeking induced by the anxiogenic drug yohimbine. Neuropsychopharmacology 36: 497–510.
20. Kenny PJ (2011) Reward mechanisms in obesity: new insights and future directions. Neuron 69: 664–679.
21. Parylak SL, Koob GF, Zorrilla EP (2011) The dark side of food addiction. Physiol Behav 104: 149–156.
22. Cottone P, Sabino V, Roberto M, Bajo M, Pockros L, et al. (2009) CRF system recruitment mediates dark side of compulsive eating. Proc Natl Acad Sci U S A 106: 20016–20020.
23. Bossert JM, Marchant NJ, Calu DJ, Shaham Y (2013) The reinstatement model of drug relapse: recent neurobiological findings, emerging research topics, and translational research. Psychopharmacology 229: 453–476.
24. Nair SG, Adams-Deutsch T, Pickens CL, Smith DG, Shaham Y (2009) Effects of the MCH1 receptor antagonist SNAP 94847 on high-fat food-reinforced operant responding and reinstatement of food seeking in rats. Psychopharmacology 205: 129–140.
25. Pickens CL, Cifani C, Navarre BM, Eichenbaum H, Theberge FR, et al. (2012) Effect of fenfluramine on reinstatement of food seeking in female and male rats: implications for the predictive validity of the reinstatement model. Psychopharmacology 221: 341–353.
26. Grimm JW, See RE (2000) Dissociation of primary and secondary reward-relevant limbic nuclei in an animal model of relapse. Neuropsychopharmacology 22: 473–479.
27. See RE, Grimm JW, Kruzich PJ, Rustay N (1999) The importance of a compound stimulus in conditioned drug-seeking behavior following one week of extinction from self-administered cocaine in rats. Drug Alcohol Depend 57: 41–49.
28. Ghitza UE, Nair SG, Golden SA, Gray SM, Uejima JL, et al. (2007) Peptide YY3-36 decreases reinstatement of high-fat food seeking during dieting in a rat relapse model. J Neurosci 27: 11522–11532.
29. Deroche V, Le Moal M, Piazza PV (1999) Cocaine self-administration increases the incentive motivational properties of the drug in rats. Eur J Neurosci 11: 2731–2736.
30. Lu L, Grimm JW, Dempsey J, Shaham Y (2004) Cocaine seeking over extended withdrawal periods in rats: different time courses of responding induced by cocaine cues versus cocaine priming over the first 6 months. Psychopharmacology 176: 101–108.
31. Shalev U, Morales M, Hope B, Yap J, Shaham Y (2001) Time-dependent changes in extinction behavior and stress-induced reinstatement of drug seeking following withdrawal from heroin in rats. Psychopharmacology 156: 98–107.
32. Shaham Y, Stewart J (1995) Stress reinstates heroin-seeking in drug-free animals: an effect mimicking heroin, not withdrawal. Psychopharmacology 119: 334–341.
33. Shaham Y, Rajabi H, Stewart J (1996) Relapse to heroin-seeking in rats under opioid maintenance: the effects of stress, heroin priming, and withdrawal. J Neurosci 16: 1957–1963.
34. Sampey BP, Vanhoose AM, Winfield HM, Freemerman AJ, Muehlbauer MJ, et al. (2011) Cafeteria diet is a robust model of human metabolic syndrome with liver and adipose inflammation: comparison to high-fat diet. Obesity 19: 1109–1117.
35. Johnson PM, Kenny PJ (2010) Dopamine D2 receptors in addiction-like reward dysfunction and compulsive eating in obese rats. Nat Neurosci 13: 635–641.
36. Deroche-Gamonet V, Belin D, Piazza PV (2004) Evidence for addiction-like behavior in the rat. Science 305: 1014–1017.
37. Nair SG, Gray SM, Ghitza UE (2006) Role of food type in yohimbine- and pellet-priming-induced reinstatement of food seeking. Physiol Behav 88: 559–566.
38. Rolls BJ, Rowe EA, Turner RC (1980) Persistent obesity in rats following a period of consumption of a mixed, high energy diet. J Physiol 298: 415–427.
39. Crespi LP (1942) Quantitative variation of incentive and performance in the white rat. American Journal of Psychology 55: 467–517.
40. Mitchell EN, Marston HM, Nutt DJ, Robinson ES (2012) Evaluation of an operant successive negative contrast task as a method to study affective state in rodents. Behav Brain Res 234: 155–160.
41. Sastre A, Reilly S (2006) Excitotoxic lesions of the gustatory thalamus eliminate consummatory but not instrumental successive negative contrast in rats. Behav Brain Res 170: 34–40.
42. Flaherty CF (1996) Incentive relativity. Cambridge, UK Cambridge University Press.
43. Vendruscolo LF, Gueye AB, Darnaudery M, Ahmed SH, Cador M (2010) Sugar overconsumption during adolescence selectively alters motivation and reward function in adult rats. PLoS One 5: e9296.
44. Berridge KC, Robinson TE (1998) What is the role of dopamine in reward: hedonic impact, reward learning, or incentive salience? Brain Res Brain Res Rev 28: 309–369.
45. Sharma S, Fulton S (2013) Diet-induced obesity promotes depressive-like behaviour that is associated with neural adaptations in brain reward circuitry. Int J Obes (Lond) 37: 382–389.
46. Yamada N, Katsuura G, Ochi Y, Ebihara K, Kusakabe T, et al. (2011) Impaired CNS leptin action is implicated in depression associated with obesity. Endocrinology 152: 2634–2643.
47. Iemolo A, Valenza M, Tozier L, Knapp CM, Kornetsky C, et al. (2012) Withdrawal from chronic, intermittent access to a highly palatable food induces depressive-like behavior in compulsive eating rats. Behav Pharmacol 23: 593–602.
48. West TE, Wise RA (1988) Effects of naltrexone on nucleus accumbens, lateral hypothalamic and ventral tegmental self-stimulation rate-frequency functions. Brain Res 462: 126–133.
49. Donahue RJ, Muschamp JW, Russo SJ, Nestler EJ, Carlezon WA Jr (2014) Effects of Striatal DeltaFosB Overexpression and Ketamine on Social Defeat Stress-Induced Anhedonia in Mice. Biol Psychiatry.
50. Stewart J, Wise RA (1992) Reinstatement of heroin self-administration habits: morphine prompts and naltrexone discourages renewed responding after extinction. Psychopharmacology 108: 79–84.
51. Funk D, Harding S, Juzytsch W, Le AD (2005) Effects of unconditioned and conditioned social defeat on alcohol self-administration and reinstatement of alcohol seeking in rats. Psychopharmacology 183: 341–349.
52. Ahmed SH, Koob GF (1997) Cocaine- but not food-seeking behavior is reinstated by stress after extinction. Psychopharmacology 132: 289–295.
53. Buczek Y, Le AD, Wang A, Stewart J, Shaham Y (1999) Stress reinstates nicotine seeking but not sucrose solution seeking in rats. Psychopharmacology 144: 183–188.
54. Pankevich DE, Teegarden SL, Hedin AD, Jensen CL, Bale TL (2010) Caloric restriction experience reprograms stress and orexigenic pathways and promotes binge eating. J Neurosci 30: 16399–16407.
55. Teegarden SL, Bale TL (2007) Decreases in dietary preference produce increased emotionality and risk for dietary relapse. Biol Psychiatry 61: 1021–1029.
56. Martire SI, Maniam J, South T, Holmes N, Westbrook RF, et al. (2014) Extended exposure to a palatable cafeteria diet alters gene expression in brain regions implicated in reward, and withdrawal from this diet alters gene expression in brain regions associated with stress. Behav Brain Res 265: 132–141.
57. South T, Westbrook F, Morris MJ (2012) Neurological and stress related effects of shifting obese rats from a palatable diet to chow and lean rats from chow to a palatable diet. Physiol Behav 105: 1052–1057.
58. Greeno CG, Wing RR (1994) Stress-induced eating. Psychol Bull 115: 444–464.
59. Heatherton TF, Herman CP, Polivy J (1991) Effects of physical threat and ego threat on eating behavior. J Pers Soc Psychol 60: 138–143.
60. Tannenbaum BM, Brindley DN, Tannenbaum GS, Dallman MF, McArthur MD, et al. (1997) High-fat feeding alters both basal and stress-induced hypothalamic-pituitary-adrenal activity in the rat. Am J Physiol 273: E1168–1177.
61. Erb S, Shaham Y, Stewart J (1996) Stress reinstates cocaine-seeking behavior after prolonged extinction and a drug-free period. Psychopharmacology 128: 408–412.
62. De Vries TJ, Schoffelmeer AN, Binnekade R, Raaso H, Vanderschuren LJ (2002) Relapse to cocaine- and heroin-seeking behavior mediated by dopamine D2 receptors is time-dependent and associated with behavioral sensitization. Neuropsychopharmacology 26: 18–26.
63. de Wit H, Stewart J (1981) Reinstatement of cocaine-reinforced responding in the rat. Psychopharmacology 75: 134–143.
64. Fuchs RA, Evans KA, Mehta RH, Case JM, See RE (2005) Influence of sex and estrous cyclicity on conditioned cue-induced reinstatement of cocaine-seeking behavior in rats. Psychopharmacology 179: 662–672.
65. Self DW, Barnhart WJ, Lehman DA, Nestler EJ (1996) Opposite modulation of cocaine-seeking behavior by D1- and D2-like dopamine receptor agonists. Science 271: 1586–1589.
66. Shaham Y, Erb S, Leung S, Buczek Y, Stewart J (1998) CP-154,526, a selective, non-peptide antagonist of the corticotropin-releasing factor1 receptor attenuates stress-induced relapse to drug seeking in cocaine- and heroin-trained rats. Psychopharmacology 137: 184–190.
67. Spealman RD, Barrett-Larimore RL, Rowlett JK, Platt DM, Khroyan TV (1999) Pharmacological and environmental determinants of relapse to cocaine-seeking behavior. Pharmacol Biochem Behav 64: 327–336.
68. Weiss F, Martin-Fardon R, Ciccocioppo R, Kerr TM, Smith DL, et al. (2001) Enduring resistance to extinction of cocaine-seeking behavior induced by drug-related cues. Neuropsychopharmacology 25: 361–372.

69. Pickens CL, Airavaara M, Theberge F, Fanous S, Hope BT, et al. (2011) Neurobiology of the incubation of drug craving. Trends Neurosci 34: 411–420.
70. Anker JJ, Carroll ME (2011) Females are more vulnerable to drug abuse than males: evidence from preclinical studies and the role of ovarian hormones. Curr Top Behav Neurosci 8: 73–96.
71. Feltenstein MW, Henderson AR, See RE (2011) Enhancement of cue-induced reinstatement of cocaine-seeking in rats by yohimbine: sex differences and the role of the estrous cycle. Psychopharmacology 216: 53–62.
72. Cifani C, Koya E, Navarre BM, Calu DJ, Baumann MH, et al. (2012) Medial prefrontal cortex neuronal activation and synaptic alterations after stress-induced reinstatement of palatable food seeking: a study using c-fos-GFP transgenic female rats. J Neurosci 32: 8480–8490.
73. Prendergast BJ, Onishi KG, Zucker I (2014) Female mice liberated for inclusion in neuroscience and biomedical research. Neurosci Biobehav Rev 40C: 1–5.

15

Application of Selection Mapping to Identify Genomic Regions Associated with Dairy Production in Sheep

Beatriz Gutiérrez-Gil[1]*, Juan Jose Arranz[1], Ricardo Pong-Wong[2], Elsa García-Gámez[1], James Kijas[3], Pamela Wiener[2]

1 Dpto. Producción Animal, Universidad de León, León, Spain, **2** The Roslin Institute and R(D)SVS, University of Edinburgh, Roslin, Midlothian, United Kingdom, **3** Animal, Food and Health Sciences, CSIRO, Brisbane, Australia

Abstract

In Europe, especially in Mediterranean areas, the sheep has been traditionally exploited as a dual purpose species, with income from both meat and milk. Modernization of husbandry methods and the establishment of breeding schemes focused on milk production have led to the development of "dairy breeds." This study investigated selective sweeps specifically related to dairy production in sheep by searching for regions commonly identified in different European dairy breeds. With this aim, genotypes from 44,545 SNP markers covering the sheep autosomes were analysed in both European dairy and non-dairy sheep breeds using two approaches: (i) identification of genomic regions showing extreme genetic differentiation between each dairy breed and a closely related non-dairy breed, and (ii) identification of regions with reduced variation (heterozygosity) in the dairy breeds using two methods. Regions detected in at least two breeds (breed pairs) by the two approaches (genetic differentiation and at least one of the heterozygosity-based analyses) were labeled as core candidate convergence regions and further investigated for candidate genes. Following this approach six regions were detected. For some of them, strong candidate genes have been proposed (e.g. *ABCG2, SPP1*), whereas some other genes designated as candidates based on their association with sheep and cattle dairy traits (e.g. *LALBA, DGAT1A*) were not associated with a detectable sweep signal. Few of the identified regions were coincident with QTL previously reported in sheep, although many of them corresponded to orthologous regions in cattle where QTL for dairy traits have been identified. Due to the limited number of QTL studies reported in sheep compared with cattle, the results illustrate the potential value of selection mapping to identify genomic regions associated with dairy traits in sheep.

Editor: Bernhard Kaltenboeck, Auburn University, United States of America

Funding: The authors gratefully acknowledge support from the Spanish Ministry of Economy and Competitiveness (Project AGL2009-07000), Institute Strategic Grant funding from the UK Biotechnology and Biological Sciences Research Council (BBSRC) and the financial support of the European Science Foundation through the GENOMIC-RESOURCES Exchange Grant awarded to Beatriz Gutierrez (EX/3723). BGG is funded through the Spanish "Ramón y Cajal" Programme from the Spanish Ministry of Economy and Competitiveness (State Secretariat for Research, Development and Innovation). The funders had no role in study design, data collection and analysis, decision to publish, or preparation of the manuscript.

Competing Interests: The authors have declared that no competing interests exist.

* E-mail: beatriz.gutierrez@unileon.es

Introduction

Since their domestication 8 000–9 000 years ago (reviewed by [1]), sheep (*Ovis aries*) have been used by humans for the production of wool, meat and milk. Adaptation to very different geographic and climatic conditions and the specialization for specific characteristics have resulted in a phenotypically highly diverse species. The first documented modifications to sheep by human-imposed selection had taken place by the time that illustrations and records first appeared c. 3 000 BC and primarily concerned morphological and coat colour traits with the initial major morphological changes including reduction in the length of the legs, lengthening of the tail and alteration of horn shape [2]. Initially, sheep were kept solely for meat, milk and skins. Archaeological evidence suggests that selection for woolly sheep may have begun around 6000 BC.

Dairy sheep are mainly found in Europe, especially in Mediterranean areas, where they have been traditionally exploited as a dual purpose species, with income from both meat and milk. Sheep milk has a higher solid content than cow or goat milk, which means that it is particularly suited to processing into cheese. Historically, most sheep milk has been produced by multipurpose local breeds with low-to-medium milk yields and raised under traditional husbandry conditions [3]. More recently, modernization of husbandry methods and the establishment of breeding schemes focused on milk production have led to the development of "dairy breeds", facilitated by the implementation of quantitative genetics-based breeding and the use of artificial insemination [2]. The market for sheep milk and sheep dairy products appears to be growing, even in those countries without a history of sheep dairying [4].

Selection sweep mapping strategies, in which regions of the genome are identified that show patterns consistent with positive selection, can be used as a complementary approach to linkage mapping and genome-wide association study (GWAS) analysis to identify regions of the genome that influence important traits in livestock. Various methods have been applied to livestock and other domesticated animals, with the aim of identifying genomic regions with characteristics that reflect the influence of selection: extended low diversity haplotypes [5], overall low heterozygosity (e.g. [6,7]), specific diversity patterns [8], extreme allele frequencies [9] and between-breed differentiation [10,11,12]. Because of their well-documented selection pressures and highly-developed genetic resources, domesticated animal species also provide a valuable resource with the potential to identify the molecular pathways underlying phenotypic traits through the use of selection mapping approaches [10,13].

To perform a search for signatures of selection related to dairy production in sheep, we used genotypes obtained with the *Illumina OvineSNP50 BeadChip* (Illumina Inc., San Diego, CA) for a number of European breeds genotyped within the framework of the Sheep HapMap Project [14]. These breeds include several selected primarily for dairy production and others not used for dairy. In order to specifically target regions under dairy-related selection and not related to other traits that may have been under selection in the sheep populations, only selection signatures commonly identified in different European dairy breeds were considered. We applied two approaches for the detection of selection sweeps: (i) we looked for regions with extreme genetic differentiation between each dairy breed and a closely related non-dairy breed, and (ii) we looked for regions of the genome with reduced heterozygosity in the dairy breeds using two methods. We then searched for candidate genes that could be selection targets within the regions that were identified in multiple breeds and using multiple analysis methods. For these regions we also looked for correspondence with previously reported QTL related to dairy production traits in cattle or sheep. Although the selection history of dairy cattle is quite different from that of dairy sheep, in particular because breeding schemes in sheep are focused on more localized (and in many cases isolated) breeds than the global dairy cattle population, comparison of our results with studies in cattle allowed us to evaluate whether some of the same regions/genes show evidence of selection in both dairy sheep and dairy cattle.

Materials and Methods

Data

Samples. We analysed a subset of the dataset generated in the Ovine HapMap project [14], which included 5 dairy and 5 non-dairy sheep breeds (Table 1).

Genotypes. After an initial quality control procedure described in detail elsewhere [14], this dataset provides the genotypes of 49,034 SNPs (using the *Illumina OvineSNP50 BeadChip*) distributed across the 26 autosomal ovine chromosomes and chromosome X (only one of the markers genotyped belongs to chromosome Y). Markers were filtered to exclude loci assigned to unmapped contigs. The analyses reported here focused on the remaining 44,545 of these SNP located on autosomes. The positions of the markers according to the Sheep Genome Assembly v2.0 (update September 2011) were used for the analyses.

Selection Sweep Mapping Analysis Methods

(i) Genetic differentiation: Pair-wise F_{ST} calculations. In order to search for genomic regions that have been under divergent selection in dairy and non-dairy breeds, we examined genetic differentiation across the genome for five breed pairs. The selection of sheep breeds to serve as non-dairy partners for dairy breeds was based on the shortest divergence time estimates reported by the Sheep HapMap project (based on the extent of haplotype sharing and correlation of linkage disequilibrium values; Supplementary Information Figure S10 and Figure 3 in [14]), and close relationships according to additional Principal Component Analyses (PCA) performed in a selection of breeds (described in detail in File S1).

The following pairs of breeds of European ancestry were considered in the differentiation analysis:

a. Chios (Greek, dairy) *vs* Sakiz (Turkey, non-specialized)
b. Churra (Spanish, dairy) *vs* Ojalada (Spanish, meat)
c. Comisana (Italian, dairy) *vs* Australian Poll Merino (Australian, originated in southwest Europe, wool)
d. East Friesian Brown (highly specialized dairy) *vs* Finnsheep (Finland, primary wool, more recently used as a meat producing breed)
e. Milk Lacaune (French, highly specialized dairy) *vs* Australian Poll Merino (Australian, originated in southwest Europe, wool)
f. Milk Lacaune (French, highly specialized dairy) *vs* Meat Lacaune (French, meat)

For each of these pairs, unbiased estimates of Weir and Cockerham's F_{ST} [15], a measure of genetic differentiation, were calculated as functions of variance components, as detailed in Akey et al. [16]. This type of approach to selection mapping, exploiting between-breed allele frequency differences, has been applied in studies of humans [16] and domesticated animals [10,11,12,17,18] where it has been demonstrated to be effective in identifying genes that are associated with breed differentiation.

(ii) Reduced diversity: Observed heterozygosity. For all the breeds included in the pair-wise F_{ST} calculations, observed heterozygosity (ObsHtz) was calculated for each SNP marker. This approach has previously been applied in selection mapping studies of chickens [6,7], pigs [19] and dogs [20].

(iii) Reduced diversity: Regression analysis for detection of regions with asymptotic heterozygosity patterns. For all the breeds included in the pair-wise F_{ST} calculations, tests of significant asymptotic relationships between heterozygosity and distance from a test position were performed across the genome based on the approach of Wiener and Pong-Wong [8]. This method detects regions with patterns of variation consistent with positive selection: an asymptotic increase in marker variation (heterozygosity; y) with increasing distance (x) from a selected locus $y = A + B R^x$ (where R is the asymptotic rate of increase; B is the difference between heterozygosity at the test position and the asymptotic level; A is the asymptotic level of heterozygosity). For each regression (performed in Genstat, [21]), we recorded the parameters of the asymptotic regression, their standard errors, the significance level associated with the regression (p) and the variance explained by the curve. Positive and increasing regressions ($0<R<1$, $B<0$) were considered as being in the direction predicted by positive selection. Analysis of simulated data suggests improved precision of this selection mapping approach compared to an alternative haplotype-based method as well as robustness to demographic influences [8].

Protocols for Selection Mapping Analyses

In order to determine appropriate parameters for the above-mentioned analyses, we investigated their behaviour on a test genomic region encompassing the myostatin (*GDF-8*) gene, which is known to have been under selection in the Texel breed (details in File S2).

Window/bracket sizes. Based on the analysis of the myostatin gene (File S2), window and bracket sizes for the three methods were established. For the differentiation and reduced heterozygosity analyses, F_{ST} and ObsHtz values, respectively, were

Table 1. Breeds included in the present study.

Group	Breed name	Number of samples	Aptitude
Dairy	Chios	23	High milk production
	Churra	96	Double purpose breed (milk and lamb production
	Comisana	24	Highly-specialized dairy breed
	East Friesian Brown	39	Highly-specialized dairy breed
	Milk Lacaune	103	Highly-specialized dairy breed
Non-dairy	Australian Poll Merino	98	Meat production
	Meat Lacaune	78	Meat production
	Ojalada	24	Meat production
	Sakiz	22	Triple-purpose (milk, meat, wool)
	Finnsheep	99	Primary used for wool production; more recently used for meat production.

The classification established into Dairy and Non-dairy groups are presented together with some details about the breed aptitude.

averaged across sliding windows of 9 SNPs (F_{ST}-9SNPW, ObsHtz-9SNPW). For the regression analysis, the test position was moved every 50 Kb across each chromosome and all markers within 10 Mb of this position (10 Mb-bracket size) were considered in the asymptotic regression. A –log(p) value was determined for each test position.

Identification of selection signals by individual methods. Evidence of positive selection was interpreted for window estimates in the extreme of the empirical distributions, as suggested by Akey et al. [10,16] and employed in various subsequent studies (e.g. [11,13]. Specifically, we considered the positions showing signatures of selection as the top 0.5th percent of the distributions for differentiation (F_{ST}) and asymptotic regression (–log(p), for regressions in the predicted direction) or the bottom 0.5th percent for observed heterozygosity. Based on the results of the analysis of the myostatin gene (File S2), a selected "region" was defined as the range of positions within 2 Mb of each other showing evidence of selection by any of the three methods. An additional criterion for selected regions was that they were identified in at least two breed pairs, for F_{ST}, or two dairy breeds, for heterozygosity-based methods (with distances up to 2 Mb allowed between the regions identified for different breeds). For genetic differentiation, we further required that regions of extreme F_{ST} must be detected in at least two different pairs of dairy – non-dairy breeds that did not share a common breed (e.g. top regions found only in the Milk Lacaune-Australian Poll Merino and Comisana-Australian Poll Merino but not in other studied pairs were not included in the list of differentiated regions). By requiring at least two breeds (or breed pairs) for the initial identification of candidate regions for each methodology, this selection mapping strategy will not identify dairy gene variants occurring in only one breed.

Criteria for Identification of Regions with Shared Selection Signals

Based on the selected "regions" identified by the individual methods through the overlapping of at least two breeds or breed pairs, and taking into account that the F_{ST}-based method is expected to specifically target traits relevant for dairy production, whereas signals detected by heterozygosity-based methods may not be specific for dairy-related selection, we defined a "convergent candidate region" (CCR) as one where a signal was identified by the pair-wise F_{ST} comparison and at least one of the reduced heterozygosity methods. Hence, a CCR was labelled where there was overlap between the position ranges of the candidate regions identified by the genetic differentiation methodology and at least one of the two heterozygosity-based methods, such that each CCR was associated with a region identified in at least two breeds (breed pairs) and using at least two different methods.

Identification of Candidate Genes within CCR Regions

We identified the genes mapping to the end of each CCR using the genome browser of the sheep genome reference sequence (v2.0; http://www.livestockgenomics.csiro.au/cgi-bin/gbrowse/oarv2.0/) and identified the corresponding orthologous regions in the bovine genome (Cow (UMD3.1) using Ensembl (http://www.ensembl.org/Bos_taurus/Info/Index). A systematic extraction of all the annotated genes contained within the orthologous genomic ranges in cattle was performed using Biomart (www.biomart.org). Subsequently, an exhaustive search was performed for candidate genes previously linked to cattle dairy traits [22]. In addition, genes not included in this database but reported as candidate genes in the literature in relation to milk production or dairy-related traits were also identified. We also looked for correspondence with genes for which signatures of selection have been reported in studies of dairy cattle [23,24,25] and sheep [14,26].

We evaluated correspondence of the CCR with QTL reported for milk production and other functional traits related to dairy production in sheep (based on the SheepQTL database, http://www.animalgenome.org/cgi-bin/QTLdb/OA/index). We also examined overlap between the CCR and QTL influencing milk-related traits, mastitis and other functional traits related to dairy production in cattle (based on the CattleQTL database; http://www.animalgenome.org/cgi-bin/QTLdb/BT/index), positioned on the bovine genome reference sequence (UMD_version 3.1).

Results

Regions Identified by Individual Methods

Genetic differentiation. The level and range of the top 0.5% of F_{ST} values averaged in sliding windows of 9 SNPs (F_{ST}-9SNPW) varied among the five breed pairs (Figure 1). The lowest genome-wide differentiation within a pair was found, as expected, for the Milk Lacaune-Meat Lacaune pair (0.076), whereas the highest levels of genetic differentiation were found for the East Friesian Brown-Finnsheep pair (0.752, for the 9SNP-window centered on marker OAR3_185527791) (Table 2).

Twenty-eight genomic regions distributed across 15 autosomes were identified in at least two dairy-non-dairy breed pairs (Table S1, where a reference number has been given to each of them: F_{ST}-CandidateRegionX, F_{ST}-CRX). The largest number of F_{ST}-based candidate regions per chromosome was found on OAR3 (5 regions). The length of the F_{ST}-based candidate regions varied from 0.215 Mb (OAR3, F_{ST}-CR8) to 9.211 Mb (OAR6, F_{ST}-CR14).

Reduced observed heterozygosity in dairy breeds. Fifty-five regions showing reduced observed heterozygosity (ObsHtz-CR1–ObsHtz-CR55) in more than one dairy breed were found across 21 of the 26 autosomes (Table S2; where a non-dairy breed showed reduced heterozygosity in the same region, this is also indicated). Eight of the candidate regions found in dairy breeds covered intervals larger than 3 Mb. The largest was that on OAR13 (ObsHtz-CR42; 56.061–63.781 Mb), followed by one on OAR6 (ObsHtz-CR27:34.576–41.863 Mb), while the smallest region was a single window centered on marker on OAR2 (ObsHtz-CR9; 211.205 Mb). A normalized observed heterozygosity (NObsHtz) (based on that introduced by Rubin et al. [6]) was also calculated for all breeds analysed, again averaged in 9-SNP windows. There were no regions in the extreme lower end of the distribution (NObsHtz<-6) in the dairy breeds although the region on OAR6 (*ABCG2* gene region) had a value of −5.99 for the Meat Lacaune breed.

Regression analysis for detection of regions with asymptotic heterozygosity patterns in dairy breeds. Three regions ranging in size from 0.1 to 4.0 Mb were identified with asymptotic heterozygosity patterns (bracket size = 10 Mb) in two or more dairy breeds (RegBrack10-CR1–RegBrack10-CR3) (Table 3, where a non-dairy breed showed reduced heterozygosity in the same region, this is also indicated).

The myostatin analysis suggested that a bracket size of 10 Mb was optimal for identification of selected region. However, because this is a new methodology, the results obtained for the dairy breeds with all three bracket sizes (5-, 10- and 20-Mb) were compared to aid interpretation of results based on this approach. The number of candidate regions identified in at least two dairy breeds decreased with increasing bracket size. For the 5-Mb bracket size, a total of seven candidate regions were observed, whereas only three and one candidate regions were observed for the 10- and 20-Mb bracket sizes, respectively (Table 3). The region commonly identified through the use of all three bracket sizes was located on OAR6 (RegBrack5-CR6, RegBrack10-CR2 and RegBrack20-CR1). The signal for this region was seen in Milk Lacaune (34.875–38.875 Mb, 10-Mb bracket) and Comisana (36.125–38.325 Mb, 10-Mb bracket) breeds. In addition, the Meat Lacaune variety also showed extreme results for this region for all three bracket sizes (34.375–38.175, 10-Mb bracket). Another region on OAR2 (104 Mb) was identified by both of the smaller bracket sizes.

Some of the inconsistencies between bracket sizes were investigated further. In several cases, where regions were not found in the top 0.5% of –log(p) values for a particular bracket size, they did appear in the top 1% of –log(p) values. Regarding the region on OAR20 (~50 Mb) that was identified in two dairy breeds using the 10-Mb bracket size (RegBrack10-CR3, Table 3) but not using the 5-Mb bracket size: for Churra, positions within this region appeared within the top 1st percent of –log(p) values for the smaller bracket size but did not reach the threshold for the top

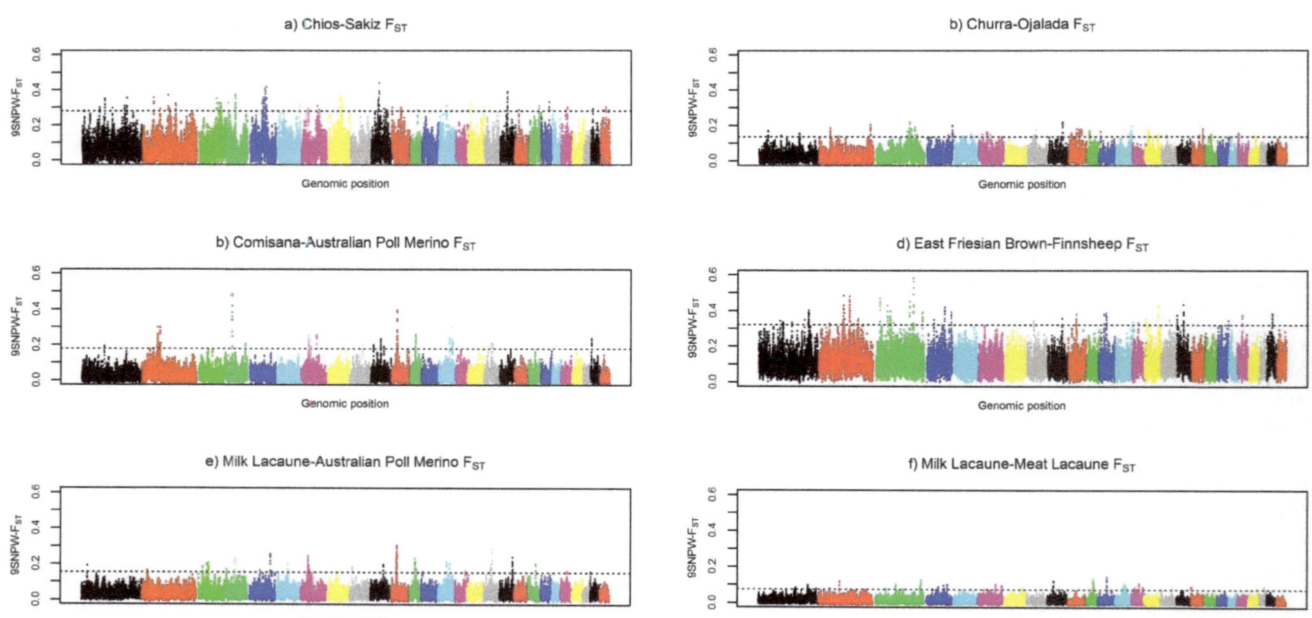

Figure 1. Genome-wide distribution of F_{ST} values for the six analysed breed pairs. The level of genetic differentiation, measured by F_{ST}, was estimated within each dairy – non-dairy breed pair[1], and averaged in sliding windows of 9 SNPs (F_{ST}-9SNPW) across the genome: The horizontal line indicates the top 0.5.th percent threshold considered for the F_{ST}-distributions. These raw results were used to identify F_{ST}-based candidate regions (F_{ST}-CRs) when overlapping significant selection signals (allowing gaps up to 2-Mb) were identified between different pairs. [1]Breed pairs analysed: a) Chios-Sakiz, b) Churra-Ojalada; c) Comisana-Australian Poll Merino; d) East Friesian Brown -Finnsheep, e) Milk Lacaune-Australian Poll Merino f) Milk Lacaune-MeatLacune.

Table 2. Maximum and minimum of the 0.005 top averaged pair-wise F_{ST} values in sliding windows of 9 SNPs (F_{ST}-9SNPW) estimated for the pairs considered in the present work to detect selection signals in dairy sheep.

Breed pair	Min. F_{ST}-9SNPW	Max. F_{ST} -9SNPW
Chios-Sakiz	0.2799	0.4392
Churra-Ojalada	0.1345	0.2193
Comisana-Australian Poll Merino	0.1781	0.4873
East Friesian Brown-Finnsheep	0.3212	0.7515
Milk Lacaune-Australian Poll Merino	0.1547	0.3071
Milk Lacaune-Meat Lacaune	0.0757	0.1449

0.5th percent, whereas for Milk Lacaune, this region was identified using both bracket sizes. Regarding the five regions (Table 3) that were identified in two dairy breeds using 5-Mb bracket size but not 10-Mb, four of the regions were in the top 1st percent of –log(p) values for one or both of the dairy breeds. Two of these regions (RegBrack5-CR1 and RegBrack5-CR3) were found in Chios and Churra, however, while these regions were found for Churra using both the 5- and 10-Mb bracket sizes, for the 10-Mb bracket size, the top –log(p) values for Chios were dominated by regions on OAR13 and OAR16, which did not feature in the top –log(p) values for the other dairy breeds. Thus, these Chios-specific signals may have overwhelmed the more general dairy signals for the larger bracket size in this breed. The region labelled as RegBrack5-CR4, identified at ~75 Mb on OAR3 for Churra and Milk Lacaune using the 5-Mb bracket size, did not feature in the top 1st percent of the –log(p) values for the 10-Mb bracket for either of these breeds. It is worth noting that regions identified using one bracket size but not a smaller one could reflect more recent selection events for which the pattern of heterozygosity with respect to distance from the selected locus appears linear rather than asymptotic in the smaller bracket.

Convergence Candidate Regions (CCR)

Six candidate regions were detected in at least two breed pairs by the pair-wise F_{ST} comparison and in at least two breeds by a heterozygosity-based analysis (Table 4). One of the regions, CCR3 (OAR6:30.367–41.863 Mb), was identified by all three analysis methods. The orthologous bovine genomic regions corresponding to each of the CCR are shown in Table 5. A total of 406 genes (positional candidate genes) were found in these six core regions (Table S3). There were three other regions where an F_{ST}-CR signals was less than 1 Mb from an ObsHtz-CR signal (OAR3:18.648–19.360 Mb, OAR3:167.711–168.959 Mb, and OAR13:95.801–98.865 Mb) but because they did not overlap, they were not considered as CCR.

Among the positional candidate genes extracted from the six CCRs, a search for functional candidates for milk production traits and mastitis was performed by comparison with the genes included in the Ogorevc et al. [22] database of cattle candidate genes for dairy-related traits. A total of 13 genes were common to these two lists (Table 5). The evidence for relationships with milk production traits for these genes was based on the different aspects considered in the Ogorevc et al. [22] database such as gene expression studies related to mammary gland (*TFAP2C, FAM110A, CD82, ABCG2*) or mastitis (*BID, MAFF, AHCY*), mouse model studies in which gene knockouts or expression of transgenes resulted in phenotypes associated with the mammary gland (*FKBP4, MKL1, POFUT1, CHUK*) and association studies of milk production traits (*ABCG2, SPP1, SCD*).

In order to assess whether there was greater overlap between the CCRs and candidate genes than expected by chance, we repeatedly (1 000 000 times) assigned regions of the same length as the CCR at random positions on the bovine genome and checked overlap with all candidate genes from the Ogorevc et al. [22] database that could be positioned on the bovine genome (423 genes). Although we could not do the test with the sheep genome as the annotation is not as complete, the length of the sheep and bovine genomes is very similar and so we expect this test would provide similar results. The number of overlaps between CCR regions and candidate genes based on a model with random positioning of CCR regions was very different from the actual situation: only 8.4% of the replicates contained any overlaps and the maximum number of overlaps was 4.

Some other positional candidate genes not included in the Ogorevc et al. [22] database were identified as possible functional candidates based on their known biological function and an exhaustive literature review of reported signatures of selection in dairy cattle (Table 5). There was also correspondence between the CCR and QTL previously reported in dairy cattle and sheep for milk production traits or functional traits related to dairy production (Table 5), which is discussed below.

Discussion

This study reports the first genome-wide analysis of regions under selection for dairy traits in sheep. For this we have used the valuable information generated in the International Sheep HapMap project [14], through the use of the *Illumina OvineSNP50 BeadChip*, to evaluate a range of European sheep breeds that have been selected for dairy production. With the aim of identifying the signatures of selection specifically due to dairy selection and not related to other traits that may have been selection target in the studied sheep populations (e.g. coat colour), we also included in our study other non-dairy European sheep breeds. Furthermore, because of the difficulties in distinguishing between the effects caused in the genome by genuine selective sweeps rather than demographic events such as population expansion or contraction [16], we used three different analysis methods and only considered for further exploration those six regions identified by the F_{ST}-based method and at least one of the two heterozygosity-based methodologies.

Candidate Dairy Selection Regions

Based on the convergence among the three different analysis methods, six core regions were identified as candidate regions under positive selection in dairy sheep. Based on the comparison

Table 3. Initial candidate regions identified on the basis of the regression analysis performed for detection of regions with asymptotic heterozygosity patterns in at least two of the dairy breeds (top 0.5% results for bracket sizes 5, 10 and 20 Mb).

Analysis	Regression-CR	Chr.	Dairy breed	Start position (Mb)	End position (Mb)	Non-dairy breed	Start position (Mb)	End position (Mb)
Regression top 0.5% bracket 5 Mb	RegBrack5-CR1	2	Churra	51.810	54.110	Ojalada	52.610	53.760
			Chios	52.860	53.410			
	RegBrack5-CR2	2	Milk Lacaune	104.360	104.560	Meat Lacaune	104.360	104.510
			Churra	104.460		Australian Poll Merino	104.410	104.460
	RegBrack5-CR3	2	Churra	122.360	122.910			
			Chios	123.010	123.210			
	RegBrack5-CR4	3	Milk Lacaune	75.192	75.292			
			Churra	75.292				
	RegBrack5-CR5	3	Milk Lacaune	168.742	168.892	Australian Poll Merino	168.692	168.942
			Churra	168.792	168.892	Meat Lacaune	168.792	168.892
	RegBrack5-CR6	6	Milk Lacaune	35.475	36.625	Meat Lacaune	34.725	36.775
			Comisana	36.625	37.325	Australian Poll Merino	35.975	37.175
	RegBrack5-CR7	11	Milk Lacaune	18.380	18.530	Ojalada	18.430	18.530
			Churra	18.430	18.480	Meat Lacaune	18.430	18.480
Regression top 0.5% bracket 10 Mb	RegBrack10-CR1	2	Milk Lacaune	104.410		Ojalada	104.410	104.460
			Churra	104.460	104.510	Meat Lacaune	104.410	104.460
						Finnsheep	104.460	104.510
	RegBrack10-CR2	6	Milk Lacaune	34.875	38.875	Meat Lacaune	34.3747	38.175
			Comisana	36.125	38.325	Australian Poll Merino	35.525	38.225
	RegBrack10-CR3	20	Churra	49.971	50.171			
			Milk Lacaune	50.071				
Regression top 0.5% bracket 20 Mb	RegBrack20-CR1	6	Milk Lacaune	34.825	38.525	Meat Lacaune	34.375	38.175
			Comisana	35.525	38.825	Australian Poll Merino	34.975	38.175

We also indicate if the same signature of selection was also identified in the non-dairy breeds.

Table 4. Convergence candidate regions (CCR) for selection signals identified for dairy sheep.

CCR	Chr.	Method	Individual method candidate region	Start marker*	Start position (Mb)	End marker*	End position (Mb)
CCR1	3	F_{ST}	F_{ST}-CR7	s51772	152.68	OAR3_165450843	154.582
		ObsHtz	ObsHtz-CR17	s26177	153.95	OAR3_165549468_X	154.679
CCR2	3	F_{ST}	F_{ST}-CR9	s34668	209.872	OAR3_234328134_X	215.814
		ObsHtz	ObsHtz-CR21	OAR3_229873996	211.624	s35739	215.403
CCR3	6	F_{ST}	F_{ST}-CR14	OAR6_34086500	30.367	OAR6_44210019	39.577
		Regression	RegBrack10-CR2	OAR6_38919831	34.875	OAR6_38919831	38.875
		ObsHtz	ObsHtz-CR27	OAR6_38585187	34.576	s38254	41.863
CCR4	13	ObsHtz	ObsHtz-CR42	OAR13_60893851	56.061	s63708	63.781
		F_{ST}	F_{ST}-CR24	s48133	62.277	OAR13_71091738	65.811
CCR5	15	F_{ST}	Fst-CR26	s31340	72.774	OAR15_80448054	74.55
		ObsHtz	ObsHtz-CR44	s02793	72.843	s28875	72.948
CCR6	22	ObsHtz	ObsHtz-CR51	OAR22_23392099	19.588	OAR22_24747565	20.991
		F_{ST}	F_{ST}-CR28	OAR22_24682845	20.925	OAR22_26951573	23.157

A CCR region was defined when overlapping selection regions identified by the genetic differentiation analysis (in at least two breed pairs), averaged for a 9-SNP window size (F_{ST}), and by at least one of the two heterozygosity-based analysis methodologies (in at least two breeds): observed heterozygosity, averaged for a 9-SNP window size (ObsHtz), and regression analysis, considering a 10-Mb bracket size (Regression).

*For Regression results, this indicates the closest marker to the Start/End position.

to predicted overlaps for randomly-positioned CCR, these regions were highly enriched for candidate dairy-related loci. We discuss further the CCR regions that meet specific criteria.

Region Identified by all the Three Methods

- **CCR3 (OAR6:30.367–41.863 Mb).** The three analysis methods identified this region of positive selection in the first half of OAR6, which includes the *ABCG2* (ATP-binding cassette, sub-family G (white), member 2) and *SPP1* (osteopontin) genes (at 36.565–36.610 Mb and 36.708–36.720 Mb respectively), and is orthologous to the region of the bovine genome on BTA6 where several QTL for milk production traits have been reported (See Table 5 for QTL identifier number in the CattleQTLdb). This region also includes the *FAM13A* (family with sequence similarity 13, member A) gene, which has been shown to be associated with mastitis in Jersey cows [27]. In dairy cattle, strong selection signals have previously been identified [23,24] in the proximity of the *ABCG2* gene, which harbors one of the few causal mutations or Quantitative Trait Nucleotide (QTN) described in livestock species [28]. In sheep, a selection signal in the *ABCG2* region has also been identified in a work focused on Altamurana sheep, where differences in allele frequencies were compared for animals with high and low milk yields [29].

The identification of a selection signature in this region of OAR6 by the pair-wise F_{ST} comparison (F_{ST}-CR14) was based on four breed pairs. For the Milk Lacaune-Australian Poll Merino and the Comisana-Australian Poll Merino pairs, the signal of genetic differentiation involved the *ABCG2* and *SPP1* genes, whereas for the two other pairs, the identified signal was upstream (Chios-Sakiz; OAR6:30.367–30.380 Mb) or downstream (Churra-Ojalada; OAR6:39.316–39.577 Mb) of these genes. The ObsHtz analysis showed a selection signal (ObsHtz-CR27) for Milk Lacaune, Comisana and Churra dairy breeds, and also for three non-dairy breeds, Australian Poll Merino, Meat Lacaune and Ojalada. Both Lacaune breeds showed low values of ObsHtz extended for long intervals (3.48 and 5.47 Mb for Milk Lacaune and Meat Lacaune, respectively). With regard to the regression-based analysis, this region was the only one detected in multiple breeds for all three bracket sizes (for Milk Lacaune, Comisana, Meat Lacaune and Australian Poll Merino breeds).

Together these results suggest that CCR3 shows selection for dairy traits in several sheep breeds, and that this signal may be related to the documented effects of the *ABCG2* [28] or *SPP1* [30] genes on milk production and lactation regulation, respectively. The selection signal positioned directly at *ABCG2* and *SPP1* was only seen in the highly specialized breeds Milk Lacaune and Comisana (F_{ST}, ObsHtz and Regression). In other dairy breeds for which the selection is more recent and less efficient (e.g. Churra and Chios), selection may not have substantially altered the frequencies of favoured alleles at these loci, which could explain why a strong selection signal directly at these genes was not observed. A previous study in Churra sheep found suggestive associations between the *ABCG2* gene and milk fat percentage and milk yield [31] while no studies to date have tested the effects of these two genes on dairy traits in the Lacaune and Comisana breeds.

The results reported in the current study also suggest that in this region of OAR6 there could be a selection signal related to meat specialized breeds such as Meat Lacaune, Australian Poll Merino and Ojalada. In this regard, it is worth noting that several QTL for growth and carcass traits have been described in the orthologous bovine region [32,33]. Hence, analogous to the observations in the orthologous bovine region, this region of the sheep genome may influence both dairy and meat production traits.

Regions with High F_{ST} in more than Two Breed Pairs

This criterion was used to highlight the CCR regions where the genetic differentiation analysis showed a particularly strong indication of a dairy selection signature, as this is possibly the most effective analysis performed in this study to detect regions specifically affected by dairy selection rather than selection acting on non-dairy-related traits. With the aim of establishing stringent criteria we consider in this section only those regions where more than two breed pairs (none sharing a common breed, as explained above) showed the selection signal. In addition to CCR3 discussed above, this category also includes the following two regions:

- **CCR1 (OAR3:152.680 to 154.679 Mb).** This core region, for which the F_{ST}-selection signals were identified for the Churra-Ojalada, Comisana-Australian Poll Merino and East Friesian Brown-Finnsheep pairs, includes *HMGA2* (high mobility group AT-hook 2), a gene associated with human stature [34]. The identification of this gene as a selection target was also found in an analysis of dogs with divergent stature [10]. The bovine region orthologous to CCR1 includes QTL related to stature (with the *HMGA2* gene suggested as a possible causative locus [35]) and rump length (see Table 5). Hence, the CCR1 signal identified in the present study might indicate selection targeting sheep body conformation traits. This hypothesis would agree with the differences in body size between some of the pairs involved in this selection signal. For example, the adult weight of Australian Poll Merino is significantly higher than that of Lacaune and Comisana; Churra and East Friesian Brown are also generally heavier than their comparison breeds. *HGMA2* has also been suggested as a candidate gene related to ear size and shape in both pigs and dogs [36,37], thus further investigation is required to assess whether there are differences in ear morphology between the sheep breeds showing this selection signal. Although the confidence interval of a QTL for protein percentage reported in Churra sheep [38] (Table 5) overlaps with CCR1, the causal mutation for that QTL was later found in the *LALBA* gene [39], which maps outside of this core region.
- **CCR2 (OAR3:209.872–215.814 Mb).** Four candidate genes in the orthologous bovine region to this CCR (distal end of BTA5) were identified from the Ogorevc et al. [22] database. Two of them were related to mastitis in a disease-induced mouse-model study [40]: *BID* (BH3 interacting domain death agonist), which is a pro-apoptotic induced gene, and *MAFF* (v-maf avian musculoaponeurotic fibrosarcoma oncogene homolog F), which is related to cell proliferation. The identification of two other genes as candidates for dairy traits in this regions, *FKBP4* (FK506 binding protein 4) and *MLK1* (mixed lineage protein kinase), was also based on mouse model studies (http://www.informatics.jax.org/). Furthermore, *FKBP4* is expressed in breast cancer tissue (Genes-to-Systems Breast Cancer database, G2SBC, http://www.itb.cnr.it/breastcancer//index.html) and *MLK1* is expressed in epithelial tumor cell lines of colonic, breast and esophageal origin [41]. QTL effects described in the bovine region orthologous to CCR2 (on BTA5) influence milk production and some conformation traits (Table 5). A previous study in dairy cows found a selection signature in this region [23]. In that case, the gene displaying the strongest evidence of selection was *CD163*, which is involved in the innate immune response and clearance of plasma hemoglobin [42]. This region also includes the gene coding for CSNK1ε (casein-kinase epsilon), which is related to

Table 5. Convergence candidate regions (CCR) for ovine dairy selection sweeps identified in this study.

Convergence candidate regions	Sheep genome range (Mb) (Oar v2.0)	Bovine genome range (Mb) (UMD 3.1)	Functional candidate genes based on Ogorevc et al. [22]	Other candidate genes[1]	QTL described in sheep	QTL described in cattle in relation to milk production and functional dairy traits (CattleQTLdb identifier[2])	Nb. of positional candidates[3]
CCR1	OAR3:152.680–154.679	BTA5:46.720–49.009		*HMGA2*	Milk protein percentage [38]	Somatic cell score (2659), Milk fat yield (4495), Milk yield (2429), Rump length (3422), Stature (16277, 16278), Clinical mastitis (4973)	11
CCR2	OAR3:209.872–215.814	BTA5:106.976–112.636	*BID, MAFF, FKBP4, MKL1*	*CSNK1E*		Milk fat yield (daughter deviation) (9995), Milk protein yield (daughter deviation) (9994), Milk fat percentage (2717), Chest width (4623), Hip height (3420)	100
CCR3	OAR6:30.367–41.863	BTA6:31.710–43.022	*ABCG2, SPP1*	*FAM13A*		Milk protein percentage (EBV) (15002, 15003), Milk fat percentage (1753, 16057), Milk protein percentage (1755, 9913, 16058, 16059), Milk protein yield (daughter deviation) (10145), Milk fat yield (EBV) (11303, 12031), Milk protein yield (EBV) (11304), Milk yield (EBV) (11302), Somatic cell score (EBV) (6165, 6164), Milk fatty acid unsaturated index (11506, 11508, 11509, 11510), Milk myristoleic acid percentage (11507), Milk palmitoleic acid percentage (11505), Teat placement (10285), Udder attachment (10284)	32
CCR4	OAR13:56.061–65.811	BTA13:57.572–67.005	*POFUT1, TFAP2C, FAM110A, AHCY*	*GHRH, ASIP*		Milk protein percentage (2672), Milk protein yield (EBV) (6090), Milk fat yield (2555), Milk protein yield (daughter deviation) (10156), Milk protein yield (2671), Milk yield (2670), Udder attachment (1584), Udder composite index (1589), Udder depth (1588), Udder height (1586), Udder width (1587), Rump angle (3429), Foot angle (1583)	172
CCR5	OAR15:72.774–74.550	BTA15:75.154–76.879	*CD82*			Teat placement (1595), Udder cleft (1600), Udder composite index (1602), Milk fat yield (4503), Milk protein yield (4502), Milk protein yield (EBV), (6103), Milk fat percentage (3452), Milk protein percentage (EBV) (11345), Milk yield (EBV) (11346)	17
CCR6	OAR22:19.587–23.157	BTA26:20.286–24.226	*CHUK, SCD*		Milk fatty acid composition [57,58], Somatic cell score [60]	Milk yield (10452), Milk protein yield (10454), Milk fat yield (3636), Milk protein yield (3638), Milk protein yield (11702), Milk yield (11701), Milk fat yield (10453), Milk fat percentage (2598), Milk fat yield (2572), Milk protein yield (2573), Milk yield (2574), Milk protein percentage (4814), Milk protein percentage (3639), Milk yield (3634), Somatic Cell Count (1503)	74

The interval of each region (in bp) is based on the sheep genome reference sequence v2.0 (http://www.livestockgenomics.csiro.au/cgi-bin/gbrowse/oarv2.0/). The corresponding orthologous bovine genomic intervals are based on the bovine genome reference sequence UMD 3.1 (http://www.ensembl.org/Bos_taurus/Info/Index). The positional candidate genes that map within the bovine candidate range and that are included as candidate genes for milk production and mastitis traits in the database provided by Ogorevc et al. [22] are indicated as functional candidate genes. The affected trait and CattleQTLdb reference for previously reported cattle QTL that map within the bovine candidate genomic regions and that influence milk production traits or other functional traits related to dairy production are also indicated.

[1]Other candidate genes. This category includes two types of genes:

–Those that although are not included in the Ogorevc et al. [22] database may be considered as candidate genes in relation to milk production related traits based on other studies.

–Those that are likely to be related to non-dairy selection signatures such as morphological traits and coat colour features.

[2]CattleQTLdb identifier: Search reference number at http://www.animalgenome.org/cgi-bin/QTLdb/BT/search to find complete details about QTL reported in the orthologous region of the corresponding sheep CCR identified in this study.

[3]Number of positional candidate genes extracted from the orthologous bovine region using BioMart for each of the labeled CCRs (based on Table S3).

circadian rhythms. In a study of the human milk fat globule transcriptome, *CSNK1ε* was identified as one of the nine core "clock" genes that showed differential expression over a 24-hour period time in lactating women [43]. Of particular interest is the finding that this OAR3 region was labelled as a CCR based on the overlap of candidate regions detected by pair-wise-F_{ST} in the pairs including the most highly specialized dairy breeds (Milk Lacaune, Comisana and East Friesian Brown), which may have been under selection for circadian-related adaptation of milk production to intensive milking.

Other Regions

- **CCR4 (OAR13:56.061 to 65.811 Mb).** Several genes included in this core candidate region were also found in the Ogorevc et al. [22] database. The *POFUT1* (protein O-fucosyltransferase 1) gene plays a crucial role in Notch signaling, which regulates mammary stem cell function and luminal cell-fate commitment [44]. *TFAP2C* (transcription factor AP-2 gamma; activating enhancer binding protein 2 gamma) is involved in mammary development, differentiation, and oncogenesis playing a critical role in gene regulation in hormone responsive breast cancer [45], and *AHCY* (adenosylhomocysteinase) has been suggested as potentially involved in mastitis defense based on its disease-associated expression [46]. Another positional candidate gene for this core region is the *GHRH* (growth hormone-releasing hormone) gene. Although the direct relationship of this gene and milk production traits is still not clear [47,48], its link to the somatotropic axis and other functional candidate genes included in the Ogorevc et al. [22] database (*GH, GHR, GHRHR*) suggest a possible influence, directly or indirectly, on dairy traits. In addition to these candidate dairy-related genes, the *ASIP* (Agouti signaling protein) gene is also located in this region (OAR13:63.028–63.033 Mb). This gene has a major role in metabolic processes [49] and coat colour pigmentation in mammalian species [50]. Based on the known associations between polymorphisms at this gene and coat colour patterns in sheep [51] it is possible that the identified selection signal results from coat colour selection. In their analysis of the complete HapMap dataset, Kijas et al. [14] also identified a selection signal near *ASIP*.
- **CCR5 (OAR15:72.774–74.550 Mb).** This region included the *CD82* (CD82 molecule) gene, which is included in the Ogorevc et al. [22] database based on its expression in the mammary gland. This gene is included in the group of genes that regulate breast cancer metastasis, as a metastasis suppressor [52]. Whereas no studies have reported an association of this gene with dairy related traits, there is a functional relationship between *CD82* and *ERBB3* (Receptor tyrosine-protein kinase erbB-3) [53], which is related to normal mammary development [54].
- **CCR6: (OAR22:19.588–23.157 Mb).** Two functional candidate genes [22] were found in this region: *SCD* (Stearoyl-CoA desaturase) and *CHUK* (conserved helix-loop-helix ubiquitous kinase). The *SCD* gene encodes a multifunctional complex enzyme important in the cellular biosynthesis of fatty acids. Several studies in different populations of dairy cattle have reported associations between polymorphisms at this gene with milk production traits [55] and milk fatty acid composition [56]. In sheep, the *SCD* gene has been suggested as positional and functional candidate gene for a QTL identified on OAR22 in a Sarda × Lacaune back-cross population for the ratio of conjugated linoleic acid to vaccenic acid in sheep milk [57]. A later study in Churra sheep also identified a QTL on OAR22 for the same trait close to the *SCD* position, although various analyses questioned this gene as responsible for the identified effect [58]. The *CHUK* gene is listed in the Ogorevc et al. [22] database because it is expressed in breast cancer tumors and is a regulator of mammary epithelial proliferation [59]. According to the SheepQTL database, this region includes a QTL for somatic cell score described in an Awassi x Merino cross population [60] and it has also been identified as a selection signal by the analysis of allele frequency differences between animals with divergent milk yields reported in Altamurana sheep [29].

The bovine region orthologous to CCR6 (on BTA26), overlaps with a region showing a selection signature in dairy cattle [23], where the *C10ORF76* (chromosome 10 open reading frame 76) gene was associated with the strongest selection signal. Although there is not a reported association of this gene with milk production traits, it is expressed in the mammary gland and it is altered in breast cancer cells, based on the G2SBC database.

Inconsistencies between this Study and Previous QTL and Selection Mapping Studies of Cattle and Sheep

Although all six CCR overlapped with QTL for dairy traits in sheep or cattle (Table 4 and discussed above), our study did not identify a selection signal close to several genes previously associated with dairy traits in sheep and cattle. For example, there were no CCR near the *LALBA* (alpha-lactalbumin) gene (OAR3:137 Mb), where a particular variant has been recently been proposed to explain a QTL for milk protein percentage identified in Churra sheep [39]. The lack of signal near this QTL in the F_{ST} analysis of Churra vs Ojalada is consistent with the fact that the causative mutation is still segregating in Churra, which allowed its identification as QTL.

In addition, in their analysis of the complete Sheep HapMap dataset, Kijas et al. [14] reported positive selection surrounding the *PRLR* gene, which is associated with milk traits in dairy cattle [61]. In our study, although none of the CCRs map to OAR16, where this gene is located (39.250–39.284 Mb), it is worth mentioning that this gene is included in the interval of F_{ST}-CR27 (OAR16:37.347–40.850 Mb), which was identified based on the signals detected in three breed pairs involving the most specialized dairy breeds in this study (East Friesian Brown-Finnsheep, Milk Lacaune-Australian Poll Merino and Comisana-Australian Poll Merino) but was not classified a CCR due to the lack of selection signals from the heterozygosity-based methods. Other regions that were detected by the F_{ST}-pairwise comparison for many breed pairs but that were not supported by the heterozygosity-based methods were found on OAR2 (F_{ST}-CR2:52.346–53.409 Mb) and OAR9 (57.363–60.849 Mb). Whereas the first region does not include any functional candidate gene for dairy traits, the region in OAR9 included three genes related to the metabolism of fatty acids (*FABP4, FABP5* and *FABP9*). *FABP4* and *FABP5* have been shown to be highly expressed in the mammary gland during lactation [62] and significant associations have been found between *FABP4* and fatty acid composition of bovine milk [63]. We acknowledge that one or more of these regions may represent false negatives that were missed by our stringent selection signal criteria. However, because of the difficulty in linking a sweep signal to a given phenotype, we suggest that application of stringent criteria in this type of study is an appropriate option to avoid reporting long lists of candidate regions based on spurious results.

We also did not find evidence of selection on some major candidate genes for milk production for which selection signatures have been observed in cattle (e.g. *DGAT1:* OAR9:13.534–13,543 Mb; *GHR:* OAR16:32.068–32.231). In contrast to our results, the *GHR* gene (BTA20) showed the largest difference in sliding window average allele frequencies in a study of divergent selection between dairy and beef cattle [24], and also showed significant extended haplotype homozygosity [25]. With regard to *DGAT1*, evidence of selection has also been identified when comparing dairy and beef cattle breeds [24].

In their study, Kijas et al. [14] also identified a strong selection signal on OAR10, associated to the presence or absence of horns and close to the gene responsible of the polled phenotype, *RXFP2* (relaxin/insulin-like family peptide receptor 2) gene (OAR10:27.602–27.646 Mb). In our study, a selection signal was identified in this region based on the ObsHtz-based method (ObsHtz-CR33:24.856–27.897 Mb, for the dairy breeds Comisana, Churra and Milk Lacaune) and the F_{ST}-based method (OAR10:25.540–28.983 Mb). However because the F_{ST} signal was due only to the two breed pairs involving the Australian Poll Merino, this was not labelled as F_{ST}-CR.

Apart from the overlap between two CCRs (CCR3 on OAR6 and CCR6 on OAR22) with the selection signals identified in Altamurana sheep for milk yield [29], we did not find evidence of selection near the signals reported for this Italian breed. This lack of correspondence may derive from breed-specific signals reported for Altamurana.

Comparison of the Three Selection Mapping Methods

From our point of view, the analysis method that involved the estimation of pair-wise F_{ST} for pairs of related breeds showing divergent specialization (one for milk production, one not) should be the most powerful analysis in terms of identifying selection specifically related to dairy production. Four out of the 28 candidate regions showing multiple pair-wise F_{ST} signals were detected in four out of the six breed pairs (F_{ST}-CR3, F_{ST}-CR9, F_{ST}-CR14 and F_{ST}-CR18). Of these, F_{ST}-CR3 (OAR2:52.346–53.409 Mb) was not included as a CCR due to the lack of consistency with the ObsHtz or 10-Mb Regression analysis results, although the same region was identified by the 5-Mb Regression analysis (RegBrack5-CR1 in Table 3) in two dairy breeds (Churra and Chios) and one non-dairy breed (Ojalada). Given that no functional candidate genes from the Ogorevc et al. [22] database were found in the orthologous bovine region, it is possible that this region underlies breed differentiation not directly related to dairy traits.

Among the 55 candidate regions identified based on the ObsHtz analysis (ObsHtz-CRs, Table S2), there were only twelve regions showing a signal in dairy but not in non-dairy breeds (ObsHtz-CR3, 7, 8, 10, 12, 25, 28, 29, 31, 41, 45 and 55). Considering that the background genome has been previously selected for meat, maternal characteristics, and other traits, whereas the development of dairy breeds is much more recent, it would be expected that the selection signals specifically related to dairy traits would not be seen in the other breeds (although Meat Lacaune could be an exception). However, as none of these regions showing a reduction of heterozygosity exclusively in dairy breeds were identified by the F_{ST}-based method, they were not identified as final core CCRs (and thus are not present in Table 4). Although the evidence linking these regions to dairy-related selection is weaker than for the CCRs, we performed an additional search for functional candidate genes and dairy-related QTL mapping within these regions, similar to that performed in the eight identified CCRs (see Table S4). A total of 118 genes were extracted from the orthologous bovine regions of these eleven dairy-breed-limited regions of reduced heterozygosity (data not shown). Among them, only the *HSPD1* (Heat shock 60 kDa protein 1; chaperonin) gene is included in the Ogorevc et al. [22] database, due to its expression in the mammary gland. This gene is also included in the G2SBC database although no studies have reported so far its association with milk production traits. Interestingly, among the dairy QTL detected in these regions there is greater overlap with ovine QTL for milk production traits (Table S4) than for the list of core CCRs. Hence, these regions identified exclusively by ObsHtz could include gene variants occurring in individual dairy breeds, as it is the case for many of the QTL described in sheep.

There were eight regions that overlapped between those identified by F_{ST} (including a full set of regions, including those that contained pairs with the same breeds that were removed from Table S1) and ObsHtz (out of 35 and 55, respectively). The explanation for the higher number of regions identified by ObsHz is that the regions identified using F_{ST} were slightly larger (incorporated more windows) than those identified using ObsHtz.

There were far fewer signals identified using the Regression approach than either F_{ST} or ObsHtz. Although the top (or bottom) 0.5th percent results were considered as signals of selection for all methods, the Regression method first filtered out the intervals with non-significant and non-asymptotic regression patterns, and thus the total number of eligible intervals was substantially reduced compared to the other approaches in which the distribution of F_{ST}/ObsHtz values for all markers (with the exception of those on the very ends of the chromosomes) was considered. Thus the implementation of Regression in this study was more stringent than the other methods.

The regions identified by the Regression method showed greater overlap with ObsHtz than F_{ST}, which is not surprising since both Regression and ObsHtz are designed to detect regions with a reduction in diversity. For the 10-Mb bracket size (results considered for the identification of CCR), all three regions identified with the Regression approach overlapped with those identified with ObsHtz while one out of the three, RegBrack10-CR2, overlapped with the regions identified with $F_{ST,}$ and was therefore considered as CCR (CCR3).

Conclusions

The results reported here provide a genome-wide map of selection signatures in the dairy sheep genome. The six core candidate regions identified are likely to influence traits of economic interest in dairy sheep production and can be considered as starting points for future studies aimed at the identification of the causal genetic variation underlying these signals. For some of these regions, strong candidate genes have been proposed (e.g. *ABCG2, SPP1*), whereas some other genes designated as candidates based on their association with sheep and cattle dairy traits (e.g. *LALBA, DGAT1A*) were not associated with a detectable sweep signal. Discrepancies between selection signals in dairy sheep and cattle may be explained either by statistical or biological factors, such as the limited statistical power of the analyses to identify effects of small magnitude or the fact that the genetic architecture of milk production and dairy-related traits substantially differs from sheep to cattle and also between the different breeds of dairy sheep, which have been subjected to different levels of selection pressure. Many of the identified regions corresponded to orthologous regions in cattle where QTL for dairy traits have been identified. Due to the limited number of QTL studies reported in sheep compared with cattle, the results illustrate the potential value of the study of selection signatures to uncover mutations with potential effects on quantitative dairy sheep traits. Additional studies are needed to confirm and refine the results reported here. To this end, the recent availability of the high-density ovine chip (700 K) will provide a valuable tool to perform more powerful and precise selection mapping studies.

Supporting Information

Table S1 Candidate regions for signatures of selection identified on the basis of the pair-wise F_{ST} analysis.
(PDF)

Table S2 Candidate regions identified based on reduced heterozygosity signals identified in at least two of the dairy breeds.
(PDF)

Table S3 List of all genes from the orthologous bovine genome regions corresponding to the six convergence candidate regions (CCR) for dairy selection sweeps identified in this study, extracted using the Biomart tool (http://www.biomart.org/).
(XLSX)

Table S4 Candidate regions identified by the analysis based on observed heterozygosity (ObsHtz-CR), averaged in sliding windows of 9 SNPs (ObsHtz-9SNPW), that were exclusively detected in dairy breeds.
(PDF)

File S1 Summary of the criteria for selection of breeds to be included in the study, including the results of a Principal Component Analysis (PCA) performed with the initial set of breeds considered.
(PDF)

File S2 Summary of the results of the analysis performed in this work in relation to the myostatin (*GDF-8*) gene region. These results were evaluated to establish criteria for the analyses performed to detect dairy selection signatures in the dairy breeds.
(PDF)

Acknowledgments

We thank Samantha Wilkinson for providing R scripts.

Author Contributions

Conceived and designed the experiments: BGG PW JJA. Analyzed the data: BGG PW. Contributed reagents/materials/analysis tools: RPW JJA EGG JK. Wrote the paper: BGG PW JJA RPW JK. Conceived the study: BGG PW.

References

1. Legge T (1996) The beginning of caprine domestication. In: Harris DR, editor. The Origins and Spread of Agriculture and Pastoralism in Eurasia. Smithsonian New York: Institution Press. pp. 238–262.
2. Maijala K (1997) Genetic aspects of domestication, common breeds and their origin. In: Piper L, Ruvinsky A, editors. The genetics of sheep. Oxford: CAB Int. pp. 539–564.
3. Barillet F (1997) Genetics of milk production. In: Piper L, Ruvinsky A, editors. The genetics of sheep. Oxford: CAB Int. pp. 539–564.
4. Ida A, Vicovan PG, Radu R, Vicovan A, Cutova N, et al. (2012) Improving the milk production at the breeds and populations of sheep from various geoclimatic zones. Lucrări Ştiinţifice - Seria Zootehnie 57: 17.
5. Gibbs RA, Taylor JF, Van Tassell CP, Barendse W, Eversole KA, et al. (2009) Genome-wide survey ofSNP variation uncovers the genetic structure of cattle breeds. Science 324: 528–532.
6. Rubin CJ, Zody MC, Eriksson J, Meadows JR, Sherwood E, et al. (2010) Whole-genome resequencing reveals loci under selection during chicken domestication. Nature 464: 587–591.
7. Elferink MG, Megens HJ, Vereijken A, Hu X, Crooijmans RP et al. (2012) Signatures of selection in the genomes of commercial and non-commercial chicken breeds. PLoS One 7: ve32720.
8. Wiener P, Pong-Wong R (2011) A regression-based approach to selection mapping. J Hered 102: 294–305.
9. Stella A, Ajmone-Marsan P, Lazzari B, Boettcher P (2010) Identification of selection signatures in cattle breeds selected for dairy production. Genetics 185: 1451–1461.
10. Akey JM, Ruhe AL, Akey DT, Wong AK, Connelly CF, et al. (2010) Tracking footprints of artificial selection in the dog genome. Proc Natl Acad Sci USA 107: 1160–1165.
11. Vaysse A, Ratnakumar A, Derrien T, Axelsson E, Rosengren Pielberg G, et al. (2011) Identification of genomic regions associated with phenotypic variation between dog breeds using selection mapping. PLoS Genet 10: e1002316.
12. Ai H, Huang L, Ren J (2013) Genetic diversity, linkage disequilibrium and selection signatures in chinese and Western pigs revealed by genome-wide SNP markers. PLoS One 8: e56001.
13. Boyko AR, Quignon P, Li L, Schoenebeck JJ, Degenhardt JD, et al. (2010) A simple genetic architecture underlies morphological variation in dogs. PLoS Biol 8: e1000451.
14. Kijas JW, Lenstra JA, Hayes B, Boitard S, Porto Neto LR, et al. (2012a) Genome-wide analysis of the world's sheep breeds reveals high levels of historic mixture and strong recent selection. PLoS Biol 10: e1001258.
15. Weir BS, Cockerham CC (1984) Estimating F-Statistics for the Analysis of Population Structure. Evolution 38: 1358–1370.
16. Akey JM, Zhang G, Zhang K, Jin L, Shriver MD (2002) Interrogating a high-density SNP map for signatures of natural selection. Genome Res 12: 1805–1814.
17. Wilkinson S, Lu ZH, Megens HJ, Archibald AL, Haley C, et al. (2013) Signatures of diversifying selection in European pig breeds. PLoS Genet 9: e1003453.
18. Barendse W, Harrison BE, Bunch RJ, Thomas MB, Turner LB (2009) Genome wide signatures of positive selection: the comparison of independent samples and the identification of regions associated to traits. BMC Genomics 10: 178.
19. Rubin CJ, Megens HJ, Martinez Barrio A, Maqbool K, Sayyab S, et al. (2012) Strong signatures of selection in the domestic pig genome. Proc Natl Acad Sci USA. 109: 19529–19536.
20. Axelsson E, Ratnakumar A, Arendt ML, Maqbool K, Webster MT, et al. (2013) The genomic signature of dog domestication reveals adaptation to a starch-rich diet. Nature 495: 360–364.
21. Payne RW, Murray DA, Harding SA, Baird DB, Soutar DM (2007) GenStat for Windows (10th Edition) Introduction. Hemel Hempstead: VSN. International.
22. Ogorevc J, Kunej T, Razpet A, Dovc P (2009) Database of cattle candidate genes and genetic markers for milk production and mastitis. Anim Genet 40: 832–851.
23. Flori L, Fritz S, Jaffrézic F, Boussaha M, Gut I, et al. (2009) The genome response to artificial selection: a case study in dairy cattle. PLoS One 4: e6595.
24. Hayes BJ, Chamberlain AJ, Maceachern S, Savin K, McPartlan H, et al. (2009) A genome map of divergent artificial selection between Bos taurus dairy cattle and Bos taurus beef cattle. Anim Genet 40: 176–184.
25. Qanbari S, Pimentel EC, Tetens J, Thaller G, Lichtner P, et al. (2010) A genome-wide scan for signatures of recent selection in Holstein cattle. Anim Genet 41: 377–389.
26. Moradi MH, Nejati-Javaremi A, Moradi-Shahrbabak M, Dodds K G, McEwan JC (2012) Genomic scan of selective sweeps in thin and fat tail sheep breeds for identifying of candidate regions associated with fat deposition. BMC Genet 13: 10.
27. Kowalewska-Łuczak I, Kulig H (2013) Polymorphism of the FAM13A, ABCG2, OPN, LAP3, HCAP-G, PPARGC1A genes and somatic cell count of Jersey cows - Preliminary study. Res Vet Sci 94: 252–255.
28. Olsen HG, Nilsen H, Hayes B, Berg PR, Svendsen M, et al. (2007) Genetic support for a quantitative trait nucleotide in the ABCG2 gene affecting milk composition of dairy cattle. BMC Genet 8: 32.
29. Moioli B1, Scatà MC, Steri R, Napolitano F, Catillo G (2013) Signatures of selection identify loci associated with milk yield in sheep. BMC Genet 14: 76.
30. Sheehy PA, Riley LG, Raadsma HW, Williamson P, Wynn PC (2009) A functional genomics approach to evaluate candidate genes located in a QTL interval for milk production traits on BTA6. Anim Genet 40: 492–498.
31. García-Fernández M, Gutiérrez-Gil B, Sánchez JP, Morán JA, García-Gámez E, et al. (2011) The role of bovine causal genes underlying dairy traits in Spanish Churra sheep. Anim Genet 42: 415–420.
32. Eberlein A, Takasuga A, Setoguchi K, Pfuhl R, Flisikowski K, et al. (2009) Dissection of genetic factors modulating fetal growth in cattle indicates a substantial role of the non-SMC condensin I complex, subunit G (NCAPG) gene. Genetics 183: 951–964.
33. Gutiérrez-Gil B, Wiener P, Williams JL, Haley CS (2012) Investigation of the genetic architecture of a bone carcass weight QTL on BTA6. Anim Genet 43: 654–661.
34. Yang TL, Guo Y, Zhang LS, Tian Q, Yan H, et al. (2010) HMGA2 is confirmed to be associated with human adult height. Ann Hum Genet 74: 11–16.
35. Pryce JE, Hayes BJ, Bolormaa S, Goddard ME (2011) Polymorphic regions affecting human height also control stature in cattle. Genetics 187: 981–984.
36. Li P, Xiao S, Wei N, Zhang Z, Huang R, et al. (2012) Fine mapping of a QTL for ear size on porcine chromosome 5 and identification of high mobility group AT-hook 2 (HMGA2) as a positional candidate gene. Genet Sel Evol 44: 6.

37. Boyko AR, Quignon P, Li L, Schoenebeck JJ, Degenhardt JD, et al. (2010) A simple genetic architecture underlies morphological variation in dogs. PLoS Biol 8: e1000451.
38. Gutiérrez-Gil B, El-Zarei MF, Alvarez L, Bayón Y, de la Fuente LF et al. (2009) Quantitative trait loci underlying milk production traits in sheep. Anim Genet 40: 423–434.
39. García-Gámez E, Gutiérrez-Gil B, Sahana G, Sánchez JP, Bayón Y, et al. (2012) GWA analysis for milk production traits in dairy sheep and genetic support for a QTN influencing milk protein percentage in the LALBA gene. PLoS One 7: e47782.
40. Zheng J, Watson AD, Kerr DE (2006) Genome-wide expression analysis of lipopolysaccharide-induced mastitis in a mouse model. Infect Immun 74: 1907–1915.
41. Dorow DS, Devereux L, Dietzsch E, De Kretser T (1993) Identification of a new family of human epithelial protein kinases containing two leucine/isoleucine-zipper domains. Eur J Biochem 213: 701–710.
42. Schaer DJ, Schaer CA, Buehler PW, Boykins RA, Schoedon G, et al. (2006) CD163 is the macrophage scavenger receptor for native and chemically modified hemoglobins in the absence of haptoglobin. Blood 107: 373–380.
43. Maningat PD, Sen P, Rijnkels M, Sunehag AL, Hadsell DL, et al. (2009) Gene expression in the human mammary epithelium during lactation: the milk fat globule transcriptome. Physiol Genomics. 37: 12–22.
44. Bouras T, Pal B, Vaillant F, Harburg G, Asselin-Labat ML, et al. (2008) Notch signaling regulates mammary stem cell function and luminal cell-fate commitment. Cell Stem Cell 3: 429–441.
45. Woodfield GW, Chen Y, Bair TB, Domann FE, Weigel RJ (2010) Identification of primary gene targets of TFAP2C in hormone responsive breast carcinoma cells. Genes Chromosomes Cancer 49: 948–962.
46. Schwerin M, Czernek-Schäfer D, Goldammer T, Kata SR, Womack JE, et al. (2003) Application of disease-associated differentially expressed genes–mining for functional candidate genes for mastitis resistance in cattle. Genet Sel Evol 35 Suppl 1: S19–34.
47. Dybus A, Grzesiak W (2006) GHRH/HaeIII gene polymorphism and its associations with milk production traits in Polish Black-and-White cattle. Arch Tierz Dummerstorf 49: 434–438.
48. Szatkowskaac I, Dybusac A, Grzesiakab W, Jedrzejczakac M, Muszyńskaac M (2009). Association between the growth hormone releasing hormone (GHRH) gene polymorphism and milk production traits of dairy cattle. J Appl Anim Res 36: 119–12.
49. Wolff GL, Roberts DW, Mountjoy KG (1999) Physiological consequences of ectopic agouti gene expression: The yellow obese mouse syndrome. Physiol Genomics 1: 151–163.
50. Bennett DC, Lamoreux ML (2003) The colour loci of mice–A genetic century. Pigment Cell Res 16: 333–344.
51. Norris BJ, Whan VA (2008) A gene duplication affecting expression of the ovine ASIP gene. Genome Res 18: 1282–1293.
52. Debies MT, Welch DR (2001) Genetic basis of human breast cancer metastasis. J Mammary Gland Biol Neoplasia 6: 441–451.
53. Odintsova E, Voortman J, Gilbert E, Berditchevski F (2003) Tetraspanin CD82 regulates compartmentalisation and ligand-induced dimerization of EGFR. J Cell Sci 116: 4557–4566.
54. Lahlou H, Müller T, Sanguin-Gendreau V, Birchmeier C, Muller WJ (2012) Uncoupling of PI3K from ErbB3 impairs mammary gland development but does not impact on ErbB2-induced mammary tumorigenesis. Cancer Res 72: 3080–3090.
55. Alim MA, Fan YP, Wu XP, Xie Y, Zhang Y, et al. (2012) Genetic effects of stearoyl-coenzyme A desaturase (SCD) polymorphism on milk production traits in the Chinese dairy population. Mol Biol Rep 39: 8733–8740.
56. Moioli B, Contarini G, Avalli A, Catillo G, Orru L, et al. (2007) Short communication: effect of stearoyl-coenzyme A desaturase polymorphism on fatty acid composition of milk. J Dairy Res 90: 3553–3558.
57. Carta A, Sechi T, Usai MG, Addis M, M Fiori, et al. (2006) Evidence for a QTL affecting the synthesis of linoleic conjugated acid cis-9, trans-11 from 11-c 18:1 acid on ovine chromosome 22. Proc. 8th World Congress on Genetics Applied to Livestock Production. Belo Horizonte, Brazil. Commun. no. 12–03. Instituto Prociencia, Belo Horizonte, Brazil.
58. García-Fernández M, Gutiérrez-Gil B, García-Gámez E, Sánchez JP, Arranz JJ (2010) Detection of quantitative trait loci affecting the milk fatty acid profile on sheep chromosome 22: role of the stearoyl-CoA desaturase gene in Spanish Churra sheep. J Dairy Sci 93: 348–357.
59. Cao Y, Luo JL, Karin M (2007) IkappaB kinase alpha kinase activity is required for self-renewal of ErbB2/Her2-transformed mammary tumor-initiating cells. Proc Natl Acad Sci USA 104: 15852–15857.
60. Raadsma HW, Jonas E, McGill D, Hobbs M, Lam MK, et al. (2009). Mapping quantitative trait loci (QTL) in sheep. II. Meta-assembly and identification of novel QTL for milk production traits in sheep. Genet Sel Evol 41: 45.
61. Viitala S, Szyda J, Blott S, Schulman N, Lidauer M, et al. (2006) The role of the bovine growth hormone receptor and prolactin receptor genes in milk, fat and protein production in Finnish Ayrshire dairy cattle. Genetics 173: 2151–2164.
62. Sumner-Thomson JM, Vierck JL, McNamara JP (2011) Differential expression of genes in adipose tissue of first-lactation dairy cattle. J Dairy Sci 94: 361–369.
63. Nafikov RA, Schoonmaker JP, Korn KT, Noack K, Garrick DJ, et al. (200 Association of polymorphisms in solute carrier family 27, isoform A6 (SLC27A6) and fatty acid-binding protein-3 and fatty acid-binding protein-4 (FABP3 and FABP4) with fatty acid composition of bovine milk. J Dairy Sci 96: 6007–6021.

16

A Major Locus for Chloride Accumulation on Chromosome 5A in Bread Wheat

Yusuf Genc[1,2], Julian Taylor[1], Jay Rongala[2], Klaus Oldach[1,2]*

1 School of Agriculture, Food and Wine, University of Adelaide, Waite Campus, Glen Osmond, South Australia, Australia, **2** South Australian Research and Development Institute, Plant Genomics Centre, Waite Campus, Glen Osmond, South Australia, Australia

Abstract

Chloride (Cl^-) is an essential micronutrient for plant growth, but can be toxic at high concentrations resulting in reduced growth and yield. Although saline soils are generally dominated by both sodium (Na^+) and Cl^- ions, compared to Na^+ toxicity, very little is known about physiological and genetic control mechanisms of tolerance to Cl^- toxicity. In hydroponics and field studies, a bread wheat mapping population was tested to examine the relationships between physiological traits [Na^+, potassium (K^+) and Cl^- concentration] involved in salinity tolerance (ST) and seedling growth or grain yield, and to elucidate the genetic control mechanism of plant Cl^- accumulation using a quantitative trait loci (QTL) analysis approach. Plant Na^+ or Cl^- concentration were moderately correlated (genetically) with seedling biomass in hydroponics, but showed no correlations with grain yield in the field, indicating little value in selecting for ion concentration to improve ST. In accordance with phenotypic responses, QTL controlling Cl^- accumulation differed entirely between hydroponics and field locations, and few were detected in two or more environments, demonstrating substantial QTL-by-environment interactions. The presence of several QTL for Cl^- concentration indicated that uptake and accumulation was a polygenic trait. A major Cl^- concentration QTL (5A; *barc56/gwm186*) was identified in three field environments, and accounted for 27–32% of the total genetic variance. Alignment between the 5A QTL interval and its corresponding physical genome regions in wheat and other grasses has enabled the search for candidate genes involved in Cl^- transport, which is discussed.

Editor: Tai Wang, Institute of Botany, Chinese Academy of Sciences, China

Funding: This work was supported by the Molecular Plant Breeding Cooperative Research Centre, the South Australian Research and Development Institute, the Grains Research and Development Corporation and the University of Adelaide, Australia. The funders had no role in study design, data collection and analysis, decision to publish, or preparation of the manuscript.

Competing Interests: The authors have declared that no competing interests exist.

* E-mail: klaus.oldach@sa.gov.au

Introduction

Worldwide, salinity poses a serious threat to agricultural production, with globally salt-affected soils (including saline and sodic soils) totalling around 830 million hectares [1]. Saline soils are generally dominated by sodium and chloride ions, and the ability of crop plants to exclude these ions is often equated to salinity tolerance-ST (i.e. improved growth or yield under salinity stress). Despite intensive research and numerous scientific reports over several decades, there is a lack of consensus on whether Na^+ exclusion is always a useful trait to select for to improve ST, at least in the case of bread wheat. Few studies have shown good phenotypic correlation between Na^+ exclusion and ST [2–5], while others have reported weak [6,7] or no correlation [8–10]. In contrast to Na^+ exclusion, there has been very little research on the role of Cl^- exclusion and its contribution to ST [3,11–13]. Similar to Na^+ exclusion, these few studies on Cl^- reported either significant phenotypic correlation or no correlation with ST. It is clear that future research needs to place equal emphasis on the impact of Cl^- in ST as not only Na^+ but also Cl^- is present at toxic concentrations in saline-affected growth media used in the assessment of ST [13,14].

In screening studies for ST, sodium chloride is the most commonly used salt. Despite both Na^+ and Cl^- ions being present at toxic concentrations in growth media, there has been a lack of interest in Cl^-, which may be attributed to the earlier reports that Na^+ was more toxic than Cl^- [15]. Although these authors cautioned about assumptions made from extrapolations of two lines of bread wheat, their findings were not verified with a large set of genotypes differing in ST. This was later questioned by Martin and Koebner [16] on the basis that while attempting to separate the toxic effects of Na^+ and Cl^-, the authors used phytotoxic concentrations of nitrate in their experiments. Martin and Koebner [16] concluded that Cl^- was more toxic than Na^+, but the full toxic effect was apparent only when Na^+ and Cl^- were present simultaneously. However, more recent studies in barley found that Na^+ and Cl^- had a similar effect upon plant growth [17]. While the issue of whether Na^+ or Cl^- is more detrimental to plant growth remains controversial, it is appropriate to measure the concentration of both ions in the plant and to determine their relevance to ST for reasons mentioned earlier. Munns and Tester [18] argued that toxicity of Na^+ versus Cl^- can be best studied through genetic approaches as the alternative method of using different salts has to date produced equivocal results. The potential of the genetic approach has not been employed extensively.

Chloride is an essential micronutrient and has several functions in plant metabolism; enzyme activation, photosynthesis, a counter ion for cation transport, osmoregulation, and movement of stomata. Like most anions, it is weakly bound to soil particles, mostly in a soluble form in soil solution, and at high concentrations can be toxic to plant growth. Critical toxicity concentration in plants was estimated at 110–200 mmol kg^{-1} DW (4,000–7,000 mg kg^{-1} DW) and 420–1400 mmol kg^{-1} DW (15,000–50,000 mg kg^{-1} DW) for sensitive and tolerant species, respectively [19]. At present there is very little information on genetic control mechanisms of Cl^- exclusion in plant species. A better understanding of genetic control of Cl^- exclusion and identification of molecular markers has the potential to speed up breeding for a complex trait such as ST. To date, rice and barley appear to be the only cereal species in which genetic control of Cl^- exclusion has been investigated. In two studies involving rice F_2 and RIL populations derived from a cross between salt tolerant and salt-sensitive varieties CSR27 and MI48 respectively, few Cl^- concentration QTL were co-located with Na^+ concentration QTL, while others mapped to different regions [20,21]. Similar findings were also reported in barley [22,23]. If QTL for Na^+ and Cl^- concentration map to different locations, this would suggest separate genetic control mechanisms for regulation of these ions. At present, we are not aware of any reports on QTL mapping of Cl^- concentration in wheat.

Screening for ST is usually conducted in one of three main environments: hydroponics, soil-based pot assays or field trials. Due to inherent difficulties with field screening such as non-uniform distribution of salinity throughout the experimental area, fluctuations in rainfall and potential nutritional deficiencies, controlled environments are often preferred. However, as reported in recent studies [24], the results of controlled environments can be quite different from those of field environments and, therefore, require verification. The only two genetic studies on Cl^- accumulation to date have been conducted in hydroponics, and how these results correlate to field environments is unknown. It is important to note that the ability of controlled environmental studies to predict yield responses in the field is rarely addressed in the scientific literature, and the validation of controlled environmental studies in the field is important for plant breeding.

In previous studies in hydroponics and field trials [24,25], we reported QTL for grain yield, grain number m^{-2}, 1000-grain weight, maturity, plant height, seedling biomass, tiller number, chlorophyll content, leaf symptoms, Na^+ and K^+ concentrations of leaves and shoots for a bread wheat mapping population (Berkut/Krichauff). With the recent renewed interest in Cl^- [13], we revisited this population to (i) elucidate the genetic control mechanisms of Cl^- homeostasis via a QTL approach, and (ii) investigate the relationships among seedling biomass, grain yield and plant Na^+, K^+ and Cl^- concentrations. Here we report for the first time identification of a major QTL for Cl^- concentration in bread wheat and discuss its importance for marker-assisted selection and fine mapping/discovery of genes involved in Cl^- transport in bread wheat. We also demonstrate that Cl^- accumulation is a polygenic trait, but does not appear to be a reliable predictor of ST based on grain yield alone.

Materials and Methods

Plant material

A doubled-haploid (DH) population (152 lines) from a cross between bread wheat (*Triticum aestivum* L.) genotypes Berkut [Irene/Babax//Pastor] and Krichauff [Wariquam//Kloka/Pitic62/3/Warimek/Halberd/4/3Ag3/Aroona] was used in this study. The rationale for screening this population for plant Cl^- concentration and subsequent QTL detection was that a previous study revealed significantly lower shoot Cl^- accumulation in the Krichauff parent than in the Berkut parent [26].

Phenotyping and trait analysis

Growth room and field studies were described previously [24,25]. The data for grain yield, grain number m^{-2}, 1000-grain weight, maturity, plant height, seedling biomass, tiller number, chlorophyll content, leaf symptoms and Na^+ and K^+ concentrations of penultimate leaves and shoots were reported earlier [24,25]. In the present study shoot and leaf Cl^- concentrations of DH population grown in hydroponics and field trials (Roseworthy, Balaklava and Georgetown in South Australia) characterised by low, moderate and high salinity [24] were determined. Either single (hydroponics, two replicates) or 15–20 plants per entry (field trials, two replicates) were sampled for elemental analysis. Shoot (hydroponics) and leaf samples (field trials) were dried at 65°C for 48 h and dry weights recorded. The dried plant samples were then ground and analysed for Cl^-, calcium (Ca^{2+}) and magnesium (Mg^{2+}) concentration using either Inductively Coupled Plasma Optical Emission Spectrometry (ICP-OES) (ARL 3580 B, Appl. Res Lab. SA, Ecublens, Switzerland) [27,28] or a chloride meter (Model 926, Sherwood, Cambridge, UK). For analysis of Cl^- using the ICP-OES method, 0.1 g of ground shoot sample was extracted with hot (95°C) 4% HNO_3 acid in 50 mL capped polypropylene tubes for 90 minutes, whereas for measurements of Cl^- using the chloride meter, 0.5 g of ground sample was digested in 40 mL of 1% HNO_3 at 85°C for 5 hours in a 54well HotBlock (Environmental Express, Mt. Pleasant, South Carolina, USA). ICP-OES was used initially for analysis of the Cl^- concentration of hydroponically-grown plants, but due to prohibitive cost, leaf samples of field-grown plants were analysed using a chloride meter. As two different analytical methods were used for determination of Cl^- concentration in plant tissues, a number of samples were analysed using both methods, and the high correlation of the measurements between the two methods (hydroponically-grown samples, $r^2 = 0.98$, $n = 45$; field-grown samples, $r^2 = 0.97$, $n = 15$) indicated that the methods were comparable. As single measurements were taken from each extraction, duplicate analysis (one sample per batch of 24) was carried out to determine the homogeneity of the samples, and relative standard deviations between the two measurements were below 5% in all cases. Chloride concentration was expressed on a dry mass basis (mmol kg^{-1} DW).

Linkage map and interval construction

Genotyping and construction of a genetic linkage map for the Berkut/Krichauff population was described earlier [24,25]. The constructed linkage map initially comprised 557 markers across 21 chromosomes. After omission of co-locating markers this was reduced to 403 markers with an average interval distance of 9.16 cM. For computational purposes the alleles of the Berkut (A)/Krichauff (B) population were then converted into 1 and -1 respectively and missing marker scores were imputed using the flanking marker method of Martinez and Curnow [29]. A total of 384 inferred interval markers were then constructed using the mid-point interval method of Verbyla et al. [30].

Multi-environment analysis

To understand the genetic relationships of the DH lines across the field trials and growth room a multi-environment trials (MET) analysis was conducted for each of the traits Na^+, K^+ and Cl^-. For grain yield the MET analysis was restricted to field sites only. The analysis approach follows Smith et al. [31] which involves a linear mixed model including the parsimonious modelling of genetic effects of the DH lines through an appropriate genotype by environment interaction model and also captures non-genetic sources of variation through the use of separate spatial models for the plot errors at each site. The method initially involves the assessment of the spatial or environmental variation occurring at each site through the investigation of the assumption of variance homogeneity, detection of outliers, and the identification of global trends that may exist across the rows or columns of the experiment. For trends existing due to adjacency of plots in a trial, the model included a separable row by column autoregressive correlation structure. Stronger linear trends in either direction are fitted as fixed effects in the model. Design parameters such as genotypic replication or blocking structures were fitted as separate random effects.

The genotype by environment interaction model involved the use of an unstructured heterogeneous correlation matrix that appropriately captures the genetic relationship of the DH lines between trials. If a strong positive genetic correlation exists between any two trials then the relative performance or rankings of the varieties at each of the trials will be similar. As a consequence these trials will most likely share common or co-locating QTL with a common parent being favoured at each locus. Trials that exhibit little or no genetic correlation between them would exhibit different relative rankings for the varieties and most likely have unshared QTL. Each multi-environment analysis was performed using residual maximum likelihood (REML) and the estimated genetic correlations between sites were extracted for interpretation.

Multivariate analysis

A multivariate linear mixed model analysis of four traits (Na^+, K^+, Cl^- and grain yield) was conducted for each field trial in order to estimate genetic correlations of the DH lines between traits. A multivariate analysis was also conducted for the traits in the growth room and included Na^+, K^+, Cl^-, and seedling biomass. For each of the trials, estimates of the genetic relationships between DH lines were modelled through the use of a trait by genotype interaction with an unstructured heterogeneous correlation matrix. The model also included a separable trait by row by column spatial model for the plot errors with an unstructured heterogeneous correlation matrix for the trait component of the model. This unstructured correlation matrix ensures that traits collected from the same trial are connected phenotypically. This separable structure for the spatial model also assumes that the traits have a common row by column separable autoregressive correlation structure. Similar to the MET models, strong trends for any given trait were captured using the appropriate fixed effects, and random effects were used to model genotypic replication as well as blocking structures existing within each trial. Each multivariate analysis was performed using REML and the estimated genetic correlations between traits were extracted for interpretation.

QTL analysis

For each of the field sites and the growth room the detection and estimation of QTL for the measured traits was accomplished using the R [32] package wgaim [33]. The package is a computational implementation of Verbyla et al. [30,34]. In this approach, an initial base linear mixed model is established that contains non-genetic effects that account for extraneous variation. These include an appropriate spatial model for the errors as well as fixed and random effects that are relevant to the trial being examined. The base model also includes a random effect term that captures the genetic variation between the DH lines. Following Verbyla et al. [34] the base model is then extended by including the complete set of inferred interval markers into the base linear mixed model as a contiguous block of random effects with a single variance parameter. The significance of this variance parameter is then checked using a simple residual likelihood ratio test. If found significant, an alternative outlier model is formulated and the inferred interval marker with the largest outlier statistic is chosen as a putative QTL. This inferred interval marker is then removed from the contiguous block of random effects and placed as a separate random covariate in the original base model as well as the extended model that includes the remaining set of inferred interval markers. The forward selection process is then repeated until the variance parameter associated with the remaining inferred interval markers is not significant. The complete set of putative QTL selected appears additively as random covariates and is summarised using the methods of Verbyla et al. [34]. The summary includes the left and right flanking markers of the individual QTL, their effect sizes, approximate LOD scores as well as individual contributions to the overall genetic variance.

For all traits analysed in the present study, the best linear unbiased predictions of the genotypes were extracted from the base linear model and were used to calculate a generalized (broad-sense) heritability using the formula developed by Cullis et al. [35].

Comparative analysis and candidate genes co-located with the 5A Cl^- concentration QTL

To align the genetic position of the 5A Cl^- QTL to its physical position in the wheat genome, the sequence of RFLP markers with nearby location to the QTL-flanking SSR markers *gwm304* and *barc141* were identified using the database GrainGenes 2.0 (wheat.pw.usda.gov). The sequences of co-located RFLP markers *bcd21* and *psr128* were 451 bp and 430 bp, respectively, and were both derived from ESTs (GrainGenes 2.0). The sequences were used for homology searches using the BLAST tool at https://urgi.versailles.inra.fr/blast/blast.php. The search was carried out against the sequences of all bread wheat chromosomes showing the best hits on 5AL, as expected. The gene sequence hits were used for synteny analysis using the Genome Zipper v5 across wheat, rice, *Brachypodium* and sorghum revealing the syntenic regions between 64 non-rendundant wheat ESTs, *Brachypodium* chromosome 4, rice chromosome 9 and sorghum chromosome 2.

To assign potential functions to the wheat genes underlying the 5A Cl^- QTL interval, all 64 non-redundant wheat ESTs were used as queries for homology searches at the National Center for Biotechnology Information (NCBI) using BLASTN against the non-redundant nucleotide database.

Results

Responses to salinity stress, distributions and relationships between traits

Data on Cl^- concentration provided an opportunity to re-examine the relationships amongst traits associated with ST such Na^+ and K^+ accumulation, seedling biomass and grain yield in low (Balaklava), moderate (Roseworthy) and high (Georgetown and growth room) saline environments [24]. Krichauff had 10–20% lower Na^+ concentration than Berkut in field trials, and these differences diminished in hydroponics, whereas Krichauff had 14–25% lower Cl^- concentration than Berkut in all environments ranging from 362–669 and 482–775 mmol kg^{-1} DW for Krichauff and Berkut, respectively (Table 1), similar to previous studies [26]. It was interesting to observe that Cl^- concentrations were much higher than Na^+ concentrations. Berkut had slightly higher K^+ concentration than Krichauff but only at low to moderately saline field trials at Roseworthy and Balaklava (812–934 and 729–882 mmol kg^{-1} DW for Berkut and Krichauff respectively; Table 1). As for seedling biomass and/or grain yield

Table 1. Parental means, population mean and range for Na^+, Cl^-, K^+, Ca^{2+} and Mg^{2+} concentrations (mmol kg^1 DW) in penultimate leaves (field trials) and whole shoots (hydroponics), seedling biomass [shoot DW (g plant^1)] and grain yield (t ha^1) in Berkut/Krichauff DH population tested for ST in hydroponics and field trials (Roseworthy, Balaklava and Georgetown).

		Parental Lines		DH population		
Test environment	**Trait**	**Berkut**	**Krichauff**	**mean**	**range**	**Heritability h^2**
Hydroponics	Na^+ conc.	298	295	270	194–361	0.58
(100 mM NaCl ~10 dS m^1)	Cl^- conc.	457	376	378	236–480	0.67
	K^+ conc.	771	779	749	661–869	0.82
	Shoot DW	1.523	1.296	1.537	1.210–1.835	0.57
	Ca^{2+} conc.	107.2	87.3	97.9	77.4–116.7	0.83
	Mg^{2+} conc.	94.7	77.5	84.1	73.2–95.1	0.77
Roseworthy	Na^+ conc.	15.2	12.6	12.4	8.8–15.9	0.57
(low salinity, ECe<4 dS m^1)	Cl^- conc.	482	362	393	272–510	0.82
	K^+ conc.	812	729	739	621–847	0.64
	Grain yield	2.237	2.392	2.116	1.451–2.489	0.76
Balaklava	Na^+ conc.	13.1	11.6	10.9	7.4–14.5	0.78
(Moderate salinity, ECe = 4–8 dS m^1)	Cl^- conc.	557	447	474	301–598	0.82
	K^+ conc.	934	882	865	749–1011	0.77
	Grain yield	2.714	2.888	2.671	1.758–3.035	0.81
	Ca^{2+} conc.	121.3	97.2	110.7	71.9–151.4	0.82
	Mg^{2+} conc.	77.2	62.2	73.5	52.0–95.1	0.79
Georgetown	Na^+ conc.	20.5	16.3	18.7	10.9–30.4	0.60
(High salinity, ECe>8 dS m^1)	Cl^- conc.	775	669	688	571–884	0.84
	K^+ conc.	1363	1332	1328	1064–1523	0.76
	Grain yield	0.645	0.686	0.573	0.277–0.792	0.72

The means represent predicted values from MET (Na^+, Cl^-, K^+) and single environment (Ca^{2+} and Mg^{2+}) analysis of each trait. Broad-sense heritability is also given for individual traits at each environment.

production under salinity stress, Berkut produced 18% higher seedling biomass than Krichauff in hydroponics, whilst Krichauff had 6–7% higher grain yield in field trials (Table 1). In all traits, there was evidence of transgressive segregation.

To determine whether selection for Na^+ and/or Cl^- exclusion or even K^+ accumulation would lead to improved ST, multivariate analysis of concentrations of Na^+, Cl^-, K^+, seedling biomass and grain yield was performed for each of the environments (Table 2). The analysis showed that there was generally a good estimated correlation between Cl^- and either Na^+ or K^+ with two exceptions: there were negligible correlations for Na^+ *vs* Cl^-, and K^+ *vs* Cl^- at Balaklava and in hydroponics respectively. A negative but moderate correlation was observed between seedling biomass and either Na^+ ($r = 0.479$) or Cl^- (0.527).

To analyse genotype by environment interaction for each of the measured traits, multi-environment analyses and genetic correlations were estimated between environments. Representing low (Balaklava) to moderate (Roseworthy) saline environments, correlations for Na^+, Ka^+, Cl^- concentrations and grain yield were consistently high between these sites whereas low to moderate correlations were observed for these traits between other higher saline environments (Table 3). Therefore, it is reasonable to assume that selection for similar trait values may not be consistent between higher saline sites, indicating environmental effects controlling ion accumulation and grain yield.

Table 2. Estimated genetic correlations between shoot DW (hydroponics), grain yield (field) Na^+, K^+, and Cl^- (field and hydroponics) extracted from the fitted multi-trait model at each environment.

Environment	Na^+ *vs* Cl^-	K^+ *vs* Cl^-	Shoot DW or yield *vs* Na^+	Shoot DW or yield *vs* K^+	Shoot DW or yield *vs* Cl^-
Hydroponics	0.875	0.195	−0.486	−0.146	−0.531
Roseworthy	0.451	0.634	0.200	0.097	0.053
Balaklava	0.122	0.517	−0.200	0.060	0.097
Georgetown	0.319	0.763	0.066	0.148	0.082

Table 3. Estimated genetic correlations extracted from the fitted multi-environment model for individual traits.

		Roseworthy	Balaklava	Georgetown
Na^+ concentration	Balaklava	0.861		
	Georgetown	0.016	0.167	
	Growth room	0.182	0.186	0.464
		Roseworthy	Balaklava	Georgetown
K^+ concentration	Balaklava	0.794		
	Georgetown	0.568	0.598	
	Growth room	0.361	0.322	0.225
		Roseworthy	Balaklava	Georgetown
Cl^- concentration	Balaklava	0.897		
	Georgetown	0.582	0.462	
	Growth room	0.276	0.427	0.339
		Roseworthy	Balaklava	
Grain yield	Balaklava	0.706		
	Georgetown	0.130	0.338	

Generalized (broad-sense) heritability (h^2)

Estimates of h^2 differed with trait and environment, ranging from moderate to high (0.6–0.8) (Table 1). Amongst the mineral elements, Na^+ concentration had the lowest h^2, while Cl^- concentration had the highest h^2. Heritability of shoot DW (0.6) was lower than that of grain yield (0.7–0.8). Heritability of individual traits across environments showed relatively consistent (Ca^{2+}, Mg^{2+} and Cl^- concentration) to inconsistent patterns (Na^+ concentration). As reported earlier [24], consistently higher h^2 values indicate greater ability for selection for the traits, while lower and variable h^2 suggest the presence of substantial environmental effects, difficulty for direct selection, and the need for more replications.

QTL for Cl^- concentration

In the initial analysis in which differences in phenology were not included, there were few Cl^- concentration QTL co-locating with QTL for maturity on 5A and 5D (data not shown). Similar to Bonneau et al. [36], after the known differences in the genetic component of the phenology were addressed by fixing the maturity genes in the analyses, 14 QTL were identified (Table 4). However, most QTL were specific to single environments, and only three QTL were detected in two or more environments (3A, 5A, 7D) indicating some genotype by environment interaction. Interestingly, there were no co-located QTL controlling trait variation from hydroponics and field trials. The most significant QTL in hydroponics on chromosome 2A explained 20% of the total genetic variance and the Krichauff allele was responsible for increased Cl^- concentration. QTL on chromosome 3A and 7D were detected from multi-location trials and explained 4–11% of the total genetic variance, while QTL on 5A accounted for 27-32% of the total genetic variance (Table 4). Either the Berkut (3A, 5A) or the Krichauff (7D) allele was associated with increased Cl^- concentration at these loci. As the two QTL on 5A appear in tandem, these loci were further investigated to determine whether there may just be one rather than two separate QTL. The plot of outlier statistics (Figure 1) shows that there is in fact just one QTL on 5A expressed at all field locations. The QTL detected at one location only accounted for a small proportion of the total genetic variance, varying from 3.6 to 9.9% with either the Berkut or Krichauff allele being associated with increased Cl^- concentration (Table 4).

Some QTL for Cl^- concentration were co-located with QTL for either Na^+ or K^+ concentration from hydroponics and field trials (Table 4). It was interesting to observe that in hydroponics QTL for Cl^- concentration were co-located with QTL for Na^+ concentration (2A, 2B, 2B, 3A, 7A), while in field trials they were co-located with both Na^+ (3A, 5A, 7D) and K^+ (5A).

QTL for calcium (Ca^{2+}) and magnesium (Mg^{2+}) concentration

As Ca^{2+} and Mg^{2+} nutrition of the plant can also be affected by salinity [26,37–40], their genetic control under salinity stress was also investigated, in a limited way, using a QTL mapping approach. A total of 13 QTL for Ca^{2+} concentration and 6 QTL for Mg^{2+} concentration were identified in hydroponics and the field (Table 5). At those loci, either the Berkut or Krichauff allele increased the concentration of these cations. The most significant QTL for Ca^{2+} concentration was the QTL in hydroponics accounting for 13% of the genetic variance (Table 5). This QTL was also co-located with the Cl^- concentration QTL detected in hydroponic conditions (Table 4). For Mg^{2+} concentration, the QTL on 3A in hydroponics was the most significant, explaining 15% of the genetic variance (Table 5). This QTL was also co-located with a QTL for Cl^- concentration detected in environments with low to moderately saline conditions (Roseworthy and Balaklava) and hydroponics e (Table 4). However, there were no common QTL that were detected under hydroponics and the field for either of these two cations.

Table 4. QTL associated with Cl^- concentration in hydroponics and field trials (Roseworthy, Balaklava and Georgetown) under varying degrees of salinity stress.

Environment	Ch	Interval	Distance (cM)	Size*	Prob.	% Var.	LOD	**Co-locations with Na^+ or K^+ in field locations and hydroponics reported earlier [24,25]
Roseworthy	2B	*cfd011- gwm374(C)*	88.0–95.8	−12.5	0.001	4.1	2.4	
	3A	*wmc343- cfa2262*	75.7–79.7	20.6	0.000	11.1	6.4	
	3B	*wPt-9049(C)- wPt-0021*	124.4–154.0	13.4	0.002	3.6	2.1	
	5A	*barc56/gwm186*	90.0–100.5	36.8	0.000	32.4	18.3	Na^+-GT, K^+-RW, K^+-BA, K^+-GT
	6D	*cfd005(C)- gpw95010(C)*	172.8–174.1	−11.7	0.001	3.9	2.4	
	7D	*barc214- gwm437*	130.8–133.5	−11.3	0.002	3.6	2.0	Na^+-RW, Na^+- RH, Na^+-WT
	7D	*wmc014a- wPt-0695*	243.5–246.4	−11.3	0.002	3.6	2.1	
Balaklava	3A	*barc324- wmc343*	67.0–75.7	9.4	0.002	4.4	2.2	
	3B	*gwm247- wPt-4412*	195.1–196.1	13.9	0.000	9.9	4.8	
	5A	*gwm156(C)- gwm304*	84.1–89.3	25.4	0.000	30.8	14.8	
Georgetown	5A	*barc56- gwm186*	90.0–100.5	30.7	0.000	27	11.1	
	7B	*6cg1- wPt-7318*	0.0–22.7	−14.5	0.000	5.4	2.9	
	7D	*barc214- gwm437*	130.8–133.5	13.2	0.001	5.7	2.6	
Hydroponics	1D	*wmc216- wPt-1799*	80.7–131.2	21.3	0.002	5.8	2.0	
	2A	*wPt-3114- wmc170(C)*	92.5–109.9	−33.5	0.000	21.1	7.1	Na^+- HYDRO, Na^+-RW, Na^+-BA
	2B	*wmc272- barc349*	106.5–112.7	−19.4	0.000	8.5	2.7	Na^+-HYDRO
	2B	*wPt-7859- wPt-7161*	198.9–200.2	18.9	0.000	8.4	2.9	Na^+-HYDRO
	3A	*barc324- wmc343*	67.0–75.7	17.4	0.001	6.7	2.3	Na^+-RW
	7A	*gwm282- wPt-0961(C)*	170.2–183.3	−19.3	0.000	7.8	2.7	Na^+-HYDRO

Only those intervals with P values ≤ 0.01 and LOD$>$2.0 are presented. Field locations Roseworthy, Balaklava and Georgetown were classified as low, moderate and high salinity, respectively. Please see Genc et al. [24] for soil salinity classification.

*Positive and negative values indicate that Berkut and Krichauff alleles increased the phenotypic values, respectively. **The same co-locations appearing at multiple environments were presented only once. Abbreviations; Hydroponics = HYDRO, Balaklava = BA; Georgetown = GT; Roseworthy = RW. QTL names with letter C indicate several co-locating markers at those loci.

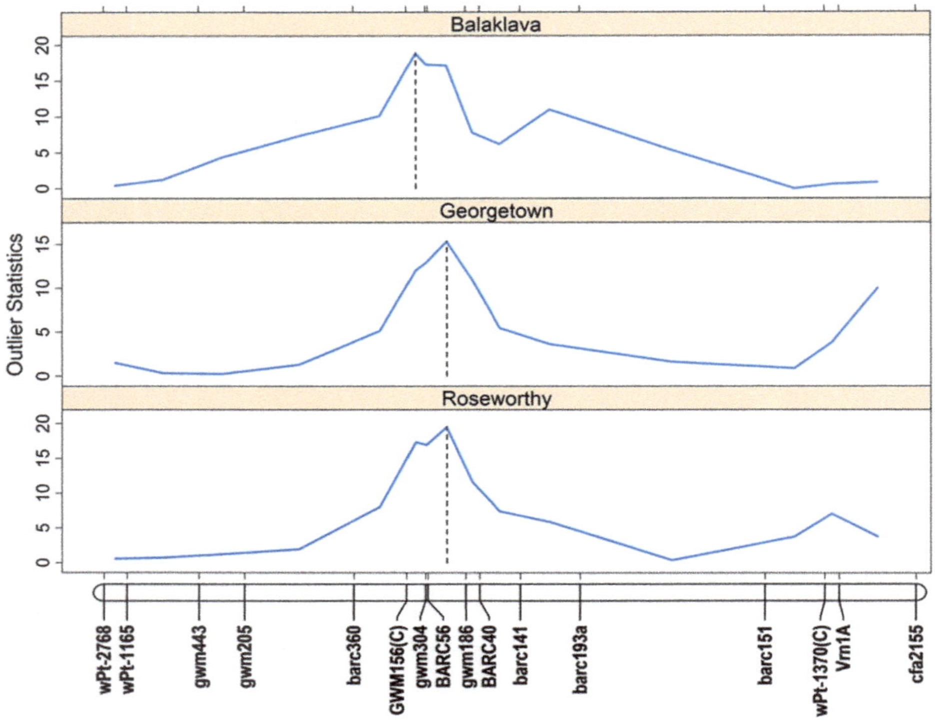

Figure 1. Location of Cl⁻ concentration QTL (*barc56*/*gwm186*) on chromosome 5A detected in field trials (Balaklava, Georgetown and Roseworthy) with varying salinity levels. The outlier statistics represent LOD scores (Table 4).

Known chloride transporters/channel in grass genomes and the 5A Cl^- QTL'

In previous studies, employing transcription analysis under salt stress, cellular localization and transgenesis for functional characterization, CLC (chloride channel) and CCC (cation chloride co-transporter) genes had been identified to play a role in Cl^- homoeostasis in plants; examples are CLC1 in tobacco and soybean [13,41,42,43] and CCC in Arabidopsis [44].

To investigate the presence of candidate genes such as CLCs, CCCs and other ion transporters within the QTL interval on chromosome 5A, we physically positioned the 5A Cl^- concentration QTL in the wheat genome sequence. For this purpose, the gene-based sequences of RFLP markers, *bcd21* and *psr128* with close linkage to the QTL-flanking SSR markers *gwm304* and *barc141* (Figure 2) were used to find wheat genome sequences. As expected, both RFLP sequences had their best hits in bread wheat chromosome 5AL and allowed to retrieve matching contigs of 4.2 kb and 9.1 kb for *bcd21* and *psr128*, respectively. As both RFLPs had originally been derived from ESTs, the corresponding wheat genome contigs (4.2 and 9.1 kb) identified gene hits in rice chromosome 9 (*Os09g0321900* and *Os09g0412200*). These rice genes functioned as borders of the physical interval in the comparative analysis between rice, *Brachypodium* and wheat using the alignment in Genome Zipper v5 (Figure 2). In rice (MSU Release 7 at rice.plantbiology.msu.edu/cgi-bin/gbrowse/rice/#search), the syntenic interval contained 547 genes.

Within the physical interval underlying the 5A Cl^- QTL, there were five different classes of genes encoding different transporters or channels: eleven ABC-transporter genes, and single genes encoding a nucleobase-ascorbate transporter, a vacuolar iron transporter (VIT1), a voltage-dependent anion channel (VDAC1) and a potassium transporter (HKT23-like) (Table 6).

Discussion

Implications of screening for Cl^- concentration in hydroponics and field environments

Phenotyping for ST is generally conducted under hydroponic conditions, and results are rarely validated in relevant field environments. Our recent studies in bread wheat demonstrated that phenotyping for Na^+ exclusion or ST in hydroponics had limited value in predicting field responses, and QTL differed vastly between hydroponics and field locations [24]. Given the renewed interest in Cl^- exclusion and ST [13], we analysed Cl^- concentration of hydroponically- and field-grown plants of Berkut/Krichauff DH population to determine the value of hydroponics for QTL analysis of Cl^- concentration, and elucidate genetic control mechanisms of Cl^- accumulation. The results demonstrated that plant Cl^- accumulation varied significantly between hydroponics and field trials and as a result, different QTL were identified between the two systems. As was the case with Na^+ concentration [24,25], this was most probably due to the two systems being vastly different [24]. These results suggest that there may be very little value in hydroponics testing to predict field responses to Cl^- concentration in bread wheat, and future studies should consider field testing or soil-based-pot assays as an alternative.

ST and Na^+ or Cl^- exclusion

In most studies to date Na^+ exclusion, and to a limited extent Cl^- exclusion, are traits contributing to ST. However, studies that also examined relationships between ST (absolute or relative growth) and Na^+ or Cl^- concentration reported inconsistent correlations [3–8,10,12,45–48]. It is noteworthy that studies reporting high correlations (r^2>0.5) analysed either a small

Table 5. QTL associated with Ca^{2+} and Mg^{2+} concentrations in hydroponics and in a field trial (Balaklava) under varying degrees of salinity stress.

Environment	Trait	Ch	Interval	distance (cM)	Size*	Prob.	% Var.	LOD
Balaklava	Ca^{2+} conc.	3A	*cfa2262-wPt-3816*	79.7–100.95	5.7	0.000	10.6	3.6
		4A	*gwm165a-wmc420*	37.8–49.4	5.1	0.000	9.9	3.2
		5B	*gwm499-wPt-5851*	43.9–46.1	−5.2	0.000	11.4	2.9
		7D	*wmc436b-barc214*	96.8–130.8	4.6	0.001	6.2	2.2
	Mg^{2+} conc.	2A	*gwm294-gdm093(C)*	113.5–150.8	2.4	0.002	6.2	2.1
		4B	*gwm149(C)-wPt-1505(C)*	48.0–48.7	2.3	0.001	9.1	2.3
		5B	*wPt-3457-wPt-1250*	51.5–54.3	−2.4	0.001	10.1	2.2
Hydroponics	Ca^{2+} conc.	1D	*wmc216-wPt-1799*	80.7–131.2	4.9	0.000	13.3	10.1
		2B	*wPt-5707-wPt-3561*	58.4–61.0	−1.9	0.001	3.9	2.5
		3B	*gwm389-wPt-8093(C)*	0.0–0.7	−1.9	0.000	4.0	3.4
		3B	*wPt-4412-wPt-8352(C)*	196.1–197.1	1.6	0.002	2.8	2.1
		4A	*wmc106-gwm165a*	28.4–37.8	2.5	0.000	6.3	4.4
		4D	*gpw95001-gwm165b*	49.7–50.5	−2.9	0.000	9.0	6.5
		5B	*gwm371-gwm499*	37.6–43.9	−2.5	0.000	6.3	3.1
		6B	*cfd076b-wPt-4924*	119.8–124.4	3.4	0.000	11.8	6.6
		7B	*wPt-6372(C)-wPt-3833*	63.2–66.8	2.2	0.000	5.1	3.4
	Mg^{2+} conc.	2A	*gwm294-gdm093(C)*	113.5–150.8	1.6	0.000	6.6	2.8
		3A	*gwm732a-barc1121(C)*	2.2–8.8	−1.4	0.000	7.6	2.9
		3A	*barc324-wmc343*	67.0–75.7	2.1	0.000	15.4	5.5
		4B	*gwm513(C)-gwm495*	43.4–44.7	1.6	0.000	9.9	3.4

Only those intervals with P values ≤0.01 and LOD>2.0 are presented. Balaklava location was classified as moderate salinity. Please see Genc et al. [24] for soil salinity classification.
*Positive and negative values indicate that Berkut and Krichauff alleles increased the phenotypic values, respectively. QTL names with letter C indicate several co-locating markers at those loci.

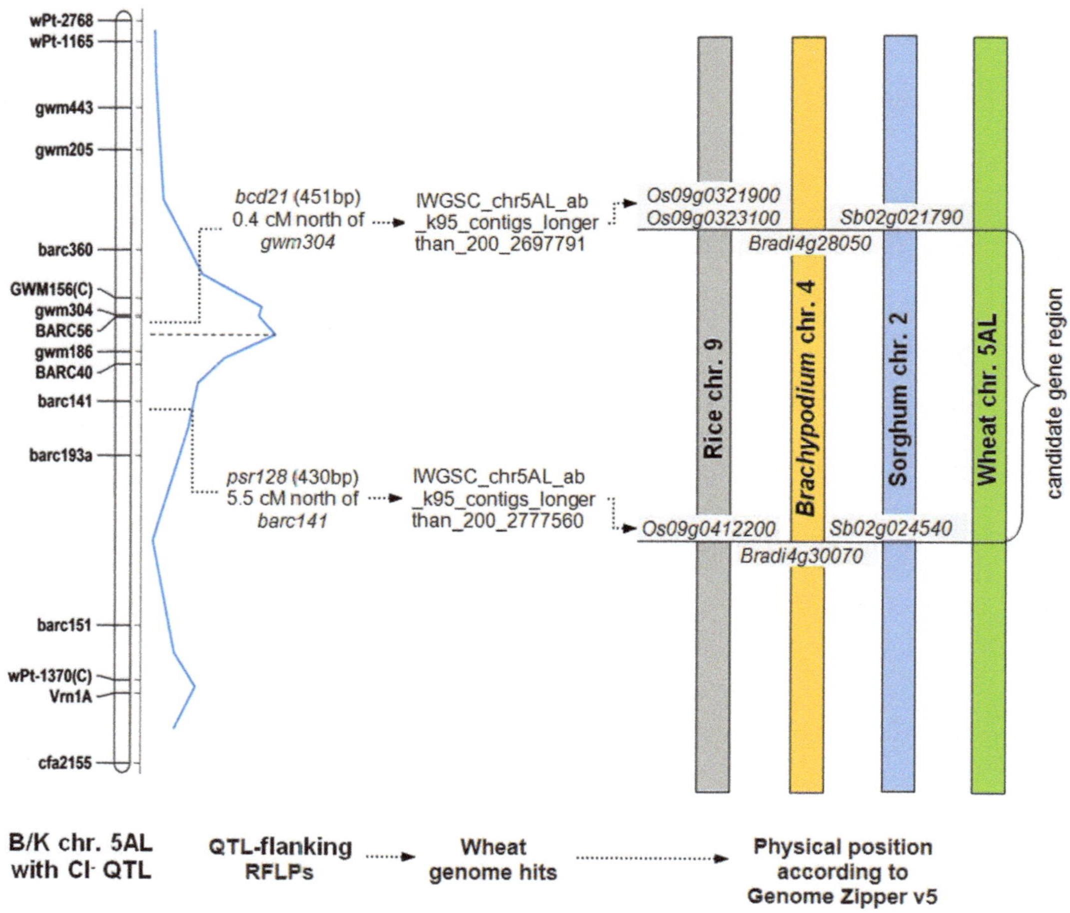

Figure 2. Inferred physical position of the Cl^- concentration QTL on 5AL in Berkut/Krichauff identified at Roseworthy field location onto 5AL in wheat.

number of genotypes or were conducted under controlled environmental conditions [4,7,12,46,49]. In the present study genetic correlations were investigated using multivariate analysis. Moderate correlations in controlled environments (generally phenotypic) are not uncommon [13,21–23,25], while such correlations involving a large number of genotypes in the field are almost non-existent [24]. The lack of genetic correlation between Na^+ and/or Cl^- exclusion and grain yield in field studies suggests that other biochemical and physiological processes need to be taken into consideration for identifying mechanisms associated with ST. These results also indicate that a reductionist approach, such as selection for Na^+ and/or Cl^- exclusion only, may not substantially improve ST in bread wheat. A more reliable approach would be to select for grain yield, unless specific physiological traits are shown to have significant and consistent correlations with grain yield under saline environments.

Ion channels and transporters involved in Na^+, K^+ and Cl^- homeostasis

Here we aim to introduce a brief discussion on transport of these ions from the soil solution into the root cell and their movements within the plant with respect to ion channels and transporters. However, a greater focus will be placed on Cl^-, and for Na^+ and K^+, readers are referred to recent reviews [41,50,51]. It is well established that the initial entry of Na^+ from the soil solution into the root cell is passive along the concentration gradient [52], and Na^+ uptake occurs primarily via non-selective cation channels and transporters [41,51,53]. However, Na^+ efflux (from cytosol into vacuole or removal from xylem) as a tolerance mechanism has to be active as it requires energy [41]. Potassium uptake from the soil solution into the root cell is an active process (i.e. moving across the membrane against its concentration gradient) and largely mediated by genes encoding channels and transporters [54]. Chloride uptake can be both active and passive depending on the external concentration. Under non-saline conditions transport of negatively charged Cl^- across negatively charged plasma membrane requires energy, therefore is an active process and mediated by transporters, while under saline conditions most Cl^- influx across the plasma membrane becomes passive [14]. However, its movement within or out of the plant must be active and aided by transporters [13]. Despite being the most abundant anion in the plant cells, compared to a number of well characterised Na^+ and K^+ transporters and encoding genes [41], very little is known about Cl^- transport mechanisms and the genes involved. To date two groups of gene families have repeatedly been discussed in relation to Cl^- homeostasis: CLCs and CCCs. From limited studies, it appears that CLCs, with their location in endomembranes, are involved in turgor regulation, stomatal movement and NO_3^- transport [55] but not root Cl^- uptake [41], while CCCs are involved in long distance transport of Na^+, K^+ and Cl^- and function as K^+:Cl^-, Na^+:Cl^- or Na^+:

Table 6. Candidate genes underlying the physical interval of the Cl^- QTL on chromosome 5A.

Brachypodium (v1.2)	Rice (Gene ID at MSU[a]/at IRGSP v2)	Sorghum (v1.4)	Wheat (v5[b])	Predicted protein function[a]
-	-	*Sb02g022750*	-	ABC transporter
Bradi4g28660	*LOC_Os09g19734/OS09G0361400*	*Sb02g022910*	*WHE0957_E03_J05ZT; Traes_5AL_99BEC1C3B*	Voltage dependent anion channel 1 (VDAC1)
Bradi4g29102	*LOC_Os09g20480/Os09g0371000*	*Sb02g023340*	*Traes_5AL_F8B48EC59*	ABC transporter
Bradi4g29110	*LOC_Os09g20490/Os09g0371100*	*Sb02g023370*	-	ABC transporter
Bradi4g29120	"	*Sb02g023380*	-	"
Bradi4g29110	*LOC_Os09g20500/Os09g0371200*	*Sb02g023370*	-	ABC transporter
Bradi4g29120	"	*Sb02g023380*	-	"
Bradi4g29140	*LOC_Os09g20510/Os09g0371300*	*Sb02g023360*	-	ABC transporter
Bradi4g29110	*LOC_Os09g20520/Os09g0371400*	*Sb02g023370*	-	ABC transporter
Bradi4g29120	"	*Sb02g023380*	-	"
Bradi4g29347	*LOC_Os09g21000/Os09g0376900*	*Sb02g023620*	*Traes_5AL_B64648FE6*	Potassium transporter family (HKT23-like)
Bradi4g29440	*LOC_Os09g21340/Os09g0381100*	*Sb02g023720*	*WHE1104_A05_B10ZS; WHE0807_A06_B11ZS; Traes_5AL_3E0C865DF*	Nucleobase-ascorbate transporter
Bradi4g29650	*LOC_Os09g23110/Os09g0394500*	*Sb02g024060*	*Traes_5AL_01A13992D; Traes_5AL_B8B668113*	ABC transporter
Bradi4g29720	*LOC_Os09g23300/Os09g0396900*	*Sb02g024130*	*WHE1787_E02_I03ZS; Traes_5AL_F80B422BA*	Vacuolar iron transporter 1 (VIT1)
Bradi4g29810	*LOC_Os09g23640/Os09g0401100*	-	*Traes_5AL_678EA44B2*	ABC transporter

[a]according to MSU Rice Genome Annotation Project release 7, Ensembl Plants release 22 or NCBI;
[b]Genome Zipper v5.

K^+:Cl^- co-transporters [44,56]. However, there may be other gene families involved in Cl^- transport, as discussed by Teakle and Tyerman [13].

Genetic control mechanisms of Na^+, K^+ and Cl^-homeostasis under salinity stress

A good understanding of inheritance of homeostasis of these ions is required for a successful breeding strategy. Our present knowledge of mechanisms of their inheritance is a mere reflection of the number of studies conducted on them. For instance, due to greater focus on Na^+, we know more about Na^+ than K^+ or Cl^-. The limited studies in rice and wheat suggest that Na^+ and K^+ homeostasis under salinity stress are under separate genetic control [25,57–59], although studies in barley [22,23] found that QTL for Na^+ co-located with QTL for K^+, suggesting one or more genes regulating Na^+ and/or K^+ transport such as vacuolar sodium-hydrogen antiporter (NHX) genes [22]. As for Cl^-, to date there have been only four quantitative genetic studies that reported QTL for Cl^- concentration; two in rice [20,21] and two in barley [22,23]. In those studies as well as in the present study, moderate correlations between Cl^- and either Na^+ or K^+, and QTL for different ions mapping to the same and/or different regions indicate the presence of common (i.e. CCCs) and specific transporters for the uptake of these ions [i.e. high-affinity potassium (HKT) and (CLCs)] which in turn suggests common and separate genetic control. For instance, in the present study, Cl^- QTL on 2A and 5A co-located with QTL for Na^+ and K^+ concentration, respectively [24]. A physiological explanation for these co-locations and correlations between cations (Na^+ and K^+) and anions (Cl^-) may be the charge balance between these two groups of ions since the net movement of ions must be balanced so that there is charge equivalence with small difference [13]. Whereas there were no CCC and CLC genes physically close to the Cl^- concentration QTL on chromosome 5A there are 15 transporter and channel genes in the physical interval as candidates for the observed Cl^- accumulation. Although we have used the latest release of the comparison between wheat ESTs and contigs with sequenced grass genomes (Genome Zipper v5), it is possible that other genes reside in this region in wheat and the microsynteny is less well preserved as it appears to be so far.

Nguyen et al. [22] recently reported a Cl^- concentration QTL under salt stress in barley but used an incorrect barley chromosome nomenclature so that the actual chromosome 5H was mislabelled as 7H (other chromosomes were also mislabelled). The physical position of the RFLP markers *ABC324* and *ABC302* that flank their barley Cl^- QTL on 5HL [22] suggest a position close to the physical chromosomal region corresponding to the 5AL Cl^- concentration QTL reported here. In fact, the physical position of the northern flanking marker *ABC324* (position chromosome 5H: 399,222,591) slightly overlaps with the position of the southern end of the5A QTL flanked by RFLP marker *psr128* (position chromosome 5H: 412,653,548). It is possible that both QTL are caused by orthologous genes in wheat and barley, although this is far from certain as the QTL intervals contain hundreds of genes and the barley QTL was identified under salt stress in a hydroponics system whereas the QTL in wheat was repeatedly observed under salt stressed field conditions but not in hydroponics. Only further work such as fine mapping and gene expression analysis of the candidate genes will prove unequivocally the identity of the underlying gene for the differential Cl^- accumulation between Berkut and Krichauff. The present study provides a compelling case that the 5A QTL contains a K^+:Cl^- co-transporter gene several other candidates capable of moving Cl^- ions across membranes. However, as this is the first report in wheat, there is clearly a need for testing other mapping populations and genetics resources to identify other Cl^- transporter gene(s) to gain a better understanding of genetic control mechanisms of Cl^- homoeostasis in crops.

Genetic control mechanisms of Ca^{2+} and Mg^{2+} accumulation under salinity stress

The inheritance of plant Ca^{2+} and Mg^{2+} accumulation was also investigated, given the reports of salinity-induced nutritional deficiencies such as Ca^{2+} and Mg^{2+} [26,37,39,40] and the importance of maintenance of adequate nutrition for these essential elements to plant growth and yield under salinity stress. To our knowledge, there have only been two studies in barley [22,23] that investigated inheritance of Ca^{2+} and Mg^{2+} uptake or accumulation under salinity stress. However, only in one study [23] QTL for Ca^{2+} and Mg^{2+} were detected under salinity stress; one QTL for Mg^{2+} concentration on 6H, and three QTL for Ca^{2+} concentration on 1H, 6H and 7H. The QTL on 6H was common not only to Ca^{2+} and Mg^{2+} but also to ST. To our knowledge, this is the first time in the literature that a QTL for a nutrient other than Na^+ was co-located with ST, providing evidence for the role of Ca^{2+} and Mg^{2+} nutrition in growth and yield under salinity stress. These results also indicate that Ca^{2+} and Mg^{2+} uptake may occur through common as well as independent pathways. In contrast to the barley study, in the present study, none of the Ca^{2+} and Mg^{2+} concentration QTL co-located with each other or ST (measured as seedling biomass or grain yield), suggesting independent genetic control. However, further studies are required to enable better understanding of their genetic control mechanisms.

Conclusions

As was the case with Na^+ [24], plant Cl^- responses and related QTL differed widely between hydroponics and field tests, indicating substantial genotype and QTL interactions with environments. The results also indicated that hydroponics-based seedling assays may be very limited in their ability to predict field responses to salinity, and soil-based assays may be the second best option after field testing. As Cl^- concentration in the plant correlated only moderately with seedling biomass and showed no correlation with grain yield in the field, it does not appear, on its own, to be a reliable physiological parameter to select for in a breeding context, at least in bread wheat. Further research involving other mapping populations/genetic resources is warranted to be definitive. In the short term, selection for grain yield, which is integrative of all tolerance mechanisms, appears a more reliable strategy, while in the long term identification of donors for various physiological traits and subsequently combining them in a genotype (pyramiding) is likely to be the way forward [60]. This latter process can be fast-tracked via marker assisted selection. Finally the presence of several QTL for Cl^- concentration indicates that Cl^- uptake/accumulation is a polygenic trait. The discovery of a major QTL for Cl^- concentration on 5A that co-locates with several candidate genes that could be involved in Cl^- transport in bread wheat provides a starting point for further analysis through fine mapping and functional studies.

Acknowledgments

We would like to thank Dr Hugh Wallwork (South Australian Research and Development Institute) for access to the Berkut/Krichauff DH population and the coordination of the field trials, the staff at Australian Grain Technologies, the LongReach Plant Breeders, the University of Adelaide Barley Breeding Program and Mr Jim Lewis (South Australian Research and Development Institute) for sowing, harvesting and general maintenance of the field trials, Mr Robin Hosking (the Australian Centre for Plant Functional Genomics) for his construction and creative modification of the supported hydroponic system and technical support throughout this project, Mrs Teresa Fowles and Mr Lyndon Palmer (the University of Adelaide) for their help with ICP-OES analysis, Prof. Mark Tester (Australian Centre for Plant Functional Genomics) for the use of a chloride meter, Drs Graham Lyons and John Harris (the University of Adelaide) for their critical review of the manuscript prior to submission, and the editor and the reviewers for their helpful comments.

Author Contributions

Conceived and designed the experiments: YG JT JR KO. Performed the experiments: YG JR KO. Analyzed the data: YG JT KO. Contributed reagents/materials/analysis tools: YG JT KO. Wrote the paper: YG JT KO.

References

1. Martinez-Beltran J, Manzur CL (2005) Overview of salinity problems in the world and FAO strategies to address the problem. In Proceedings of the international salinity forum; Riverside, California. pp. 311–313.
2. Schachtman DP, Munns R, Whitecross MI (1991) Variation in sodium exclusion and salt tolerance in *Triticum tauschii*. Crop Science 31: 992–997.
3. Ashraf M, O'Leary JW (1996) Responses of newly developed salt-tolerant genotype of spring wheat to salt stress: yield components and ion distribution. Journal of Agronomy and Crop Science 176: 91–101.
4. Rashid A, Querishi RH, Hollington PA, Wyn Jones RG (1999) Comparative responses of wheat cultivars to salinity at the seedling stage. Journal of Agronomy and Crop Science 182: 199–207.
5. Poustini K, Siosemardeh A (2004) Ion distribution in wheat cultivars in response to salinity stress. Field Crops Research 85: 125–133.
6. Hollington PA (2000) Technological breakthroughs in screening/breeding wheat varieties for salt tolerance. In: Gupta SK, Sharma SK, Tyagi NK, editors. National Conference on Salinity Management in Agriculture. Central Soil Salinity Research Institute, Karnal, India. pp. 273–289.
7. Huang Y, Zhang G, Wu F, Chen J, Zhou M (2006) Differences in physiological traits among salt-stressed barley genotypes. Communications in Soil Science and Plant Analysis 37: 567–570.
8. Ashraf M, McNeilly T (1988) Variability in salt tolerance of nine spring wheat cultivars. Journal of Agronomy and Crop Science 160: 14–21.
9. Bagci SA, Ekiz H, Yilmaz A (2007) Salt tolerance of sixteen wheat genotypes during seedling growth. Turkish Journal of Agriculture and Forestry 31: 363–372.
10. Genc Y, McDonald GK, Tester M (2007) Reassessment of tissue Na^+ concentration as a criterion for salinity tolerance in bread wheat. Plant, Cell and Environment 30: 1486–1498.
11. Royo A, Aragüés R (1999) Salinity-yield response functions on barley genotypes assessed with a triple line source sprinkler system. Plant and Soil 209: 9–20.
12. El-Hendawy S, Hu Y, Schmidhalter U (2005) Growth, ion content, gas exchange and water relations of wheat genotypes differing in salt tolerances. Australian Journal of Agricultural Research 56: 123–134.
13. Teakle NL, Tyerman SD (2010) Mechanisms of Cl^- transport contributing to salt tolerance. Plant, Cell and Environment 33: 566–589.
14. White PJ, Broadley MR (2001) Chloride in soils and its uptake and movement within the plant: A Review. Annals of Botany 88: 967–988.
15. Kingsbury R, Epstein E (1986) Salt sensitivity in wheat. A case for specific ion toxicity. Plant Physiology 80: 651–654.
16. Martin P, Koebner R (1995) Sodium and chloride ions contribute synergistically to salt toxicity in wheat. Biologia Plantarum 37: 265–271.
17. Tavakkoli E, Rengasamy P, McDonald GK (2010) The response of barley to salinity stress differs between hydroponics and soil systems. Functional Plant Biology 37: 621–633.
18. Munns R, Tester M (2008) Mechanisms of salinity tolerance. Annual Review of Plant Biology 59: 651–681.

19. Xu G, Magen H, Tarchitzky J, Kafkafi U (2000) Advances in chloride nutrition. Advances in Agronomy 68: 96–150.
20. Ammar MHM, Pandit A, Singh RK, Sameena S, Chaucan MS, et al. (2009) Na^+, K^+ and Cl^- ion concentrations in salt tolerant *Indica* rice variety CSR27. Journal of Plant Biochemistry and Biotechnology 18: 139–150.
21. Pandit A, Rai V, Bal S, Sinha S, Kumar V, et al. (2010) Combining QTL mapping and transcriptome profiling of bulked RILs for identification of functional polymorphism for salt tolerance genes in rice (*Oryza sativa* L.). Molecular Genetics and Genomics 284: 121–136.
22. Nguyen VL, Ribot SA, Dolstra O, Niks RE, Visser RGF, et al. (2013) Identification of quantitative trait loci for ion homeostasis and salt tolerance in barley (*Hordeum vulgare* L). Molecular Breeding 31: 137–152.
23. Nguyen VL, Dolstra O, Malosetti M, Kilian B, Graner A, et al. (2013) Association mapping of salt tolerance in barley (*Hordeum vulgare* L). Theoretical and Applied Genetics. DOI.10.1007/s00122-013-2139-0.
24. Genc Y, Oldach K, Gogel B, Wallwork H, McDonald GK, et al. (2013) Quantitative trait loci for agronomical and physiological traits for a bread wheat population grown in environments with a range of salinity levels. Molecular Breeding 32: 39–59. DOI: 10.1007/s110320139851y.
25. Genc Y, Oldach K, Verbyla A, Lott G, Hassan M, et al. (2010) Sodium exclusion QTL associated with improved seedling growth in bread wheat under salinity stress. Theoretical and Applied Genetics 121: 877–894.
26. Genc Y, Tester M, McDonald GK (2010) Calcium requirement of wheat in saline and non-saline conditions. Plant and Soil 327: 331–345.
27. Wheal MS, Palmer LT (2010) Chloride analysis of botanical samples by ICPOES. Journal of Analytical Atomic Spectrometry 25: 1946–1952.
28. Wheal MS, Fowles TO, Palmer LT (2011) A cost effective acid digestion method using closed polypropylene tubes for inductively coupled plasma optical emission spectrometry (ICP-OES) analysis of plant essential elements. Analytical Methods 3: 2854–2863.
29. Martinez O, Curnow RN (1992) Estimating the locations and sizes of the effects of quantitative trait loci using flanking markers. Theoretical and Applied Genetics 85: 480–488.
30. Verbyla AP, Cullis BR, Thompson R (2007) The analysis of QTL by simultaneous use of the of the full linkage map. Theoretical and Applied Genetics 116: 95–111.
31. Smith A, Cullis BR, Thompson R (2001) Analysing variety by environment data using multiplicative mixed models. Biometrics 57: 1138–1147.
32. R Development Core Team (2013) R: A language and environment for statistical computing, R Foundation for Statistical Computing. Vienna, Austria.
33. Taylor JD, Diffey S, Verbyla AP, Cullis BC (2013) wgaim: Whole Genome Average Interval Mapping for QTL detection using mixed models, R package version 1.3–0.
34. Verbyla AP, Taylor JD, Verbyla KL (2012) RWGAIM: An efficient high dimensional random whole average (QTL) interval mapping approach. Genetics Research 94: 291–306.
35. Cullis BR, Smith AB, Coombes NE (2006) On the design of early generation variety trials with correlated data. Journal of Agricultural, Biological and Environmental Statistics 11:381–393.
36. Bonneau J, Taylor J, Parent B, Bennett D, Reynolds M, et al. (2013) Multi-environment analysis and improved mapping of a yield-related QTL on chromosome 3B of wheat. Theoretical and Applied Genetics 126: 747–761.
37. Ehret DI, Redmann RE, Harvey BL, Cipywnyk A (1990) Salinity-induced calcium deficiencies in wheat and barley. Plant and Soil 128: 143–151.
38. Bergmann W (1992) Nutritional disorders of plants: Developments, visual and analytical diagnosis. Gustav Fisher, Jena, Stuttgart, New York.
39. Cramer GR (2002) Sodium-calcium interactions under salinity stress. In: Lauchli A, Luttge U, editors. Salinity: Environment- plants- molecules. Kluwer, Dordrecht. pp. 205–227.
40. Adcock KG, Gartrell JW, Brennan RF (2001) Calcium deficiency of wheat grown in acidic sandy soil from Southwestern Australia. Journal of Plant Nutrition 24: 1217–1227.
41. Mian AA, Senadheera P, Maathuis FJ (2011) Improving crop salt tolerance: anion and cation transporters as genetic engineering targets. Plant Stress 5: 64–72.
42. Lurin C, Geelen D, Barbier-Brygoo H, Guern J, Maurel C (1996) Cloning and functional expression of a plant voltage-dependent chloride channel. Plant Cell 8: 701–711.
43. Wong TH, Li MW, Yao XQ, Lam HM (2013) The GmCLC1 protein from soybean functions as a chloride ion transporter. Journal of Plant Physiology 170: 101–104.
44. Colemenero-Flores JM, Martinez G, Gamba G, Vazuez N, Iglesias DJ, et al. (2007) Identification and functional characterization of cation-chloride cotransporters in plants. Plant Journal 50: 278–292.
45. Isla R, Royo A, Aragüés R (1997) Field screening of barley cultivars to soil salinity using a sprinkler and a drip irrigation system. Plant and Soil 197: 105–117.
46. Khan MA, Shirazi MU, Khan MA, Mujtaba SM, Islam E, et al. (2009) Role of proline, K/Na ratio and chlorophyll content in salt tolerance of wheat (*Triticum aestivum* L.). Pakistan Journal of Botany 41: 633–638.
47. Rawson HM, Richards RA, Munns R (1988) An examination of selection criteria for salt tolerance in wheat, barley and triticale genotypes. Australian Journal of Agricultural Research 39: 759–772.
48. Salam A, Hollington PA, Gorham J, Wyn Jones RG, Gliddon C (1999) Physiological genetics of salt tolerance in wheat (*Triticum aestivum* L): Performance of wheat varieties, inbred lines and reciprocal F_1 hybrids under saline conditions. Journal of Agronomy and Crop Science 183: 145–156.
49. Munns R, James RA (2003) Screening methods for salinity tolerance: a case study with tetraploid wheat. Plant and Soil 253: 201–218.
50. Maathuis FJM, Amtmann A (1999) K^+ Nutrition and Na^+ Toxicity: The Basis of Cellular K^+/Na^+ Ratios. Annals of Botany 84: 123–133.
51. Tester M, Davenport R (2003) Na^+ tolerance and Na^+ transport in higher plants. Annals of Botany 91: 503–527.
52. Cheeseman JM (1982) Pump-leak sodium fluxes in low salt corn roots. Journal of Membrane Biology 70: 157–164.
53. Byrt CS, Platten JD, Spielmeyer W, James RA, Lagudah ES, et al. (2007) HKT1;5-like cation transporters linked to Na^+ exclusion loci in wheat, *Nax2* and *Kna1*. Plant Physiology 143: 1918–1928.
54. Horie T, Brodsky DE, Costa A, Kaneko T, Schiavo FL, et al. (2011) K^+ transport by the OsHKT2;4 transporter from rice (*Oryza sativa*) with atypical Na^+ transport properties and competition in permeation of K^+ over Mg^{2+} and Ca^{2+} ions. Plant Physiology 156: 1493–1507.
55. Hechenberger M, Schwappach B, Fischer WN, Frommer WB, Jentsch TJ, et al. (1996) A family of putative chloride channels from Arabidopsis and functional complementation of a yeast strain with a CLC gene disruption. Journal of Biological Chemistry 271: 33632–33638.
56. Kong X-Q, Gao X-H, Sun W, An J, Zhao Y-X, et al. (2011) Cloning and functional characterization of a cation-chloride cotransporter gene OsCCC1. Plant Molecular Biology 75: 567–578.
57. Garcia A, Rizzo CA, Ud-Din J, Bartos SL, Senadhira D, et al. (1997) Sodium and potassium transport to the xylem are inherited independently in rice and the mechanisms of sodium: potassium selectivity differs between rice and wheat. Plant, Cell and Environment 20: 1167–1174.
58. Koyama ML, Levesley A, Koebner RMD, Flowers TJ, Yeo AR (2001) Quantitative trait loci for component physiological traits determining salt tolerance in rice. Plant Physiology 125: 406–422.
59. Lin HX, Zhu MZ, Yano M, Gao JP, Liang ZW, et al. (2004) QTLs for Na^+ and K^+ uptake of the shoots and roots controlling rice salt tolerance. Theoretical and Applied Genetics 108: 253–260.
60. Peng S, Ismail AM (2004) Physiological basis of yield and environmental adaptation in rice. In: Nguyen HT, Blum A, editors. Physiology and biotechnology integration for plant breeding. CRC Press, New York, Basel. pp. 72–118.

17

Discontinuity of Human Presence at Atapuerca during the Early Middle Pleistocene: A Matter of Ecological Competition?

Guillermo Rodríguez-Gómez[1]*, Ana Mateos[1], Jesús Angel Martín-González[2], Ruth Blasco[3], Jordi Rosell[4,5], Jesús Rodríguez[1]

1 Paleofisiología y Ecología Social de homínidos, Centro Nacional de Investigación sobre la Evolución Humana (CENIEH), Burgos, Spain, **2** Departamento de Matemáticas y Computación, Universidad de Burgos, Burgos, Spain, and temporarily assigned to CENIEH, Burgos, Spain, **3** The Gibraltar Museum, Gibraltar, Gibraltar, **4** Àrea de Prehistòria, Universitat Rovira i Virgili (URV), Tarragona, Spain, **5** Institut Català de Paleoecologia Humana i Evolució Social (IPHES), Tarragona, Spain

Abstract

Increasing evidence suggests that the European human settlement is older than 1.2 Ma. However, there is a fierce debate about the continuity or discontinuity of the early human settlement of Europe. In particular, evidence of human presence in the interval 0.7–0.5 Ma is scarce in comparison with evidence for the previous and later periods. Here, we present a case study in which the environmental conditions at Sierra de Atapuerca in the early Middle Pleistocene, a period without evidence of human presence, are compared with the conditions in the previous period, for which a relatively intense human occupation is documented. With this objective in mind, the available resources for a human population and the intensity of competition between secondary consumers during the two periods are compared using a mathematical model. The Gran Dolina site TD8 level, dated to 0.7–0.6 Ma, is taken as representative of the period during which Atapuerca was apparently not occupied by humans. Conditions at TD8 are compared with those of the previous period, represented by the TD6-2 level, which has yielded abundant evidence of intense human occupation. The results show that survival opportunities for a hypothetical human population were lower at TD8 than they were at TD6-2. Increased resource competition between secondary consumers arises as a possible explanation for the absence of human occupation at Atapuerca in the early Middle Pleistocene.

Editor: David Caramelli, University of Florence, Italy

Funding: This research was funded by the MINECO project, CGL2012-38434-C03-02, CGL2012-38434-C03-03, CGL2012-38358 and CGL-BOS-2012-34717. G. Rodríguez-Gómez is the beneficiary of a predoctoral FPI Grant from the Spanish MICINN. The fieldwork at the Atapuerca sites was funded by the Junta de Castilla y León. R. Blasco is a Beatriu de Pinós postdoctoral scholarship recipient from Generalitat de Catalunya and was co-financed by the European Union through Marie Curie Actions, FP7. The funders had no role in study design, data collection and analysis, decision to publish, or preparation of the manuscript.

Competing Interests: The authors have declared that no competing interests exist.

* Email: guillermo.rodriguez@cenieh.es

Introduction

The current paleoanthropological scenario shows an increasingly complex human population dynamic for the Pleistocene period. Some phenomena, such as migrations, replacements of species and abandonment of territories with unfavourable conditions for human colonization, seem to have played significant role in the evolution of the genus *Homo*. From this perspective, one of the most interesting subjects is the continuity or discontinuity between the hominins of the Early and Middle Pleistocene in Western Europe and the origin of the Neandertal lineage [1]. This topic has been treated from different perspectives and by different disciplines. Several authors have proposed the existence of migration waves during the Early Pleistocene taking into account different evidence [2–13]. Bermúdez de Castro and Martinón-Torres [14] suggest a theoretical evolutionary scenario for the Early Pleistocene based on isolation processes and intermittent contacts between the Eurasian populations, as previously proposed by Dennell et al [15] for the Middle Pleistocene. According to their hypotheses, the hominins from Eurasia lost contact with Africa after the first *Out of Africa* because of the formation and evolution of significant biogeographical barriers between the two continents, such as the Negev desert [16,17]. From this point forward, Eurasian populations followed an independent evolutionary process in which the same phenomena of climatic and geographical barriers caused periods of disconnection between some regions [13,18]. Apparently, these frontiers mainly affected the European populations, producing alternating episodes of isolation with population fluxes and refluxes. This dynamic seems to have also occurred during the Middle Pleistocene and may help to explain some significant changes that occurred in Western Europe during this period. An alternative explanation relates human dispersal in Europe to climate change [12] and links the permanence of humans Oldowan technology in Europe to faunal continuity, and specifically to the presence of the sabertooth *Megantereon whitei*, a hypercarnivorous predator which, presumably, provided hominins with large amounts of scavengable carcasses [13]. Arribas and Palmqvist [13] suggest that there was isolation between Europe and Africa between 1.8 Ma until 0.6 Ma, when Achelean populations expanded from Africa into Western Europe.

Currently, human settlement during the Early Pleistocene is represented in Western Europe by a short list of sites, such as Fuente Nueva 3 [19,20], Barranco León [21], Vallparadís [22,23] but see also [24], Sima del Elefante and Gran Dolina in Spain [25], Pirro Nord [26] and Ca'Belvedere di Monte Poggiolo [27] in Italy, Le Vallonet [28], Saint-Hilaire-la Gravelle [29,30] and Pont de Lavaud [31] in France, Happisburgh [32] in England and Untermassfeld [33] and Dorn-Dürkheim 3 [34] in Germany. The site of Pakefield (England), which dates to the beginning of the Middle Pleistocene (0.7 Ma) [35], can also be considered in this list. Lézignan le Cèbe, in southern France, has been proposed as one of the oldest sites documenting human occupation in Europe [36], but this interpretation is controversial. Technologically, all of these archaeological locations can be classified as Oldowan Technological Complexes or Mode 1 [11,37]. *Homo antecessor*, described from level TD6 of Gran Dolina, seems to have inhabited this area at least between the Jaramillo Subchron and the Matuyama-Brunhes Boundary [38]. Human remains older than the Jaramillo Subchron have been found at Sima del Elefante (1.2 Ma) [39] and Barranco León (1.4 Ma) [21], but see also Muttoni et al. [40]. Unfortunately, these fossil remains do not meet enough taxonomic criteria to establish possible relationships with other species such as *H. antecessor* and to describe the human scenario at this early time. In the absence of other data, these fossils have been classified as *Homo* sp. [21,38].

Mosquera et al. [11] postulated a general continuity in the hominin occupation of Sierra de Atapuerca with the exception of a gap between 0.9 and 0.5 Ma at the Gran Dolina site, based on the archaeological evidence. These authors suggest that this depopulation was not a local phenomenon but a European event. During this period, evidence of human presence is scarce in Western Europe. Although no human remains have been recovered between OIS18 and OIS16, some isolated lithic assemblages have been dated to the beginning of this period, such as those found at the Middle Loire River Basin [41] and at Caune de l'Arago [42] in France. In contrast, the number of archaeological sites increases significantly in approximately 0.6–0.5 Ma, revealing new palaeoanthropological and cultural features that mark the European Middle Pleistocene [12,43,44]. New lithic assemblages with early Acheulean industries seem to appear in Western Europe at the end of the Early Pleistocene ([11] and reference therein) although the dates of some sites are debatable [12]. In any case, Acheulean technology arrived in Europe around or before 0.6–0.5. Ma. The new settlers, with full Acheulean Mode 2 technology, occupied the European landscapes intensely at this time, as shown by the increasing number of sites. The sparsely populated northern latitudes began to be systematically occupied. Examples of this phenomenon can be found at Boxgrove in England [45], and at Bilzingsleben [46] and Schöningen [47] in Germany. Interestingly, the oldest European hearths have been dated to approximately 400 ka (Terra Amata, Beeches Pit, Schöningen or Bilzingsleben) [11,48]. The hominin fossil evidence is currently the focus of an intense debate concerning the evolutionary relationships of the Early and Middle Pleistocene European hominins [1,15,49–53] and references therein.

Given the shortage of sites and the sparse anthropic evidence from the beginning of the European Middle Pleistocene, three possible scenarios may be considered. In the first scenario, a discontinuity occurred between the Early and Middle Pleistocene human populations, and thus, Europe was almost depopulated at this time. Alternatively, if continuity between the Early and Middle Pleistocene human populations occurred, the scarcity of evidence might be explained by a contraction of the human populations as a response to adverse environmental conditions. In this latter case, the Early Pleistocene hominins would have survived in some refuges where the environment remained more consistent and eventually evolved into the new Middle Pleistocene forms, both anatomical and culturally. A third possible scenario is that the Early Pleistocene human populations survived in some refuges from OIS18 to OIS14 but were eventually substituted by the Acheulean immigrants approximately 0.5 Ma. Alternatively, it could be argued that the scarcity of evidence of human presence is just a consequence of the low completeness of the fossil record. Although this possibility may not be definitively ruled out, the scarcity of lithic record in this period, in comparison to the previous one, is striking, since stone tools are abundantly produced by humans and they have a high probability of being preserved in the archaeological record.

Here, we focus on the critical period 0.7–0.5 Ma to test whether the lack of evidence of human presence is related to adverse ecological conditions during this period. Resource availability and competition with carnivores have been repeatedly proposed as key limiting factors for Early Pleistocene European hominin populations [4,13,54–59]. Thus, a key question is whether resource availability was lower in the period between OIS18 and OIS12 than at the end of the Early Pleistocene. Rodríguez-Gómez et al. [60] presented a model to study predator-prey relationships and estimate resource availability on a local scale. This model is used here to test the hypothesis that the absence of human settlement was coincident with a period of low resource availability.

The Gran Dolina site in the Sierra de Atapuerca (in northern Spain) provides a unique opportunity to test this hypothesis on a local scale. This site has a long stratigraphic sequence that dates from the Jaramillo Subchron to the end of the Middle Pleistocene. Evidence of human presence at Sierra de Atapuerca before and after the critical period 0.7–0.5 Ma has been registered at different sites and stratigraphic levels. Human settlement in the 1.2–0.7 Ma period is documented at the TE9 level at Sima del Elefante, and the TD3-TD4 and TD6 levels at Gran Dolina, while the GII, GIIIa, GIIIb units of Galería, the TD10-2 and TD10-1 levels of Gran Dolina and the Sima de los Huesos site document human settlement during the period 0.5–0.25 Ma [61–64]. The interval between OIS18 and OIS16 (roughly from 0.7 to 0.5 Ma) is represented at Atapuerca by the TD7, TD8 and TD9 levels of Gran Dolina, all of which lack evidence of human presence in the Atapuerca area [25]. This archaeological gap in Atapuerca has been discussed taking as a perspective the technological evidence [11,43]. The TD8 level provides the richer faunal assemblage of this period at Atapuerca [62,63]; thus, it has been selected for the study of this critical period.

The aim of this study is to compare competition intensity and resource availability at Atapuerca during the period for which evidence of human presence is lacking, represented by the TD8 assemblage, with the conditions at the end of the Early Pleistocene, represented by the TD6-2 assemblage, a period of intense human occupation at Atapuerca. We introduce in this analysis an index of intraguild carnivore competition to compare the changes in the local conditions between these two periods. These data will provide us which information about the main features of the palaeoecosystem and the survival opportunities for a hypothetical human population at the Sierra de Atapuerca during this period.

Materials and Methods

The Atapuerca Gran Dolina TD8 Level

The Sierra de Atapuerca is located 15 km east of Burgos, in the north of the Iberian Peninsula. This Cretaceous limestone massif has various cavities filled with well-stratified Pleistocene sediments, known from south to north as Sima del Elefante (TE), Galería (G) and Gran Dolina (TD). These sites have been excavated since 1981 by Atapuerca Team with permission of the Consejería de Cultura y Turismo de la Junta de Castilla y León. Gran Dolina (TD) (3°31′08 W, 42°21′09 N; UTM coordinates: X = 457279, Y = 4689172) is a cavity approximately 18 m in height that was filled with Lower and Middle Pleistocene sediments. Its stratigraphic sequence was initially divided into 11 stratigraphic levels (TD1-TD11 from bottom to top) and revised in subsequent studies; e.g., [25].

The TD8 level was formed by a succession of brecciated flows of red lutites with boulders and gravels [65]. Its sedimentation is composed of overlapping cones with main vertexes at the north of the site. The vertical positions of these vertexes and their proximity to the roof suggest a small entrance into the cave during the TD8 formation. The ESR and U-series dates taken from the middle part of the sedimentary deposit suggest an average age of 600 kyr (602±52 kyr) [63]. The result obtained by TL from one sample collected at the base of TD8 correlates with the Matuyama-Brunhes boundary when the range of error is taken into account (820±140 kyr) [62]. From an archaeological perspective, evidence of human presence was not documented at TD8, as noted above. It might be argued that the small entrance and the general conditions (humidity and darkness) of the cave prevented a continuous access by a hypothetical human population, although the evidence available is not conclusive on this respect.

Taking into account the species of carnivores recovered at the TD8 level (see below) and the taphonomic characteristics identified in the faunal assemblage (e.g., tooth-mark dimensions), hyena is proposed as the main agent responsible for the ungulate accumulations [66]. However, a certain degree of variability with respect to those features traditionally used to define carnivore dens can be observed at TD8 (e.g., an absence of immature carnivore remains, a low proportion of coprolites, few marks related to the end stages of carnivore consumption, the absence of an attritional age profile and large quantities of whole bones and epiphyses) (see [67]). According to Blasco et al. [66], this variability seems to be the result of a combination of several types of dwellings (dens and refuges) and the occasional access of other carnivores during the formation of the TD8 deposit.

The TD8 Faunal assemblage

The faunal list for TD8 was obtained from Rodríguez et al. [25], Blasco et al. [66], and van der Made [68]. We restricted our analysis to mammal species of weighing more than 10 kg because these include the main sources of meat and fat, as well as the main potencial competitors and predators of a hunter-gatherer population [69,70]. This size interval includes small to medium-sized predators such as the lynx that may prey on small ungulates that are potentially important in a human diet. Rodríguez [71] provides estimations for the body mass of the mammal species identified at Gran Dolina based on the few fossils available at that time and using allometric equations. However, excavation of Gran Dolina in subsequent years increased the fossil sample from TD8. Gran Dolina TD8 site contains 899 remains that belong to mammal species of more than 10 kg. No specific permits are required for this study, which complied with all relevant regulations. The current regulation is Decreto 37/2007, 25th of April 2007, Junta de Castilla y León Cultural Heritage (BOCyL 79, 25/05/2007). The material revised is temporary housed at Institut Català de Paleoecologia Humana i Evolució Social (IPHES) at Tarragona (Spain). This research is under the frame of the Research Project CGL2012-38434-C03-02 from Spanish MINECO. The specimen numbers are provided in (Table S1).

Thus, we analysed the entire TD8 fossil assemblage and reviewed the body size estimations provided by Rodriguez [71], recalculating the body masses with allometric equations [72] when new data were available. There are eleven primary consumer species in TD8 weighing more than 10 kg: *Bison voigtstedtensis, Cervus elaphus* (red deer), *Dama vallonetensis, Equus altidens, Eucladoceros giulii, Hippopotamus* sp., *Macaca* sp., *Megaloceros solilhacus, Stephanorhinus etruscus, Sus scrofa* (wild boar) and *Ursus* sp. The bear, *Ursus* sp., is considered to be an omnivore, and in this study, it was included as both a potential prey and a potential predator. Five large predators were identified in the TD8 assemblage: *Canis mosbachensis, Crocuta crocuta* (spotted hyaena), *Hyaena* sp. (considered analogous to striped hyaena), *Lynx* sp., *Panthera gombaszoegensis and Ursus* sp. The small canid *Vulpes* sp. was not included in the analyses because its diet was presumed to be composed of small mammals, as discussed by Rodríguez-Gómez et al. [60]. The families Viverridae and Mustelidae were also excluded because their diets are also based mainly on small mammals. The TD8 fossil assemblage lacks adequate elements to estimate the body masses of *Hippopotamus* sp., *Hyaena* sp., *Macaca* sp., *Megaloceros solilhacus*, *Panthera gombaszoegensis* and *Sus scrofa* using allometric equations. Thus, for these species, we used the body masses provided by Rodríguez [71] and Blasco et al [66], except for *Hippopotamus* sp., for which the body mass for *Hippopotamus* gr. *H. antiquus* provided by Mazza and Bertini [73] was used. The body masses used are shown in Table 1.

Although we lack evidence of human presence at TD8, *Homo* sp. has been included in the analyses as a hunter-gatherer to estimate competition and resource availability for a hypothetical human population living in Atapuerca at that time. We assume for *Homo* sp. the same trophic behaviour inferred for *Homo antecessor* in the TD6-2 assemblage. Hunting has been interpreted as the main food procurement strategy at TD6-2 [74,75], although other Early Pleistocene sites like Fuente Nueva-3 evidence a predominantly scavenging behaviour of early *Homo* [55].

Thus, we analysed the distribution of resources between secondary consumers for two different scenarios and examined the effects of these different configurations of the TD8 paleoecommunity: 1) a TD8 assemblage and 2) a TD8 assemblage + *Homo* sp.

Rodríguez Gómez et al. [60] used a mathematical model to quantify the resources available for a human population in the ecosystem represented at TD6-2. TD6-2 is another level at the Gran Dolina site, lately dating to approximately 0.9 Ma [61]. This level has yielded abundant faunal remains [25,76,77] and Mode 1 stone tools, together with a large assemblage of human fossils attributed to *Homo antecessor* [8]. The study by Rodríguez-Gómez et al. [60] on the TD6-2 assemblage, suggests the existence of a rich environment, abundant in trophic resources for a hominin population, at Atapuerca at the end of the Early Pleistocene.

To make the results for TD6-2 and TD8 directly comparable we also ran the model for TD6-2, including *Homo antecessor* as a secondary consumer, because it was not included in [60]. Two different levels of animal food in the diet of *Homo* were tested to represent either a diet with a low (30%, H_{min}) or high (60%, H_{max}) meat component. In addition, we included two scenarios for TD6-2, adding a large felid to its carnivore guild, although none was recorded in the fossil assemblage. Thus, we repeated our analyses,

Table 1. Estimated body masses of the species in the TD8 assemblage.

Species	Estimated Body Mass (kg)
Bison voigtstedtensis	397
Cervus elaphus	163
Dama vallonetensis	84
Equus altidens	324
Eucladoceros giulii	360
Hippopotamus sp.	2,225
Megaloceros solilhacus	383
Macaca sylvanus	18
Stephanorhinus struscus	1,400
Sus scrofa	85
Ursus sp.	282
Canis mosbachensis	12
Crocuta crocuta	75
Hyaena sp.	50
Lynx sp.	10
Panthera gombaszoegensis	90

Weights of *Hyaena* sp., *Macaca* sp., *Megaloceros solilhacus, Panthera gombaszoegensis* and *Sus scrofa* were taken from Rodríguez [71] and Blasco et al [66]. To *Hippopotamus* sp. weight was taken from [73].

including *Homotherium latidens* as a member of the TD6-2 predatory guild, to evaluate the effect of its possible presence on our results, as explained in Rodríguez-Gómez [60].

The model

We investigated the distribution of resources, primary consumer biomass, among secondary consumers in different scenarios. On the one hand, it is necessary to estimate resource availability, i.e., the biomass of primary consumers available to secondary consumers or total available biomass (TAB). On the other hand, the requirements of secondary consumers (TBD) should also be estimated (Figure 1) [78]. A summary description of the model components is provided below; for a detailed formal description of this model see Rodríguez-Gómez et al. [60]. The model was written and executed in Matlab R2009b.

Total Available Biomass

Our model was developed on the basis of the assumption that all of the variations in population size and composition may be taken as oscillations around a mean value that is constant through time-an assumption that is widely accepted in population dynamics studies [79]. We represented the average long-term condition of every population using a Leslie Matrix [80,81]. Leslie Matrices are used in population dynamics to represent a population structure at different times and to describe its oscillations (Figures 1 and 2A). We sought the Leslie Matrix that represented the average structure over time by introducing two additional conditions:

1. - The population should be stable (i.e., population size should be constant from year to year).
2. - The population should be stationary (i.e., the age structure should be constant from year to year).

Input data are physical and physiological variables (adult body mass, body mass at birth, litter size, breeding interval, age at reproductive maturity, growth rate and lifespan) that are species specific. For species with living representatives, such as *Sus scrofa* and *Cervus elaphus*, the values of these physiological variables were taken directly from the literature. For species without living representatives, the values reported in the literature for closely related living species of similar body mass were used (e.g., *Equus zebra* was used as an analogue for *Equus altidens*). For species defined to genus level such as *Macaca* sp., we used values for species of similar size, as *Macaca sylvanus*. In the cases of *Bison voigtstedtensis*, *Dama vallonetensis*, *Eucladoceros giulii*, *Hippopotamus* sp., *Stephanorhinus etruscus* and *Ursus* sp., which lack closely related living species of similar size, we computed a least square regression equation for each physiological variable with respect to mean body weight using data for species in the same family; see further details in Supplementary Material, Table S3 in [60].

The population profiles obtained from this model for every primary consumer population provide estimates of the average sustainable biomass output by age classes, which were eventually translated into body size intervals. Biomass output by age interval was obtained from the annual mortality rates obtained from the Leslie Matrix (Figure 2B). Each dead individual of a primary consumer species was assigned to one of six size categories according to its average body mass at the age of death: 10–45 kg, 45–90 kg, 90–180 kg, 180–360 kg, 360–1,000 kg or >1,000 kg (see [57]). The biomass made available for secondary consumers by each single primary consumer population was obtained as the sum of the biomass of all dead individuals (Figure 2C).Total biomass output (TBO) was obtained as the sum of the biomass outputs in each size category from each primary consumer population (Figure 1). The distribution of sustainable TBO by size category is an important feature of the model, because prey body size is a main selection factor for predators [82–84]. With this treatment of the data it is then possible to represent features such as the hunting of sub-adults in species with very low adult mortality rates and very low predation at the adult stage, such as rhinos and hippos. This model may overestimate TBO because it

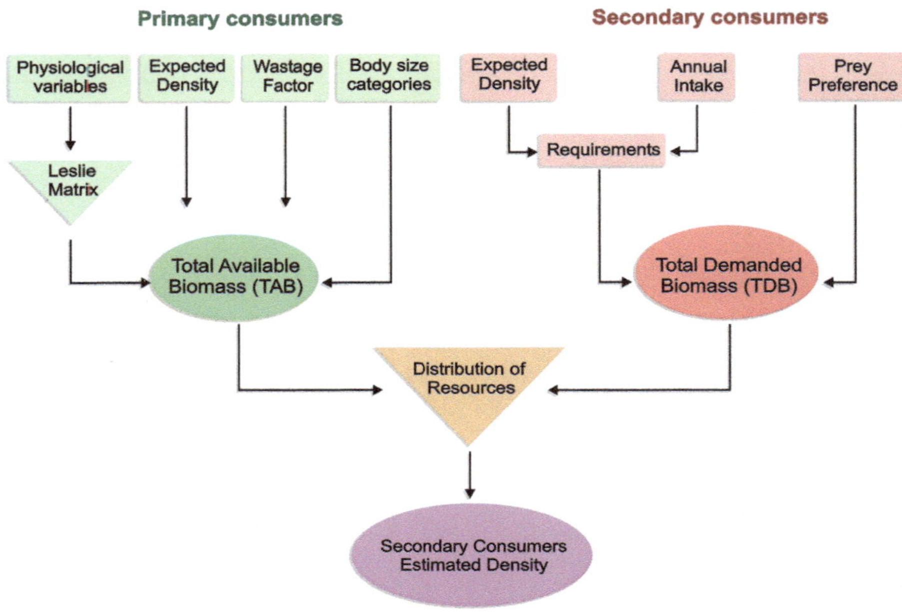

Figure 1. Flow diagram showing the components of the model used to evaluate trophic resource availability and intraguild competition (modified from [78]).

considers that all the available biomass was consumed exclusively by mammals. The role of other secondary consumers, like vultures is not been considered in the model, although we acknowledge its relevance in actual ecosystems. There is not way to estimating the amount of TBO consumed by non-mammalian secondary consumers in the past, but it is reasonable to assume that it was similar in both levels (TD6-2 and TD8), an assumption that strengthens the null hypothesis of the absence of ecological differences between both assemblages.

Only female individuals are represented in a Leslie Matrix. Thus, we assumed the sex ratio was equal to 1:1, that the population profile was the same for males and females and that the survival rate was equal for both sexes. A further assumption is that the sub-adult survival rate should be lower than the adult survival rate [60].

The model solutions are not dependent on population size: thus, an estimate of population density is needed to estimate the sustainable biomass output. Mediterranean taxa dominate the TD8 pollen spectrum [25]; thus, we used the equation provided by Damuth [85] to estimate the density of primary consumers in a European mixed temperate forest:

$$\log(D) = -0.79 * \log(m) + 4.33$$

where D is the population density in number of individuals per square kilometre and *m* is the body mass in grams.

Combining the mortality profiles obtained from the Leslie Matrix with the mean body size per age class and the estimated population density of the species, the sustainable biomass output can be computed. Because a carcass includes a variable amount of non-edible tissues (horns, bones, hide, etc.), this sustainable biomass output cannot be fully used by secondary consumers. The percentage of non-edible TBO is represented in the model by a size-specific "wastage factor" [86]. Once this percentage has been subtracted, the final amount of biomass available to secondary consumers or total available biomass (TAB) is obtained. TAB is also distributed by body mass classes (Figure 1).

Our model yields several population profiles for each species, corresponding to different mortality rates. We selected extreme values with maximum and minimum pressure on sub-adults (or maximum and minimum mortality rates) that produce minimum and maximum TAB levels, respectively (TAB-m and TAB-M, respectively). We limited the results to those solutions for which sub-adult mortality rates were higher than adult mortality rates because this is the pattern usually observed in natural populations [87].

Total Demanded Biomass (TDB)

Carnivore-demanded resources should be estimated as a first step in evaluating resource distribution among secondary consumers. The carnivore intake rate was estimated using the equation reported by Farlow [88]:

$$\log I = 0.69686 \log(m) + 0.27747;$$

$$r^2 = 0.96758;\ F_{1;100} = 2{,}984.773;\ p < .01$$

where *I* is the intake rate in kcal per day and *m* is the body mass in grams. Some adjustments were made for each secondary consumer according to its inferred dietary preferences. Taking the coyote as an analogue, we estimated that large mammal flesh represented only 20% of the energetic requirements of *Canis mosbachensis* and that it was primarily consumed as carrion [57]. The spotted hyena, *Crocuta crocuta*, is able to exploit bone marrow thanks to its bone-crashing abilities. We assumed that approximately 2% of the total energetic requirements of the spotted hyaena were satisfied by bone marrow, and consequently, its energetic requirements were reduced by a factor of 0.02 [89,90]. In the case of *Hyena* sp., by analogy with the striped

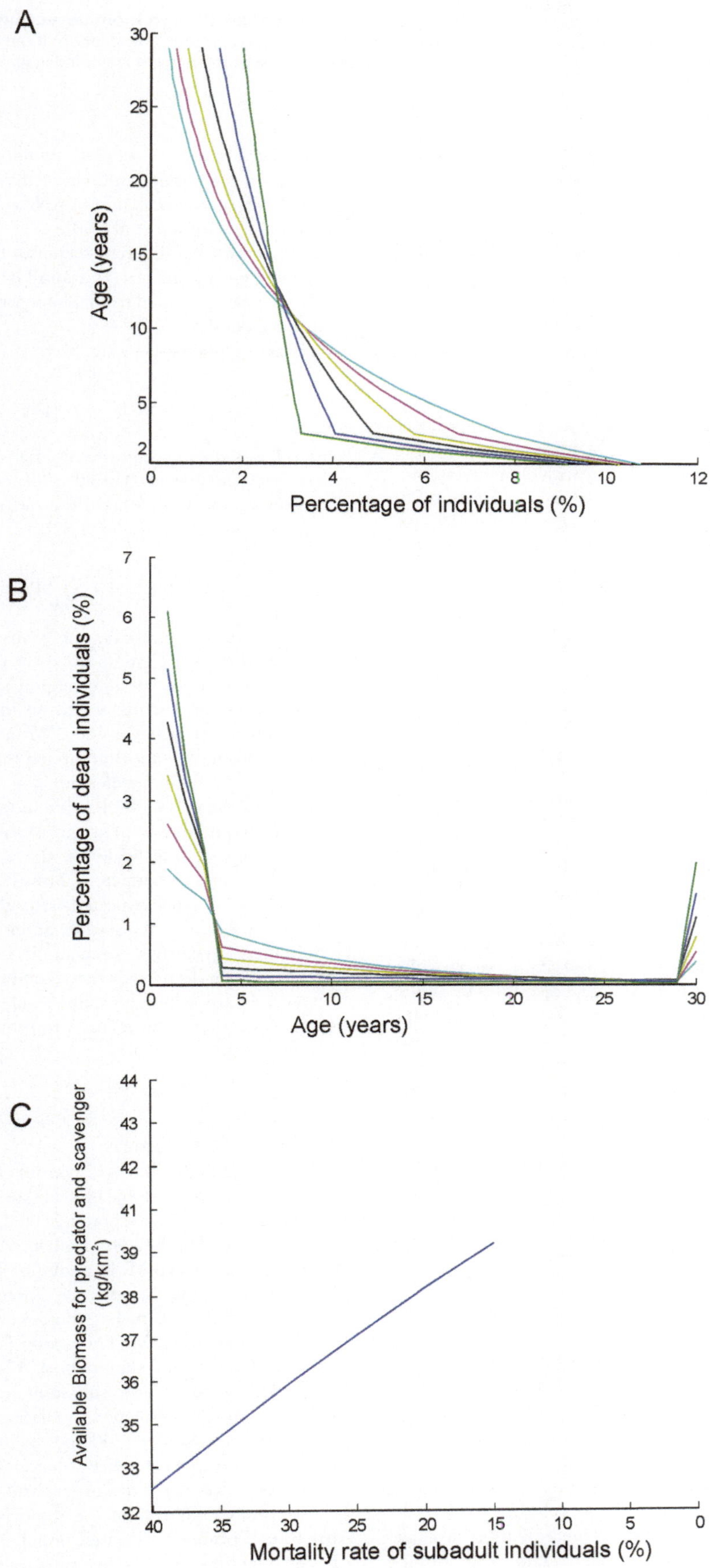

A
Age (years)
30
25
20
15
10
5
2
0
2
4
6
8
10
12
Percentage of individuals (%)
B
Percentage of dead individuals (%)
7
6
5
4
3
2
1
0
0
5
10
15
20
25
30
Age (years)
C
Available Biomass for predator and scavenger (kg/km²)
44
43
42
41
39
38
37
36
35
33
32
40
35
30
25
20
15
10
5
0
Mortality rate of subadult individuals (%)

Figure 2. Graphical representation of population profiles (A), mortality profiles (B) and biomass output available for secondary consumers (C) at different sub-adult mortality rates for *Equus altidens*. Each line represents the solution of the model for a different level of sub-adult mortality. The percentage of dead individuals in the mortality profiles represents the percentage of individuals in the population that died at age *i*.

hyaena, carrion of large mammals would represent approximately 75% of its diet; the remainder could be invertebrates, vegetable food and small vertebrates [91]. The diet of the TD8 lynx (*Lynx* sp.), was presumed to be similar to that of the recent Iberian Lynx (*Lynx pardina*) [57]. Thus, it was assumed that species between 10 and 90 kg represented only 5% of the lynx diet [92–94], lagomomorphs and other small mammals making up the bulk of its diet. Because *Ursus* sp. was likely to have been highly omnivorous, it was assumed that meat represented only 10% of its energetic requirements as in recent European brown bears (*Ursus arctos*) [95,96]. Likely, fish was also an important component of its diet as suggested by the nitrogen-isotope values obtained for the Venta Micena bears [97].

The annual energetic requirements of a carnivore population by km^2 are obtained multiplying the individual annual intake by the population density (Figure 1). The equation provided by Damuth [98] for African flesh-eaters was used to estimate the typical carnivore density:

$$\log(D) = -0.64 * \log(m) + 2.33$$

where *D* is the population density in number of individuals per square kilometre and *m* is the body mass in grams. In the case of *Ursus* sp., the equation for carnivores was used instead of the equation for primary consumers because it predicts the population densities of recent bear species more accurately [99–101].

The requirements of *Homo* sp. were estimated to be similar to those of recent hunter-gatherer populations, with a mean daily requirement of 3,000 kcal per individual [102]. The average body mass was considered to be 76 kg, based on pelvis and femur estimates for *Homo heidelbergensis* from the Sima de los Huesos site [103,104]. Studies of recent hunter-gatherer populations have shown that animal resource consumption represents between 30% and 60% of their nutritional intake [105,106]. Thus, we modelled *Homo* sp. as a species that meets 30% (H_{min}) or 60% (H_{max}) of its energetic requirements (3,000 kcal/day) by consuming the meat of large mammals. Population densities and diet compositions observed for recent hunter-gatherers populations are shown for comparison in Table 2 (extracted from [107]).

As in the case of TAB, TDB was distributed over the same six body size categories based on the inferred prey size preferences of each predator, on the basis of the behaviour of their living relatives (Table 3 and Figure 1) [57]. The preference of a predator for a body size category is represented by the percentage of predation (PD) that this size category was presumed to represent in its diet. If a predator was presumed to be unable to kill prey in a given size category and to not consume carrion, a PD of 0 was assigned to the predator in that size category.

Distribution of TAB between secondary consumers

The distribution of TAB between secondary consumers is based on the proportional predation pressure (PPP_{ij}) of each species in each body size category. PPP_{ij} represents the relative amount of biomass demanded by the *jth* carnivore species from the *ith* prey body size category and is calculated as the proportion of the total amount of biomass demanded from a prey body size category by all carnivores that corresponds to the requirements of a single carnivore species. PPP_{ij} incorporates intraguild competition in the model because the resources obtained by a carnivore species depends on the number and characteristics of its competitors. See a detailed formal description of resource distribution computation in Rodríguez-Gómez et al. [60].

To compare the different scenarios considered in our analysis, we generated two indices (SCI and GCI) that relate the estimated and expected (estimated from allometric equations [98]) secondary consumer densities.

Species competition index (SCI):

$$SCI_i = 1 - (Ds_i / Dx_i)$$

where Dx_i is the expected density for species *i* obtained from the allometric equation in Damuth [98]. Ds_i is the estimated density for species *i* and is obtained from our model.

Global competition index (GCI):

$$GCI = 1 - (\sum Ds / \sum Dx)$$

where $\sum Ds$ is the summation of estimated densities for all species and $\sum Dx$ is the summation of expected densities for all species.

These indices provide information about competition intensity in the ecosystem with regard to an ideal condition in which all species reach optimal densities. We assume that if the densities estimated from our model approach these thresholds densities, all species would fulfil needs with the have plenty of resources available to them. The SCI index shows to what degree a species fulfils its requirements in a given environment. GCI performs similarly but at the scale of the whole guild of secondary consumers guild. In both cases, however, if the estimated densities were closer to the expected densities or optimal ones, we considered that resources were abundant when compared with requirements (i.e. that competition is low). Conversely, if our model results indicate that the secondary consumers were able to coexist only at low densities, this would be so because there was a scarcity of resources in relation to requirements, which implies a high competition.

Results

Total Available Biomass

The minimum TAB, corresponding to the maximum sub-adult mortality rate, was 496,814 kcal/km^2*year (TAB-m), and the maximum TAB, corresponding to the minimum sub-adult mortality rate, was 643,968 kcal/km^2*year (TAB-M). TAB-m is 23% lower than TAB-M. In addition, the distributions of TAB-M and TAB-m by size category are different (Table 4 and Figure 3), mainly because TAB-m has more biomass in the first category (10–45 kg) than TAB-M. The reason for the different distribution is that both adults and sub-adults of *Macaca* sp. are present in this category and with a low sub-adult mortality rate, the biomass output of macaques is higher, increasing TAB in this size category. For the rest of species considered, adult and sub-adult individuals belong to different body mass categories, and biomass increases in larger body size categories as sub-adult mortality rate decreases. These results demonstrate the importance of including the age structure of primary consumer populations in the model, because the distribution of TAB in size categories is not homogeneous, and

Table 2. Population densities and food resource use observed in recent hunter-gatherer populations [107].

Group	Area	Density ind./km^2	Gathering%	Hunting%	Fishing%
Punan	29.6	0.118	65.00	30	5
Siberian Eskimo	274.9	0.047	1.00	30	60
Guayaki-Ache	28.7	0.0348	30.00	62	10
Efe	47.0	0.1596	88.20	11	0,8
Hadza	25.0	0.240	60.00	40	0
!Kung	110.0	0.066	67.00	33	0
G/Wi	180.0	0.0293	55.00	45	0
Mardudjara	226.0	0.0075	70.00	30	0
Kiowa	280.0	0.014	20.00	80	0
Caribou Inuit	2365.0	0.003	0.10	55	44.9
Nunamiut Inuit	249.0	0.0096	0.10	89	10.9
Polar Inuit	731.0	0.0041	0.01	30	69.99

prey body size is a key factor in prey selection by most predators. Thus, the TAB of a prey size category is not equally available for all secondary consumers.

Requirements of the secondary consumers

The energy necessary to maintain the species of the TD8 carnivore guild (first scenario) at their ecological densities is 693,725 kcal/km^2*year (Table 5). This energy requirement exists if all species fulfil all of their expected requirements. The species with higher energetic requirements are *Crocuta crocuta* and *Panthera gombaszoegensis*, approximately 222,000 kcal/km^2*year each, or 32% of total requirements. Next is *Hyaena* sp., which accounts for approximately 160,000 kcal/km^2*year or 23% of the total. *Canis mosbachensis* accounts for approximately 40,000 kcal/km^2*year or 6% of the total. *Lynx* sp. and *Ursus* sp. account for approximately 20,000 kcal/km^2*year. However, these are estimates, and to establish whether all of the requirements of the secondary consumers are fulfilled, the distribution of TAB by size category and the prey preferences of the carnivores should be taken into consideration.

Comparing different scenarios and conditions

Two scenarios were considered for TD8: only the species in the TD8 assemblage and the TD8 assemblage plus *Homo* sp. In addition, we considered two other factors: TAB (TAB-m or TAB-M) and *Homo* sp. requirements (H_{min} or H_{max}). Thus, we had six different scenarios for TD8 (Table S2 and Figure 4). Comparing the scenarios, we found the worst case to be the hypothetical assemblage of TD8 with *Homo* sp. meeting 60% of its energetic requirements from meat (H_{max}) and TAB at a minimum (TAB-m). The scenario with less competition between secondary consumers occurs when TAB is at a maximum (TAB-M). As might be expected, the parameter with the greatest effect is TAB (Table 6 and Figure 4).

Distribution of resources

The distribution of resources in all scenarios yield viable ecosystems with regard to the minimun viable population density (MVPD) of the species involved, estimated using equations provided by Silva and Downing [108] (Table 6 and Figure 4). Nevertheless, it should be noted that the MVPD corresponds to

Table 3. Percentage of predation (PD) of the TD8 carnivores plus *Homotherium latidens* and *Homo* sp. by body mass category.

Species	Body size range (kg)					
	10–45	45–90	90–180	180–360	360–1,000	>1,000
Canis mosbachensis	17	17	17	17	17	17
Crocuta crocuta	21	32	26	11	5	5
Homo sp.	24	29	19	14	10	5
Homotherium latidens	6	6	28	33	22	6
Hyaena sp.	17	17	17	17	17	17
Lynx sp.	75	25	0	0	0	0
Panthera gombaszoegensis	6	6	31	38	19	0
Ursus sp.	17	17	17	17	17	17

The scores represent the relative importance that animals in each body size category had in the carnivore's diet. The sum of the scores in a row is 1. A score of 0 indicates no consumption of mammals in that body size category.

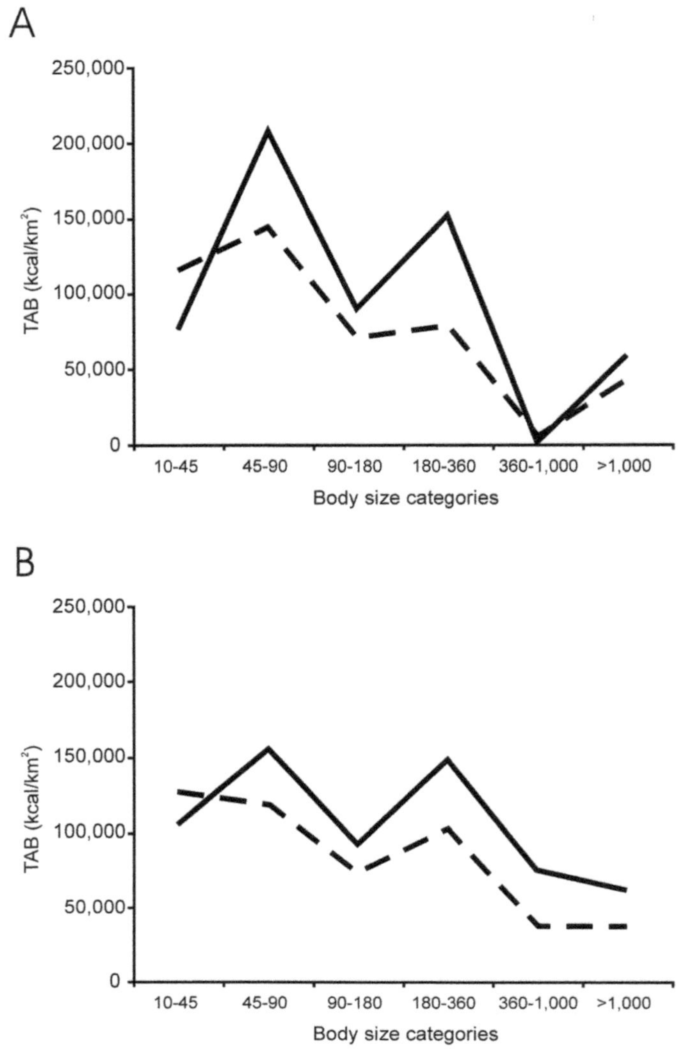

Figure 3. Biomass output distributed among six body size categories (see text). Dashed line: maximum sub-adult mortality rate for all primary consumer species or TAB-m; solid line: minimum sub-adult mortality rate (greater than or equal to the adult mortality rate) or TAB-M. A: TD6-2 available biomass; B: TD8 available biomass.

populations living in extreme conditions and prone to extinction because MVPD is estimated on the basis of populations classified as "endangered", "vulnerable", or "close to extinction" by the IUCN [109].

With respect to the energy requirements met, mainly the species that satisfies a smaller percentage of its energy requirement in all cases is *Panthera gombaszoegensis* while *Lynx* sp. is the least affected by the competition for resources (Table S2). Even with the inclusion of *Homo* sp. all species reach viable densities, slightly higher when *Homo* sp. has minor requirements. We used as reference density for *Homo* sp. 0.24 individuals per square kilometre, the highest density observed in recent hunter-gatherers (Table 2). In the worst case, scenario with *Homo* sp. and TAB-m condition, *Panthera gombaszoegensis* met 49% of their requirements with 0.06 individuals per square kilometre; *Canis mosbachensis*, *Ursus* sp. and *Hyaena* sp. met 71% of their requirements with 0.24, 0.03 and 0.09 individuals per square kilometre, respectively; *Crocuta crocuta* met 61% of its requirements with a density of 0.08 individuals per square kilometre; and *Lynx* sp. met 81% of its requirements with a density of 0.38 individuals per square kilometre. *Homo* sp. met 60% of its requirements with a density of 0.15 individuals per square kilometre for TAB-m (see SCI in Table S2).

Comparison between TD8 and TD6-2

We take the conditions for the human groups inhabiting Atapuerca 900,000 years ago, represented by the TD6-2 assemblage, as a reference against which resource availability and competition between carnivores in TD8 may be compared (Figure 4). TAB varies in TD6-2 from a minimum of 457,693 kcal/km^2*year to a maximum of 583,638 kcal/km^2*year (see Table 3 in [57]), in both of which are below the respective values observed for TD8 (496,659 and 643,201 kcal/km^2*year, respectively). Moreover, in the TD6-2 assemblage, the maximum available resources (TAB-M) are higher than the maximum consumer requirements (TDB-M = 461,028 kcal/km2*year when

Table 4. Maximum and minimum total available biomass (TAB) in kcal/km^2*yr, distributed over the six body size categories for the TD8 assemblage.

Body size range (kg)	10–45	45–90	90–180	180–360	360–1,000	>1,000	Total
TAB-M	106,512	155,722	92,136	149,351	76,849	62,630	643,201
TAB-m	126,928	118,768	72,589	102,942	38,128	37,304	496,659

The maximum TAB (TAB-M) is obtained when the sub-adult mortality rate is 0, while the minimum TAB (TAB-m) is obtained when all populations sustain the maximum possible sub-adult mortality rate while simultaneously satisfying the premises of stability and stationarity.

Homo antecessor consumes more meat) and thus, all species are able to fulfil their requirements. Meat resources were high enough at TD6-2 to sustain the expected densities, even in excess (Table S3), except in the case of the most unfavourable scenario with TAB-m and the diet of *Homo antecessor* including a high amount of meat. Conversely, in the case of the TD8 assemblage, this does not occur, and TAB-M (643,201 kcal/km^2*year) is insufficient to satisfy the secondary consumers' requirements (TBD is equal to 689,279 kcal/km^2*year). Despite that TAB being lower in TD6-2 than in TD8, TD6-2-TAB meets the carnivores' requirements and TD8-TAB does not. This implies a higher degree of competition between secondary consumers in TD8 than in TD6-2. When the global competition indices are compared (Figure 4), we found that TD8 had a higher GCI than TD6-2, whether *Homo antecessor* is assumed to be highly dependent on animal resources (H_{max}) or not (H_{min}) for TAB-M condition but not for H_{max} with TAB-m. In addition, we evaluated two hypothetical scenarios: the TD6-2 assemblage with a large felid such as *Homotherium latidens* [60] and TD8 with *Homo* sp. In the hypothetical scenario of the TD6-2 assemblage with *Homotherium latidens* and TAB-m, TD8-GCI is similar to TD6-2-GCI with *Homo antecessor* consuming H_{min}. When *Homo antecessor* is considered to be more dependent on meat resources (H_{max}), TD6-2-GCI is slightly higher than TD8-GCI. However, if *Homo* sp. is included in the TD8 assemblage, both for H_{min} and H_{max} scenarios, competition increases to a level higher than observed in TD6-2 with *Homotherium latidens* (Figure 4 and Table 6). As it might be expected, the highest competition is observed when *Homo* is included in the TD8 assemblage with high meat consumption requirements (H_{max}). Under these conditions, GCI is 0.35 for TAB-m and greater than 0.2 for TAB-M (Figure 4 and Table 6). It is worth noting that the inclusion of *Homo* sp. and *Homotherium latidens* in TD8 and TD6-2 levels softens the differences between both macromammal guilds.

Discussion

Evidence of human presence in Europe during the period 0.5–0.7 Ma is very scarce. Although several European sites provide abundant evidence of human presence before and after this period, the European continent was apparently depopulated during the 0.5–0.7 Ma interval. The results presented here suggest that during this period, the environment was more hostile to a hominin population than it was previously. The Atapuerca environment was able to sustain the expected population densities of a diverse carnivore guild, including *Homo antecessor*, 0.9 Ma, as shown by the application of the model to the TD6-2 assemblage, even with the inclusion of a large felid not recorded in the fossil assemblage. In contrast, the higher values of the global competition index (GCI) obtained for TD8 in comparison to TD6-2 suggest an environment with a higher intraguild competition for resources at Atapuerca 0.6 Ma. Consequently, survival opportunities for *Homo* at Atapuerca would have been higher in the late Early Pleistocene than in the early Middle Pleistocene. Certainly the value of the population density obtained for *Homo* at TD8 is higher than the minimum viable population size (MVPS) for these species, according to the equation provided by Silva and Downing [108]. Nevertheless, the value of MVPD should be considered an absolute minimum and not an average for a sustainable population. For this reason, we focus our interpretation on the relative values of GCI in concluding that the conditions for a human population were worse at TD8 than at TD6-2 and that the Atapuerca environment was less suitable for a permanent human settlement at 0.6 Ma than at 0.9 Ma. These results support the

Table 5. Requirements of the secondary consumers in the TD8 assemblage plus *Homo* sp.

Species	W (kg)	D (ind/km²)	Requirements (kcal/km²/year)	Percentage requirement (%)	Percentage requirement with a less *Homo* sp. hunter (%)	Percentage requirement with a more *Homo* sp. hunter (%)
Canis mosbachensis	12	0.42	40,062	0.06	0.05	0.05
Crocuta crocuta	75	0.13	217,864	0.32	0.28	0.26
Lynx sp,	10	0.47	19,825	0.03	0.03	0.02
Hyaena sp,	50	0.17	162,932	0.24	0.21	0.19
Panthera gombaszoegensis	90	0.11	224,627	0.33	0.29	0.27
Ursus dolinensis	282	0.06	23,970	0.03	0.03	0.03
Homo sp. (30%)	76	0.24	78,840	-	0.10	-
Homo sp. (60%)	76	0.24	157,680	-	-	0.19

Two different levels of meat consumption were tested for *Homo* sp. In the first case, meat represents 30% of the energy intake, while in the second case, meat represents up to 60% of energy intake.

hypothesis that the human absence from TD8 was related to a more hostile environment during this period at Atapuerca, characterised by a higher competition and less access to resources than in the previous period. These results support the interpretation of Blain et al. [110] that the Atapuerca area was not necessarily always a suitable place for human settlement.

The differences between TD6-2 and TD8 are due to different community structures. Cuenca-Bescós and García [111] and Cuenca-Bescós et al. [112] differentiate several faunal units (FU) in Gran Dolina and separate TD6-2 and TD8 assemblages into two different faunal units FU4 and FU5, respectively. FU4 is characterised by the presence of *Homo antecessor* and the large red-toothed shrew *Dolinasorex glyphodon*, and FU5 is considered the local range zone of *Microtus ratticepoides* and *Blanus cinereus*

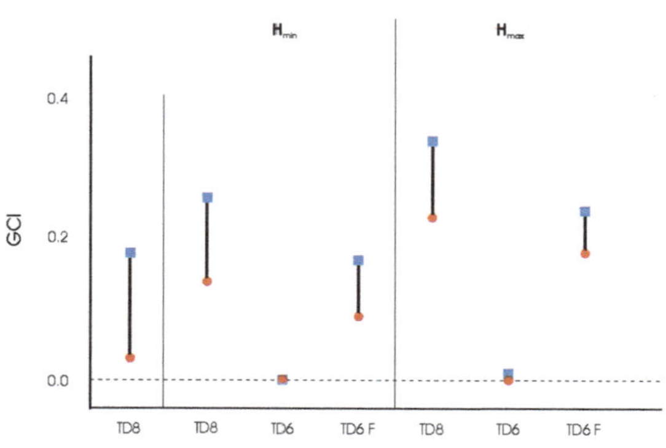

Figure 4. Graphical representation of the global competition index (GCI) for different scenarios. H_{min} denotes the scenarios that include human presence and assume low animal resource requirements for the human population, while H_{max} denotes the scenarios that include human presence and assume high animal resource requirements. TD8: TD8 assemblage; TD6: TD6-2 assemblage. TD6 F: TD6-2 assemblage plus *Homotherium latidens*. GCI takes values from 0 to 1, 0 being minimum competition and 1 being maximum competition. The solid circles represent the condition of maximum total available biomass (TAB-M). The solid squares represent the condition of minimum total available biomass (TAB-m). The black bars represent the range of values between TAB-m and TAB-M.

[25,111,112]. With respect to large primary consumer mammals, it can be observed that the differences between TD6-2 and TD8 are reflected in *Castor fiber* and *Mammuthus* sp. which do not appear in the TD8 assemblage, and *Macaca* sp., *Megaloceros solilhacus* and *Hippopotamus* sp., which do not appear in TD6-2 assemblage. The rest of the species are equal in both assemblages. As *Castor fiber* and *Mammuthus* sp. are approximately equivalent in terms of biomass to *Macaca* sp. and *Hippopotamus* sp., respectively (because these species belong to the same body mass categories) the main change between both assemblages is the presence of *Megaloceros solilhacus*. This species provides biomass to the categories of 45 to 90 kg, 180 to 360 kg and 360 to 1,000 kg. As shown in Figures 3A and 3B, the patterns of biomass output distribution are different in both assemblages. In the TD8 assemblage, the fourth (180–360 kg) and fifth (360–1,000 kg) categories contain higher proportion of biomass than in TD6-2. TD8 presents a more balanced biomass distribution than TD6-2, with a trapezoidal form rather than a triangular form.

The differences between TD6-2 and TD8 are larger for the secondary consumer group. *Canis mosbachensis*, *Crocuta crocuta*, *Lynx* sp. and *Ursus* sp. (*Ursus dolinensis* to TD6-2 level) are present in both assemblages. The TD8 level marks the last occurrence of *Canis mosbachensis* and *Crocuta crocuta* in the Gran Dolina sequence [112]. The main difference between TD8 and TD6-2 is the absence of *Homo antecessor* and the presence of *Panthera gombaszoegensis* and *Hyaena* sp. in the younger assemblage. *Panthera gombaszoegensis* is recorded at Atapuerca in the lower levels of Gran Dolina in TD3-TD4 and TD5 and also in Sima del Elefante in TE9 and TE12, all of which are older than 0.7 Ma [25]. If *Homo antecessor* were considered an effective hunter, the main difference between the TD6-2 and TD8 palaeoecosystems would be the presence of the scavenger *Hyaena* sp. In addition, it may be assumed that Middle Pleistocene human groups also used scavenging as a feeding strategy and were competitors of *Hyaena* sp., which might also be considered a partial ecological equivalent of *Homo*. In this interpretation, *Homo* would be replaced in the TD8 assemblage by two competitors: *Hyaena* sp. and *Panthera gombaszoegensis*. Alternatively, the absence of *Homo* may be interpreted as a key factor in determining the structure of the TD8 carnivore guild, allowing the presence of certain species that would be competitively displaced if a human population, absent for reasons other than competition, were

Table 6. Global competition index (GCI) for TD8 and TD6-2 assemblages and several hypothetical scenarios.

	TAB-m	TAB-M
TD8	0.19	0.04
TD8 H_{min}	0.27	0.14
TD6 H_{min}	0.00	0.00
TD6 F H_{min}	0.17	0.09
TD8 H_{max}	0.35	0.23
TD6 H_{max}	0.01	0.00
TD6 F H_{max}	0.24	0.18

TAB-m: minimum total available biomass; TAB-M: maximum total available biomass; H_{min}: meat represents 30% of the energy intake; H_{max}: meat represents 60% of the energy intake; F: scenario with a large felid such as *Homotherium latidens*.

present in the area. In this alternative interpretation, the absence of human settlement at Atapuerca 0.6 Ma would not be the consequence but the cause of the community structure observed in the TD6-2 assemblage.

Although the results presented here suggest more adverse conditions in TD8 than in TD6-2 other possible explanations for the absence of hominins at TD8 should be considered. The Gran Dolina cave and its sedimentation dynamics constituted a favourable environment for the establishment of carnivore dens and shelters 0.6 Ma [66], but may not have been favourable for human access, unlike TD6-2, because the entrance into the cave was smaller during the deposition of TD8 [66]. The possible effect of an accumulation bias in the TD8 fossil assemblage against certain species should also be considered because the main accumulation agents were hyaenas [66]. Proboscideans were a common faunal element in the Iberian Peninsula during the late Early, Middle and Late Pleistocene [113], but their remains are rarely transported to dens and carnivore shelters, except maybe in the case of *Homotherium* [114,115]. However, because the secondary consumers present at TD8 were not able to prey on proboscideans, their presence at Atapuerca 0.6 Ma would have had little effect on the intensity of competition and thus would not affect our results. The hypothetical presence of the sabertooth *Homotherium latidens*, a large predator that has been recorded at Gran Dolina in level TD5 (Early Pleistocene) and in level TD10-3 (Middle Pleistocene) [25] would have significantly increased intraguild competition. Given that saberthooths were likely able to kill juvenile, and very old proboscideans [55,57], if both *Homotherium latidens* and a proboscidean species were present at Atapuerca 0.9 Ma, biomass output would have been increased in the heavier body mass categories, but little of this additional biomass could have been consumed by predators. The presence of a proboscidean would increase resource availability carrion, which would have reduced competition among scavengers. Conversely, competition between predators would be increased by the presence of a top predator like *Homotherium*. Thus, the presence of these species at Atapuerca in the early Middle Pleistocene would change the values of the results presented here, but not their meaning nor our interpretation.

With respect to the debate about the continuity or discontinuity of the peopling of Europe in the early Middle Pleistocene, the results presented here show that a discontinuity in hominin occupation existed at Gran Dolina that coincided with an increase in carnivore competition. According to this interpretation, at approximately 0.6 Ma the TD8 palaeoecosystem was not as favourable to maintaining a hominin settlement as it was at 0.9 Ma, and Atapuerca had no conditions that made it favourable as refuge for human populations, thus representing a "bottleneck" [49] to the human population at the Sierra de Atapuerca. Finlayson et al. [116] propose that *Homo* preferred mosaic landscapes and that homogeneous habitats were ignored by humans throughout the Palaeolithic. Although the Palaeolithic human groups were able to adapt to a wide range of environments [117], they required heterogeneous habitats [116]. If the Atapuerca palaeoecosystem were more homogenous 0.6 than 0.9 Ma, the absence of hominins at TD8 could be explained by their inability to settle homogeneous environments. With respect to vegetation, and according to Rodríguez et al. [25], TD8 presents a high dominance of Mediterranean taxa, while in TD6-2, Mediterranean taxa occur together with cold and dry adapted species, suggesting the existence of a mosaic habitat with areas of steppe vegetation. The preference of *Homo* for heterogeneous environments could indicate its inability to directly compete against specialist species, like open habitat cursorial predators [118], and its need for high environmental diversity to obtain resources using a generalist strategy.

It is likely, environmental conditions for *Homo* were better 0.9 Ma than in later periods, due to higher resource availability and less competition with other carnivores. A faunal turnover occurred in Europe at the beginning of the Middle Pleistocene [4,54,58], marked by the appearance of new carnivores and increased herbivore richness [4,57], that changed the structure of mammalian communities throughout Europe.

This dramatic change in the ecological scenario at the beginning of the Middle Pleistocene might be linked to the appearance in Europe of behavioral and technological improvements and innovations that increased the hunting abilities and survival opportunities of hominins. The use of fire for food processing improved the palatability and edibility of foods and increased energy gain [119]. Interestingly, both technology and hominin populations were completely different before and after the critical interval of the alleged European depopulation. Nevertheless, the subsistence strategies of human groups were successful in both the Early and Middle Pleistocene [120,121]. Roebroeks [67] suggests a demographic population increase and a human expansion in the Middle Pleistocene on the basis of the technological improvements that occurred during this time.

It is difficult to point towards a unique explanation for the absence of humans from TD8, but what can be said is that survival opportunities for a human population were worse at TD8 than at

TD6-2 because intraguild competition was higher. Nevertheless, it is necessary to take into account that the excavation of TD8 affected an area of only 24 m^2 [122]. It is expected that future excavation of a larger area of this level will provide more faunal remains and other evidence to shed light on the hominin population continuity or discontinuity debate.

The structure of the mammalian palaeocommunity and the intensity of competition in the predatory guild likely constrained human ecodynamics in the Pleistocene. This study provides a new avenue for evaluating the relative suitability of a palaeoenvironment for a human hunter-gatherer population, taking into consideration resource availability and competition intensity. Fossil assemblages with and without evidence of human presence may be compared providing a different way to approach the study of variations in human presence in the Palaeolithic. Although this approach does not provide information about the mechanisms that may have produced changes from one community structure to another, it quantifies changes in trophic relationships using the global competition index (GCI). Investigation of more European sites using a similar approach will help to test whether the apparent discontinuity in the peopling of Europe is related to more adverse environmental conditions or decreased survival opportunities at the beginning of the Middle Pleistocene (0.7−0.5 Ma), as suggested by the Atapuerca record, or whether other mechanisms are implicated.

Conclusions

The reconstruction of trophic relationships in palaeocommunities and the comparison of the intensities of intraguild competition, using the global competition index (GCI) presented here make it possible to evaluate the relative suitability of past ecosystems for hominins. Increased intraguild competition made conditions at Atapuerca more adverse for secondary consumers at 0.6 than 0.9 Ma. This increased competition is a possible cause of the apparent depopulation of the Atapuerca area in the early Middle Pleistocene. Nevertheless, more sites of this period should be studied with a similar approach to determine whether increased intraguild competition for resources played a role in changes in the distribution of *Homo* in Europe in the 0.5–0.7 Ma interval. Both sites with and without evidence of human presence should be compared to shed light on the fiercely debated question of the continuity *vs.* discontinuity of human occupation in Europe at the beginning of the Middle Pleistocene. This study demonstrates that mathematical modeling is a helpful tool in addressing this topic.

Supporting Information

Table S1 Specimen Number.
(XLSX)

Table S2 Sustainable densities of the TD8 secondary consumers for six different scenarios (see text) for maximum and minimum total available biomass (TAB). Estimated density of carnivores (individuals per square kilometre), nutritional requirements (kilocalories per year), total intake (kilocalories per year), unsatisfied requirements (kilocalories per year), sustainable density (individuals per square kilometre), Species Competition Index (SCI). Total intake is defined as the biomass (in kcal) consumed by the species after dividing TAB among the secondary consumers, taking into account the distribution of TAB by body size category (Table 4) and the carnivore preferences (Table 3).
(DOCX)

Table S3 Sustainable densities of TD6-2 secondary consumers for eight different scenarios (see text) for maximum and minimum total available biomass (TAB). Estimated density of carnivores (individuals per square kilometre), nutritional requirements (kilocalories per year), total intake (kilocalories per year), unsatisfied requirements (kilocalories per year), sustainable density (individuals per square kilometre), Species Competition Index (SCI), Total intake is defined as the biomass (in kcal) consumed by the species after dividing TAB among the secondary consumers, taking into account the distribution of TAB by body size category (Table 4) and the carnivore preferences (Table 3).
(DOCX)

Acknowledgments

We are grateful to P. Palmqvist and the Academic Editor for their useful comments and suggestions on a previous version of this manuscript. An anonymous editor from Elsevier's Language services improved the English of the original manuscript. We also thank Estefanía Pérez Fernández for her suggestions and support in the revision of the manuscript. We are very grateful to the participants in the fieldwork and all of the members of the Atapuerca Research Team.

Author Contributions

Conceived and designed the experiments: AM J. Rodríguez. Performed the experiments: GRG. Analyzed the data: GRG AM J. Rodríguez. Contributed reagents/materials/analysis tools: JAMG. Wrote the paper: GRG AM JAMG RB J. Rosell J. Rodríguez. Discussion: GRG AM JAMG RB J. Rosell J. Rodríguez.

References

1. Gómez-Robles A, Bermúdez de Castro JM, Arsuaga J-L, Carbonell E, Polly PD (2014) No known hominin species matches the expected dental morphology of the last common ancestor of Neanderthals and modern humans. Proc Natl Acad Sci. In press.
2. Bermúdez de Castro JM, Martinón-Torres M, Blasco R, Rosell J, Carbonell E (2013) Continuity or discontinuity in the European Early Pleistocene human settlement: the Atapuerca evidence. Quat Sci Rev 76: 53–65.
3. Muttoni G, Scardia G, Kent DV (2010) Human migration into Europe during the late Early Pleistocene climate transition. Palaeogeogr Palaeoclimatol Palaeoecol 296: 79–93.
4. Palombo MR (2010) A scenario of human dispersal in the northwestern Mediterranean throughout the Early to Middle Pleistocene. Quatern Int 223–224: 179–194.
5. O'Regan HJ (2008) The Iberian Peninsula – corridor or cul-de-sac? Mammalian faunal change and possible routes of dispersal in the last 2 million years. Quat Sci Rev 27: 2136–2144.
6. O'Regan HJ, Turner A, Bishop LC, Lamb AL (2011) Hominins without fellow travellers? First appearances and inferred dispersals of Afro-Eurasian large-mammals in the Plio-Pleistocene. Quat Sci Rev 30: 1343–1352.
7. Made Jvd, Mateos A (2010) Longstanding biogeographic patterns and the dispersal of early Homo out of Africa and into Europe. Quatern Int 223–224: 195–200.
8. Carbonell E, Sala Ramos R, Rodríguez XP, Mosquera M, Ollé A, et al. (2010) Early hominid dispersals: A technological hypothesis for "out of Africa". Quatern Int 223–224: 36–44.
9. Palombo MR (2013) What about causal mechanisms promoting early hominin dispersal in Eurasia? A research agenda for answering a hotly debated question. Quatern Int 295: 13–27.
10. Agustí J, Blain H-A, Cuenca-Bescós G, Bailon S (2009) Climate forcing of first hominid dispersal in Western Europe. J Hum Evol 57: 815–821.
11. Mosquera M, Ollé A, Rodríguez XP (2013) From Atapuerca to Europe: Tracing the earliest peopling of Europe. Quatern Int 295: 130–137.
12. Jiménez-Arenas JM, Santonja M, Botella M, Palmqvist P (2011) The oldest handaxes in Europe: fact or artefact? J Archaeol Sci 38.
13. Arribas A, Palmqvist P (1999) On the Ecological Connection Between Sabre-tooths and Hominids: Faunal Dispersal Events in the Lower Pleistocene and a Review of the Evidence for the First Human Arrival in Europe. J Archaeol Sci 26: 571–585.

14. Bermúdez de Castro JM, Martinón-Torres M (2013) A new model for the evolution of the human Pleistocene populations of Europe. Quatern Int 295: 102–112.
15. Dennell RW, Martinón-Torres M, Bermúdez de Castro JM (2011) Hominin variability, climatic instability and population demography in Middle Pleistocene Europe. Quat Sci Rev 30: 1511–1524.
16. Almogi-Labin A (2011) The paleoclimate of the Eastern Mediterranean during the transition from early to mid Pleistocene (900 to 700 ka) based on marine and non-marine records: An integrated overview. J Hum Evol 60: 428–436.
17. Amit R, Enzel Y, Sharon D (2006) Permanent Quaternary hyperaridity in the Negev, Israel, resulting from regional tectonics blocking Mediterranean frontal systems. Geology 34: 509–512.
18. Rodríguez J, Martín-González JA, Goikoetxea I, Rodríguez-Gómez G, Mateos A (2013) Mammalian paleobiogeography and the distribution of Homo in early Pleistocene Europe. Quatern Int 295: 48–58.
19. Duval M, Falguères C, Bahain J-J (2012) Age of the oldest hominin settlements in Spain: Contribution of the combined U-series/ESR dating method applied to fossil teeth. Quat Geochronol 10: 412–417.
20. Duval M, Falguères C, Bahain J-J, Grün R, Shao Q, et al. (2012) On the limits of using combined U-series/ESR method to date fossil teeth from two Early Pleistocene archaeological sites of the Orce area (Guadix-Baza basin, Spain). Quatern Res 77: 482–491.
21. Toro-Moyano I, Martínez-Navarro B, Agustí J, Souday C, Bermúdez de Castro JM, et al. (2013) The oldest human fossil in Europe dated to ca. 1.4 Ma at Orce (Spain). J Hum Evol 65: 1–9.
22. Martínez K, Garcia J, Carbonell E, Agustí J, Bahain J-J, et al. (2010) A new Lower Pleistocene archeological site in Europe (Vallparadís, Barcelona, Spain). Proc Natl Acad Sci 107: 5762–5767.
23. Duval M, Moreno D, Shao Q, Voinchet P, Falguères C, et al. (2011) Datación por ESR del yacimiento arqueológico del Pleistoceno inferior de Vallparadís (Terrassa, Cataluña, España). Trabajos de Prehistoria 68: 7–24.
24. Madurell-Malapeira J, Alba DM, Minwer-Barakat R, Aurell-Garrido J, Moyà-Solà S (2012) Early human dispersals into the Iberian Peninsula: A comment on Martínez et al. (2010) and Garcia et al. (2011). J Hum Evol 62: 169–173.
25. Rodríguez J, Burjachs F, Cuenca-Bescós G, García N, Made Jvd, et al. (2011) One million years of cultural evolution in a stable environment at Atapuerca (Burgos, Spain). Quat Sci Rev 30: 1396–1412.
26. Arzarello M, Marcolini F, Pavia G, Pavia M, Petronio C, et al. (2007) Evidence of earliest human occurrence in Europe: the site of Pirro Nord (Southern Italy). Naturwissenschaften 94: 107–112.
27. Bahain J-J, Falguères C, Voinchet P, Duval M, Dolo J-M, et al. (2007) Electron Spin Resonance (ESR) dating of some European Late Lower Pleistocene Sites. Quaternaire 18: 175–186.
28. de Lumley H, Kahlke H-D, Moigne A-M, Moulle P-E (1988) Les faunes de grands mammifères de la grotte du Vallonnet, Roquebrune-Cap-Martin, Alpes-Maritimes. L' Anthropologie 92: 465–495.
29. Voinchet P (2002) Datations par résonance paramagnétique électronique (RPE) de quartz blanchis extraits de sédiments fluviatiles pléistocènes: contribution méthodologique et application aux systèmes de la Creuse, du Loir et de l'Yonne. Paris.
30. Despriée J, Gageonnet R (2003) La très haute nappe alluviale d'âge pléistocène inférieur de la vallée de la Creuse à Eguzon (Indre): figures de cryoturbations, habitats préhistoriques et datations absolues. Bulletin de la Société géologique de France 174: 383–400.
31. Despriée J, Gageonnet R, Voinchet P, Bahain J-J, Falguères C, et al. (2006) Une occupation humaine au Pléistocène inférieur sur la bordure nord du Massif central. C R Palevol 5: 821–828.
32. Parfitt SA, Coope GR, Field MH, Peglar SM, Preece RC, et al. (2010) Middle Pleistocene biota of the early Anglian 'Arctic Fresh-water Bed' at Ostend, Norfolk, UK. Proc Geol Assoc 121: 55–65.
33. Parés JM, Duval M, Arnold L (2013) New views on an old move: Hominin migration into Eurasia. Quatern Int 295: 5–12.
34. Fiedler L, Franzen JL (2002) Artefakte vom altpleistozänen Fundplatz "Dorn-Dürkheim 3" am nördlichen Oberrhein. Germania 80: 421–440.
35. Stuart AJ, Lister AM (2001) The mammalian faunas of Pakefield/Kessingland and Corton, Suffolk, UK: evidence for a new temperate episode in the British early Middle Pleistocene. Quat Sci Rev 20: 1677–1692.
36. Crochet J-Y, Welcomme J-L, Ivorra J, Ruffet G, Boulbes N, et al. (2009) Une nouvelle faune de vertébrés continentaux, associée à des artefacts dans le Pléistocène inférieur de l'Hérault (Sud de la France). C R Palevol 8: 725–736.
37. Barsky D, Garcia J, Martínez K, Sala R, Zaidner Y, et al. (2013) Flake modification in European Early and EarlyeMiddle Pleistocene stone tool assemblages. Quatern Int 316: 140–154.
38. Bermúdez de Castro JM, Martinón-Torres M, Gómez-Robles A, Prado-Simón L, Martín-Francés L, et al. (2011) Early Pleistocene human mandible from Sima del Elefante (TE) cave site in Sierra de Atapuerca (Spain): A comparative morphological study. J Hum Evol 61: 12–25.
39. Carbonell E, Bermúdez de Castro JM, Parés JM, Pérez-González A, Cuenca-Bescós G, et al. (2008) The first hominin of Europe. Nature 452.
40. Muttoni G, Scardia G, Kent DV (2013) A critique of evidence for human occupation of Europe older than the Jaramillo subchron (wl Ma): Comment on 'The oldest human fossil in Europe from Orce (Spain)' by Toro-Moyano et al. (2013). J Hum Evol 65: 746–749.
41. Despriée J, Voinchet P, Tissoux H, Bahain J-J, Falguères C, et al. (2011) Lower and Middle Pleistocene human settlements recorded in fluvial deposits of the middle Loire River Basin, Centre Region, France. Quat Sci Rev 30: 1474–1485.
42. Barsky D, de Lumley H (2010) Early European Mode 2 and the stone industry from the Caune de l'Arago's archeostratigraphical levels "P". Quatern Int 223–224: 71–86.
43. Ollé A, Mosquera M, Rodríguez XP, Lombera-Hermida Ad, García-Antón MD, et al. (2013) The Early and Middle Pleistocene technological record from Sierra de Atapuerca (Burgos, Spain). Quatern Int 295: 138–167.
44. Doronichev V, Golovanova L (2010) Beyond the Acheulean: A view on the Lower Paleolithic occupation of Western Eurasia. Quatern Int 223–224: 327–344.
45. Roberts MB, Parfitt SA (2000) Boxgrove: A Middle Pleistocene Hominid Site at Eartham Quarry, Boxgrove, West Sussex. Geoarchaeology: An International Journal, 15: 819–822.
46. Mania D, Vlcek E (1999) The Bilzingsleben site: Homo erectus, his culture and his ecosphere. In: Ullrich H, editor. Hominid Evolution: Lifestyles and Survival Strategies: Archaea. pp. 293–314.
47. Thieme H (1997) Lower Palaeolithic hunting spears from Schöningen, Germany. Nature 358: 807–810.
48. Roebroeks W, Villa P (2011) On the earliest evidence for habitual use of fire in Europe. Proc Natl Acad Sci 108: 5209–5214.
49. Bennett KD, Provan J (2008) What do we mean by 'refugia'? Quat Sci Rev 27: 2449–2455.
50. Tattersall I (2011) Before the Neanderthals: Hominid Evolution in Middle Pleistocene Europe. In: Condemi S, Weniger G-C, editors. Continuity and Discontinuity in the Peopling of Europe: One Hundrer Fifty Years of Neanderthal Study: Vertebrate Paleobiology and Paleoanthropology - Springer.
51. Hublin JJ (2009) The origin of Neandertals. Proc Natl Acad Sci 106: 16022–16027.
52. Mallegni F (2011) The Earliest European Human Peopling After the Recent Discoveries: Early Neanderthals or Different Lineages? In: Condemi S, Weniger G-C, editors. Continuity and Discontinuity in the Peopling of Europe: One Hundrer Fifty Years of Neanderthal Study: Vertebrate Paleobiology and Paleoanthropology - Springer.
53. Stringer C (2012) The Status of Homo heidelbergensis (Schoetensack 1908). Evol Anthropol 21: 101–107.
54. Turner A (1992) Large carnivores and earliest European hominids: changing determinants of resource availability during the Lower and Middle Pleistocene. J Hum Evol 22: 109–126.
55. Espigares MP, Martínez-Navarro B, Palmqvist P, Ros-Montoya S, Toro I, et al. (2013) *Homo* vs. *Pachycrocuta*: Earliest evidence of competition for an elephant carcass between scavengers at Fuente Nueva-3 (Orce, Spain). Quatern Int 295: 113–125.
56. Palmqvist P, Martínez-Navarro B, Pérez-Claros JA, Torregrosa V, Figueirido B, et al. (2011) The giant hyena Pachycrocuta brevirostris: Modelling the bone-cracking behavior of an extinct carnivore. Quatern Int 243: 61–79.
57. Rodríguez J, Rodríguez-Gómez G, Martín-González JA, Goikoetxea I, Mateo A (2012) Predator–prey relationships and the role of *Homo* in Early Pleistocene food webs in Southern Europe. Palaeogeogr Palaeoclimatol Palaeoecol 365–366: 99–114.
58. Palombo MR (2007) What is the Boundary for the Quaternary Period and Pelistocene Epoch? The Contribution of Turnover Patterns in Large Mammalian Complexes from North-Western Mediterranean to the Debate. Quaternaire 18: 35–53.
59. Martínez-Navarro B, Palmqvist P (1996) Presence of the African Sabertoothed Felid *Megantereon whitei* (Broom, 1937) Mammalia, Carnivora, Machair-odontinae in Apollonia-1 (Mygdonia Basin, Macedonia, Greece). J Archaeol Sci 23: 869–872.
60. Rodríguez-Gómez G, Rodríguez J, Martín-González JA, Goikoetxea I, Mateos A (2013) Modeling trophic resource availability for the first human settlers of Europe: The case of Atapuerca-TD6. J Hum Evol 64: 645–657.
61. Parés JM, Arnold L, Duval M, Demuro M, Pérez-González A, et al. (2013) Reassessing the age of Atapuerca-TD6 (Spain): New paleomagnetic results. J Archaeol Sci 40: 4586–4595.
62. Berger GW, Pérez-González A, Carbonell E, Arsuaga JL, Bermúdez de Castro JM, et al. (2008) Luminescence chronology of cave sediments at the Atapuerca paleoanthropological site, Spain. J Hum Evol 55: 300–311.
63. Falguères C, Bahain J-J, Yokoyama Y, Arsuaga JL, Bermúdez de Castro JM, et al. (1999) Earliest humans in Europe: the age of TD6 Gran Dolina, Atapuerca, Spain. J Hum Evol 37: 343–352.
64. Bischoff JL, Williams RW, Rosenbauer RJ, Aramburu A, Arsuaga JL, et al. (2007) High-resolution U-series dates from the Sima de los Huesos hominids yields 600 kyrs: implications for the evolution of the early Neanderthal lineage. J Archaeol Sci 34: 763–770.
65. Parés JM, Pérez-González A (1999) Magnetochronology and stratigraphy at Gran Dolina section, Atapuerca (Burgos, Spain). J Hum Evol 37: 325–342.
66. Blasco R, Rosell J, Made Jvd, Rodríguez J, Campeny G, et al. (2011) Hiding to eat: the role of carnivores in the early Middle Pleistocene from the TD8 level of Gran Dolina (Sierra de Atapuerca, Burgos, Spain). J Archaeol Sci 38: 3373–3386.

67. Palmiqvist P, Arribas A (2001) Taphonomic decoding of the paleobiological information locked in a lower Pleistocene assemblage of large mammals. Paleobiology 27: 512–530.
68. Made Jvd (2013) First description of the large mammals from the locality of Penal, and updated faunal lists for the Atapuerca ungulates Equus altidens, Bison; and human dispersal into Western Europe. Quatern Int 295: 36–47.
69. Owen-Smith N, Mills MGL (2008) Predator–prey size relationships in an African large-mammal food web. Journal of Animal Ecology 77: 173–183.
70. Roebroeks W (2001) Hominid behaviour and the earliest occupation of Europe: an exploration. J Hum Evol 41: 437–461.
71. Rodríguez J (1997) Análisis de la estructura de las comunidades de mamíferos del Pleistoceno de la Sierra de Atapuerca. Revisión de metodologías. Madrid: Universidad Autónoma de Madrid.
72. Damuth JD, MacFadden BJ (1990) Body Size in Mammalian Paleobiology: estimations and Biological Implications: Cambridge University Press.
73. Mazza PPA, Bertini A (2013) Were Pleistocene hippopotamuses exposed to climate-driven body size changes? Boreas 42: 194–209.
74. Díez JC, Fernández-Jalvo Y, Rosell J, Cáceres I (1999) Zooarchaeology and taphonomy of Aurora Stratum (Gran Dolina, Sierra de Atapuerca, Spain). J Hum Evol 37: 623–652.
75. Saladié P, Huguet R, Díez C, Rodríguez-Hidalgo A, Cáceres I, et al. (2011) Carcass transport decisions in *Homo antecessor* subsistence strategies. J Hum Evol 61: 425–446.
76. Carbonell E, Bermúdez de Castro JM, Arsuaga JL, Allue E, Bastir M, et al. (2005) An Early Pleistocene hominin mandible from Atapuerca-TD6, Spain. Proc Natl Acad Sci 102: 5674–5678.
77. Carbonell E, Bermúdez de Castro JM, Arsuaga JL, Díez JC, Rosas A, et al. (1995) Lower Pleistocene Hominids and Artifacts from Atapuerca-TD6 (Spain). Science 269: 826–830.
78. Rodríguez-Gómez G, Martín-González JA, Goikoetxea I, Mateos A, Rodríguez J (2014) A New Mathematical Approach to Model Trophic Dynamics of Mammalian Palaeocommunities. The Case of Atapuerca-TD6. In: Pardo-Igúzquiza E, Guardiola-Albert C, Heredia J, Moreno-Merino L, Durán JJ et al., editors. 15th Annual Conference of the International Association for Mathematical Geosciences. Madrid: Lectures Notes in Earth System Sciences - Springer. pp. 739–745.
79. Owen-Smith N (2010) Dynamics of Large Herbivore Populations in Changing Environments: Towards Appropriate Models. Malaysia: Blackwell Publishing Ltd.
80. Leslie PH (1945) On the use of matrices in certain population mathematics. Biometrika 33: 183–212.
81. Leslie PH (1948) Some further notes on the use of matrices in population mathematics. Biometrika 35: 213–245.
82. Levinton JS (1982) The body size-prey size hypothesis: the adequacy of body size as a vehicle for character displacement. Ecology 63: 869–872.
83. Carbone C, Mace GM, Roberts SC, Macdonald DW (1999) Energetic constraints on the diet of terrestrial carnivores. Nature 402: 286–288.
84. Radloff FGT, Toit JTD (2004) Large predators and their prey in a southern African savanna: a predator's size determines its prey size range. Journal of Animal Ecology 73: 410–423.
85. Damuth J (1981) Population density and body size in mammals. Nature 290: 699–700.
86. Viljoen PC (1993) The effects of changes in prey availability on lion predation in a natural ecosystem in northern. Zoological symposium 65: 193–213.
87. Gaillard J-M, Festa-Bianchet M, Yoccoz NG, Loison A, Toïgo C (2000) Temporal variation in fitness components and population dynamics of large herbivores. Annual Review of Ecology Systems 31: 367–393.
88. Farlow JO (1976) A Consideration of the Trophic Dynamics of a Late Cretaceous Large-Dinosaur Community (Oldman Formation). Ecology 57: 841–857.
89. Blumenschine RJ, Madrigal TC (1993) Variability in Long Bone Marrow Yields of East African Ungulates and its Zooarchaeological Implications. J Archaeol Sci 20: 555–587.
90. Outram A, Rowley-Conwy P (1998) Meat and Marrow Utility Indices for Horse (Equus). J Archaeol Sci 25: 839–849.
91. Holekamp KE, Kolowski JM (2009) Family Hyaenidae (Hyaenas). In: Wilson DE, Mittermeier RA, editors. Handbook of the mammals of the world. Barcelona: Lynx Ediciones. pp. 234–262.
92. Beltrán JF, Sanjosé C, Delibes M, Braza F (1985) An analysis of the Iberian lynx predation upon fallow deer in the coto Doñana, SW Spain. XVIIth Congress of the International Union of Game Biologist: 961–967.
93. Delibes M (1980) El lince ibérico. Ecologia y comportamientos alimenticios en el Coto de Doñana, Huelva. Doñana, Acta Vertebrata 7: 1–128.
94. Rodríguez A (2008) Lince ibérico – Lynx pardinus (Temminck, 1827). Enciclopedia virtual de los vertebrados españoles.
95. Bocherens H, Argant A, Argant J, Billiou D, Crégut-Bonnoure E, et al. (2004) Diet reconstruction of ancient brown bears (Ursus arctos) from Mont Ventoux (France) using bone collagen stable isotope biogeochemistry (13C, 15N). Can J Zool 82: 576–586.
96. Parde J-M, Camarra J-J (1992) Encyclopédie des Carnivores de France, Part 5: L'Ours: (Ursus arctos, Linnaeus, 1758): Société Française Pour L'Etude et la Protection des Mammifères.
97. Palmqvist P, Pérez-Claros JA, Janis CM, Figueirido B, Torregrosa V, et al. (2008) Biogeochemical and ecomorphological inferences on prey selection and resource partitioning among mammalian carnivores in an Early Pleistocene community. PALAIOS 23: 724–737.
98. Damuth J (1993) Copes rule, the island rule and the scaling of mammalian population density. Nature 365: 748–750.
99. DeMaster DP, Stirling I (1981) Ursus maritimus. Mammalian Species 145: 1–7.
100. Larivière S (2001) Ursus americanus. Mammalian Species 647: 1–11.
101. Pasitschniak-Arts M (1993) Ursus arctos. Mammalian Species 439: 1–10.
102. Eaton SB, Eaton III SB, Konner MJ (1997) Paleolithic nutrition revisited: A twelve-year retrospective on its nature and implications. Nature 51: 207–216.
103. Carretero JM, Arsuaga JL, Martínez I, Quam R, Lorenzo C, et al. (2002) Los humanos de la Sima de los Huesos (Sierra de Atapuerca) y la evolución del cuerpo en el género Homo. In: Baquedano E, Rubio Jara S, editors. Miscelánea Homenaje a Emiliano Aguirre. Madrid: Paleoantropología. Museo Arqueológico Regional. pp. 120–134.
104. Bonmatí A, Arsuaga JL (2005) Inventory and preliminary description of Middle Pleistocene pelvis remains from the site of Sima de los Huesos, Atapuerca (Spain). Am J Phys Anthropol Res 126 (Suppl 40): 76.
105. Jenike MR (2001) Nutritional ecology: diet, physical activity and body size. In: Panter-Brick C, Layton RH, Rowley-Conwy P, editors. Hunter-gatherers An interdisciplinary perspective: Cambridge University Press.
106. Leonard WR, Robertson ML, Snodgrass JJ (2007) Energetic Models of Human Nutritional Evolution. In: Ungar PS, editor. Evolution of the human diet The Known, the Unknown, and the Unknowable: Oxford University Press. pp. 344–359.
107. Binford LR (2001) Constructing frames of reference. An analytical method for archaeological theory building using ethnographic and environmental data sets: University of California Press. 118–129 p.
108. Silva M, Downing JA (1994) Allometric Scaling of Minimal Mammal Densities. Conserv Biol 8: 732–743.
109. Thornback J, Jenkins M (1982) The IUCN mammal red data book. Gland, Switzerland: International Union for the Conservation of Nature.
110. Blain H-A, Cuenca-Bescós G, Burjachs F, López-García JM, Lozano-Fernández I, et al. (2013) Early Pleistocene palaeoenvironments at the time of the Homo antecessor settlement in the Gran Dolina cave (Atapuerca, Spain). J Quaternary Sci 28: 311–319.
111. Cuenca-Bescós G, García N (2007) Biostratigraphic succession of the Early and Middle Pleistocene mammal faunas of the Atapuerca cave sites (Burgos, Spain). Cour Forsch-Inst Senckenberg 255: 99–110.
112. Cuenca-Bescós G, Rofes J, López-García JM, Blain H-A, De Marfá RJ, et al. (2010) Biochronology of Spanish Quaternary small vertebrate faunas. Quatern Int 212: 109–119.
113. Made Jvd, Mazo AV (2001) Spanish Pleistocene Proboscidean diversity as a function of climate. The World of Elephants: Proceedings of the 1st International Congress Rome. pp. 214–218.
114. Antón M, Galobart A, Turner A (2005) Co-existence of scimitar-toothed cats, lions and hominins in the European Pleistocene. Implications of the post-cranial anatomy of Homotherium latidens (Owen) for comparative palaeoecology. Quat Sci Rev 24: 1287–1301.
115. Meade GE (1961) The saber toothed cat, *Dinoblastis serus*. Texas Memorial Museum 3: 23–60.
116. Finlayson C, Carrión J, Browna K, Finlayson G, Sánchez-Marco A, et al. (2011) The Homo habitat niche: Using the avian fossil record to depict ecological characteristics of Palaeolithic Eurasian hominins. Quat Sci Rev 30: 1525–1532.
117. Carrión JS, Rose J, Stringer CB (2011) Early Human Evolution in the Western Palaearctic: Ecological Scenarios. Quat Sci Rev 30: 1281–1295.
118. Saladié P, Rodríguez-Hidalgo A, Huguet R, Cáceres I, Díez C, et al. (2014) The role of carnivores and their relationship to hominin settlements in the TD6-2 level from Gran Dolina (Sierra de Atapuerca, Spain). Quat Sci Rev 93: 47–66.
119. Carmody RN, Weintraub GS, Wrangham RW (2011) Energetic consequences of thermal and nonthermal food processing. Proc Natl Acad Sci 108: 19119–19203.
120. Huguet R, Saladié P, Cáceres I, Díez C, Rosell J, et al. (2013) Successful subsistence strategies of the first humans in south-western Europe. Quatern Int 295: 168–182.
121. Blasco R, Rosell J, Fernández Peris J, Arsuaga JL, Bermúdez de Castro JM, et al. (2013) Environmental availability, behavioural diversity and diet: a zooarchaeological approach from the TD10-1 sublevel of Gran Dolina (Sierra de Atapuerca, Burgos, Spain) and Bolomor Cave (Valencia, Spain). Quat Sci Rev 70: 124–144.
122. Rosell J, Blasco R, Made Jvd, Cáceres I, Campeny G, et al. (2010) Acumulaciones producidas por carnívoros en el Pleistoceno medio inicial: una reconstrucción a partir del conjunto faunístico del nivel TD8 de Gran Dolina (Sierra de Atapuerca, Burgos). Zona arqueológica 13: 158–172.

18

Tualang Honey Improves Human Corneal Epithelial Progenitor Cell Migration and Cellular Resistance to Oxidative Stress *In Vitro*

Jun Jie Tan[1]*, Siti Maisura Azmi[1], Yoke Keong Yong[2], Hong Leong Cheah[1], Vuanghao Lim[1], Doblin Sandai[1], Bakiah Shaharuddin[1¤]

1 Advanced Medical and Dental Institute, Universiti Sains Malaysia, Kepala Batas, Penang, Malaysia, **2** Department of Human Anatomy, Faculty of Medicine and Health Sciences, Serdang, Selangor Darul Ehsan, Malaysia

Abstract

Stem cells with enhanced resistance to oxidative stress after *in vitro* expansion have been shown to have improved engraftment and regenerative capacities. Such cells can be generated by preconditioning them with exposure to an antioxidant. In this study we evaluated the effects of Tualang honey (TH), an antioxidant-containing honey, on human corneal epithelial progenitor (HCEP) cells in culture. Cytotoxicity, gene expression, migration, and cellular resistance to oxidative stress were evaluated. Immunofluorescence staining revealed that HCEP cells were holoclonal and expressed epithelial stem cell marker p63 without corneal cytokeratin 3. Cell viability remained unchanged after cells were cultured with 0.004, 0.04, and 0.4% TH in the medium, but it was significantly reduced when the concentration was increased to 3.33%. Cell migration, tested using scratch migration assay, was significantly enhanced when cells were cultured with TH at 0.04% and 0.4%. We also found that TH has hydrogen peroxide (H_2O_2) scavenging ability, although a trace level of H_2O_2 was detected in the honey in its native form. Preconditioning HCEP cells with 0.4% TH for 48 h showed better survival following H_2O_2-induced oxidative stress at 50 μM than untreated group, with a significantly lower number of dead cells (15.3±0.4%) were observed compared to the untreated population (20.5±0.9%, $p<0.01$). Both TH and ascorbic acid improved HCEP viability following induction of 100 μM H_2O_2, but the benefit was greater with TH treatment than with ascorbic acid. However, no significant advantage was demonstrated using 5-hydroxymethyl-2-furancarboxaldehyde, a compound that was found abundant in TH using GC/MS analysis. This suggests that the cellular anti-oxidative capacity in HCEP cells was augmented by native TH and was attributed to its antioxidant properties. In conclusion, TH possesses antioxidant properties and can improve cell migration and cellular resistance to oxidative stress in HCEP cells *in vitro*.

Editor: Xuefeng Liu, Georgetown University, United States of America

Funding: This project was supported by the Universiti Sains Malaysia Short Term Grant (304/CIPPT/6311032)(http://www.research.usm.my/?tag = 22) and Advanced Medical and Dental Institute. The funders had no role in study design, data collection and analysis, decision to publish, or preparation of the manuscript.

Competing Interests: The authors have declared that no competing interests exist.

* E-mail: jjtan@amdi.usm.edu.my

¤ Current address: Institute of Genetic Medicine, Newcastle University, International Centre for Life, Newcastle Upon Tyne, United Kingdom

Introduction

The cornea, which is a transparent and tough tissue that covers the anterior segment of the eye, is responsible for transmitting and reflecting light onto the retina. As the first layer of defence against external insults and oxidative insult from the sunlight, the corneal epithelium possesses mechanisms to maintain its cellular homeostasis. These mechanisms are orchestrated by a population of self-renewing stem cells that reside in the basal limbal epithelium, which is a niche area situated at the peripheral edge of the cornea called the limbus [1]. These cells express keratinocyte stem cell markers (p63, EGFR, K19, ABCG2 and integrin β1) and exhibit low expression of corneal differentiation markers (K3, involucrin, and connexin-43) [2], and they are responsible for sustaining the clarity and integrity of the corneal epithelium required for normal vision. Complete depletion or dysfunction of the corneal epithelial stem cells that occurs in some severe ocular surface abnormalities as a result of caustic injuries such as burns, inflammatory conditions, or hereditary genetic disorders such as aniridia [3,4] will lead to conjunctivalisation, keratinisation, and opacification and result in impaired vision or blindness. Under these circumstances, visual acuity can only be restored by transplanting corneal epithelial stem cells onto the injured cornea. To minimise the risk of immune rejection, autologous stem cell transplantation may be the only option. Hence, culturing corneal epithelial stem cells and preserving their stemness and functions *in vitro* are pivotal for ensuring successful regeneration following transplantation.

Reactive oxygen species (ROS) are common metabolic by-products of aerobic metabolism, and their level is maintained through intrinsic antioxidant mechanisms in healthy cells. When maintained at the appropriate physiological level, ROS are vital in modulating several cellular signalling pathways that affect cell growth and function, including the phosphoinositide 3-kinase (PI3K) [5] and mitogen-activated protein kinase (MAPK) pathways [6]. In addition, ROS have the capability to dictate stem cell

Table 1. Dilution factor for Tualang honey supplemented medium.

Tualang honey concentrations (%)	20% Tualang honey: KSFM
0.004%	1:5000
0.04%	1:500
0.4%	1:50
3.33%	1:5

Abbreviation: KSFM, keratinocyte-serum free medium.

fate at physiological levels [7–9]. However, abnormal redox homeostasis involving ROS overproduction can induce oxidative stress, a physiological condition that renders cells susceptible to damage. Studies have confirmed that overproduction of ROS can compromise genomic stability [10] and trigger mutations and promote cancer growth [11]. High ROS levels also contribute to poor cell engraftment and viability, which impede regeneration after transplantation [12]. Although stem cells have greater antioxidant capacity compared to differentiated cells [13,14], they can exhibit telomere shortening-induced replicative senescence and reduced self-renewal capability under oxidative stress [15]. Hence, protecting stem cells from oxidative damage may help to promote cell survival, homing, and regeneration after transplantation. This protection could be achieved by maintaining a reduced environment at the site of transplantation through adjunctive therapy with dietary antioxidant [16] or by adding an antioxidant supplement to cells during *in vitro* expansion prior to transplantation. The efficacy of the latter strategy is supported by studies showing the potential for supplemental antioxidant in the culture medium to enhance the intracellular antioxidant activity of stem cells [15], prevent cellular damage, and salvage culture-induced loss of stemness [17].

Tualang honey is a medicinal honey that is collected from the honeycomb of *Apis dorsata*, the bees that built their hives on the Tualang tree (*Koompassia excels*) that is common in tropical forests in Malaysia. This honey has been extensively studied and has been found to have therapeutic benefits in treating various medical conditions, including protecting post-menopausal bone structure [18], promoting burn wound contraction with antibacterial effects [19,20], enhancing post-tonsillectomy healing [21], and inhibiting the growth of various cancer cells [22–24]. Generally, honey has been traditionally used to treat eye-related diseases [25,26]. Uwaydat et al. (2011) recently showed that raw honey accelerated healing of corneal abrasions and attenuated the inflammatory response and angiogenesis in endotoxin-induced keratitis [27]. Similar to other types of honey, previous studies of Tualang honey have also described its anti-inflammatory and antioxidant properties in treating alkali-induced eye injury *in vivo* [28] and its ability to save keratinocytes from inflammation and DNA damage as a result of ultraviolet radiation *in vitro* [29].

Although many *in vivo* studies of the effects of Tualang honey have been conducted, the potential for using Tualang honey in the cultivation of stem cells has not been investigated. To date, only one study described the use of Tualang honey to supplement the culture medium when cultivating a human osteoblast cell line (CRL1543) [30]. Although many studies have shown the therapeutic benefits of Tualang honey in treating cornea injury [28,29], its effects on corneal epithelial stem cells have yet to be evaluated. Herein we characterised the effects of Tualang honey on cytotoxicity, gene expression, and migration of human corneal epithelial progenitor (HCEP) cells and assessed its potential for improving cell resistance to oxidative stress.

Methodology

HCEP cell culture and expansion

HCEP cells were purchased from Gibco (Invitrogen Life Technologies Co., Carlsbad, CA, US) and ATCC (Manassas, VA, US). Cells were expanded in standard keratinocyte serum-free medium (KSFM, Gibco) that was supplemented with 5 ng/ml recombinant epidermal growth factor (rEGF) and 50 µg/ml bovine pituitary tissue extracts (Invitrogen Life Technologies Co., Carlsbad, CA, US). Passage 2–5 HCEP cells were used in all of the experiments.

Preparation of Tualang honey

Tualang honey used in this experiment was from Federal Agriculture Marketing Authorities of Malaysia (FAMA) and was a gift from Professor Siti Amrah Sulaiman, Universiti Sains Malaysia. Tualang honey was diluted to 20% in serum-free DMEM/F12 (Gibco, Invitrogen Life Technologies Co., Carlsbad, CA, US) and filtered through a 0.2 µm syringe filter (Pall Co., Port Washington, NY, US) prior to use in cell culture. Filtered Tualang honey was further diluted in KSFM according to the dilution factor described in Table 1.

Table 2. Sequences of primers used in this study.

Primers	Sequence (5′ - 3′)	Accession Number	PCR product (bp)
Beta-actin-F	GAGGCGTACAGGGATAGCA	NM_001101.3	302
Beta-actin-R	GTGGGCATGGGTCAGAAG		
ABCG2-F	GAGCTCGTCCCCTGGATGT	NM_004827.2	186
ABCG2-R	CGGAACCTTTTGAGTGGGCA		
Connexin43-F	CAAAATCGAATGGGGCAGGC	NM_000165.3	136
Connexin43-R	GCTGGTCCACAATGGCTAGT		
K12-F	CTCGCAGAGTGTGATAGGCA	NM_000223.3	146
K12-R	CCCCAAAGCCGGAACTAGAA		

Abbreviations: F, forward primer; R, reverse primer; PCR, polymerase chain reaction.

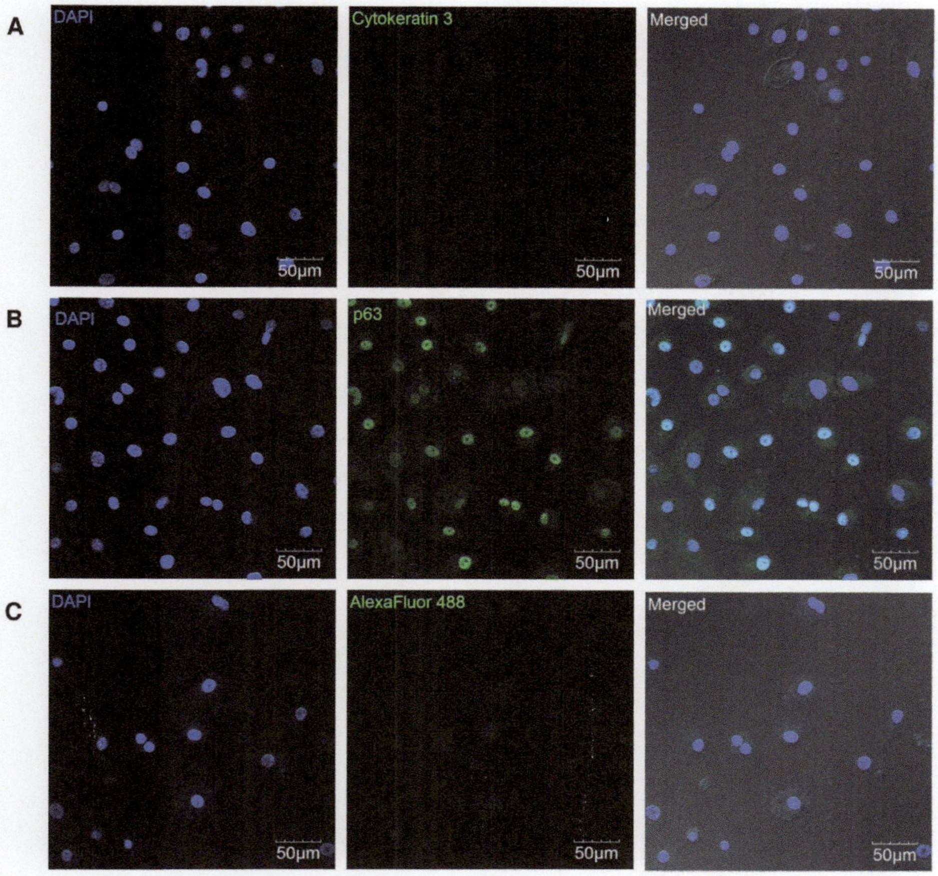

Figure 1. Representative confocal images of immunofluorescence-labelled HCEP cells. HCEP cells did not express the cornea-specific marker cytokeratin 3 (green) (A) but did express nuclear p63 transcription factor (green) (B). HCEP cells stained with AlexaFluor488 secondary antibody without any primary antibody were served as the negative control (C). Abbreviations: DAPI, 4′,6-diamidino-2-phenylindole.

Immunofluorescence labelling

HCEP cells were seeded onto Lab-Tek8 well-chamber slides (ThermoSci., Logan, UT, USA) using honey supplemented medium. Cells were fixed with 4% paraformaldehyde at 4°C for 10 min and then permeabilised with phosphate buffered saline containing 0.1% Triton-X and 0.1% Tween-20 (all from Sigma, St Louis, MO, USA). Cell samples were washed with PBS and blocked with 10% goat serum (Cedarlane Lab, Ontario, Canada) for 1 h. The cells then were incubated with rabbit anti-p63 (Santa Cruz Biotechnology, Heidelberg, Germany) and mouse anti-keratin 3 (Clone AE5, Millipore, Billerica, MA, USA) primary antibodies overnight at 4°C. Samples were washed thrice with PBS and incubated with AlexaFluor488 goat anti-rabbit secondary antibody at 37°C for 2 h. Samples were then counterstained with DAPI and imaged using a confocal microscope (Olympus, Japan).

RNA extraction and cDNA synthesis

The total RNA was isolated using the RNeasy Mini Kit (Qiagen, Hilden, Germany) according to the manufacturer's instructions. The isolated RNA was treated with DNase I (Sigma, St. Louis, MO, USA) to ensure the absence of genomic DNA contamination. Total RNA samples were quantitatively and qualitatively assessed using UV-spectrophotometric measurement and agarose gel electrophoresis, respectively. The cDNA was synthesised using the QuantiTect Reverse Transcription Kit (Qiagen, Hilden, Germany) according to manufacturer's protocol.

Primer design

Full-length exon spanning gene sequences were obtained from the NCBI GenBank Database (http://www.ncbi.nlm.nih.gov/genbank/). All primers were designed from the gene sequences using Primer-BLAST online software (NCBI, NIH, USA). All primers are listed in Table 2. The sequences of the primers were compared to the GenBank Database using BLAST in order to

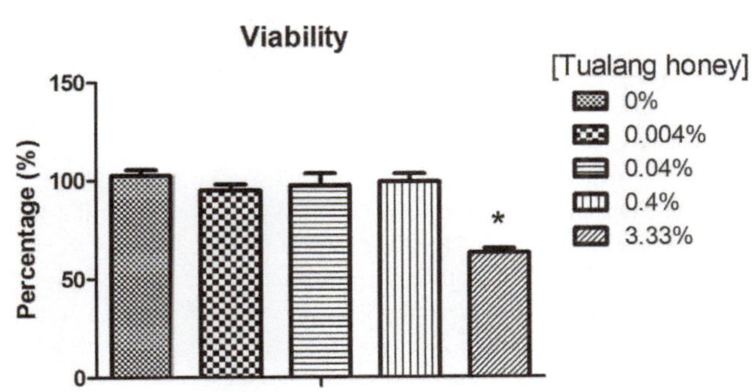

Figure 2. HCEP cell viability after treatment with 0, 0.004, 0.04, 0.4, and 3.33% Tualang honey for 48 h. Significant lower viability was observed in HCEP cells treated with 3.33% Tualang honey compared to the other treatments. ***$p<0.001$.

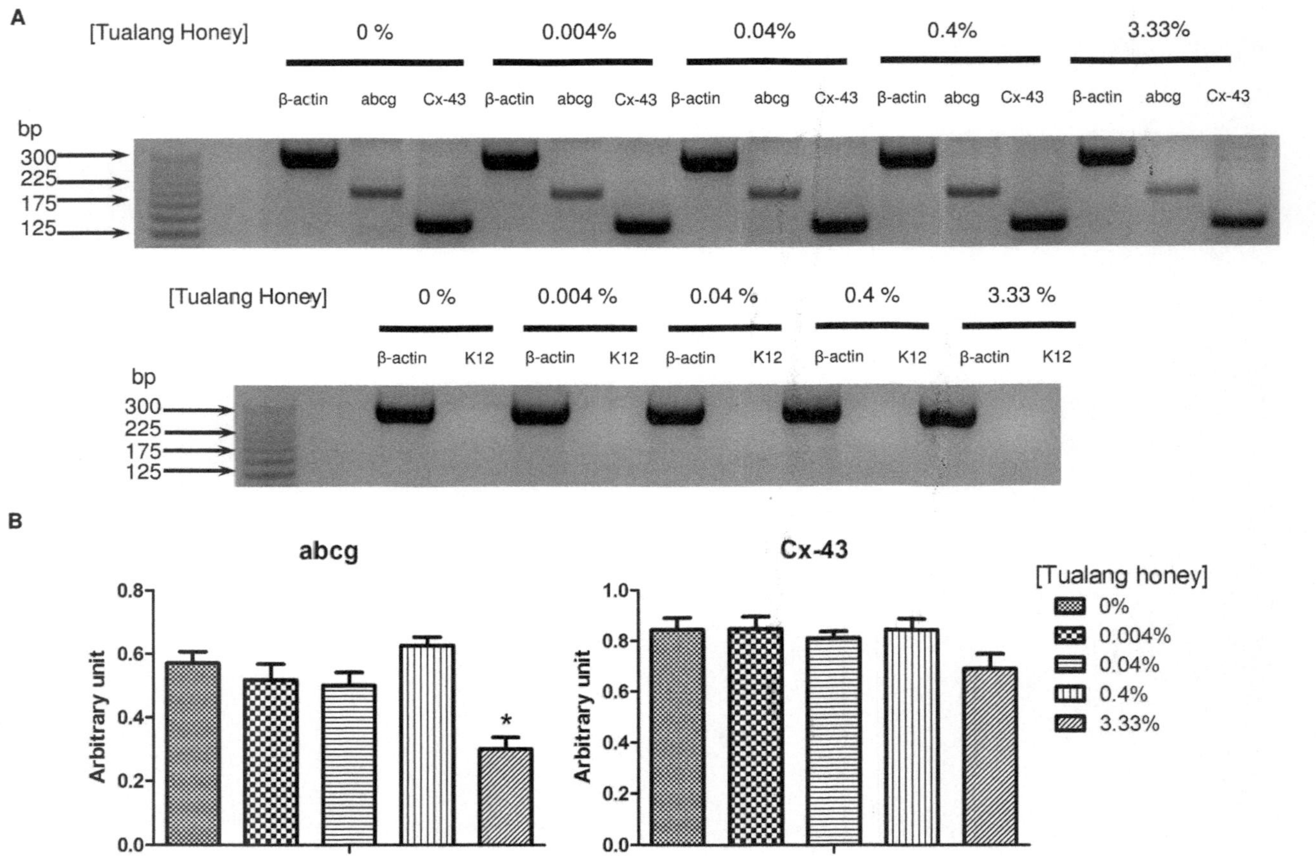

Figure 3. mRNA expression of Tualang honey treated HCEP cells. (A) RTPCR showed abcg and connexion-43 mRNA expressions (normalised to β-actin expression) but not cytokeratin-12 expression in HCEP cells. (B) abcg mRNA expression was down-regulated in HCEP cells treated with 3.33% Tualang honey, but the mRNA for connexin-43 remained unchanged in all groups. *$p<0.05$ compared to untreated control (0%). Abbreviations: abcg, ATP-binding cassette transporter; Cx-43, connexion-43.

determine their specificity. Primers that could have resulted in non-specific signals were excluded. All primers were purchased from BioBasic Inc. (Ontario, Canada).

Polymerase chain reactions (PCR)

PCR amplification was performed using the MyCycler Thermal Cycler (Bio-Rad, Hercules, CA, USA). All PCR reagents used in this study were purchased from Biotools B&M Labs (S.A., Madrid, Spain). Total cDNA used in each reaction was 1 μL unless specified otherwise. Reaction buffer (1 X), 1.5 mM $MgCl_2$, 1.75 mM of each dNTP, 0.5 μM of each primer, 100 ng of cDNA, and 1 U of DNA Taq Polymerase were added to all samples to reach a final volume of 20 μl in each reaction. A negative control (sample without template) was also included. PCR was performed at 95°C for 2 min as initial denaturation followed by 35 cycles of 30 sec at 95°C, 30 sec at 60°C, and 30 sec at 72°C, and then at 72°C for another 2 min. The PCR products were loaded with gel loading dye (Promega, Madison, WI, USA) onto 4% agarose gel in 1X TAE buffer and electrophoresed for 60 min at 80 V. A 25 base pair molecular ladder (Promega, Madison, WI, USA) was used. Subsequently, the gel was stained with ethidium bromide (Bio-Rad, Hercules, CA, USA) to visualize the presence of PCR amplicons.

Cytotoxicity assay

HCEP cells were seeded at 5000 cells/well onto a 96-well plate and left in an incubator with 5% CO_2 at 37°C overnight. The culture medium then was changed to test medium supplemented with Tualang honey at various concentrations (Table 1), and the cells were incubated for 48 h. Cell viability was tested using AlamarBlue (Molecular Probes, Invitrogen Life Technologies Co., Carlsbad, CA, USA) according to the manufacturer's protocol. After 3 h of incubation with AlamarBlue, the fluorescence intensity of each sample was read using a FLUOstar Omega multi-mode microplate reader (BMG Labtech, Germany) with an excitation wavelength of 570 nm and an emission wavelength of 585 nm. Controls were HCEP cells in regular medium without Tualang honey. Cell viability was expressed as a percentage using the following formula:

$$\text{Viability} = \frac{FI_{\text{treated}}}{FI_{\text{non-treated}}} \times 100\%$$

Where

FI_{treated} = Fluorescence intensity of test samples (Tualang honey treated HCEP cells)

$FI_{\text{non-treated}}$ = Fluorescence intensity of control samples (non-treated HCEP cells)

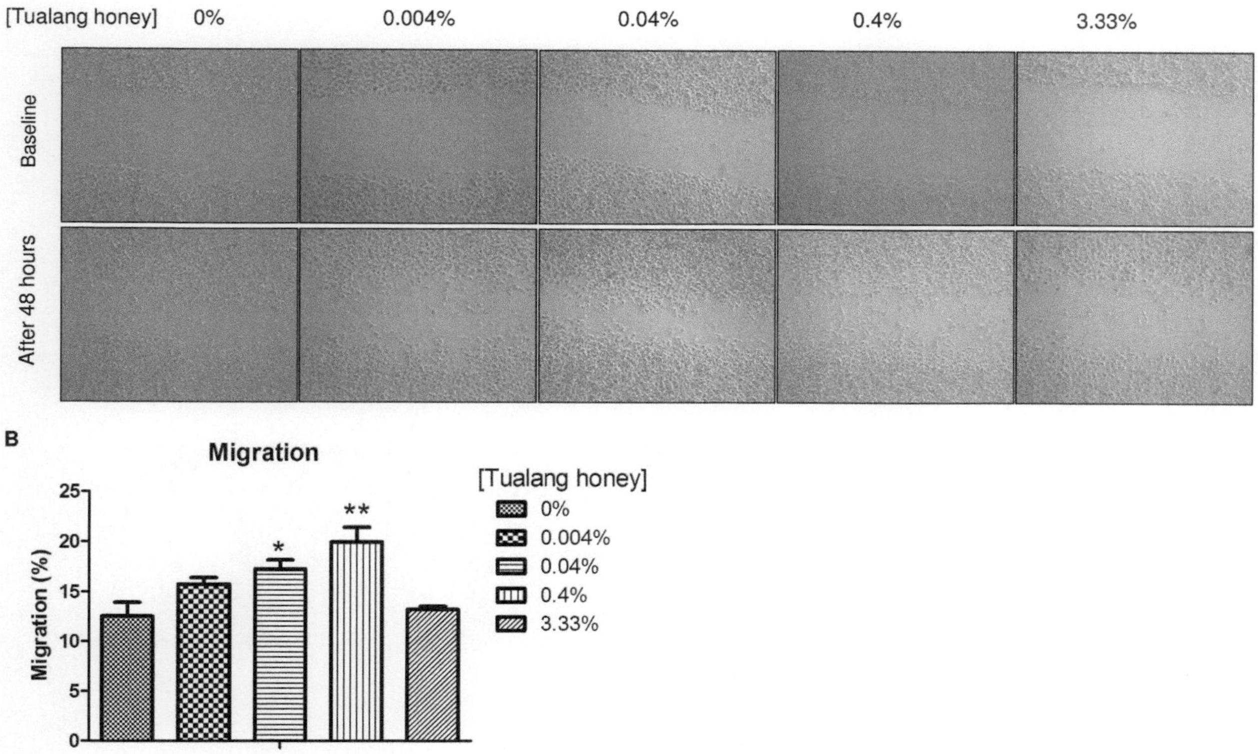

Figure 4. HCEP cell migration following treatment with Tualang honey. (A) Representative images of the HCEP cell scratch migration assay at baseline and after 48 h. (B) The gap size occupied by HCEP cells after 48 h was largest in the 0.4% Tualang honey treatment (*$p<0.05$; **$p<0.01$ compared to untreated control).

Scratch migration assay

HCEP cells were seeded onto a 6-well plate and allowed to expand and reach 90% confluence. A scratch was made onto each HCEP cell-containing well using a 200 µl pipette tip. The culture medium then was changed to standard KSFM supplemented with 0.004, 0.04, 0.4, or 3.33% (v/v) Tualang honey, and the cells were incubated at 37°C for 2 days. Ten representative images were taken using a charge-coupled device camera under an inverted light microscope pre- and post-treatment. Images obtained were analysed for wound closure using ImageJ software (NIH). All experimental samples were compared to a control (i.e., HCEP cells without Tualang honey treatment). The percentage of closure of the gap area was calculated using the following formula:

$$\text{Gap}_{\Delta}(\%) = \text{Gap}_{48}(\%) - \text{Gap}_{0}(\%)$$

Where

Gap_{Δ} = Occupied gap area after 48 h

Gap_{48} = Gap area at 48 h

Gap_{0} = Gap area at baseline

Hydrogen peroxide inhibition assay

Tualang honey was prepared at 0.04, 0.4, and 4% and added to wells containing 5, 10, 20, 30, and 40 µM hydrogen peroxide (H_2O_2). The concentration of H_2O_2 was assessed using the Amplex Red hydrogen peroxide assay kit (Molecular Probes, Invitrogen Life Technologies Co., Carlsbad, CA, USA) after 30 min of incubation at room temperature according to the manufacturer's protocol. The excitation and emission wavelengths were set at 544 and 590 nm, respectively, to obtain the fluorescence reading using FLUOstar Omega multi-mode microplate reader.

Oxidative stress assay

HCEP cells were cultured with 0.004, 0.04, 0.4, and 3.33% (v/v) Tualang honey in supplemented KSFM for 48 h. Treated cells then were exposed to 50 µM H_2O_2 for 24 h. The number of dead cells in treated groups after H_2O_2 exposure was measured using propidium iodide staining (BD Bioscience Franklin Lakes, NJ, USA) and quantified using a flow cytometer (FACS Canto, BD Bioscience Franklin Lakes, NJ, USA). Untreated HCEP cells served as the negative control. Ascorbic acid, a potent anti-H2O2 agent used as a positive control and 5-hydroxymethyl-2-furancarboxaldehyde were both purchased from Sigma, St Louis, MO, USA.

Gas Chromatography-Mass Spectrometry (GC-MS) analysis

GC-MS analysis of the honey was conducted using a Shimadzu system (Japan) consisting of a GC-MS-QP2010 gas chromatograph and a quadrupole mass spectrometer. The interface and source temperatures were 280°C and 250°C, respectively. Electron impact mass spectra were recorded in the 20–650 amu range at 70 eV ionization energy. Separation was performed on a fused-silica bonded-phase capillary column BP X5 (30 mx0.25 mm ID and 0.25 µm film thickness). The injector temperature was set at 250°C; and the samples were run in split mode with the ratio being adjusted to 25:1 and an injection volume of 1 µL. The temperature program was isothermal at

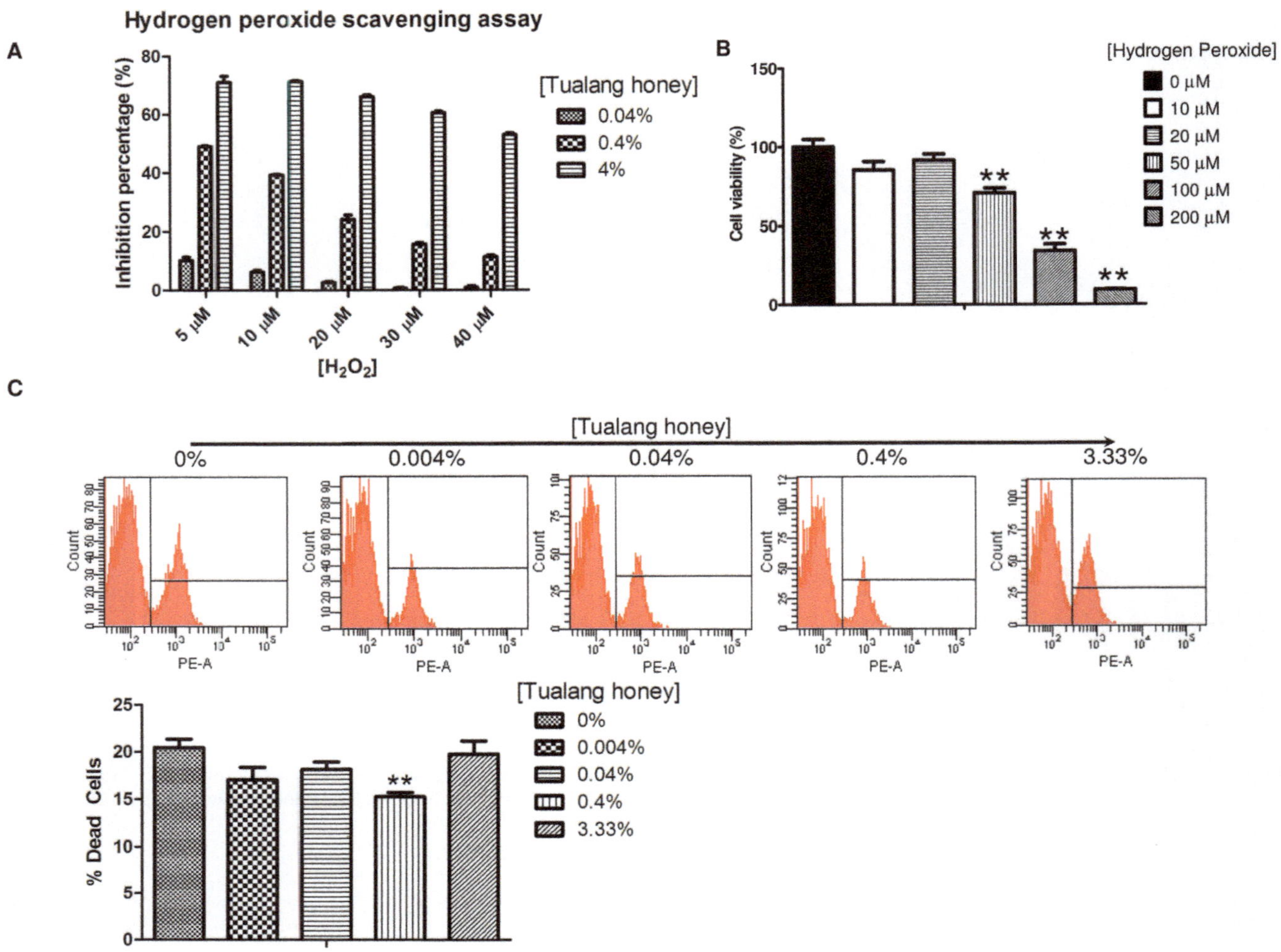

Figure 5. Effects of Tualang honey on hydrogen peroxide and HCEP cell resistance to oxidative stress. (A) *In vitro* inhibitory effects of Tualang honey at 0.04, 0.4, and 4% (v/v) against 5, 10, 20, 30, and 40 µM H_2O_2. (B) HCEP viability in response to H_2O_2 induction at 0, 10, 20, 50, 100 and 200 µM after 24 hours using AlamarBlue assay. (C) Flow cytometric analysis showed the total number of PI-stained dead cells in Tualang honey treated HCEP cells in response to exposure to 50 µM H_2O_2 after 24 h (**$p<0.01$ compared to untreated control). Abbreviation: PI, propidium iodide.

35°C for 1 min, then it was raised to 280°C at 25°C/min and to 310°C at 10°C/min. This temperature was held for 2 min. Samples in the chromatograms were identified by comparing their mass spectra with NIST08 library data as well as the retention times against known standards.

Statistical analysis

All experiments were repeated three times and data were expressed as mean ± standard error (SEM). All statistical analyses were performed using Graphpad Prism (La Jolla, CA, USA). The differences between groups were analysed using one-way ANOVA with Dunnett post-hoc test. Differences were considered significant at $p<0.05$.

Results

Cultured HCEP cells possessed stem cell characteristics

The cultured HCEP cells were highly proliferative and capable of forming holoclones. Immunofluorescence staining confirmed that the cultured HCEP cells used in this study expressed nuclear p63 but not cytokeratin 3/12 (Figure 1), suggesting a keratinocyte stem cell phenotype. However, the cultured HCEP cells exhibited signs of replicative senescence as soon as they reached passage 5 or 6.

Low levels of Tualang honey favoured HCEP cell viability, gene expression, and migration

Viability of HCEP cells was assessed after 24 h and no sign of cytotoxicity was observed in groups treated with 0.004, 0.04, or 0.4%Tualang honey (Figure 2). However, cell viability was significantly reduced to 63.1±2.1% at the concentration of 3.33% compared to the untreated control ($p<0.001$). We also sought to investigate whether Tualang honey could affect HCEP cell stemness or trigger corneal epithelial differentiation. To do this, the mRNA level of ATP-binding cassette transporter 2 (abcg2), a marker which was found to express in human corneal epithelial stem cells, and corneal epithelial differentiation marker connexin-43 and cytokeratin-12, were examined. RTPCR revealed that the mRNA expression for connexin-43 and abcg2 were detected in all groups, but expression of cytokeratin-12 was not (Figure 3A). Semi-quantitative analysis of the expressed mRNA revealed that connexin-43 mRNA remained unaffected by

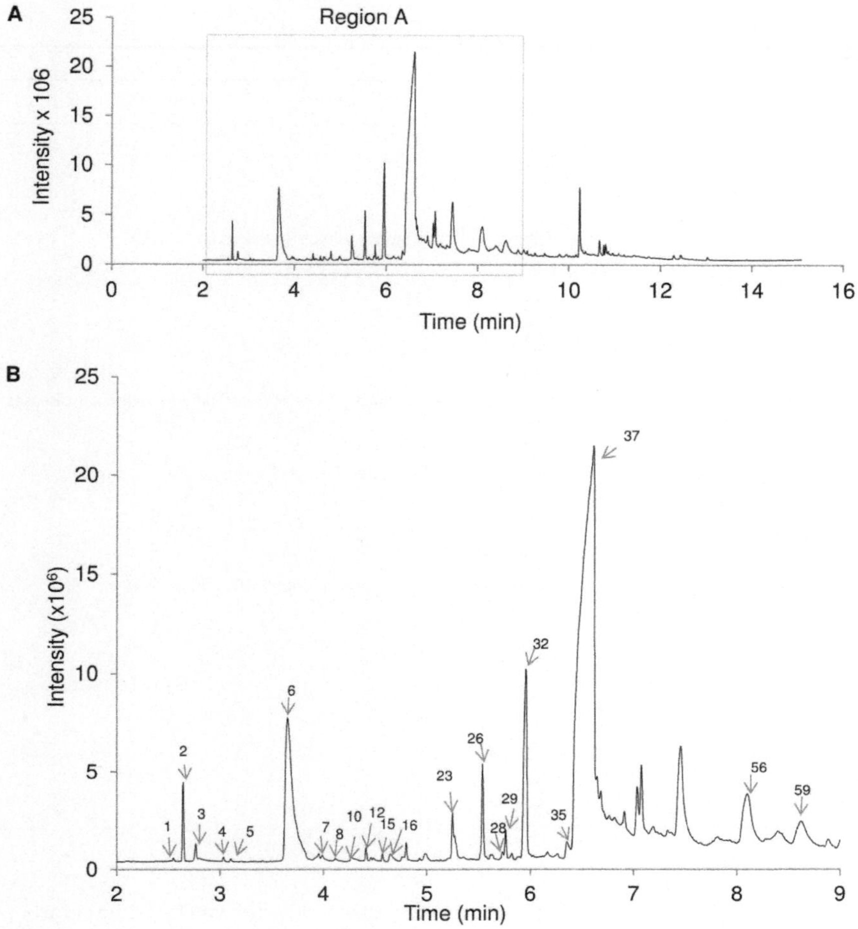

Figure 6. GC-MS analysis of Tualang honey. (A) Region A in the chromatogram of 20% Tualang honey diluted in distilled water. (B) Region A was enlarged and analysed further to identify the phytochemical constituents in Tualang Honey based on the NIST08 Mass Spectral Library.

Tualang honey in all groups, which also indicates that Tualang honey had minimal or no potential in triggering corneal epithelial differentiation. However, a significant down-regulation of abcg2 mRNA was found in HCEP cells treated with 3.33% Tualang honey; this represents a decrease of 47% when compared with the expression in untreated cells ($p<0.05$) (Figure 3B). These results suggest that Tualang honey did not affect the HCEP stemness and differentiation at non-cytotoxic level.

The *in vitro* scratch migration assay showed that the percentage of gap area covered by migrated HCEP cells after 48 h of treatment increased in a dose-dependent manner (Figure 4). HCEP cells treated with 0.04 and 0.4% Tualang honey occupied 17.3±0.9% ($p<0.05$) and 20±1.5% ($p<0.01$) of the gap area, respectively, compared to 12±6% in the untreated group. In the 3.33% Tualang honey treatment, only 13.3±0.3% of the gap area was occupied after 48 h.

Tualang honey scavenged H_2O_2 in a dose-dependent manner and enhanced HCEP cell resistance to oxidative stress

When Tualang honey was tested for its H_2O_2 scavenging ability, the level of inhibition was found to increase with increasing Tualang honey concentration (Figure 5A). This result suggests that Tualang honey is a source of anti-H_2O_2 antioxidant. Notably, only negligible scavenging effects were observed at 30 and 40 µM H_2O_2 when the Tualang honey was diluted to 0.04%. This indicates that over-dilution of Tualang honey may compromise its H_2O_2 scavenging ability. To identify the cytotoxicity of H_2O_2, HCEPs were exposed to 10, 20, 50, 100 and 200 H_2O_2 and the viability was assessed after 24 h using AlamarBlue assay. As shown in Figure 5B, HCEP viability was reduced by H_2O_2 in a dose-dependent manner, and the difference became apparent and statistically significant when H_2O_2 level was increased to ≥50 µM ($p<0.01$).

This study was extended to investigate the potential for Tualang honey to improve HCEP cell resistance to H_2O_2-induced oxidative stress. Interestingly, HCEP cells treated with 0.4% honey had a higher survival rate than the untreated HCEP cells, with a significantly lower number of dead cells (15.3±0.4%) compared to the control (20.5±0.9%, $p<0.01$) (Figure 5C).

Tualang honey contains active compounds with known antioxidant properties

The chromatogram of filtered 20% Tualang honey diluted in distilled water revealed the presence of several volatile compounds (Figure 6). Of those, only 20 chemical constituents were identified (Table 3). The major constituent in Tualang honey was 5-hydroxymethyl-2-furancarboxaldehyde (5HMF), a five carbon ring aromatic aldehyde antioxidant that accounted for a relative peak area of 36.21% [31]. Other known antioxidants, such as 3-

Table 3. Phytochemical constituents detected in Tualang honey.

Peak	Area (%)	Phytochemical	Activity
37	36.21	5-(hydroxymethyl) 2-Furancarboxaldehyde,	Antioxidant [31]
6	7.46	3-Furaldehyde	Antioxidant [32]
56	4.73	Beta.-D-Glucopyranose, 1,6-anhydro-	-
32	4.23	4H-Pyran-4-one, 2,3-dihydro-3,5-dihydroxy-6-methyl-	Antimicrobial, anti-inflammatory [60,61]; antioxidant [62–64]
59	3.06	1,6-Anhydro-.beta.-D-glucofuranose	-
26	1.18	Methyl 2-furoate	-
23	1.13	Phenylacetaldehyde	Antioxidant [65]
2	0.71	Formic acid	-
29	0.33	Levoglucosenone	Anticancer, treatment for autoimmune system and cardiovascular diseases [66]
16	0.2	2-Furancarboxaldehyde, 5-methyl-	-
3	0.16	Acetic acid	Antihistamine [67]
12	0.14	2(5H)-Furanone	-
7	0.13	2-Furanmethanol	Antioxidant [68–70]
28	0.12	Maltol	Antioxidant [71,72], anticonvulsant, depressant [73], anti-aging [74]
35	0.1	2(3H)-Furanone, dihydro-4-hydroxy-	-
8	0.09	Propanoic acid, 2-hydroxy-, ethyl ester	-
15	0.09	2(5H)-Furanone, 5-methyl-	-
10	0.08	2-Propanone, 1,3-dihydroxy-	-
4	0.04	2-Propanone, 1-hydroxy- (CAS) Acetol	-
1	0.03	Hydrogen chloride	-
5	0.02	Propanoic acid, 2-oxo- (CAS) Pyruvic acid	-

furaldehyde (7.46%), phenylacetaldehyde (1.13%), 2-furanmethanol (0.13%), and maltol (0.12%), were also present in Tualang honey [31,32], albeit at lower percentages.

The improvement in HCEP resistance to H_2O_2-induced oxidative stress was attributed to the antioxidant properties of Tualang honey at its native form

To test whether the observed improvement in HCEP resistance to H_2O_2-induced oxidative stress following the treatment with Tualang honey was attributed to 5-hydroxymethyl-2-furancarboxaldehyde (5HMF), the viability of HCEPs treated with 100 μM of 5HMF for 48 h were examined with AlamarBlue after exposed to 50 and 100 μM H_2O_2 for 24 h. As shown in Figure 7, HCEP viability was significantly decreased after treated with 5HMF for 48 h compared to the untreated group ($p<0.05$). However, the viability became comparable to that of untreated control after 24 h induction of H_2O_2 at 50 and 100 μM. This indicates that although 5HMF had little effects in improving HCEP resistance to H_2O_2, the benefit was nullified by its mild cytotoxicity.

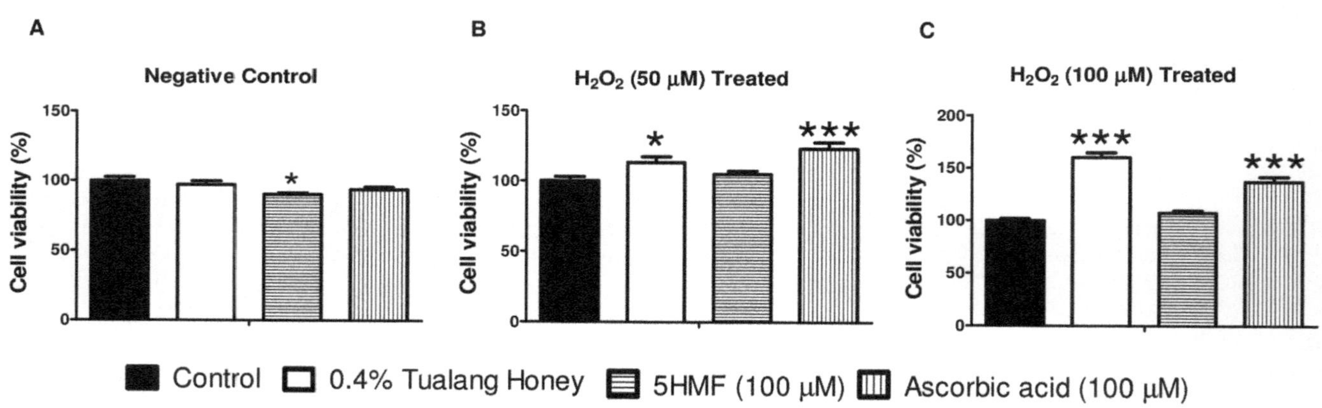

Figure 7. AlamarBlue cell viability assay of Tualang honey (0.4%), ascorbic acid (100 μM) and 5HMF(100 μM) treated HCEP cells after H_2O_2 induction. The resistance of treated cells against H_2O_2 was tested at (A) 0, (B) 50 and (C) 100 μM for 24 h. Significant difference in viability was found between Tualang honey and ascorbic acid-treated group using ANOVA with Tukey multiple comparisons test (*$p<0.05$; ***$p<0.01$ compared to untreated control). Abbreviation: 5HMF, 5-hydroxymethyl-2-furancarboxaldehyde.

Table 4. pH values of HCEP cell culture medium after supplementation with Tualang honey at various concentrations.

Tualang Honey concentrations	0%	0.004%	0.04%	0.4%	3.33%	5.0%	10.0%
pH	7.65	7.67	7.58	7.59	7.17	5.83	4.81

To assess whether the antioxidant property of Tualang honey was responsible for the elevated resistance to H_2O_2-induced oxidative stress, HCEPs treated with 100 μM ascorbic acid, a known powerful antioxidant, was included as the positive control. AlamarBlue assay showed better HCEP survival following H_2O_2 insults at 50 μM and 100 μM after treated with ascorbic acid or Tualang honey as compared to the untreated group. More importantly, the resistance to 100 μM H_2O_2 was found significantly greater in Tualang honey-treated HCEP cells than that of ascorbic acid-treated (Figure 7C). Taken together, these results confirm that the enhanced HCEP resistance to oxidative stress is conferred by the antioxidant property of Tualang honey in its native form.

Discussion

Tualang honey has been used to treat bacterial infections [33], promote burn wound healing [19,34], and protect bone in post-menopausal women [18]. However, its potential as a supplement in cell culture medium for stem cell expansion has not been studied, and little is known about the effects of honey on cells at the cellular level. This is the first study to evaluate the use of Tualang honey in culturing HCEP cells and its effects in enhancing cell function *in vitro*. Thus, it is a pivotal study for exploring the potential of this honey and its application in corneal regeneration.

The ATP binding cassette transport 2 (abcg2) is known for its capability to efflux Hoechst 33342 and has been used as a marker to identify side population cells [35]. This marker was also found to present in clonogenic human limbal-derived epithelial stem cells [36]. A study by Kubota et al. (2010) suggested that abcg2 has a vital role in maintaining endogenous anti-oxidative capacity in HCEPs [37]. Here, the cultured human corneal epithelial cells used in this study expressed mRNA for abcg2 and nuclear p63 protein, the putative corneal epithelial stem cell markers [38,39]. However, significant downregulation of abcg2 mRNA was detected when Tualang honey was introduced to the cells at cytotoxic level, 3.33%. This may also suggest that the cytotoxicity of Tualang honey in HCEP cells is via the downregulation of abcg2 expression, reduces the cell anti-oxidative capacity which renders the cells susceptible to oxidative damage. Although no terminal corneal epithelial differentiation was detected (based on the lack of cytokeratin 3 protein and cytokeratin 12 mRNA expression), we found that the cells constantly expressed gap junction protein connexin-43 mRNA, a negative marker for corneal epithelial stem cells [40]. This suggests that the cells had partial commitment to the corneal epithelial lineage. Hence, in order to accurately describe the cell population, we called them human corneal epithelial progenitor cells (i.e., HCEPs).

Previous studies showed that the bactericidal effects of honey were partly, if not entirely, due to its acidity, high osmolality, and H_2O_2 content [41,42]. These characteristics could also be cytotoxic to cells. We addressed the cytotoxicity of Tualang honey to cultured HCEP cells by lowering the concentration to a level that favoured cell growth (≤0.4%). Our data show that the pH of the culture medium was not altered by Tualang honey at low concentration (0.004–0.4%), but the medium became acidic at high concentration (3.33%) (Table 4). Furthermore, a high level of honey supplementation could produce a hyperosmotic culture medium, which could induce ROS generation and apoptosis in corneal epithelial cells [43]. In contrast to our finding, Ghashm *et al.* (2010) reported that the pH of the culture medium remained suitable for cell culture after adding Tualang honey at high concentrations (3.5–20%) compared to the control medium without Tualang honey [23]. This discrepancy may be due to differences in preparation and storage conditions of the Tualang honey used in the experiments, as storage conditions can alter the content and properties of the honey [44].

We also found that Tualang honey diluted to 0.04% did not affect gene expression and was favourable to HCEP cells, as shown by the enhanced cell migration *in vitro* in this treatment. This result suggests that dilution of Tualang honey does not hamper its beneficial effects on HCEP cells. These data coincide with a past study that showed improvement in proliferation of human osteoblast cells (CRL 1543) when the culture medium was supplemented with 0.0195% Tualang honey [30]. The underlying mechanism for the observed improvements is unknown, but it could be related to the active compounds present in Tualang honey or to the presence of H_2O_2, a ROS that is essential for modulating stem cell behaviours at the physiological level [45–47]. Pan *et al.* (2011) recently suggested that low levels of H_2O_2 (10–50 μM) could promote rabbit corneal epithelial cell attachment, mobility, and wound repair [48]. This contradicts our findings using human cells that H_2O_2 showed significant cytotoxicity at 50 μM and no noticeable changes in cell number at 10 and 20 μM when compared with the untreated control. Nonetheless, this discrepancy may due to the difference in the species of origin of corneal epithelial cells used in the experiments.

Furthermore, we also found that H_2O_2 was present in Tualang honey, but only at a negligible level of <2 μM after dilution to ≤ 0.4%. This finding suggests that the H_2O_2 level may not be sufficient to exert significant changes in cell behaviours. Although H_2O_2 is present in naturally occurring Tualang honey, it also contains several phytochemical compounds with antioxidant properties that are capable of mitigating H_2O_2. The predominant phytocompound identified in Tualang honey was 5-hydroxy-methyl-2-furancarboxaldehyde, which is a five carbon ring aromatic aldehyde antioxidant that is commonly found in fruits [49] and marine products [50]. Compared to other types of honey, Tualang honey had been identified as a new source of antioxidant with superior activity that is attributed to its high phenolic content [51].

Oxidative stress has been shown to cause chromosomal instability, shortened telomeres, and cellular replicative senescence in stem cells *in vitro* [52,53], all of which hamper cell function and limit the therapeutic outcome of cell transplantation. Accumulating evidence supports the premise that cellular antioxidant levels in stem cells play a vital role in dictating their fate, regenerative capability, and therapeutic outcome after transplantation [54,55]. Overexpression of cellular redox regulators such as Cu/Zn superoxide dismutase enzymes and nuclear factor erythroid 2-

related factor-2 (Nrf-2) has been shown to improve stem cell functions [56]. The oxidative stress tolerance of stem cells can also be augmented by the addition of exogenous catalase [57] or antioxidants from natural products [16,58,59]. Herein, Tualang honey at 0.4% was found to improve HCEP cell resistance to oxidative stress, as shown by the significantly lower number of dead cells after treatment with 50 μM H_2O_2 in the treatment versus control group. This indicates that Tualang honey can be used as a source of antioxidant for preconditioning HCEP cells prior to transplantation. However, more evidence is needed to confirm the changes in HCEP cell antioxidant enzyme levels that likely account for the Tualang honey-induced enhancement of the oxidative stress tolerance of HCEP cells.

In summary, this study describes a novel approach to integrating the application of natural products to the process of corneal regeneration. Our data indicate that Tualang honey is an antioxidant and contains active phytocompounds that enhance HCEP cell migration and resistance to oxidative stress *in vitro* in a dose-dependent manner. The beneficial effects, however, are offset by the cytotoxicity of Tualang honey at high concentration. In-depth studies to isolate and identify the active components in Tualang honey and to identify the mechanism responsible for the observed benefits *in vitro* and *in vivo* are needed to enable use of this natural product for the treatment of corneal diseases.

Acknowledgments

The authors thank Dr. Gary Yam (Singapore Eye Research Institute), Dr. Fam Pei Shan, Nur Hikmah binti Ramli, and Noraida binti Zakaria (Universiti Sains Malaysia) for their technical help with this project, and special appreciation goes to David Lyn (Matrix Optics) for his assistance with confocal microscopy.

Author Contributions

Conceived and designed the experiments: JJT BS. Performed the experiments: JJT SMA HLC VL. Analyzed the data: JJT YKY VL. Contributed reagents/materials/analysis tools: JJT DS BS. Wrote the paper: JJT.

References

1. Chen Z, de Paiva CS, Luo L, Kretzer FL, Pflugfelder SC, et al. (2004) Characterization of putative stem cell phenotype in human limbal epithelia. Stem Cells 22: 355–366.
2. Kim HS, Jun Song X, de Paiva CS, Chen Z, Pflugfelder SC, et al. (2004) Phenotypic characterization of human corneal epithelial cells expanded ex vivo from limbal explant and single cell cultures. Exp Eye Res 79: 41–49.
3. He Y, Pan Z, Luo F (2012) A Novel PAX6 Mutation in Chinese Patients with Severe Congenital Aniridia. Current Eye Research 37: 879–883.
4. Smith W, Lange J, Sturm A, Tanner S, Mauger T (2012) Familial peripheral keratopathy without PAX6 mutation. Cornea 31: 130–133.
5. Le Belle JE, Orozco NM, Paucar AA, Saxe JP, Mottahedeh J, et al. (2011) Proliferative neural stem cells have high endogenous ROS levels that regulate self-renewal and neurogenesis in a PI3K/Akt-dependant manner. Cell Stem Cell 8: 59–71.
6. Ito K, Hirao A, Arai F, Takubo K, Matsuoka S, et al. (2006) Reactive oxygen species act through p38 MAPK to limit the lifespan of hematopoietic stem cells. Nat Med 12: 446–451.
7. Li TS, Marban E (2010) Physiological levels of reactive oxygen species are required to maintain genomic stability in stem cells. Stem Cells 28: 1178–1185.
8. Chaudhari P, Ye Z, Jang YY (2012) Roles of Reactive Oxygen Species in the Fate of Stem Cells. Antioxid Redox Signal.
9. Pendergrass KD, Boopathy AV, Seshadri G, Maiellaro-Rafferty K, Che PL, et al. (2013) Acute Preconditioning of Cardiac Progenitor Cells with Hydrogen Peroxide Enhances Angiogenic Pathways Following Ischemia-Reperfusion Injury. Stem Cells Dev.
10. Limoli CL, Giedzinski E (2003) Induction of chromosomal instability by chronic oxidative stress. Neoplasia 5: 339–346.
11. Kryston TB, Georgiev AB, Pissis P, Georgakilas AG (2011) Role of oxidative stress and DNA damage in human carcinogenesis. Mutat Res 711: 193–201.
12. Song H, Cha MJ, Song BW, Kim IK, Chang W, et al. (2010) Reactive oxygen species inhibit adhesion of mesenchymal stem cells implanted into ischemic myocardium via interference of focal adhesion complex. Stem Cells 28: 555–563.
13. Dernbach E, Urbich C, Brandes RP, Hofmann WK, Zeiher AM, et al. (2004) Antioxidative stress-associated genes in circulating progenitor cells: evidence for enhanced resistance against oxidative stress. Blood 104: 3591–3597.
14. Urish KL, Vella JB, Okada M, Deasy BM, Tobita K, et al. (2009) Antioxidant levels represent a major determinant in the regenerative capacity of muscle stem cells. Mol Biol Cell 20: 509–520.
15. Ko E, Lee KY, Hwang DS (2012) Human umbilical cord blood-derived mesenchymal stem cells undergo cellular senescence in response to oxidative stress. Stem Cells Dev 21: 1877–1886.
16. Gurusamy N, Ray D, Lekli I, Das DK (2010) Red wine antioxidant resveratrol-modified cardiac stem cells regenerate infarcted myocardium. J Cell Mol Med 14: 2235–2239.
17. Alves H, Mentink A, Le B, van Blitterswijk CA, de Boer J (2013) Effect of antioxidant supplementation on the total yield, oxidative stress levels, and multipotency of bone marrow-derived human mesenchymal stromal cells. Tissue Eng Part A 19: 928–937.
18. Mohd Effendy N, Mohamed N, Muhammad N, Mohamad IN, Shuid AN (2012) The effects of tualang honey on bone metabolism of postmenopausal women. Evid Based Complement Alternat Med 2012: 938574.
19. Khoo YT, Halim AS, Singh KK, Mohamad NA (2010) Wound contraction effects and antibacterial properties of Tualang honey on full-thickness burn wounds in rats in comparison to hydrofibre. BMC Complement Altern Med 10: 48.
20. Nasir NA, Halim AS, Singh KK, Dorai AA, Haneef MN (2010) Antibacterial properties of tualang honey and its effect in burn wound management: a comparative study. BMC Complement Altern Med 10: 31.
21. Mat Lazim N, Abdullah B, Salim R (2013) The effect of Tualang honey in enhancing post tonsillectomy healing process. An open labelled prospective clinical trial. Int J Pediatr Otorhinolaryngol 77: 457–461.
22. Yaacob NS, Nengsih A, Norazmi MN (2013) Tualang honey promotes apoptotic cell death induced by tamoxifen in breast cancer cell lines. Evid Based Complement Alternat Med 2013: 989841.
23. Ghashm AA, Othman NH, Khattak MN, Ismail NM, Saini R (2010) Antiproliferative effect of Tualang honey on oral squamous cell carcinoma and osteosarcoma cell lines. BMC Complement Altern Med 10: 49.
24. Fauzi AN, Norazmi MN, Yaacob NS (2011) Tualang honey induces apoptosis and disrupts the mitochondrial membrane potential of human breast and cervical cancer cell lines. Food Chem Toxicol 49: 871–878.
25. Albietz JM, Lenton LM (2006) Effect of antibacterial honey on the ocular flora in tear deficiency and meibomian gland disease. Cornea 25: 1012–1019.
26. Mansour AM (2002) Epithelial corneal oedema treated with honey. Clinical & experimental ophthalmology 30: 149–150.
27. Uwaydat S, Jha P, Tytarenko R, Brown H, Wiggins M, et al. (2011) The use of topical honey in the treatment of corneal abrasions and endotoxin-induced keratitis in an animal model. Current eye research 36: 787–796.
28. Bashkaran K, Zunaina E, Bakiah S, Sulaiman SA, Sirajudeen K, et al. (2011) Anti-inflammatory and antioxidant effects of Tualang honey in alkali injury on the eyes of rabbits: experimental animal study. BMC Complement Altern Med 11: 90.
29. Ahmad I, Jimenez H, Yaacob NS, Yusuf N (2012) Tualang honey protects keratinocytes from ultraviolet radiation-induced inflammation and DNA damage. Photochem Photobiol 88: 1198–1204.
30. Kannan TP, Ali AQ, Abdullah SF, Ahmad A (2009) Evaluation of Tualang honey as a supplement to fetal bovine serum in cell culture. Food Chem Toxicol 47: 1696–1702.
31. Mohamed SA, Khan JA (2013) Antioxidant capacity of chewing stick miswak Salvadora persica. BMC Complementary and Alternative Medicine 13: 40.
32. Frankel EN (1985) Chemistry of autoxidation: mechanism, products and flavor significance. American Oil Chemists' Society, Champaign.
33. Tan HT, Rahman RA, Gan SH, Halim AS, Hassan SA, et al. (2009) The antibacterial properties of Malaysian tualang honey against wound and enteric microorganisms in comparison to manuka honey. BMC Complement Altern Med 9: 34.
34. Sukur SM, Halim AS, Singh KK (2011) Evaluations of bacterial contaminated full thickness burn wound healing in Sprague Dawley rats Treated with Tualang honey. Indian J Plast Surg 44: 112–117.
35. Zhou S, Schuetz JD, Bunting KD, Colapietro AM, Sampath J, et al. (2001) The ABC transporter Bcrp1/ABCG2 is expressed in a wide variety of stem cells and is a molecular determinant of the side-population phenotype. Nat Med 7: 1028–1034.
36. de Paiva CS, Chen Z, Corrales RM, Pflugfelder SC, Li DQ (2005) ABCG2 transporter identifies a population of clonogenic human limbal epithelial cells. Stem Cells 23: 63–73.
37. Kubota M, Shimmura S, Miyashita H, Kawashima M, Kawakita T, et al. (2010) The anti-oxidative role of ABCG2 in corneal epithelial cells. Invest Ophthalmol Vis Sci 51: 5617–5622.
38. Priya CG, Prasad T, Prajna NV, Muthukkaruppan V (2013) Identification of human corneal epithelial stem cells on the basis of high ABCG2 expression

combined with a large N/C ratio. Microscopy research and technique 76: 242–248.
39. Arpitha P, Prajna NV, Srinivasan M, Muthukkaruppan V (2005) High expression of p63 combined with a large N/C ratio defines a subset of human limbal epithelial cells: implications on epithelial stem cells. Investigative ophthalmology & visual science 46: 3631–3636.
40. Chen Z, Evans WH, Pflugfelder SC, Li DQ (2006) Gap junction protein connexin 43 serves as a negative marker for a stem cell-containing population of human limbal epithelial cells. Stem Cells 24: 1265–1273.
41. Mavric E, Wittmann S, Barth G, Henle T (2008) Identification and quantification of methylglyoxal as the dominant antibacterial constituent of Manuka (Leptospermum scoparium) honeys from New Zealand. Mol Nutr Food Res 52: 483–489.
42. Cheng G, He Y, Xie L, Nie Y, He B, et al. (2012) Development of a reduction-sensitive diselenide-conjugated oligoethylenimine nanoparticulate system as a gene carrier. Int J Nanomedicine 7: 3991–4006.
43. Chen Y, Li M, Li B, Wang W, Lin A, et al. (2013) Effect of reactive oxygen species generation in rabbit corneal epithelial cells on inflammatory and apoptotic signaling pathways in the presence of high osmotic pressure. PloS one 8: e72900.
44. Brudzynski K, Kim L (2011) Storage-induced chemical changes in active components of honey de-regulate its antibacterial activity. Food Chem 126: 1155–1163.
45. Daniels-Wells TR, Helguera G, Rodriguez JA, Leoh LS, Erb MA, et al. (2013) Insights into the mechanism of cell death induced by saporin delivered into cancer cells by an antibody fusion protein targeting the transferrin receptor 1. Toxicol In Vitro 27: 220–231.
46. Cho KA, Woo SY, Seoh JY, Han HS, Ryu KH (2012) Mesenchymal stem cells restore CCl4-induced liver injury by an antioxidative process. Cell Biol Int 36: 1267–1274.
47. Ding H, Keller KC, Martinez IK, Geransar RM, zur Nieden KO, et al. (2012) NO-beta-catenin crosstalk modulates primitive streak formation prior to embryonic stem cell osteogenic differentiation. J Cell Sci 125: 5564–5577.
48. Pan Q, Qiu WY, Huo YN, Yao YF, Lou MF (2011) Low levels of hydrogen peroxide stimulate corneal epithelial cell adhesion, migration, and wound healing. Investigative ophthalmology & visual science 52: 1723–1734.
49. Palma M, Taylor LT (2001) Supercritical fluid extraction of 5-hydroxymethyl-2-furaldehyde from raisins. J Agric Food Chem 49: 628–632.
50. Kulkarni A, Suzuki S, Etoh H (2008) Antioxidant compounds from Eucalyptus grandis biomass by subcritical liquid water extraction. J Wood Sci 54: 153–157.
51. Kishore RK, Halim AS, Syazana MS, Sirajudeen KN (2011) Tualang honey has higher phenolic content and greater radical scavenging activity compared with other honey sources. Nutr Res 31: 322–325.
52. Liu AM, Qu WW, Liu X, Qu CK (2012) Chromosomal instability in in vitro cultured mouse hematopoietic cells associated with oxidative stress. Am J Blood Res 2: 71–76.
53. Richter T, von Zglinicki T (2007) A continuous correlation between oxidative stress and telomere shortening in fibroblasts. Exp Gerontol 42: 1039–1042.
54. Abasi M, Massumi M, Riazi G, Amini H (2012) The synergistic effect of beta-boswellic acid and Nurr1 overexpression on dopaminergic programming of antioxidant glutathione peroxidase-1-expressing murine embryonic stem cells. Neuroscience 222: 404–416.
55. Sakata H, Niizuma K, Wakai T, Narasimhan P, Maier CM, et al. (2012) Neural stem cells genetically modified to overexpress cu/zn-superoxide dismutase enhance amelioration of ischemic stroke in mice. Stroke 43: 2423–2429.
56. Chatterjee S, Browning EA, Hong N, DeBolt K, Sorokina EM, et al. (2012) Membrane depolarization is the trigger for PI3K/Akt activation and leads to the generation of ROS. Am J Physiol Heart Circ Physiol 302: H105–114.
57. Urtasun R, Lopategi A, George J, Leung TM, Lu Y, et al. (2012) Osteopontin, an oxidant stress sensitive cytokine, up-regulates collagen-I via integrin alpha(V)beta(3) engagement and PI3K/pAkt/NFkappaB signaling. Hepatology 55: 594–608.
58. Schauen M, Spitkovsky D, Schubert J, Fischer JH, Hayashi J, et al. (2006) Respiratory chain deficiency slows down cell-cycle progression via reduced ROS generation and is associated with a reduction of p21CIP1/WAF1. J Cell Physiol 209: 103–112.
59. Esteban MA, Wang T, Qin B, Yang J, Qin D, et al. (2010) Vitamin C enhances the generation of mouse and human induced pluripotent stem cells. Cell Stem Cell 6: 71–79.
60. Ragupathi Raja Kannan R, Arumugam R, Anantharaman P (2012) Chemical composition and antibacterial activity of Indian seagrasses against urinary tract pathogens. Food chemistry 135: 2470–2473.
61. Kumar PP, Kumaravel S, Lalitha C (2010) Screening of antioxidant activity, total phenolics and GC-MS study of Vitex negundo. African Journal of Biochemistry Research 4: 191–195.
62. Xiangying Y, Zhao M, Fei L,Shitong Z,Jun H (2013) Identification of 2,3-dihydro-3,5-dihydroxy-6-methyl-4H-pyran-4-one as a strong antioxidant in glucose–histidine Maillard reaction products. Food Research International 51: 397–403.
63. Čechovská L, Cejpek K, Konečný M, Velíšek J (2011) On the role of 2,3-dihydro-3,5-dihydroxy-6-methyl-(4H)-pyran-4-one in antioxidant capacity of prunes. European Food Research and Technology 233: 367–376.
64. Osada Y, Shibamoto T (2006) Antioxidative activity of volatile extracts from Maillard model systems. Food chemistry 98: 522–528.
65. Nam S, Jang HW, Shibamoto T (2012) Antioxidant Activities of Extracts from Teas Prepared from Medicinal Plants, Morus alba L., Camellia sinensis L. and Cudrania tricuspidata and Their Volatile Components. Journal of Agricultural and Food Chemistry 60: 9097–9105.
66. Westman J, Wiman K, Mohell N (2007) Levoglucosenone derivatives for the treatment of disorders such as cancer, autoimmune diseases and heart diseases. In: W. I. P. . Organization, editor editors. Geneva Switzerland.
67. Ruiz CM, Gomes JC (2000) Effects of ethanol, acetaldehyde, and acetic acid on histamine secretion in guinea pig lung mast cells. Alcohol 20: 133–138.
68. Wei A, Mura K, Shibamoto T. (2001) Antioxidative activity of volatile chemicals extracted from beer. Journal of Agricultural and Food Chemistry 49: 4097–4101.
69. Fuster MD, Mitchell AE, Ochi H, Shibamoto T (2000) Antioxidative activities of heterocyclic compounds formed in brewed coffee. Journal of Agricultural and Food Chemistry 48: 5600–5603.
70. Yanagimoto K, Lee KG, Ochi H, Shibamoto T. (2002) Antioxidative activity of heterocyclic compounds found in coffee volatiles produced by Maillard reaction. Journal of Agricultural and Food Chemistry 50: 5480–5484.
71. Suh DY, Han YN, Han BH (1996) Maltol, an antioxidant component of Korean red ginseng, shows little prooxidant activity. Archives of Pharmacal Research 19: 112–115.
72. Lee KG, Shibamoto T (2000) Antioxidant properties of aroma compounds isolated from soybeans and mung beans. Journal of Agricultural and Food Chemistry 48: 4290–4293.
73. Aoyagi N, Kimura R, Murata T (1974) Studies on Passiflora incarnata dry extract. I. Isolation of maltol and pharmacological action of maltol and ethyl maltol. Chemical & pharmaceutical bulletin 22: 1008–1013.
74. Choi KT (2008) Botanical characteristics, pharmacological effects and medicinal components of Korean Panax ginseng CA Meyer. Acta Pharmacologica Sinica 29: 1109–1118.

Permissions

All chapters in this book were first published in PLOS ONE, by The Public Library of Science; hereby published with permission under the Creative Commons Attribution License or equivalent. Every chapter published in this book has been scrutinized by our experts. Their significance has been extensively debated. The topics covered herein carry significant findings which will fuel the growth of the discipline. They may even be implemented as practical applications or may be referred to as a beginning point for another development.

The contributors of this book come from diverse backgrounds, making this book a truly international effort. This book will bring forth new frontiers with its revolutionizing research information and detailed analysis of the nascent developments around the world.

We would like to thank all the contributing authors for lending their expertise to make the book truly unique. They have played a crucial role in the development of this book. Without their invaluable contributions this book wouldn't have been possible. They have made vital efforts to compile up to date information on the varied aspects of this subject to make this book a valuable addition to the collection of many professionals and students.

This book was conceptualized with the vision of imparting up-to-date information and advanced data in this field. To ensure the same, a matchless editorial board was set up. Every individual on the board went through rigorous rounds of assessment to prove their worth. After which they invested a large part of their time researching and compiling the most relevant data for our readers.

The editorial board has been involved in producing this book since its inception. They have spent rigorous hours researching and exploring the diverse topics which have resulted in the successful publishing of this book. They have passed on their knowledge of decades through this book. To expedite this challenging task, the publisher supported the team at every step. A small team of assistant editors was also appointed to further simplify the editing procedure and attain best results for the readers.

Apart from the editorial board, the designing team has also invested a significant amount of their time in understanding the subject and creating the most relevant covers. They scrutinized every image to scout for the most suitable representation of the subject and create an appropriate cover for the book.

The publishing team has been an ardent support to the editorial, designing and production team. Their endless efforts to recruit the best for this project, has resulted in the accomplishment of this book. They are a veteran in the field of academics and their pool of knowledge is as vast as their experience in printing. Their expertise and guidance has proved useful at every step. Their uncompromising quality standards have made this book an exceptional effort. Their encouragement from time to time has been an inspiration for everyone.

The publisher and the editorial board hope that this book will prove to be a valuable piece of knowledge for researchers, students, practitioners and scholars across the globe.

List of Contributors

Peter A. Lindsey
Panthera, New York, New York, United States of America
Mammal Research Institute, Department of Zoology and Entomology, University of Pretoria, Pretoria, Gauteng, South Africa

Vincent R. Nyirenda
Zambia Wildlife Authority, Chilanga, Lusaka, Zambia

Jonathan I. Barnes
Design & Development Services, Windhoek, Namibia

Matthew S. Becker
Department of Ecology, Montana State University, Bozeman, Montana, United States of America
Zambian Carnivore Programme, Mfuwe, Zambia

Rachel McRobb
South Luangwa Conservation Society, Mfuwe, Zambia

Craig J. Tambling
Centre for African Conservation Ecology, Department of Zoology, Nelson Mandela Metropolitan University, Port Elizabeth, South Africa

W. Andrew Taylor
Centre for Veterinary Wildlife Studies, Faculty of Veterinary Science, University of Pretoria, Pretoria, South Africa

Frederick G. Watson
Zambian Carnivore Programme, Mfuwe, Zambia
Division of Science and Environmental Policy, California State University Monterey Bay, Seaside, California, United States of America

Michael t'Sas-Rolfes
Cape Town, South Africa

Alisa L. Gallant
United States Geological Survey, Earth Resources Observation and Science Center, Sioux Falls, South Dakota, United States of America

Ned H. Euliss Jr.
United States Geological Survey, Northern Prairie Wildlife Research Center, Jamestown, North Dakota, United States of America

Zac Browning
Browning's Honey Company, Inc., Jamestown, North Dakota, United States of America

Michael J. Gill
Department of Psychology, Lehigh University, Bethlehem, Pennsylvania, United States of America

Michael R. Andreychik
Department of Psychology, Fairfield University, Fairfield, Connecticut, United States of America

Véronique Bach, Erwan Stéphan-Blanchard and Karen Chardon
Laboratoire PériTox, Unité mixte Université - INERIS (EA 4285-UMI 01), Université de Picardie Jules Verne, Amiens, France

Thierry Berton
Laboratoire PériTox, Unité mixte Université - INERIS (EA 4285-UMI 01), Université de Picardie Jules Verne, Amiens, France
Unité NOVA, Institut National de l'Environnement Industriel et des Risques, Verneuil en Halatte, France

Caroline Deguines
Laboratoire PériTox, Unitémixte Université- INERIS (EA 4285-UMI 01), Université de Picardie Jules Verne, Amiens, France
Médecine Néonatale, Pôle Femme-Couple-Enfant, Centre Hospitalier Universitaire d'Amiens, Amiens, France

Flora Mayhoub
Laboratoire PériTox, Unitémixte Université - INERIS (EA 4285-UMI 01), Université de Picardie Jules Verne, Amiens, France
Faculty of Medicine, Tishreen University, Latakia, Syria

Adeline Floch- Barneaud
Laboratoire PériTox, Unitémixte Université- INERIS (EA 4285-UMI 01), Université de Picardie Jules Verne, Amiens, France
UnitéISAE, Institut National de l'Environnement Industrielet des Risques, Verneuil en Halatte, France

Sophie Desmots
Laboratoire PériTox, Unitémixte Université - INERIS (EA 4285-UMI 01), Université de Picardie Jules Verne, Amiens, France
Unité TOXI, Institut National de l'Environnement Industriel et des Risques, Verneuil en Halatte, France

Karine Tack
Unité NOVA, Institut National de l'Environnement Industriel et des Risques, Verneuil en Halatte, France

Martin Patenaude-Monette and Jean-François Giroux
Groupe de recherche en écologie comportementaleet animale, Département des sciences biologiques, Université du Québec á Montréal, Montréal, Québec, Canada

Marc Bélisle
Département de biologie, Université de Sherbrooke, Sherbrooke, Québec, Canada

Vincent Bonhomme, Srinivasan Prasad, Cédric Gaucherel and Krishnamurthy Anupama
Department of Ecology, French Institute of Pondicherry, UMIFRE 21 CNRS-MAEE/USR 3330, Pondicherry, India

Raja Ponnuchamy
Department of Ecology, French Institute of Pondicherry, UMIFRE 21 CNRS-MAEE/USR 3330, Pondicherry, India
Department of Botany, Kanchi Mamunivar Centre for Post-Graduate Studies, Pondicherry, India

Arunachalam Pragasam
Department of Botany, Kanchi Mamunivar Centre for Post-Graduate Studies, Pondicherry, India

Lipi Das and Prakash Patel
Sri Aurobindo International Centre of Education, Pondicherry, India

Forough Aghili, Hannes A. Gamper and Emmanuel Frossard
Institute of Agricultural Sciences, Department of Environmental Systems Science, Swiss Federal Institute of Technology (ETH) Zürich, Switzerland

Jost Eikenberg
Paul Scherrer Institute (PSI), Radioanalytics Laboratory, Villigen, Switzerland

Amir H. Khoshgoftarmanesh and Majid Afyuni
College of Agriculture, Department of Soil Sciences, Isfahan University of Technology, Isfahan, Iran

Rainer Schulin
Institute of Terrestrial Ecosystems, Department of Environmental Systems Science, Swiss Federal Institute of Technology (ETH) Zürich, Switzerland

Jan Jansa
Institute of Microbiology, Academy of Sciences of the Czech Republic, Prague, Czech Republic

Thomas Van Hecke, Els Vossen and Stefaan De Smet
Laboratory for Animal Nutrition and Animal Product Quality, Department of Animal Production, Faculty of Bioscience Engineering, Ghent University, Melle, Belgium

Julie Vanden Bussche and Lynn Vanhaecke
Laboratory of Chemical Analysis, Department of Veterinary Public Health and Food Safety, Faculty of Veterinary Medicine, Ghent University, Merelbeke, Belgium

Katleen Raes
Laboratory for Food Microbiology and Biotechnology, Department of Industrial Biological Sciences, Faculty of Bioscience Engineering, Ghent University - Campus Kortrijk, Kortrijk, Belgium

Sarah Bortolamiol
UMR 7533 Laboratoire Dynamiques Sociales et Recomposition des Espaces, Paris Diderot University (Sorbonne Paris Cité), Paris, France
UMR 7206 Eco-Anthropologieet Ethnobiologie (MNHN/CNRS/Paris Diderot), Paris, France
Great Ape Conservation Project (PCGS), Sebitoli UWA Station in Kibale National Park, Fort Portal, Uganda

Marianne Cohen
UMR 7533 Laboratoire Dynamiques Sociales et Recomposition des Espaces, Paris Diderot University (Sorbonne Paris Cité), Paris, France
Pole Image, Paris Diderot University (Sorbonne Paris Cité), Paris, France

Flora Pennec
UMR 7206 Eco-Anthropologieet Ethnobiologie (MNHN/CNRS/Paris Diderot), Paris, France

Quentin Vignaud
UMR 7206 Eco-Anthropologieet Ethnobiologie (MNHN/CNRS/Paris Diderot), Paris, France
Pole Image, Paris Diderot University (Sorbonne Paris Cité), Paris, France

Sabrina Krief
UMR 7206 Eco-Anthropologieet Ethnobiologie (MNHN/CNRS/Paris Diderot), Paris, France
Great Ape Conservation Project (PCGS), Sebitoli UWA Station in Kibale National Park, Fort Portal, Uganda

Kevin Potts
Department of Biology, Augsburg College, Minneapolis, Minnesota, United States of America

Protase Rwaburindore and John Kasenene
Department of Botany, Makerere University, Kampala, Uganda

Andrew Seguya
Uganda Wildlife Authority, Kampala, Uganda

Fabio L. Lobato, Alexandre C. Siqueira, Ana M. R. Liedke, Alberto Lindner and Sergio R. Floeter
Departamento de Ecologia e Zoologia, Universidade Federal de Santa Catarina, Florianó polis, SC, Brazil

Diego R. Barneche
Department of Biological Sciences, Macquarie University, Sydney, NSW, Australia

Marcio R. Pie
Setor de Ciências Biológicas, Universidade Federal do Paraná, Curitiba, PR, Brazil

David R. Bellwood
Australian Research Council Centre of Excellence for Coral Reef Studies, and School of Marine and Tropical Biology, James Cook University, Townsville, QLD, Australia

Marine Jacquier and Fabien Crauste
Université de Lyon, Université Lyon 1, CNRS UMR 5208, Institut Camille Jordan, Villeurbanne-Cedex, France
Inria Team Dracula, Inria Center Grenoble Rhône-Alpes, Grenoble Rhône-Alpes, France

Christophe O. Soulage
CarMeN, INSERM U1060, Université de Lyon, INSA-Lyon, Univ. Lyon-1, Villeurbanne, France

Hédi A. Soula
CarMeN, INSERM U1060, Université de Lyon, INSA-Lyon, Univ. Lyon-1, Villeurbanne, France
Project-Team Beagle, Inria Center Grenoble Rhône-Alpes, Grenoble Rhône-Alpes, France

Christian M. Gallardo, Cynthia T. Hsu and Keith M. Gunapala
Division of Biology, California Institute of Technology, Pasadena, California, United States of America

Maksim Parfyonov and Ralph E. Mistlberger
Department of Psychology, Simon Fraser University, Burnaby, British Columbia, Canada

Chris H. Chang
W.M. Keck Science Department, Claremont McKenna College, Pitzer College, Scripps College, Claremont, California, United States of America

Andrew D. Steele
Division of Biology, California Institute of Technology, Pasadena, California, United States of America
Biological Sciences Department, California State Polytechnic University Pomona, Pomona, California, United States of America

Timothy South and Margaret J. Morris
Department of Pharmacology, School of Medical Sciences, University of New South Wales, Sydney, Australia

Nathan M. Holmes, Sarah I. Martire and R. Frederick Westbrook
Department of Psychology, University of New South Wales, Sydney, Australia

Yu-Wei Chen, Kimberly A. Fiscella, Samuel Z. Bacharach and Donna J. Calu
Intramural Research Program, NIDA/NIH, Baltimore, Maryland, United States of America

Beatriz Gutiérrez-Gil, Juan Jose Arranz and Elsa García-Gámez
Dpto. Producción Animal, Universidad de León, León, Spain

Ricardo Pong-Wong and Pamela Wiener
The Roslin Institute and R(D)SVS, University of Edinburgh, Roslin, Midlothian, United Kingdom

James Kijas
Animal, Food and Health Sciences, CSIRO, Brisbane, Australia

Julian Taylor
School of Agriculture, Food and Wine, University of Adelaide, Waite Campus, Glen Osmond, South Australia, Australia

Yusuf Genc and Klaus Oldach
School of Agriculture, Food and Wine, University of Adelaide, Waite Campus, Glen Osmond, South Australia, Australia
South Australian Research and Development Institute, Plant Genomics Centre, Waite Campus, Glen Osmond, South Australia, Australia

Jay Rongala
South Australian Research and Development Institute Plant Genomics Centre, Waite Campus, Glen Osmond, South Australia, Australia

Guillermo Rodríguez-Gómez, Ana Mateos and Jesús Rodríguez
Paleofisiología y Ecología Social de homínidos, Centro Nacional de Investigación sobre la Evolución Humana (CENIEH), Burgos, Spain

Jesús Angel Martín-González
Departamento de Matemáticas y Computación, Universidad de Burgos, Burgos, Spain, and temporarily assigned to CENIEH, Burgos, Spain

Ruth Blasco
The Gibraltar Museum, Gibraltar, Gibraltar

Jordi Rosell
Área de Prehistória, Universitat Rovirai Virgili (URV), Tarragona, Spain
Institut Catalá de Paleoecologia Humanai Evolució Social (IPHES), Tarragona, Spain

Jun Jie Tan, Siti Maisura Azmi, Hong Leong Cheah, Vuanghao Lim,
Doblin Sandai and Bakiah Shaharuddin
Advanced Medical and Dental Institute, Universiti Sains Malaysia, Kepala Batas, Penang, Malaysia

Yoke Keong Yong
Department of Human Anatomy, Faculty of Medicine and Health Sciences, Serdang, Selangor Darul Ehsan, Malaysia

Index